Textbook of Medical Pharmacology

Second Edition

Professor and Head
Department of Pharmacology
Fr. Muller Medical College
Mangalore

CBS

CBS Publishers & Distributors

New Delhi • Bangalore

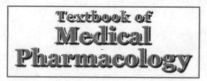

First Edition: 2004
Second Edition: 2006

Production Director : Vinod K. Jain

Published by :
Satish Kumar Jain for CBS Publishers & Distributors,
4596/1-A, 11 Darya Ganj, New Delhi - 110 002 (India)
E-mail : cbspubs@vsnl.com
Website : www.cbspd.com

Branch Office :
Seema House, 2975, 17th Cross, K.R. Road,
Bansankari 2nd Stage, Bangalore - 560070
Fax : 080-6771680 • E-mail : cbsbng@vsnl.net

Printed at
Swastik Packagings,
Delhi-92 (India)

Dedicated

to

my dear

students

Textbook of
Medical
Pharmacology

Second Edition

Foreword

$\mathcal{M}$edical education has become more and more information-oriented and is overloaded with too many subjects that the students find it very difficult to keep pace with all the information that they are supposed to cram up for the end year examinations. This is more obvious in the undergraduate days. In this scenario larger textbooks of yesteryears do not find favour with students. Graduate students are looking for examination-oriented, easy to read, shorter textbooks that cover the subject comprehensively helping them to pass the examinations without much effort.

In this background Padmaja's *Textbook of Pharmacology for Medical Students* finds a special niche. The book reads well and is very lucid with all the basic knowledge of pharmacology needed for a graduate student. Even the postgraduates might find it handy for examination time revision. With student medical education becoming an important part of the large pharmaceutical industry's hidden agenda, a good pharmacology background is all the more important these days. The budding doctor should be able to take the wheat from the chaff of all that is fed to him/her by the industry as practising doctors later in life. Most of what is given in the company literature is not based on hard scientific facts. Every doctor should be able to assess the basic pharmacological aspects of every new drug introduced to him/her later in life in practice. This book eminently serves that purpose.

I have known Dr. Padmaja for a very long time; almost from the time she started to become a pharmacologist. When I first set up a clinical pharmacology department in our medical college I used to encourage pharmacology staff to get trained in clinical pharmacology and Padmaja was one of those pioneers in that effort. I have a very high opinion of her intellectual capabilities.

This book is very well brought out by the publishers and deserves all the encouragement from the students and junior staff alike. I am sure this will happen. I wish the young lady and her book all success. I foresee frequent revisions of the text in future as pharmacology is a very rapidly growing area of medical research. May this book help all graduate students to become responsible clinicians who would know for certain when not to prescribe a drug. A recent report from the US has shown that in that country over 100,000 people die annually due to adverse drug reactions. We owe it to the public to be responsible clinicians.

This book gets very high marks in my assessment.

Prof. B.M. Hegde MD
FRCP (London), FRCP (Edinburgh), FRCP (Glasgow)
FRCPI (Dublin), FACC, FAMS
Visiting Professor of Cardiology, London University,
Affiliate Professor of Human Health,
University of Northern California,
Visiting Professor, Institute of Advanced Studies, Shimla.
MBBS, MD, Ph.D., MRCP(UK) & MRCPI examiner.
Chairman, Bharatiya Vidya Bhavan, Mangalore

`Manjunath'
Pais Hills, Bejai
Mangalore 575004. India.

Preface

Pharmacology is a rapidly expanding field. Frequent editions of the book is the only way one can keep pace with the growing field of pharmacology. Mechanisms of action of many important, commonly used drugs have been elaborated and the subject is updated. More figures, flow charts and tables have been included. In revising the topics, expert opinion has been taken from the respective subject experts including physicians, gynecologist, oncologist, anaesthetist, psychiatrist, etc. Care has been taken to structure the matter within the framework of MCI curriculum and made exam-oriented. New topics, viz. rational drug use, drugs of abuse, intravenous fluids, drugs used in scabies and pediculosis, minerals, sclerosing agents, treatment of poisoning, geriatric pharmacology and an appendix on syringes and needles have been added.

Very often drugs have been inappropriately used or even wrong drugs given by mistake. Such incidences are black marks on the noble medical profession. Moreover, in the present days when medical care has been brought under the preview of the Consumer's Act, awareness of such mistakes is all the more relevant. Some such real-life incidences have been mentioned in separate boxes with the dual intention of *(i)* warning the students so that they 'do not repeat them' and *(ii)* helping the students to remember at least some actions and adverse effects of those drugs.

I hope the book serves the purpose it is designed for.

Dr. Padmaja Udaykumar
Professor and Head
Department of Pharmacology
Fr. Muller Medical College
Mangalore

Please e-mail your feedback to raaguday@rediffmail.com

Opinion

*P*resentation of topics is very good; practical and common sense approach is given in the chapters. Tables and figures have enhanced the richness of the text and make it user-friendly. Choice of drugs given in various conditions truly fills the role of a handbook for clinicians. Prof. Padmaja's efforts are appreciated by seeing the editorial fineness, truly a ladies touch. Tables for quick reference of drug, dosage, duration of action, presentation, brand names are useful and well thought out presentation of this book. It is a student-friendly textbook. This book is not only meant for undergraduate medical students but can be a ready-reckoner for the clinicians and pharmacologists.

Dr. B. Sanjeev Rai
Dean, Fr. Muller Medical College
Mangalore

Acknowledgments

- I thank Prof. B.M. Hegde for writing the *Foreword* to this book and Dr. Neelima Ksheersagar, Dr. Sanjeev Rai and Dr. Meenakshiammal for giving their opinion on the book.

- I place on record my sincere thanks to Dr. Gopalan Kutty for proofreading the text of the book.

- I am thankful to Prof Nataraj, BMC, Bangalore, Prof Elsy I, Thrissur Medical College; Prof. Vijayaraghavan, MMC, Mysore, and Prof D.R. Kulkarni, Bijapur, for their encouragement.

- I am sincerly thankful to the following doctors for reviewing the chapters of their respective specialities: Dr. Krishnaprasad, oncologist; Dr. Raveesh Tunga, psychiatrist; Dr. Sujaya V. Rao, obstetrician and gynecologist; Dr. Preethi Jain, anaesthetist; Dr. Rammohan Rao, ophthalmologist; and Dr. Prabha Adhikari, Dr. Narasimha Hegde and Dr. Sreenivas Kakkilaya, physicians.

- I wholeheartedly thank the management of Fr. Muller Medical College: Director, Rev. Fr. Baptist Menezes; Administrator, Rev. Fr. Lawrence D'Souza; and Dean, Dr. Sanjeev Rai; for their encouragement and support.

- I am thankful to Prof. M.C. Alwar and Prof. M.R.S.M. Pai, KMC, Mangalore; Prof. Parvathi Bhat, A.J. Shetty Medical College; Prof. K.S. Karanth, KSHEMA; Prof. T. Venkatadri, Yenepoya Medical College, for their encouragement; and my colleagues Dr. Vijayalaxmi, Dr. Princy Palatty, Dr. Prasannalakshmi and Dr. Manohar for their support.

- My sincere thanks are due to my husband Prof. Udaykumar K. for his constant encouragement, suggestions, help and guidance in bringing out this book.

- I also thank Mr. Manoj Machado and Mr. Wilfred Lobo, Mangalore, for the meticulous DTP work and CBS Publishers, New Delhi, for publishing this book.

Dr. Padmaja Udaykumar

Contents

SECTION 1

GENERAL PHARMACOLOGY

SECTION 2

AUTONOMIC NERVOUS SYSTEM

SECTION 3

DRUGS ACTING ON THE KIDNEY

SECTION 7

RESPIRATORY SYSTEM

SECTION 8

BLOOD

SECTION 9

GASTROINTESTINAL TRACT

SECTION 10

CHEMOTHERAPY

SECTION 11

HORMONES

SECTION 12

MISCELLANEOUS DRUGS

APPENDICES

INDEX

GENERAL PHARMACOLOGY

- Introduction
- Routes of drug administration
- Pharmacokinetics
- Pharmacodynamics
- Adverse drug reactions and Drug interactions
- Drug development, Drug assay, Nomenclature and Essential Drugs Concept

1 *Introduction*

- **Historical aspects**
- **Definitions**
- **Sources of drugs**

HISTORICAL ASPECTS

Pharmacology is the science that deals with the study of drugs and their interaction with the living systems.

The useful and toxic effects of many plant and animal products were known to man since ancient times. The earliest writings on drugs are the Egyptian Medical Papyrus (1600 BC). The largest of them, Ebers Papyrus lists some 800 preparations.

In early days there was a close relationship between religion and treatment of diseases. The knowledge of the use of drugs often rested with the priest or holyman. Drugs were thought to be magical in their actions.

Several cultures like the Chinese, Greek, Indian, Roman, Persian, European and many others contributed a great deal to the development of medicine in early times. The drug prescriptions included preparations from herbs, plants, animals and minerals. In the middle ages many herbal gardens were cultivated, particularly by monasteries.

Though medicine developed simultaneously in several countries, the spread of knowledge was limited because of poorly developed communication across the world.

India's earliest pharmacological writings are from the 'Vedas'. An ancient Indian physician Charaka, and then, Sushruta and Vagbhata, described many herbal preparations included in 'Ayurveda' (meaning the science of life). Indians practiced vaccination as early as 550 BC.

Various other traditional systems of medicine

were practiced in different parts of the world - like Homeopathy, Unani, Siddha system and Allopathy.

Allopathy means 'the other suffering'. This word, still being used for the modern system of medicine, is a misnomer. Homeopathy meaning 'similar suffering' was introduced by Samuel Hahnemann. The principles of this system include 'like cures like' and 'dilution enhances the potency of drugs'.

Thus several systems of medicine were introduced, of which only a few survived. The basic reason for the failure of these systems is that man's concepts about diseases were incorrect and baseless in those days. By the end of the 17th century the importance of experimentation, observation and scientific methods of study became clear. Francois Magendie and Claude Bernard popularised the use of animal experiments to understand the effects of drugs. Simultaneous development of other branches of science *viz* botany, zoology, chemistry and physiology helped in the better understanding of pharmacology.

The last century has seen a rapid growth of the subject with several new drugs, new concepts and techniques being introduced. We now know much more about receptors and molecular mechanisms of action of many drugs. Several diseases, which were considered incurable and fatal, can now be completely cured with just a few tablets.

DEFINITIONS

The word pharmacology is derived from the Greek word - *Pharmacon* meaning an active principle and *logos* meaning a discourse.

Drug (Drogue - a dry herb in French) is a substance used in the diagnosis, prevention or treatment of a disease. WHO definition - "A drug is any substance or product that is used or intended to be used to modify or explore physiological systems or pathological states for the benefit of the recipient."

Pharmacokinetics is the study of the absorption, distribution, metabolism and excretion of drugs, *i.e.* what the body does to the drug (in Greek *Kinesis* = movement).

Pharmacodynamics is the study of the effects of the drugs on the body and their mechanisms of action, *i.e.* what the drug does to the body.

Therapeutics deals with the use of drugs in the prevention and treatment of disease.

Pharmacoeconomics deals with the cost *i.e.* economic aspects of drugs used therapeutically.

Pharmacogenomics is a branch of pharmaco-genetics and deals with the use of genetic information to guide the choice of drugs in a person.

Pharmacoepidemiology is the study of both the useful and adverse effects of drugs on large numbers of people. **Pharmacovigilance** is a branch of pharmacoepidemiology which deals with the epidemiologic study of adverse drug effects.

Toxicology deals with the adverse effects of drugs and also study of poisons, i.e detection, prevention and treatment of poisonings. *(Toxicon = poison in Greek)*

Chemotherapy is the use of drugs and chemicals for the treatment of infections. The term now also includes the use of chemical compounds to treat malignancies.

Pharmacopoeia *(in Greek, Pharmacon* = drug; *poeia*=to make)* is the official publication containing a list of drugs and medicinal preparations approved for use, their formulae and other information needed to prepare a drug; their physical properties, tests for their identity, purity and potency. Each country may follow its own pharmacopoeia to guide its physicians and pharmacists. We thus have the Indian

Pharmacopoeia (IP), the British Pharmacopoeia (BP), United States Pharmacopoeia (USP), Japanese Pharmacopoeia and others brought out by different countries. The International Pharmacopoeia is published by WHO in many languages like English, French and Spanish. The list is revised at regular periods to delete obselete drugs and to include newly introduced ones.

Pharmacy is the science of identification, compounding and dispensing of drugs. It also includes collection, isolation, purification, synthesis and standardisation of medicinal substances.

SOURCES OF DRUGS

The sources of drugs could be **natural** or **synthetic**.

Natural sources

Drugs can be obtained from

1. *Plants*, *e.g.* atropine, morphine, quinine, and digoxin, pilocarpine, physostigmine.

2. *Animals*, *e.g.* insulin, heparin, gonadotrophins and antitoxic sera.

3. *Minerals*, *e.g.* magnesium sulphate, aluminium hydroxide, iron, gold, sulphur and radioactive isotopes.

4. *Microorganisms* - antibacterial agents are obtained from some bacteria and fungi. We thus have penicillin, cephalosporins, tetracyclines and other antibiotics.

5. *Human* - some drugs are obtained from human source *e.g.* immunoglobulins from blood, growth hormone from anterior pituitary and chorionic gonadotrophins from the urine of pregnant women.

Synthetic

Most drugs used now are synthetic *e.g.* quinolones, omeprazole, sulfonamides, pancuronium, neostigmine.

- Many drugs are obtained by *cell cultures*, *e.g.* urokinase from cultured human kidney cells.

- Some are now produced by **recombinant DNA technology**, *e.g.* human insulin, tissue plasminogen activator. Haematopoietic growth factors like erythropoietin, filgrastim, sergramastim.

- Certain drugs are now obtained by **hybridoma technique** - eg. monoclonal antibodies like rituximab.

Plant products may be grouped on the basis of their physical and chemical properties as follows-

1. Alkaloids - are basic substances which combine with an acid to form a salt. They are insoluble in water and have a bitter taste but their salts are water soluble. Eg. Morphine, quinine, caffeine, atropine, pilocarpine, emetine - their names end with 'ine'. Many alkaloids are now synthesized in the laboratory.

2. Glycosides - are combination of sugars with other organic substances. On heating they split into a sugar and a non-sugar (aglycone) component. Sugar component determines some of the pharmacokinetic properties while aglycon is responsible for the pharmacological actions of the glycoside.

3. Oils - may be volatile or fixed oils. They are volatalised by heat and have aromas.

- **Volatile oils** are obtained from leaves, flowers, seeds or fruits of plants by distillation. They are not fats and have no food value. They are used as flavouring agents (peppermint oil), carminatives (oil of eucalyptus), antiseptics (thymol), counter irritants (terpentine oil) or to relieve pain (clove oil in toothache)

- **Fixed oils** are glycerides of oliec, palmitic and stearic acids obtained from the seeds. They are fats and have food value and are used in cooking Eg. groundnut oil, sunflower oil.

- **Mineral oils** are a mixture of dehydrocarbons obtained from petroleum. Eg. Liquid paraffin is used as a laxative while soft paraffin is used as ointment base.

Tannins are non-nitrogenous compounds. They are astringents and precipitate surface protiens and harden the skin and mucous membrane exert a protective effect.

Resins are solids which are insoluble in water but soluble in alcohol and chloroform eg. Jalap. *Some resins* - Oleoresin is (oil + resin). Gum resin is asafoetida. Gums are secreted from the barks of some trees. They are polysaccharides. They hold water eg. Gum acacia and gum tragacanth are used as emulsifying agents in the preparation of emulsions.

2 Routes of Drug Administration

- Enteral Route
- Parenteral Route
  - Injections
  - Inhalation
  - Transdermal
  - Transmucosal
- Topical

Drugs may be administered by various routes. The choice of the route in a given patient depends on the properties of the drug and the patient's requirements. A knowledge of the advantages and disadvantages of the different routes of administration is essential.

The routes can be broadly divided into

- Enteral (Oral)
- Parenteral
- Local

ENTERAL ROUTE (ORAL INGESTION)

Enteral route is the most commonly used, oldest and safest route of drug administration. The large surface area of the gastrointestinal tract, the mixing of its contents and the differences in pH at different parts of the gut facilitate effective absorption of the drugs given orally. However, the acid and enzymes secreted in the gut and the biochemical activity of the bacterial flora of the gut can destroy some drugs before they are absorbed.

Advantages

- Safest route
- Most convenient
- Most economical
- Drugs can be self-administered
- Non-invasive route.

Disadvantages

- Onset of action is slower as absorption needs time.

- Irritant and unpalatable drugs cannot be administered.

- Some drugs may not be absorbed due to certain physical and chemical characteristics, e.g. streptomycin is not effective orally.

- Irritation to the gastrointestinal tract may lead to vomiting.

- There may be irregularities in absorption.

- Some drugs may be destroyed by gastric juices, e.g. insulin.

- Oral preparations cannot be given to unconscious and uncooperative patients.

- Some drugs may undergo extensive first pass metabolism in the liver.

To overcome some of the disadvantages, irritants are given in capsules, while bitter drugs are given as sugar coated tablets. Sometimes drugs are coated with substances like synthetic resins, gums, sugar, colouring and flavouring agents making them more acceptable.

Enteric Coated Tablets

Some tablets are coated with substances like cellulose-acetate, phthalate, gluten, etc. which are not digested by the gastric acid but get disintegrated in the alkaline juices of the intestine. This will:

- Prevent gastric irritation

- Avoid destruction of the drug by the stomach

- Provide higher concentration of the drug in the small intestine

- Retard the absorption, and thereby prolong the duration of action

But if the coating is inappropriate, the tablet may be expelled without being absorbed at all.

Similarly controlled-release or sustained-release preparations are designed to prolong the rate of absorption and thereby the duration of action of drugs. This is useful for short-acting drugs. In newer controlled release formulations, the tablet is coated with a semipermeable membrane through which water enters and displaces the drug out.

Advantages

- Frequency of administration may be reduced.

- Therapeutic concentration may be maintained specially when nocturnal symptoms are to be treated.

Disadvantages

- There may be 'failure of the preparation' resulting in release of the entire amount of the drug in a short time, leading to toxicity.

- Enteric coated tablets are more expensive.

Certain precautions are to be taken during oral administration of drugs - capsules and tablets should be swallowed with a glass of water with the patient in upright posture either sitting or standing. This facilitates passage of the tablet into the stomach and its rapid dissolution. It also minimises chances of the drug getting into the larynx or behind the epiglottis. Recumbent patient should not be given drugs orally as some drugs may remain in the oesophagus due to the absence of gravitational force facilitating the passage of the drug into the stomach. Such drugs can damage the oesophageal mucosa, e.g. iron salts, tetracyclines.

Though enteral route mainly includes oral ingestion, sublingual and rectal administration may also be considered as enteral route.

PARENTERAL ROUTE

Routes of administration other than the enteral (intestinal) route are known as parenteral routes.

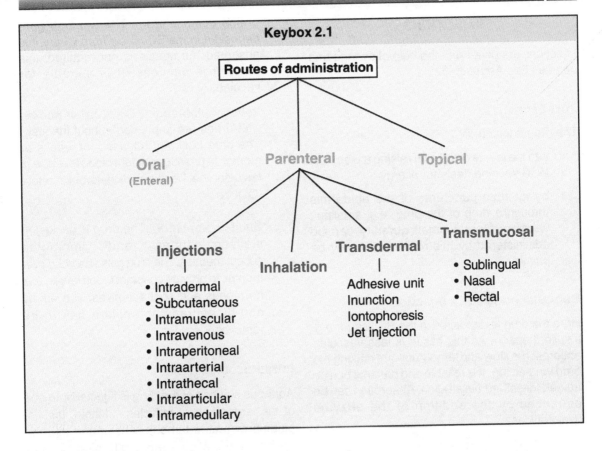

Here the drugs are directly delivered into tissue fluids or blood.

Advantages

- Action is more rapid and predictable than oral administration.

- These routes can be employed in an unconscious or uncooperative patient.

- Gastric irritants can be given parenterally and therefore irritation to the gastrointestinal tract can be avoided.

- It can be used in patients with vomiting or those unable to swallow.

- Digestion by the gastric and intestinal juices and the first pass metabolism are avoided.

Therefore, in emergencies parenteral routes are very useful for drug administration as the action is rapid and predictable and are useful even in unconscious patients.

Disadvantages

- Asepsis must be maintained
- Injections may be painful
- More expensive, less safe and inconvenient
- Injury to nerves and other tissues may occur

Parenteral routes include

1. Injections
2. Inhalation
3. Transdermal route
4. Transmucosal route

INJECTIONS

Injections are given with the help of syringe and needle - See Appendix 1.

Intradermal

The drug is injected -

- into the layers of the skin raising a bleb, *e.g.* BCG vaccine, tests for allergy

- by multiple punctures of the epidermis through a drop of the drug, *e.g.* smallpox vaccine. Only a small quantity can be administered by this route and it may be painful.

Subcutaneous (SC) Injection

Here the drug is deposited in the SC tissue, *e.g.* insulin, heparin. As this tissue is less vascular, absorption is slow and largely uniform making the drug long-acting. It is reliable and patients can be trained for self-administration. Absorption can be enhanced by the addition of the enzyme hyaluronidase.

Disadvantages

- As SC tissue is richly supplied by nerves, irritant drugs cannot be injected because they can cause severe pain.

- In shock, absorption is not dependable because of vasoconstriction.

- Repeated injections at the same site can cause lipoatrophy resulting in erratic absorption.

Hypodermoclysis is the subcutaneous administration of large volumes of saline employed in paediatric practice.

Drugs can also be administered subcutaneously as compared to oral route:

1. Dermojet: In this method, a high velocity jet of drug solution is projected from a fine orifice using a 'gun'. The solution gets deposited in the SC tissue from where it is absorbed. As needle is not required, this method is painless. It is suitable for vaccines.

2. Pellet implantation: Small pellets packed with drugs are implanted subcutaneously. The drug is slowly released for weeks or months to provide constant blood levels, *e.g.* testosterone, Desoxycorticosterone acetate (DOCA).

3. Sialistic implants: The drug is packed in sialistic tubes and implanted subcutaneously. The drug gets absorbed over months to provide constant blood levels, *e.g.* hormones and contraceptives. The empty non-biodegradable implant has to be removed.

Intramuscular (IM)

Aqueous solution of the drug is injected into one of the large skeletal muscles - deltoid, triceps, gluteus or rectus femoris. Absorption into the plasma occurs by simple diffusion. Larger molecules enter through the lymphatic channels. As the muscles are vascular, absorption is rapid and quite uniform. Drugs are absorbed faster from the deltoid region than gluteal region especially in women. The volume of injection should not exceed 10 ml. For infants, rectus femoris is used instead of gluteus because gluteus is not well-developed till the child starts walking. If the drug is injected as oily solution or suspension, absorption is slow and steady.

Advantages

- Intramuscular route is reliable.

- Absorption is rapid.

- Soluble substances, mild irritants, depot preparations, suspensions and colloids can be injected by this route.

Disadvantages

- Intramuscular injection may be painful and may even result in an abscess.

- Nerve injury should be avoided - irritant solutions can damage the nerve if injected near a nerve.

- Local infection and tissue necrosis are possible.

Intravenous (IV)

Here, the drug is injected into one of the superficial veins so that it directly reaches the circulation and is immediately available for action.

Drugs can be given IV as

1. A bolus - where an initial large dose is given, *e.g.* heparin. The drug is dissolved in a suitable amount of the vehicle and injected slowly.

2. Slow injection - over 15-20 minutes, *e.g.* aminophylline.

3. Slow infusion - when constant plasma concentrations are required, *e.g.* oxytocin in labour or when large volumes have to be given, *e.g.* dextrose, saline. Generally about one litre of solution is infused over 3 to 4 hours. However the patient's condition and the drug factors like the onset and duration of action of the drug dictates the rate of infusion.

Advantages

- Most useful route in emergencies as the drug is immediately available for action.

- Provides predictable blood concentrations with 100% bioavailability.

- Large volumes of solutions can be given.

- Irritants can be given by this route as they get quickly diluted in blood.

- Rapid dose adjustments are possible - if unwanted effects occur, infusion can be stopped; if higher levels are required, infusion rate can be increased - specially for short-acting drugs.

Disadvantages

- Once injected, the drug cannot be withdrawn.

- Irritation of the veins may cause thrombophlebitis.

- Extravasation of some drugs may cause severe irritation and sloughing.

- Only aqueous solutions can be given IV but not suspensions, oily solutions and depot preparations.

- Self medication is difficult.

Intraperitoneal

Peritoneum offers a large surface area for absorption. Fluids are injected intraperitoneally in infants. This route is also used for peritoneal dialysis.

Intrathecal

Drugs can be injected into the subarachnoid space for action on the CNS, *e.g.* spinal anaesthetics. Some antibiotics and corticosteroids are also injected by this route to produce high local concentrations. Strict aseptic precautions are a must.

Drugs are also given extradurally. Morphine can be given epidurally to produce analgesia. Direct intraventricular administration of drugs may be employed in brain tumors.

Intra-articular

Drugs are injected directly into a joint for the treatment of arthritis and other diseases of the joints. *e.g.* in rheumatoid arthritis hydrocortisone is injected into the affected joint. Strict aseptic precautions are required.

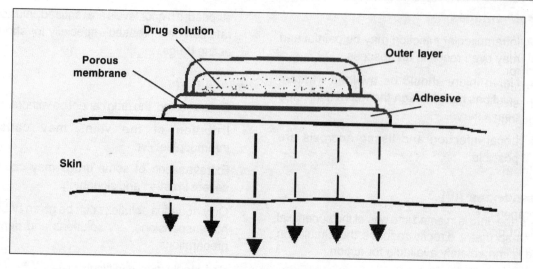

Fig 2.1 Transdermal adhesive unit

Intra-arterial

Here the drug is injected directly into the arteries. It is used only in the treatment of -

1. Peripheral vascular diseases
2. Local malignancies
3. Diagnostic studies like angiograms.

Intramedullary

Injection into a bone marrow - now rarely used.

INHALATION

Lungs offer a large surface area for absorption of drugs. Volatile liquids and gases are given by inhalation, *e.g.* general anaesthetics. In addition, drugs can be administered as solid particles, *i.e.* solutions of drugs can be atomised and the fine droplets are inhaled as aerosol, *e.g.* salbutamol. These inhaled drugs and vapours may act locally on the pulmonary epithelium and mucous membranes of the respiratory tract or may also be absorbed through these membranes.

Advantages

- Almost instantaneous absorption of the drug is achieved because of
  - the large suface area of the lungs.
  - thin alvealar membrane
  - high vascularity
- In pulmonary diseases, it serves almost as a local route as the drug is delivered at the desired site making it more effective and less harmful.
- Hepatic first pass metabolism is avoided.
- Blood levels of volatile anaesthetics can be conveniently controlled as their absorption and excretion through the lungs are governed by the laws of gases.

Disadvantage

- Irritant gases may enhance pulmonary secretion - should be avoided.
- Drug particles may induce cough e.g. Cromolyn sodium.

This is an important route of entry of certain drugs of abuse.

TRANSDERMAL

Highly lipid soluble drugs can be applied over the skin for slow and prolonged absorption, *e.g.* nitroglycerine ointment in angina pectoris. Adhesive units, inunction, iontophoresis and jet injection are some forms of transdermal drug delivery.

Adhesive units

Transdermal adhesive units (transdermal therapeutic systems) are adhesive patches (Fig 2.1) of different sizes and shapes made to suit the area of application. The drug is held in a reservoir between an outer layer and a porous membrane. This membrane is smeared with an adhesive to hold on to the area of application. The drug slowly diffuses through the membrane and percutaneous absorption takes place. The rate of absorption is constant and predictable. Highly potent drugs (because small quantity is sufficient) and short acting drugs (because effect terminates quickly after the system is removed) are suitable for use in such systems.

Sites of application are chest, abdomen, upper arm, back or mastoid region; testosterone patch is applied over the scrotum

Examples: hyoscine, nitroglycerin, testosterone, estrogen and fentanyl transdermal patches.

Advantages

- Duration of action is prolonged
- Provides constant plasma drug levels
- Patient compliance is good.

Inunction

The route where a drug rubbed into the skin gets absorbed to produce systemic effects is called inunction.

Iontophoresis

In this procedure, galvanic current is used for bringing about penetration of lipid insoluble drugs into the deeper tissues where its action is required, *e.g.* Salicylates. Fluoride iontophoresis is used in the treatment of dental hypersensitivity.

Jet injection

As absorption of drug occurs across the layers of the skin, dermojet may also be considered as a form of transdermal drug administration (See page 9).

TRANSMUCOSAL

Drugs are absorbed across the mucous membranes. Transmucosal administration includes sublingual, nasal and rectal routes.

Sublingual

Here, the tablet or pellet containing the drug is placed under the tongue. As the drug dissolves it is absorbed across the sublingual mucosa, *e.g.* nitroglycerin, nifedipine, buprenorphine. The formulation should be so designed that it quickly dissolves in the saliva. The buccal mucosa is rich in blood supply. This allows quick absorption of the drug.

Advantages

- Absorption is rapid - within minutes the drug reaches the circulation.
- First pass metabolism is avoided.
- After the desired effect is obtained, the drug can be spat out to avoid the unwanted effects.

Disadvantages

- Buccal ulceration can occur

- Lipid insoluble drugs cannot be given

Nasal

Drugs can be administered through nasal route either for systemic absorption or for local effects.

e.g. for systemic absorption - oxytocin spray is used .

For local effect - decongestant nasal drops, *e.g.* oxymetazoline; budesonide nasal spray for allergic rhinitis.

Rectal

Rectum has a rich blood supply and drugs can cross the rectal mucosa to be absorbed for systemic effects. Drugs absorbed from the upper part of the rectum are carried by the superior haemorrhoidal vein to the portal circulation (can undergo first pass metabolism), while that absorbed from the lower part of the rectum is carried by the middle and inferior haemorrhoidal veins to the systemic circulation. Drugs like indomethacin, chlorpromazine, diazepam and paraldehyde can be given rectally.

Some irritant drugs are given rectally as **suppositories.**

Advantages

- Gastric irritation is avoided.
- Can be administered by unskilled persons
- Useful in geriatric patients; patients with vomiting, those unable to swallow and after gastro intestinal surgery.
- Also useful in unconscious and uncooperative patients.

Disadvantages

- Irritation of the rectum can occur
- Absorption may be irregular and unpredictable.

Drugs may also be given by rectal route as enema.

Enema is the administration of a drug in a liquid form into the rectum. Enema may be evacuant or retention enema.

Evacuant enema: In order to empty the bowel, about 600 ml of soap water is administered per rectum. Water distends and thus stimulates the rectum while soap lubricates. Enema is given prior to surgeries, obstetric procedures and radiological examination of the gut.

Retention enema: The drug is administered with about 100 ml of fluids and is retained in the rectum for local action, *e.g.* prednisolone enema in ulcerative colitis.

TOPICAL

Drugs may be applied on the skin for local action as ointment, cream, gel, powder, paste, etc. Drugs may also be applied on the mucous membrane as in the eyes, ears and nose as ointment, drops and sprays.

Drugs may be administered as **suppository** for rectum, **bougie** for urethra and **pessary** and **douche** for vagina. Pessaries are oval shaped tablets to be placed in the vagina to provide high local concentrations of the drug at the site, *e.g.* antifungal pessaries in vaginal candidiasis.

Douche is an aqueous solution used for rinsing a body cavity. Though the word 'douche' is generally used for vaginal solutions, it can also be used for solutions meant for bladder or the rectum.

SPECIAL DRUG DELIVERY SYSTEMS

In order to improve drug delivery, to prolong duration of action and thereby improve patient compliance, special drug delivery systems are being tried. Drug targeting, *i.e.* to deliver drugs at the site where it is required to act is also being aimed at, especially for anticancer drugs. Some such systems are ocuserts, progestaserts, transdermal adhesive units, prodrugs, osmotic pumps, computerised pumps and methods using monoclonal antibodies and liposomes as carriers.

Ocusert

Ocusert systems are thin elliptical units that contain the drug in a reservoir which slowly releases the drug through a membrane by diffusion at a steady rate, *e.g.* pilocarpine ocusert used in glaucoma is placed under the lid and can deliver pilocarpine for 7 days.

Progestasert

Progestasert is inserted into the uterus where it delivers progesterone constantly for over one year.

Transdermal adhesive units (See page 13)

Prodrug

Prodrug is an inactive form of a drug which gets metabolised to the active derivative in the body. A prodrug may overcome some of the disadvantages of the conventional forms of drug administration, *e.g.* dopamine does not cross the BBB; levodopa, a prodrug crosses the BBB and is then converted to dopamine in the CNS. Prodrugs may also be used to achieve longer duration of action, *e.g.* Bacampicillin (a prodrug of ampicillin) is longer acting than ampicillin. Cyclophosphamide - an anticancer drug - gets converted to its active metabolite aldophosphamide in the liver. This allows oral administration of cyclophosphamide without causing much gastrointestinal toxicity. Zidovudine is taken up by virus infected cells and gets activated in these cells. This results in selective toxicity to infected cells. A prodrug

may be more stable at gastric pH. eg. aspirin is converted to salicylic acid which is the active drug and aspirin is better tolerated than salicylic acid.

Osmotic pumps

These are small tablet shaped units consisting the drug and an osmotic substance in two different chambers. The tablet is coated with a semipermeable membrane in which a minutelaser-drilled hole is made. When the tablet is swallowed and reaches the gut, water enters into the tablet through the semipermeable membrane. The osmotic layer swells and pushes the drug slowly out of the laser-drilled orifice. This allows slow and constant delivery of the drug over a long period of time. It is also called **Gastrointestinal Therapeutic System (GITS).** Some drugs available in this formulation are iron and prazosin.

Computerised miniature pumps

These are programmed to release drugs at a definite rate either continuously as in case of insulin or intermittently in pulses as in case of GnRH.

Various methods of drug targeting are tried especially for anticancer drugs to reduce toxicity.

Monoclonal antibodies

Monoclonal antibodies against the tumor specific antigens are used to deliver anticancer drugs to specific tumor cells.

Liposomes

Liposomes are phospholipids suspended in aqueous vehicles to form minute vesicles. Drugs encapsulated in liposomes are taken up mainly by the reticuloendothelial cells of the liver and are also concentrated in malignant tumors. Thus site-specific delivery of drugs may be possible with the help of liposomes.

3

Pharmacokinetics

- **Mechanisms of transport of drugs across biological membranes**
    - **Passive transfer**
    - **Carrier mediated transport**
    - **Endocytosis & exocytosis**
- **Absorption**
- **First Pass Metabolism**
- **Bioavailability**
- **Distribution**
- **Biotransformation**
- **Excretion**
- **Clinical Pharmacokinetics**
- **Methods of prolonging drug action**

Pharmacokinetics is the study of the absorption, distribution, metabolism and excretion of drugs, *i.e.* the movement of the drugs into, within and out of the body. For a drug to produce its specific response, it should be present in adequate

concentrations at the site of action. This depends on various factors apart from the dose. Once the drug is administered, it is absorbed, *i.e.* enters the blood, is distributed to different parts of the body, reaches the site of action, is metabolised and excreted (Fig. 3.1). All these processes involve passage of the drug molecules across various barriers - like the intestinal epithelium, cell membrane, renal filtering membrane, capillary barrier and so on. To cross these barriers the drug has to cross the cell membrane or pass in-between the epithelial or endothelial cells.

The cell membrane/biological membrane is made up of two layers of phospholipids with intermingled protein molecules. All lipid soluble substances get dissolved in the cell membrane and readily permeate into the cells.

The junctions between adjacent epithelial or endothelial cells have pores through which small water-soluble molecules can pass. Movement of some specific substances is regulated by special carrier proteins. The passage of drugs across

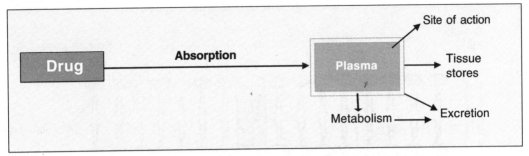

Fig. 3.1 Schematic representation of movement of drug in the body

biological membranes involves processes like passive (filtration, diffusion) and active transport.

Mechanisms of transport of drugs across biological membranes

1. Passive transfer

- Simple diffusion
- Filtration

2. Carrier-mediated transport

- Active transport
- Facilitated diffusion

3. Endocytosis & exocytosis

Passive Transfer

The drug moves across a membrane without any need for energy.

Simple diffusion

Simple diffusion is the transfer of a drug across the membrane in the direction of its concentration gradient. The speed of diffusion depends on the degree of concentration gradient. Higher the concentration gradient, faster is the diffusion across the membrane. Lipid soluble drugs are transferred across membranes by simple diffusion - after dissolving in the lipids of the cell membrane. The rate of diffusion depends on the concentration gradient - higher the gradient faster is the diffusion. Most drugs follow simple diffusion.

Filtration

Filtration is the passage of drugs through aqueous pores in the membrane. Water-soluble drugs with molecular size (mol.wt.<100) smaller than the diameter of the pores (7° A) cross the biological membranes by filtration. The movement is along the concentration gradient. *e.g.* urea.

Carrier-mediated Transport

Transport of certain substances, which cannot move by diffusion, is aided by specific carriers.

Active transport

Active transport is the transfer of drugs against a concentration gradient and needs energy. It is carried by a specific carrier protein. Only drugs related to natural metabolites are transported by this process, *e.g.* levodopa, iron, sugars amino acids. The compound binds to a specific carrier on one side of the membrane and moves across the cell. At the other side of the cell, the complex dissociates and the carrier moves back to transport another molecule. Other substances competing for the same mechanism for transport may interfere with drug movement because this process is saturable, *e.g.* when penicillin and probenecid are administered together, the duration of action of penicillin is prolonged because both of them compete for renal tubular secretion.

Facilitated diffusion

Facilitated diffusion is a unique form of carrier transport which differs from active transport in

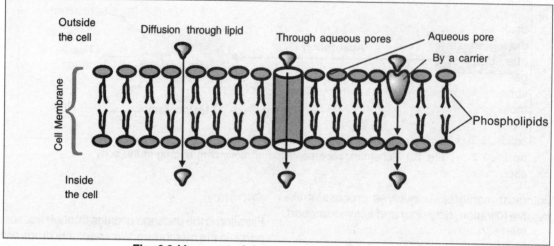

Fig. 3.2 Movement of drugs across biological membrane.

that it is not energy dependent and the movement occurs in the direction of the concentration gradient. The carrier facilitates diffusion and is highly specific for the substance, *e.g.* uptake of glucose by cells, vitamin B_{12} from intestines.

Endocytosis and exocytosis

Endocytosis is the process where small droplets are engulfed by the cell. Some proteins are taken up by this process (like pinocytosis in amoeba). This process is currently being tried for delivery of some anticancer drugs to the tissues. The reverse process - exocytosis is responsible for secretion of many substances from cells, *e.g.* neurotransmitters stored in nerve endings.

ABSORPTION

Absorption is defined as the passage of the drug from the site of administration into the circulation. For a drug to reach its site of action, it must pass through various membranes depending on the route of administration. Absorption occurs by one of the processes described above, *i.e.* passive diffusion or carrier-mediated transport. Thus except for intravenous route, the drug needs to be absorbed from all other routes of administration.

The rate and extent of absorption varies with the route of administration.

Absorption from the gut - medication taken orally may be absorbed from any part of the gut. Highly lipid soluble drugs may be absorbed from the buccal cavity from where it directly enters the systemic circulation. Acidic drugs are absorbed from the stomach, while basic drugs get ionised and are not absorbed from the stomach (see below). Basic drugs given intravenously may diffuse from blood into the stomach because of the pH and may ionise quickly. This is known as 'ion trapping'.

Intestines have a large surface area and most drugs are absorbed from the proximal part of the jejunum. Basic drugs are absorbed from the intestines because of the favorable pH. Various factors like intestinal motility and pH influence absorption from the gut.

It has now been found that drugs may be transported out from the cells of the intestinal wall back into the gut lumen. This is done with a reverse transporter or efflux transporter - P- glycoprotein. Absorption from the large intestine is negligible.

Several factors influence the rate and extent of absorption of a drug given orally (Fig. 3.3). They are:

1. **Disintegration and dissolution time:** The drug taken orally should break up into individual particles (disintegrate) to be absorbed. It then has to dissolve in the gastrointestinal fluids. In case of drugs given subcutaneously or intramuscularly, the drug molecules have to dissolve in the tissue fluids. Liquids are absorbed faster than solids. Delay in disintegration and dissolution as with poorly water-soluble drugs like aspirin, result in delayed absorption.

2. **Formulation:** Pharmaceutical preparations are formulated to produce desired absorption. Inert substances used with drugs as diluents like starch and lactose may sometimes interfere with absorption.

3. **Particle size:** Small particle size is important for better absorption of drugs. Drugs like corticosteroids, griseofulvin, digoxin, aspirin and tolbutamide are better absorbed when given as small particles. On the other hand, when a drug has to act on the gut and its absorption is not desired, then particle size should be kept large, *e.g.* anthelmintics like bephenium hydroxy-naphthoate.

4. **Lipid solubility:** Lipid soluble drugs are absorbed faster and better by dissolving in the phospholipids of the cell membrane.

5. **PH and ionisation:** Ionised drugs are poorly absorbed while unionised drugs are lipid soluble and are well absorbed. Most drugs are weak electrolytes and exist in both ionized and unionized forms. But the degree of ionisation depends on the pH. Thus acidic drugs remain unionised in acidic medium of the stomach and are rapidly absorbed from the stomach. *e.g.* aspirin, barbiturates. Basic drugs are unionised when they reach the alkaline medium of intestine from where they are rapidly absorbed, *e.g.* pethidine, ephedrine. Basic drugs given intravenously may diffuse from blood into the stomach because of acidic pH and may ionise quickly. This is known as 'ion trapping'.

Strong acids and bases are highly ionised and therefore poorly absorbed, *e.g.* heparin, streptomycin.

6. **Area and vascularity of the absorbing surface** The larger the area of absorbing surface and more the vascularity - better is the absorption. Thus most drugs are absorbed from the small intestine.

7. **Gastrointestinal motility**

   Gastric emptying time - if gastric emptying is faster, the passage of the drug to the intestines is quicker and hence absorption is faster.

   Intestinal motility - when highly increased as in diarrhoeas, drug absorption is reduced.

8. **Presence of food** delays gastric emptying, dilutes the drug and delays absorption. Drugs may form complexes with food constituents and such complexes are poorly absorbed, *e.g.* tetracyclines chelate calcium present in the food - hence their bio-availability is decreased. Moreover, certain drugs like ampicillin, roxithromycin and rifampicin are well absorbed only on empty stomach.

9. **Diseases** of the gut like malabsorption and achlorhydria result in reduced absorption of drugs.

10. **Metabolism:** Some drugs may be degraded in the GI tract, first pass metabolism *e.g.* nitroglycerine, insulin (see below). Such drugs should be given in higher doses or by alternative routes.

FIRST PASS METABOLISM

First pass metabolism is the metabolism of a drug during its passage from the site of absorption to the systemic circulation. It is also called presystemic metabolism or first pass effect and is an important feature of oral route of administration. Drugs given orally may be metabolised in the gut wall and in the liver before reaching the systemic circulation. The extent of first pass

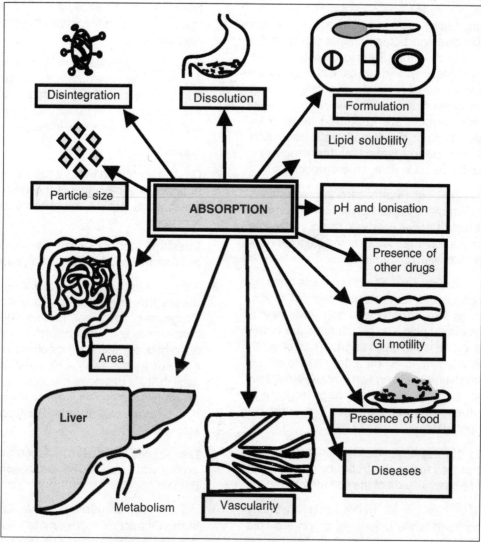

Fig. 3.3 Factors affecting absorption of drugs

metabolism differs from drug to drug and among individuals from partial to total inactivation. When it is partial, it can be compensated by giving higher dose of the particular drug, *e.g.* nitroglycerine, propranolol, salbutamol. But for drugs that undergo complete first pass metabolism, the route of administration has to be changed, *e.g.* isoprenaline, hydrocortisone, insulin. Bioavailability of many drugs is increased in patients with liver disease due to reduction in hepatic metabolism.

Absorption from parenteral routes - On intravenous administration the drug directly reaches the circulation (Fig. 3.4). On intramuscular injection, the drug molecules should dissolve in the tissue fluids and then be absorbed. Since muscles have a rich blood supply, absorption is fast. Drug molecules diffuse through the capillary membrane and reach the circulation. Lipid soluble drugs are absorbed faster. Absorption from subcutaneous administration is slower but rate of absorption is somewhat steady.

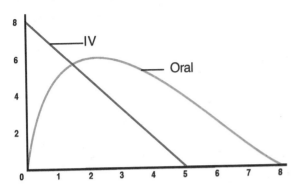

Fig. 3.4 Plasma concentration-Time curve of a drug following oral and IV administration.

Inhaled drugs are rapidly absorbed from the pulmonary epithelium particularly the lipid soluble ones.

On topical application, highly lipid soluble drugs are absorbed from the intact skin. *e.g.*: nitroglycerine; but absorption is relatively slow because of the multiple layers of closely-packed cells in the epidermis. Most drugs are readily absorbed from the mucous membranes.

BIOAVAILABILITY

Bioavailability is the fraction of the drug that reaches the systemic circulation following administration by any route. Thus, when a drug given intravenously, the bioavailability is 100 percent. On IM/SC injection and sublingual administration, drugs are almost completely absorbed (bioavailability >75%) while by oral route, bioavailability may be low due to incomplete absorption and first pass metabolism. *e.g.* bioavailability of chlortetracycline is 30%, carbamazepine - 70%, chloroquine- 80%, minocycline and diazepam almost 100%.

Factors that influence bioavailability In fact, all the ten factors which influence the absorption of a drug also alter bioavailability.

Transdermal preparations are absorbed systemically and may have 80-100% bioavailability. Large biovailability variations of a drug, particularly when it is unpredictable, can

---

Key Box 3.1
FIRST PASS METABOLISM

- First pass metabolism is the metabolism of a drug during its first passage through gut wall and liver

- Reduces bioavailability

- Extent of metabolism depends on the drug and individuals

- Measures to compensate first pass effect
  - Dose has to be increased for some drugs like propranolol
  - Route has to be changed for some others like hydrocortisone

- Examples: morphine, chlorpromazine, nitroglycerine, verapamil, testosterone, insulin, lignocaine

---

result in toxicity or therapeutic failure as in case of halofantrine (Page 416).

Determining bioavailability The drug is injected intravenously and its plasma concentration is measured at one hourly intervals. The plasma concentration is plotted against time on a graph paper. Similarly Plasma concentration - Time graph is also obtained, after oral administration of the same dose of the drug. Once these curves are obtained, the area under the curve (AUC) is measured.

Bioavailability is calculated by the formula -

$$\text{Bioavailability} = \frac{\text{AUC (oral)}}{\text{AUC (IV)}} \times 100$$

Bioequivalence

Comparison of bioavailability of different formulations of the same drug is the study of bioequivalence. Often oral formulations containing the same amount of a drug from different manufacturers may result in different plasma concentrations, *i.e.* there is no bioequivalence

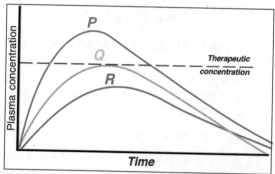

Fig 3.5: Study of bioequivalence. Three different oral formulations - P,Q & R of the same drug yield different bioavailability values. The area under each curve (AUC) gives the bioavailability of the respective formulation

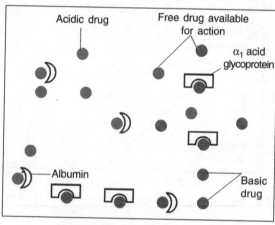

Fig. 3.6 Plasma Protein Binding

among them (Fig. 3.5). Such differences occur with poorly soluble, slowly absorbed drugs, mainly due to differences in the rate of distintegration and dissolution. Variation in bioavailability (nonequivalence) can result in toxicity or therapeutic failure in drugs that have low safety margin like digoxin and drugs that need precise dose adjustment like anticoagulants and corticosteroids. For such drugs, in a given patient, the preparations from a single manufacturer should be used.

DISTRIBUTION

After a drug reaches the systemic circulation, it gets distributed to other tissues. It should cross several barriers before reaching the site of action. Like absorption, distribution also involves the same processes, i.e. filtration, diffusion and specialised transport. Various factors determine the rate and extent of distribution, viz, lipid

solubility, ionisation, blood flow and binding to plasma proteins and cellular proteins. Unionised lipid soluble drugs are widely distributed throughout the body.

Plasma Protein Binding

On reaching the circulation most drugs bind to plasma proteins; acidic drugs bind mainly albumin and basic drugs to alpha-acid glycoprotein (Fig. 3.6). The free or unbound fraction of the drug is the only form available for action, metabolism and excretion while the protein bound form serves as a reservoir. The extent of protein binding varies with each drug, e.g. warfarin is 99% and morphine is 35% protein bound while binding of ethosuximide and lithium is 0%, i.e. they are totally free. (Table 3.1)

Clinical Significance of Plasma Protein Binding

1. Only free fraction is available for action,

TABLE 3.1 Some highly protein bound drugs		
Warfarin	Tolbutamide	Phenytoin
Frusemide	Clofibrate	Sulfonamides
Diazepam	Salicylates	Phenylbutazone
Indomethacin		

metabolism and excretion. When the free drug levels in the plasma fall, bound drug is released.

2. Protein binding serves as a store (reservoir) of the drug and the drug is released when free drug levels fall.

3. Protein binding prolongs the duration of action of the drug.

4. Many drugs may compete for the same binding sites. Thus one drug may displace another from the binding sites and result in displacement interactions, *e.g.* warfarin is 99% protein bound (*i.e.* free fraction is 1%). If another drug like indomethacin reduces its binding to 95%, the free form then becomes 5% which means, there is a 5-fold increase in free warfarin levels which could result in toxicity. Fortunately the body largely compensates by enhancing metabolism and excretion.

5. Chronic renal failure and chronic liver disease result in hypoalbuminaemia with reduced protein binding of drugs. Highly protein bound drugs should be carefully used in such patients.

Tissue binding

Some drugs get bound to certain tissue constituents because of special affinity for them. Tissue binding delays elimination and thus prolongs duration of action of the drug. For example, lipid soluble drugs are bound to adipose tissue. Tissue binding also serves as a reservoir of the drug.

Redistribution

When some highly lipid soluble drugs are given intravenously or by inhalation, they get rapidly distributed into highly perfused tissues like brain, heart and kidney. But soon they get redistributed

Key Box 3.2	
Tissue	**Binding Drugs**
Adipose tissue	Thiopentone sodium, benzodiazepines
Muscles	Emetine
Bone	Tetracyclines, Lead
Retina	Chloroquine
Thyroid	Iodine

into less vascular tissues like the muscle and fat resulting in termination of the action of these drugs. The best example is the intravenous anaesthetic thiopental sodium which induces anaesthesia in 10-20 seconds but the effect ceases in 5-15 minutes due to redistribution.

Blood-brain barrier (BBB)

The endothelial cells of the brain capillaries lack intercellular pores and instead have tight junctions. Moreover, glial cells envelope the capillaries and together these form the BBB. Only lipid soluble, unionised drugs can cross this BBB. During inflammation of the meninges, the barrier becomes more permeable to drugs, *e.g.* penicillin readily penetrates during meningitis. The barrier is weak at some areas like CTZ, posterior pituitary and parts of hypothalamus and allows some compounds to diffuse.

Placental barrier

Lipid soluble, unionised drugs readily cross the placenta while lipid insoluble drugs cross to a much lesser extent. Thus drugs taken by the mother can cause several unwanted effects in the foetus. (Table 3.5). Lipid soluble drugs with molecular weight of about 200-500 can easily cross the placenta while those with large molecular size (mol.wt > 1000) can hardly cross the placenta. These require transporters for crossing the placenta.

VOLUME OF DISTRIBUTION (V_d)

For the purpose of pharmacokinetic studies, body can be considered as a single compartment into which drugs are distributed uniformly. Each drug actually follows its own pattern of distribution from plasma to other body fluids and tissues.

Apparent volume of distribution

This is defined as the volume necessary to accommodate the entire amount of the drug administered, if the concentration throughout the body were equal to that in plasma. It relates the amount of the drug in the body to the concentration of the drug in plasma. It is calculated as

$$V_d = \frac{\textit{Amount of drug in the body}}{\textit{Plasma concentration}}$$

e.g. if the dose of a drug given is 500 mg and attains a uniform concentration of 10 mg/litre of plasma in the body, its V_d = 50 litres.

Important facts about V_d are:

- If a drug is retained mostly in the plasma, its V_d is small (*e.g.* aspirin, aminoglycosides) while if it is distributed widely in other tissues then its V_d is large (*e.g.* pethidine)

- The knowledge of V_d of drugs is clinically important in the treatment of poisoning. Drugs with large V_d like pethidine are not easily removed by haemodialysis because such drugs are widely distributed in the body.

- V_d may vary with changes in tissue permeability and protein binding as seen in some diseases.

- Drugs extensively bound to plasma proteins have a low V_d - eg. phenylbutazone.

- Low V_d drugs like aminoglycosides may have a larger V_d in presence of edema or ascitis.

BIOTRANSFORMATION (METABOLISM)

Biotransformation is the process of biochemical alteration of the drug in the body. Body treats most drugs as foreign substances and tries to inactivate and eliminate them by various biochemical reactions. These processes convert the drugs into more polar, water-soluble compounds so that they are easily excreted through the kidneys. Some drugs may be excreted largely unchanged in the urine, *e.g.* frusemide, atenolol.

Site

The most important organ of biotransformation is the liver. But drugs are also metabolised by the kidney, gut mucosa, lungs, blood and skin.

Consequences of biotransformation

Though biotransformation generally inactivates the drug, some drugs may be converted to metabolites which are also active or more active than the parent drug. Biotransformation may also activate an inactive drug (Table 3.2). When the metabolite is active, the duration of action gets prolonged (Table 3.3). **Prodrug** is an inactive drug which gets converted into an active form in the body. In case of some drugs, the active metabolite

Active drug to inactive metabolite	Active drug to active metabolite	Inactive drug to active metabolite (prodrug)
e.g. Morphine Chloramphenicol	e.g. Primidone ▶ Phenobarbitone Digitoxin ▶ Digoxin Diazepam ▶ Oxazepam	e.g. Levodopa ▶ Dopamine Prednisone ▶ Prednisolone Enalapril ▶ Enalaprilat

TABLE 3.2 Consequences of biotransformation

TABLE 3.3 Biotransformation

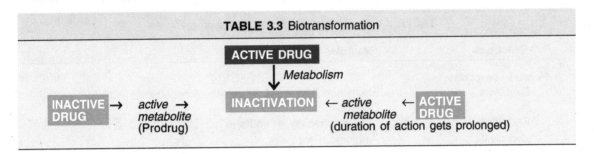

may be toxic. Eg. Paracetamol is converted to n-acetyl-p-benzoquinoneimine which causes hepatotoxicity; cyclophosphamide is converted to acrolein which causes bladder toxicity.

Enzymes in biotransformation

The biotransformation reactions are catalysed by specific enzymes located either in the liver microsomes (microsomal enzymes) or in the cytoplasm and mitochondria of the liver cells and also in the plasma and other tissues (non-microsomal enzymes).

The chemical reactions of biotransformation can take place in two phases (Fig. 3.6).

1. Phase I (Non-synthetic reactions)
2. Phase II (Synthetic reactions).

Phase I reactions

Phase I reactions convert the drug to a more polar metabolite by oxidation, reduction or hydrolysis.

Oxidation is the process of addition of oxygen (or a negatively charged radical) to a drug molecule or removal of hydrogen (or a positively charged radical) from a drug molecule. Oxidation reactions are the most important metabolising reactions, mostly catalysed by mono-oxygenases present in the liver. (See Table 3.4). They are carried on by a system which includes cytochrome P450,

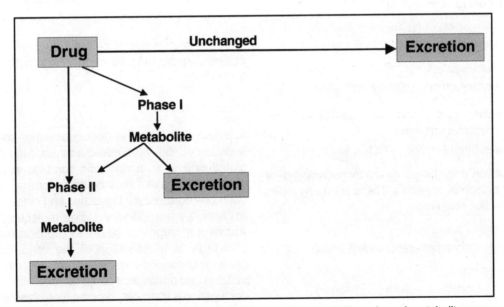

Fig. 3.6 Phases in metabolism of drugs. A drug may be excreted as phase I metabolite or as phase II metabolite. Some drugs may be excreted as such

TABLE 3.4 Important drug biotransformation reactions	
Reactions	**Examples of drugs**
Phase I - reactions	
Oxidation	Phenytoin, Diazepam, Ibuprofen, Amphetamine, Chlorpromazine, Dapsone
Reduction	Chloramphenicol, Halothane
Hydrolysis	Pethidine, Procaine
Phase II - Conjugation reactions	
Glucuronide conjugation	Chloramphenicol, Morphine, Diazepam, Aspirin
Acetylation	Sulfonamides, Isoniazid
Methylation	Adrenaline, Noradrenaline, Dopamine, Histamine
Glutathione conjugation	Paracetamol
Sulfate conjugation	Paracetamol, Steroids
Aminoacid conjugation	Salicylic acid, Benzoic acid

NADPH and molecular oxygen. There are several types of oxidation reactions like

- **Hydroxylation**
  Salicylic acid → gentisic acid
  Phenytoin → hydroxyphenytoin

- **Dealkylation**
  Imipramine → desmethylimipramine
  Codeine → morphine

- **S – oxidation** (sulfoxide formation)
  Cimetidine → cimetidine sulfoxide

- **Deamination**
  Amphetamine → Benzylmethylketone

Oxidation can also be catalysed by nonmicrosomal enzymes.

e.g. Ethyl alcohol → CO_2 + H_2O

Reduction may be catalysed by microsomal or nonmicrosomal enzymes. There are many types of reduction reactions.

1. Nitro reduction
   e.g. Chloramphenicol → Arylamine

2. Keto reduction
   e.g. Cortisone → hydrocortisone

Disulfiram and nitrites are reduced by non-microsomal enzymes.

Hydrolysis - is the process where a drug molecule is 'split' by the addition of a molecule of water. (Both microsomal and non-microsomal enzymes may be involved). Esterases, amidases and peptidases catalyse hydrolytic reactions.

Eg: Acetylcholine + H_2O → Choline + Acetic acid

Other drugs like procaine, atropine, pethidine and neostigmine are metabolized by hydroxylation.

If the metabolite of phase I reaction is not sufficiently polar to be excreted, it undergos phase II reactions.

Phase II reactions

In phase II reactions, endogenous water-soluble substances like glucuronic acid, sulfuric acid, glutathione or an amino acid combine with the drug or its phase I metabolite to form a highly polar conjugate which is inactive and gets readily excreted by the kidneys. Large molecules are excreted through the bile. Conjugation results invariably in inactivation of the drug. Some products of conjugation are glucuronides, ethereal sulfates and amino acid conjugates. Glucuronide conjugation is the most common type of metabolic reaction. Endogenous substances like bilirubin and steroid hormones also undergo conjugation.

- Glucuronide conjugation

  e.g. Morphine + Glucuronic acid → Morphine
  glucuronide

- Aminoacid conjugation

  e.g. Benzoic acid + Glycine → Hippuric acid.

Drugs like sulfonamides and isoniazid undergo conjugation with acetylcoenzyme A (acetylation) while some like adrenaline undergo methylation. Glutathione conjugation inactivates highly reactive intermediates formed during the metabolism of drugs like paracetamol.

ENZYME INDUCTION

Microsomal enzymes are located in the microsomes that line the smooth endoplasmic reticulum of the liver cells. The synthesis of these enzymes, mainly cytochrome P450 can be enhanced by certain drugs and environmental pollutants. This is called *enzyme induction* and this process speeds up the biotransformation of the inducing drug itself and other drugs metabolised by the microsomal enzymes, *e.g.* phenobarbitone, rifampicin, alcohol, cigarette smoke, DDT, griseofulvin, carbamazepine and phenytoin are some enzyme inducers.

Clinical relevance of microsomal enzyme induction:

1. Drug interactions

   a. *Therapeutic failure* - By speeding up metabolism, enzyme induction may reduce the duration of action of some other drugs which can result in therapeutic failure. *e.g.* failure of oral contraceptives in patients taking rifampicin.

   b. *Toxicity* - Enzyme induction may result in toxicity due to production of higher amounts of the toxic intermediate metabolites. *e.g.* a patient undergoing treatment with rifampicin is likely to develop hepatotoxicity with paracetamol because a higher amount of the toxic

intermediate metabolite of paracetamol is formed due to enzyme induction.

2. Tolerance to drugs may develop as in case of carbamazepine since it induces its own metabolism called *autoinduction.*

3. Result in disease: Antiepileptics enhance the breakdown of vitamin D resulting in osteomalacia on long term administration.

4. Variable response: In chronic smokers and alcoholics, enzyme induction may result in failure to achieve the expected response to some drugs metabolised by the same enzymes.

5. Therapeutic application of enzyme induction: Neonates are deficient in both microsomal and nonmicrosomal enzymes. Hence their capacity to conjugate bilirubin is low which results in jaundice. Administration of phenobarbitone - an enzyme inducer, helps in rapid clearance of the jaundice in them by enhancing bilirubin conjugation.

ENZYME INHIBITION

Some drugs inhibit cytochrome P450 enzyme activity. Drugs like cimetidine and ketoconazole bind to cytochrome P450 and thus competitively inhibit the metabolism of endogenous substances like testosterone and other drugs given concurrently. Enzyme inhibition by drugs is the basis of several drug interactions. Chloramphenicol, erythromycin, ketoconazole, cimetidine, ciprofloxacin and verapamil are some enzyme inhibitors.

Factors that influence biotransformation

- *Genetic variation* results in altered metabolism of drugs, *e.g.* succinylcholine is metabolised very slowly in people with defective pseudocholinesterase resulting in prolonged apnoea.

- *Environmental pollutants* like cigarette smoke cause enzyme induction.

- *Age* At extremes of age, the activity of metabolic enzymes in the liver are low and hence there is increased risk of toxicity with drugs.

- *Diseases* of the liver markedly affect metabolism of drugs.

Drugs are excreted from the body after being converted to water-soluble metabolites while some are directly eliminated without metabolism. The major organs of excretion are the kidneys, the intestine, the biliary system and the lungs. Drugs are also excreted in small amounts in the saliva, sweat and milk.

EXCRETION

Renal Excretion

Kidney is the most important organ of drug excretion. The three processes involved in the elimination of drugs through kidneys are glomerular filtration, active tubular secretion and passive tubular reabsorption.

Glomerular filtration

The rate of filtration through the glomerulus depends on GFR, concentration of free drug in the plasma and its molecular weight. Ionised drugs of low molecular weight (< 10,000) are easily filtered through the glomerular membrane.

Active tubular secretion

Cells of the proximal tubules actively secrete acids and bases by two transport systems. Thus acids like penicillin, salicylic acid, probenecid, frusemide; bases like amphetamine and histamine are so excreted. Drugs may compete for the same transport system resulting in prolongation of action of each other, *e.g.* penicillin and probenecid.

Passive tubular reabsorption

Passive diffusion of drug molecules can occur in either direction in the renal tubules depending on the drug concentration, lipid solubility and pH. As highly lipid soluble drugs are largely reabsorbed, their excretion is slow. Acidic drugs get ionised in alkaline urine and are easily excreted while bases are excreted faster in acidic urine. This property is useful in the treatment of poisoning. In poisoning with acidic drugs like salicylates and barbiturates, forced alkaline diuresis (Diuretic + sodium bicarbonate + IV fluids) is employed to hasten drug excretion. Similarly, elimination of basic drugs like quinine and amphetamine is enhanced by forced acid diuresis.

Faecal and Biliary Excretion

Unabsorbed portion of the orally administered drugs are eliminated through the faeces. Liver transfers acids, bases and unionised molecules into bile by specific acid transport processes. Large water-soluble conjugates are excreted in the bile. Some drugs may get reabsorbed in the lower portion of the gut and are carried back to the liver. Such recycling is called *enterohepatic circulation* and it prolongs the duration of action of the drug; examples are chloramphenicol, tetracycline, oral contraceptives & erythromycin.

Pulmonary Excretion

The lungs are the main route of elimination for gases and volatile liquids viz general anaesthetics and alcohol. This also has legal implications in medicolegal practice.

Other Routes of Excretion

Small amounts of some drugs are eliminated through the sweat and saliva. Excretion in saliva may result in a unique taste of some drugs like phenytoin, clarithromycin; metallic taste with metronidazole, metoclopramide and disulfiram.

TABLE 3.5: Example of drugs that could be toxic to the suckling infant when taken by the mother

Sulphasalazine	Doxepin
Theophylline	Amiodarone
Anticancer drugs	Primidone
Salicylates	Ethosuximide
Chloramphenicol	Phenobarbitone
Nalidixic acid	Phenothiazines

Drugs like iodide, rifampicin and heavy metals are excreted through sweat.

The excretion of drugs in the **milk** is in small amounts and is of no significance to the mother. But, for the suckling infant, it may be sometimes important especially because of the infant's immature metabolic and excretory mechanisms. Though most drugs can be taken by the mother without significant toxicity to the child, there are a few exceptions (Table 3.5).

CLINICAL PHARMACOKINETICS

The knowledge of pharmacokinetics is clinically useful for several purposes including selection and adjustment of the dosage regimen, and to obtain optimum effects from a drug. The three most important pharmacokinetic parameters are **bioavailability** (page 18), **volume of distribution** (page 20) and **clearance.**

Clearance (CL)

Clearance is the volume of plasma freed completely of the drug in unit time. It can be calculated by the ratio of the rate of elimination to the plasma concentration.

$$\text{Thus, CL} = \frac{\text{Rate of elimination}}{\text{Plasma concentration}}$$

Clearance is expressed as ml/litre/ unit time.

Clearance is the most important factor determining drug concentration and should be considered when any drug is intended for long-term administration.

Drugs are metabolised/eliminated from the body by:

1. First-order kinetics

In first order kinetics, a constant *fraction* of the drug is metabolised/eliminated per unit time. Most drugs follow first order kinetics and the rate of

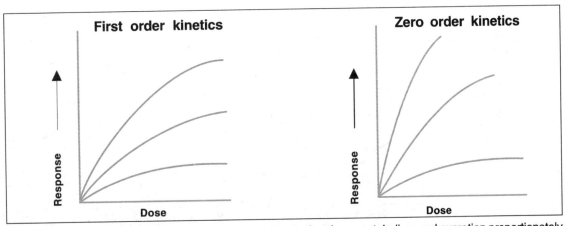

Fig. 3.7   First order kinetics - As the plasma concentration rises, metabolism and excretion proportionately increase. **Zero order kinetics -** In higher doses, the drug accumulates and the plasma concentration rises resulting in toxicity

metabolism/excretion is dependent on their concentration (exponential) in the body (Fig 3.7). It also holds good for absorption of drugs.

2. Zero order kinetics (Saturation kinetics)

Here a constant *amount* of the drug present in the body is metabolised/eliminated per unit time. The metabolic enzymes get saturated and hence with increase in dose, the plasma drug level increases disproportionately resulting in toxicity.

Some drugs like phenytoin and warfarin are eliminated by both processes, *i.e.* by first order initially and by zero order at higher concentrations.

Example of drugs that follow zero order kinetics:

- Alcohol
- Phenytoin
- Aspirin
- Heparin
- Phenylbutazone.

Plasma Half-life and Steady State Concentration

Plasma half-life ($t\frac{1}{2}$) is the time taken for the plasma concentration of a drug to be reduced to half its value (Fig. 3.8). For example If a particular dose of drug is injected intravenously and its plasma concentration is found to be 100 mcg/ml. The plasma concentration is estimated every hour and at the end of four hours it falls to 50 mcg/ml, then the plasma half life of the drug is four hours. Four to five half-lives are required for the complete elimination of a drug. Each drug has its own $t\frac{1}{2}$ and is an important pharmacokinetic parameter that guides the dosing regimen eg. esmolol has a $t\frac{1}{2}$ of 10 minutes, zolpidem 2 hours, aspirin 4 hours, chloroquine 10-24 days.

Significance of plasma $t\frac{1}{2}$

Plasma $t\frac{1}{2}$ is necessary to know -
- The duration of action of the drug
- The frequency of administration
- The time needed for action - steady state concentration.

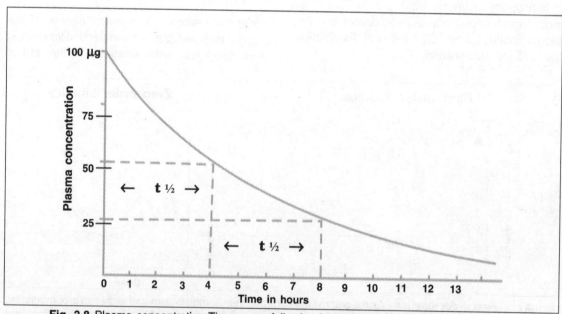

Fig. 3.8 Plasma concentration-Time curve following intravenous administration of a drug. Plasma $t\frac{1}{2}$ of the drug = 4 hours.

- To calculate the loading and maintenance doses of the drug.

Factors influencing plasma t½

1. Plasma protien binding - drugs which are extensively bound to plasma protiens have a longer t½ .

2. Enterohepatic circulation - increases the t½ of the drug.

3. Metabolism - faster the metabolism of a drug, shorter is its plasma t½ .

4. Tissue storage - drugs which are sequestered in the tissues have a longer t½ .

5. Clearance of the drug - drugs which are cleared faster have a shorter t½ .

Biological half-life is the time required for total amount of the drug in the body to be reduced to half.

Biological effect half-life is the time required for the biological effect of the drug to reduce to half. With some drugs like propranolol the pharmacological effect of the drug may last much longer, *i.e.* even after its plasma levels fall. In such drugs, biological effect half life gives an idea of the duration of action of the drug.

If a drug is administered repeatedly at short intervals before complete elimination, the drug accumulates in the body and reaches a 'state' at which the rate of elimination equals the rate of administration. This is known as the *'Steady-state'* or plateau level (Fig. 3.9). After attaining this level, the plasma concentration fluctuates around an average steady level. It takes 4-5 half-lives for the plasma concentration to reach the plateau level. Steady state plasma concentration (C_{PSS}) can be obtained as follows:

$$C_{PSS} = \frac{\text{Dose rate}}{\text{Clearance}}$$

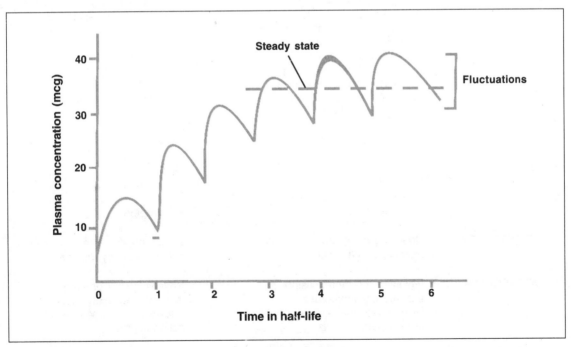

Fig. 3.9 Drug accumulation and attainment of steady state concentration on oral administration

DRUG DOSAGE

Depending on the patient's requirements and the characteristics of the drug, drug dosage can be of the following kinds -

Fixed dose

In case of reasonably safe drugs, a fixed dose of the drug is suitable for most patients, e.g. analgesics like paracetamol - 500 mg to 1000 mg 6 hourly is the usual adult dose.

Individualised dose

For some drugs especially the ones with low safety margin, the dose has to be 'tailored' to the needs of each patient, e.g. anticonvulsants, antiarrhythmic drugs.

Loading dose

In situations when target plasma concentrations have to be attained rapidly, a loading/bolus dose of the drug is given at the beginning of the treatment. A loading dose is a single large dose

Processes	Methods	Examples
TABLE 3.6: Methods of prolonging duration of action of drugs		
ABSORPTION		
Oral	Sustained release preparation, coating with resins, etc.	Iron, deriphylline
Parenteral	1. Reducing solubility - Oily suspension 2. Altering particle size large crystals that are slowly absorbed 3. Pellet implantation - Sialistic capsules 4. Reduction in vascularity of the absorbing surface 5. Combining with protein 6. Chemical alteration - Esterification	Procaine + Penicillin Depot progestins Insulin zinc suspension as DOCA Testosterone Adrenaline + lignocaine (vasoconstrictor) Protamine + zinc + insulin Estrogen Testosterone
Dermal	Transdermal adhesive patches, Ointments Ocuserts (Transmucosal) - used in eye	Scopolamine Nitroglycerin Pilocarpine
DISTRIBUTION	Choosing more protein bound member of the group	Sulfonamides - like sulfamethoxypyridazine
METABOLISM	Inhibiting the metabolising enzyme cholinesterase By inhibiting the enzyme peptidase in renal tubular cells	Physostigmine prolongs the action of acetylcholine Cilastatin - prolongs the action of imipenem
EXCRETION	Competition for same transport system - for renal tubular secretion	Probenecid prolongs the action of penicillin & ampicillin

or a series of quickly repeated doses given to rapidly attain target concentration, *e.g.* heparin given as 5000 IU bolus dose. Once the target level is reached, a *maintenance dose* is sufficient to 'maintain the drug level' and to balance the elimination.

The disadvantage with the loading dose is that the patient is rapidly exposed to high concentrations of the drug which may result in toxicity.

Therapeutic drug monitoring

The response to a drug depends on the plasma concentration attained in the patient. This in turn depends on the bioavailability, volume of distribution and clearance. As these parameters vary among individuals, there is a wide variation in the plasma concentration attained from patient to patient. Hence in some situations it may be necessary to monitor treatment by measuring plasma drug concentrations. Such situations are:

1. While using drugs with low safety margin - to avoid therapeutic failure, *e.g.* digoxin, theophylline, lithium.

2. To reduce the risk of toxicity, *e.g.* aminoglycosides.

3. When there are no reliable methods to assess benefit, *e.g.* antidepressants.

4. To treat poisoning

5. When there is unexplainable therapeutic failure - to check patient compliance.

But, for drugs whose response can be easily measured, *e.g.* blood pressure for antihypertensives and for 'hit and run' drugs whose effects persist for a long time even after the drug is eliminated, monitoring of plasma drug concentration is not required.

METHODS OF PROLONGING DRUG ACTION

(Table 3.6)

In several situations it may be desirable to use long-acting drugs. But when such drugs are not available, the duration of action of the available drugs may be prolonged.

The duration of action of drugs can be prolonged by interfering with the pharmacokinetic processes, *i.e.* by

1. Slowing absorption

2. Using a more plasma protein bound derivative

3. Inhibiting metabolism

4. Delaying excretion.

4 Pharmacodynamics

- **Mechanisms of drug action**
- **Receptor**
    - **Functions of receptors**
    - **Receptor families**
    - **Receptor regulation**
- **Dose response relationship**
- **Drug synergism and antagonism**
- **Factors that modify the effects of drugs**

1. Stimulation
2. Depression
3. Irritation
4. Replacement
5. Anti-infective or cytotoxic action
6. Modification of the immune status

Pharmacodynamics is the study of actions of the drugs on the body and their mechanisms of action, *i.e.* to know what drugs do and how they do it.

Drugs produce their effects by interacting with the physiological systems of the organisms. By such interaction, drugs merely modify the rate of functions of the various systems. But they cannot bring about qualitative changes, *i.e.* they cannot change the basic functions of any physiological system. Thus drugs act by:

Stimulation is the increase in activity of the specialised cells, *e.g.* adrenaline stimulates the heart.

Depression is the decrease in activity of the specialised cells, *e.g.* quinidine depresses the heart; barbiturates depress the central nervous system. Some drugs may stimulate one system and depress another, *e.g.* morphine depresses the CNS but stimulates the vagus.

Irritation This can occur on all types of tissues in the body and may result in inflammation, corrosion and necrosis of cells.

Replacement: Drugs may be used for replacement when there is deficiency of natural substances like hormones, metabolites or nutrients, *e.g.* insulin in diabetes mellitus, iron in anaemia, vitamin C in scurvy.

Anti-infective and cytotoxic action: Drugs may act by specifically destroying infective organisms, *e.g.* penicillins, or by cytotoxic effect on cancer cells, *e.g.* anticancer drugs.

Modification of immune status: Vaccines and sera act by improving our immunity while immuno-suppressants act by depressing immunity, *e.g.* glucocorticoids.

MECHANISMS OF DRUG ACTION

Most drugs produce their effects by binding to specific target proteins like receptors, enzymes and ion channels. Drugs may act *on* the cell membrane, *inside* or *outside* the cell to produce their effect. Drugs may act by one or more complex mechanisms of action. Some of them are yet to be understood. But the fundamental mechanisms of drug action may be:

1. Through receptors
2. Through enzymes and pumps
3. Through ion channels
4. By physical action
5. By chemical interaction
6. By altering metabolic processes.

1. **Through Receptors:** Drugs may act by interacting with specific receptors in the body (see below).

2. **Through Enzymes and Pumps:** Drugs may act by inhibition of various enzymes, thus altering the enzyme-mediated reactions, *e.g.* allopurinol inhibits the enzyme xanthine oxidase; acetazolamide inhibits carbonic anhydrase, enalapril inhibits angiotensin converting enzyme, aspirin inhibits cyclooxygenase, neostigmine inhibits acetylcholinesterase.

Membrane pumps like $H^+ K^+$ ATPase and $Na^+ K^+$ ATPase may be inhibited by drugs like omeprazole and digoxin respectively.

3. **Through Ion Channels:** Drugs may interfere with the movement of ions across specific channels, *e.g.* calcium channel blockers, sodium channel blockers, potassium channel openers and GABA gated chloride channel modulators.

4. **Physical Action:** The action of a drug could result from its physical properties like:

   - Adsorption
     Activated charcoal in poisoning
   - Mass of the drug
     Bulk laxatives like psyllium, bran
   - Osmotic property
       Osmotic diuretics - Mannitol
       Osmotic purgatives - Magnesium
                                  sulphate
   - Radioactivity - ^{131}I
   - Radio-opacity
     Barium sulphate contrast media.

5. **Chemical Interaction:** Drugs may act by chemical reaction.

   - Antacids - neutralise gastric acids
   - Oxidising agents - like potassium permanganate is germicidal
   - Chelating agents - bind heavy metals making them nontoxic.

6. **Altering Metabolic Processes:** Drugs like antimicrobials alter the metabolic pathway in the microorganisms resulting in destruction of the microorganism, *e.g.* sulfonamides interfere with bacterial folic acid synthesis.

RECEPTOR

The works of Langley and Ehrlich put forth the concept of a 'receptor substance.' In the late 19th century, Langley noted that curare could oppose contraction of skeletal muscles caused by nicotine but did not block contraction due to electrical stimulation. Paul Ehrlich observed that some organic chemicals had antiparasitic activity while others with slightly different structures did not have such activity. Clark put forward a theory to explain the drug action based on the drug-receptor occupation.

Last three decades have seen an explosion in our knowledge of the receptors. Various receptors have been identified, isolated and extensively studied.

Definition

A receptor is a macromolecular site on the cell with which an agonist binds to bring about a change.

Affinity

Affinity is the ability of a drug to bind to a receptor.

Intrinsic activity or efficacy

Intrinsic activity is the ability of a drug to elicit a response after binding to the receptor.

Agonist

An agonist is a substance that binds to the receptor and produces a response. It has affinity and intrinsic activity e.g. adrenaline is an agonist at α and β adrenergic receptors; morphine is an agonist at m opioid receptors.

Antagonist

An antagonist is a substance that binds to the receptor and prevents the action of agonist on the receptor. It has affinity but no intrinsic activity. Naloxone is an antagonist at m opioid receptors; tubocurarine is an antagonist at nicotinic receptors.

Partial agonist

A partial agonist binds to the receptor but has low intrinsic activity. Pentazocine is a partial agonist at μ opioid receptors.

Inverse agonist

Some drugs, after binding to the receptors produce actions opposite to those produced by a pure agonist. They are known as inverse agonists, e.g. Diazepam acting on benzodiazepine receptors produces sedation, anxiolysis, muscle relaxation and controls convulsions, while the inverse agonists β-carbolines bind to the same receptors to cause arousal, anxiety, increased muscle tone and convulsions.

Ligand

Ligand is a molecule which binds selectively to a specific receptor.

Spare receptors

Some experiments showed that high concentration of an agonist can still produce maximal response in presence of an irreversible antagonist and this was because of the presence of 'spare' or reserve receptors. Thus it is possible to stimulate the myocardium even when 90% of the cardiac β adrenergic receptors are blocked by an irreversible β blocker.

Silent receptors

These are receptors to which an agonist binds but does not produce a response. Presence of such silent receptors may explain the phenomenon of tolerance.

Site

The receptors may be present in the cell membrane, in the cytoplasm or on the nucleus.

Nature of receptors

Receptors are proteins.

Synthesis and life-span

Receptor proteins are synthesized by the cells. They have a definite life span after which the receptors are degraded by the cell and new receptors are synthesized.

Functions of Receptors

The two functions of receptors are -

- Recognition and binding of the ligand.
- Propagation of the message.

For the above functions, the receptor has two functional domains (areas):

- *A ligand binding domain* - the site to bind the drug molecule
- *An effector domain* - which undergoes a change to propagate the message.

Several **theories** have been proposed to explain drug receptor interaction. Drug-receptor interaction has been considered to be similar to 'lock and key' relationship where the drug specifically fits into the particular receptor (lock) like a key. The **rate theory** proposes that the magnitude of response depends on the rate of agonist - receptor association and dissociation. The rate of receptor- binding is more initially but after it reaches the peak, there is a decrease.

The **occupation theory** suggests that the magnitude of drug response depends on the proportion of the receptors occupied by the drug. Interaction of the agonist with the receptor brings about changes in the receptor which in turn conveys the signal to the effector system. The final response is brought about by the effector system through second messengers. The agonist itself is the first messenger. The entire process involves a chain of events triggered by drug receptor interaction.

Receptor Families

On stimulation of a receptor, the time required to elicit the response varies largely from a fraction of a second in some receptors to hours and days in others. This difference is because of the variation in mechanisms involved in linking the receptor and the effector systems (transduction mechanisms). Based on this, four types or super families of cell surface receptors are identified. They are best understood with the help of Figure 4.1. The receptor types are:

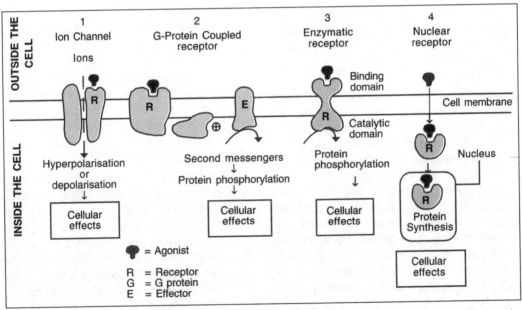

Fig. 4.1 (1) Binding of the agonist directly regulates the opening of the ion channel. **(2)** Agonist binding activates the receptor linked to an effector system by a G protein. **(3)** Agonist binding to extracellular domain activates enzymatic activity of its catalytic domain. **(4)** Agonist binds to the intracellular receptor, the complex moves to the nucleus and directs protein synthesis

1. Ion channels (ionotropic receptor)

2. G-protein coupled receptors (metabotropic receptor)

3. Enzymatic receptors (kinase linked receptor)

4. Nuclear receptors (Transcription factors or receptors that regulate gene transcription).

Receptor families and their transduction mechanisms

1. **Ion Channels** or receptor channels are proteins present on the cell surface. Binding of the agonist opens the channel allowing ions to cross the membrane. These are called ligand-gated ion channels. Depending on the ion and the channel, depolarisation/ hyperpolarisation occurs, *e.g.* nicotinic cholinergic receptor channel permits passage of Na^+ ions resulting in depolarisation.

2. **G-protein Coupled Receptors** are proteins spanning the plasma membrane. The G-proteins are bound to the inner face of the plasma membrane. The G-proteins consist of three subunits viz., α, β and γ. When a ligand binds to the G-protein coupled receptor, the associated G-protein gets activated. This in turn activates adenyl cyclase or phospholipase C to generate the respective second mesengers. These second messenger systems are called effector pathways. G-proteins acting through second messengers, bring about a chain of intracellular changes. Thus G-proteins act as a link or mediator between the receptors and the effector systems. They are called G-proteins because of their interaction with the guanine nucleotides, GTP and GDP. G-proteins are of different classes like G_S, G_I, G_Q, G_O and G_{13} - G_S is stimulatory and G_i is inhibitory. The second messengers include cAMP, IP_3, DAG, Ca^{++} and cGMP. Adrenergic receptors and muscarinic cholinergic receptors are examples of G-protein coupled receptors.

Effector pathways through which the G-protein coupled receptors work are:

- Adenylcyclase/cAMP pathway
- Phospholipase C/IP_3-DAG pathway
- Ion channel regulation.

- **Adenylyl cyclase pathway** (Fig 4.2): Stimulation of adenylcyclase results in the formation and accumulation of cAMP within the cell. This cAMP acts through protein kinases which phosphorylate various proteins to regulate the cell function. The response may be contraction, relaxation, lipolysis or hormone synthesis.

- **PhospholipaseC/IP_3-DAG pathway** (Fig 4.3): Activation of phospholipase C results in the formation of second messengers IP_3 and DAG from the membrane phospholipids phospho inositol pyrophosphate (PIP_2). IP_3 mobilises Ca^{++} from intracellular depots and this Ca^{++} mediates responses like secretion, contraction, metabolism and hyperpolarisation. DAG activates protein kinase C which regulates cell function.

- **Ion channel regulation:** The activated G-proteins can directly (without the help of second messengers) convey the signal to some ion channels causing opening or closing of the channels. The resulting responses include depolarisation/ hyperpolarisation.

3. **Enzymatic Receptors** are transmembrane proteins with an extracellular domain (site) for ligand binding and intracellular domain to carry out the catalytic activity and the two domains are linked by a single peptide chain. They are protein kinases and hence are also known as **kinase linked** receptors. Binding of the agonist to the ligand binding domain results in autophosphorylation of the intracellular domain. This in turn triggers phosphorylation of various intracellular proteins resulting in the characteristic response. *e.g.* receptors of insulin, leptin and

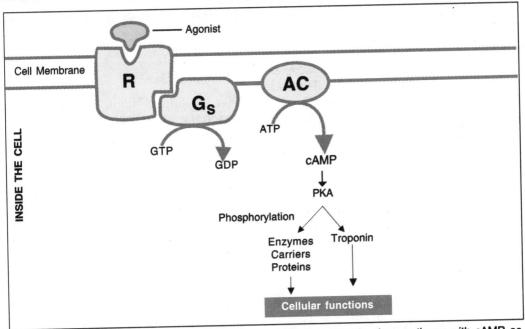

Fig 4.2 G Protein coupled receptor - transduction through adenylylcyclase pathway with cAMP as second messenger. R = Receptor, G_s = G Protein (Stimulatory).

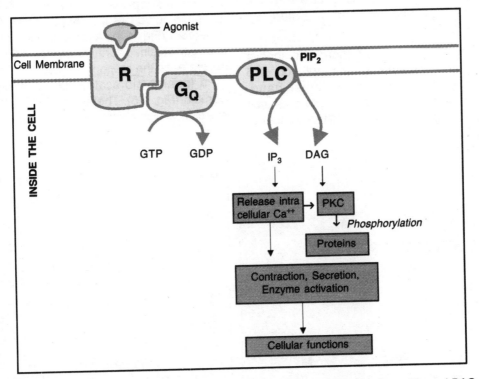

Fig 4.3 G Protein coupled receptor acting through the second messengers IP_3 and DAG

growth factors including epidermal growth factors and platelet derived growth factors.

4. **Receptors that Regulate Gene Transcription** are also called transcription factors or **nuclear receptors**. They are intracellular proteins which are in an inactive state. Binding of the agonist activates the receptor. The agonist-receptor complex moves to the nucleus where it interacts with DNA, regulates gene transcription and thereby directs the synthesis of specific proteins to regulate the activity of target cells. Examples are receptors for steroidal hormones, thyroid hormones, vitamin D and retinoids.

Receptor Regulation

The number of receptors (density) and their sensitivity can be altered in many situations. Denervation or prolonged deprivation of the agonist or constant action of the antagonist all result in an increase in the number and sensitivity of the receptors. This phenomenon is called '**up regulation.**'

Prolonged use of a β adrenergic antagonist like propranolol results in up regulation of β adrenergic receptors. On the other hand, continued stimulation of the receptors causes desensitisation and a decrease in the number of receptors - known as '**down regulation**' of the receptors.

Clinical consequences and implications of receptor regulation

After prolonged administration, a receptor antagonist should always be tapered. For example, if propranolol - a β adrenoceptor blocker is suddenly withdrawn after long-term use, it precipitates angina.

Constant use of β adrenergic agonists in bronchial asthma results in reduced therapeutic response due to down regulation of β_2 receptors.

DOSE RESPONSE RELATIONSHIP

The clinical response to the increasing dose of the drug is defined by the shape of the dose response curve (DRC). Initially the extent of response increases with increase in dose till the maximum response is reached. The dose response curve has the shape of a rectangular hyperbola (Fig. 4.4). After the maximum effect has been obtained, further increase in doses does not increase the response. If the dose is plotted on a logarithmic scale, the curve becomes sigmoid (Fig. 4.5). The slope of DRC (Fig. 4.6) has clinical significance. A steep slope indicates

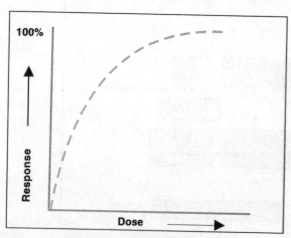

Fig. 4.4 Dose response curve

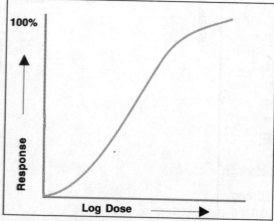

Fig. 4.5 Log dose response curve

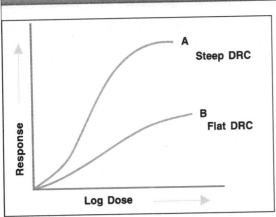

Fig.4.6 Steep and flat dose response curves

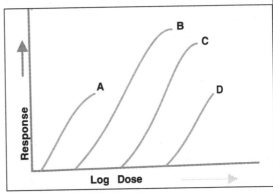

Fig. 4.7 Dose response curves of four drugs showing different potencies and maximal efficacies. Drug A is more potent but less efficacious than B and C. Drug D is less potent and less efficacious than drugs B and C

that a small increase in dose produces a large increase in response, *e.g.* loop diuretics. Such drugs are more likely to cause toxicity and therefore, individualisation of dose is required. A relatively flat DRC indicates that with an increase in dose, there is little increase in the response, *e.g.* thiazide diuretics. For such drugs standard doses can be given to most patients.

Drug Potency and Maximal Efficacy

The amount of drug required to produce a response indicates the **potency**. For example, 1 mg of bumetanide produces the same diuresis as 50 mg of frusemide. Thus bumetanide is more potent than frusemide. In Figure 4.7, drugs A and B are more potent than drugs C and D, drug A being the most potent and drug D - the least potent. Hence higher doses of drugs C and D are to be administered as compared to drugs A and B. Generally potency is of little clinical significance unless very large doses of the drug needs to be given due to low potency.

Maximal efficacy

Efficacy indicates the maximum response that can be produced by a drug, *e.g.* frusemide produces powerful diuresis, not produced by any dose of amiloride. In Figure 4.7, drugs B and C

are more efficacious than drugs A and D. Drug A is more potent but less efficacious than drugs B and C. Such differences in efficacy are of great clinical importance.

Therapeutic index

The dose response curves for different actions of a drug could be different. Thus salbutamol may have one DRC for bronchodilation and another for tachycardia. The distance between beneficial effect DRC and unwanted effect DRC indicates the safety margin of the drug (Fig. 4.8).

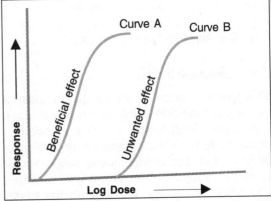

Fig. 4.8 The distance between the curves A and B indicates safety margin of the drug. The greater the distance, more selective is the drug

Median lethal dose (LD$_{50}$)

Dose which is lethal to 50% of the population.

Median effective dose (ED$_{50}$)

Dose that produces a desired effect in 50% of the test population.

Therapeutic index (TI) is the ratio of the median lethal dose to the median effective dose.

$$\text{Therapeutic index} = \frac{LD_{50}}{ED_{50}}$$

- TI gives an idea about the safety of the drug.
- The higher the therapeutic index, the safer is the drug
- TI varies from species to species
- For a drug to be considered reasonably safe, its TI must be > 1
- Penicillin has a high TI while lithium and digoxin have low TI.
- TI may be different for each action of a drug. For *eg.*, TI of aspirin used for headache is different from its TI for inflammation.

Limitations of TI

Therapeutic Index does not consider idiosyncratic responses that result in toxicity. Moreover, the data are based on animal studies which may be difficult to apply on human beings.

Therapeutic Window

Therapeutic wndow is the range of plasma concentrations below which the drug is ineffective and above which toxicity appears. Hence it is desirable to have the plasma concentration of drugs within this optimal therapeutic range in order to derive therapeutic effect without significant toxic effect. Some drugs like those with low therapeutic index have a narrow therapeutic window. *e.g.* digoxin 0.8-0.2 ng/ml. lithium 0.5 - 1.3 m Eq/l, carbamazepine 3-10 mcg/ml. Clonidine

0.2-2ng/ml. Imipramine produces optimum therapeutic effect only when its plasma levels are maintained between 50 to 200 ng/ml. Doses of such drugs must be titrated carefully.

DRUG SYNERGISM AND ANTAGONISM

When two or more drugs are given concurrently the effect may be additive, synergistic or antagonistic.

Additive Effect

The effect of two or more drugs get added up and the total effect is equal to the sum of their individual actions. Examples are ephedrine with theophylline in bronchial asthma; nitrous oxide and ether as general anaesthetics.

Synergism

When the action of one drug is enhanced or facilitated by another drug, the combination is synergistic. In Greek, ergon = work; syn = with. Here, the total effect of the combination is greater than the sum of their independent effects. It is often called 'potentiation' or 'supra-additive' effect.

Examples are -

- Acetylcholine + physostigmine
- Levodopa + carbidopa.

Antagonism

One drug opposing or inhibiting the action of another is antagonism. Based on the mechanisms, antagonism can be

- Chemical antagonism
- Physiological antagonism
- Antagonism at the receptor level
  - Reversible (Competitive)
  - Irreversible
- Non-competitive antagonism.

Chemical antagonism

Two substances interact chemically to result in inactivation of the effect, *e.g.* chelating agents inactivate heavy metals like lead and mercury to form inactive complexes; antacids like aluminium hydroxide neutralize gastric acid.

Physiological antagonism

Two drugs act at different sites to produce opposing effects. For example, histamine acts on H_1 receptors to produce bronchospasm and hypotension while adrenaline reverses these effects by acting on adrenergic receptors.

Insulin and glucagon have opposite effects on the blood sugar level.

Antagonism at the receptor level

The antagonist inhibits the binding of the agonist to the receptor. Such antagonism may be reversible or irreversible.

• *Reversible or competitive antagonism*

The agonist and antagonist compete for the same receptor. By increasing the concentration of the agonist, the antagonism can be overcome. It is thus *reversible antagonism*. The same maximal response can still be obtained by increasing the dose of the agonist. It is also called surmountable or equilibrium type of antagonism. Acetylcholine and atropine compete at muscarinic receptors. The antagonism can be overcome by increasing the concentration of acetylcholine at the receptor. d-tubocurarine and acetylcholine compete for the nicotinic receptors at the neuromuscular junction. The dose response curve shifts to the right (Fig.4.9) in the presence of competitive antagonists.

• *Irreversible antagonism*

The antagonist binds so firmly by covalent bonds to the receptor that it dissociates very slowly or not at all. Thus it blocks the action of the agonist and the blockade *cannot* be overcome by increasing the dose of the agonist and hence it is irreversible antagonism, *e.g.* adrenaline and phenoxybenzamine at alpha adrenergic receptors. This antagonism is also called non-equilibrium type of antagonism.

There is progressive flattening of the dose response curve (Fig. 4.10).

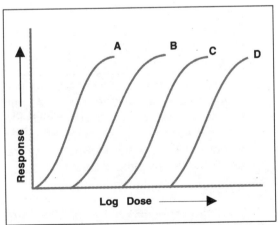

Fig. 4.9 Dose response curves of an agonist: A in the absence of competitive antagonist; B, C and D in the presence of increasing doses of a reversible competitive antagonist

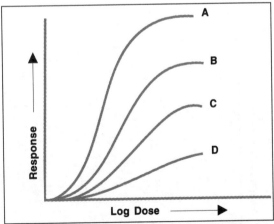

Fig. 4.10 Dose response curves of an agonist: A in the absence of antagonist. B, C, and D in the presence of increasing doses of an irreversible antagonist

Noncompetitive antagonism

The antagonist blocks at the level of receptor-effector linkage *i.e.*, at a different site beyond the receptor and not on the receptor. There is flattening as well as some rightward shift of the dose response curve (Fig. 4.11). For example verapamil blocks the cardiac calcium channels and inhibits the entry of Ca^{++} during depolarisation. It thereby antagonises the effect of cardiac stimulants like isoprenaline and adrenaline.

FACTORS THAT MODIFY THE EFFECTS OF DRUGS

The same dose of a drug can produce different degrees of response in different patients and even in the same patient under different situations. Various factors modify the response to a drug. They are:

1. **Body weight**

   The recommended dose is calculated for medium built persons. For the obese and underweight persons, the dose has to be calculated individually. Though body surface area is a better parameter for more accurate

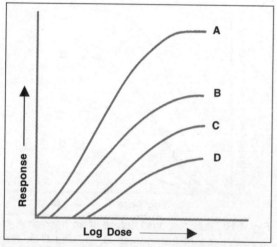

Fig. 4.11 Non-competitive antagonism - there is flattening as well as some rightward shift of DRC

calculation of the dose, it is inconvenient and hence not generally used.

Formula

$$\text{Dose} = \frac{\text{Body weight (kg)}}{70} \times \text{average adult dose}$$

2. Age

   The pharmacokinetics of many drugs change with age resulting in altered response in extremes of age.

   New born and infants7 In the newborn, the liver and kidneys are not fully mature to handle the drugs, *e.g.* chloramphenicol can produce grey baby syndrome. The blood-brain barrier is not well-formed and drugs can easily reach the brain. The gastric acidity is low, intestinal motility is slow, skin is delicate and permeable to drugs applied topically. Hence calculation of the appropriate dose, depending on body weight is important to avoid toxicity. Also pharmacodynamic differences could exist, *e.g.* barbiturates which produce sedation in adults may produce excitation in children.

   Formula for calculation of dose for children.

   Young's formula

   $$\text{Child's dose} = \frac{\text{Age (years)}}{\text{Age} + 12} \times \text{Adult dose}$$

   In the elderly, the capacity of the liver and kidney to handle the drug is reduced and they are more susceptible to adverse effects. Hence lower doses are recommended, *e.g.* elderly are at a higher risk of ototoxicity and nephrotoxicity by streptomycin.

3. Sex

   The hormonal effects and smaller body size may influence drug response in women. Special care is necessary while prescribing for pregnant and lactating women and during menstruation.

4. Species and race

Response to drugs may vary with species and race. For example, rabbits are resistant to atropine. Such variation makes it difficult to extrapolate the results of animal experiments. Blacks need higher doses of atropine to produce mydriasis.

5. Diet and environment

Food interferes with the absorption of many drugs. For example, tetracyclines form complexes with calcium present in the food and are poorly absorbed.

Polycyclic hydrocarbons present in the cigarette smoke may induce microsomal enzymes resulting in enhanced metabolism of some drugs.

6. Route of administration

Occasionally route of administration may modify the pharmacodynamic response, *e.g.* magnesium sulfate given orally is a purgative. But given IV it causes CNS depression and has anticonvulsant effects. Applied topically (poultice), it reduces local edema. Hypertonic magnesium sulfate retention enema reduces intracranial tension.

7. Genetic factors

Variations in an individual's response to drugs could be genetically mediated. **Pharmacogenetics** is concerned with the genetically mediated variations in drug responses. The differences in response is most commonly due to variations in the amount of drug metabolising enzymes since the production of these enzymes is genetically controlled.

Examples

a. **Acetylation of drugs:** The rate of drug acetylation differs among individuals who may be fast or slow acetylators, *e.g.* INH, sulfonamides and hydralazine are acetylated. Slow acetylators treated with hydralazine are more likely to develop lupus erythematosus.

b. **Atypical pseudocholinesterase:** Succinylcholine is metabolised by the enzyme pseudocholinesterase. Some people inherit an atypical pseudocholinesterase which cannot quickly metabolise succinyl choline. When succinyl choline is given to such people, they develop a prolonged apnoea due to persistant action of succinyl choline.

c. **G_6PD deficiency:** Primaquine, sulphones and quinolones can cause hemolysis in such people.

d. **Malignant hyperthermia:** Halothane and succinylcholine can trigger malignant hyperthermia in some genetically predisposed individuals (See page 86).

e. **Hepatic porphyrias:** Some people lack an enzyme required for haeme synthesis, and this results in accumulation of porphyrin-containing haeme precursors. Some drugs like barbiturates, griseofulvin and carbamazepine induce the enzyme required for porphyrin synthesis resulting in accumulation of porphyrins. In both the above cases neurological, gastrointestinal and behavioural abnormalities can occur due to excess porphyrins.

8. Dose

It is fascinating that the response to a drug may be modified by the dose administered. Generally as the dose is increased, the magnitude of the response also increases proportionately till the 'maximum' is reached. Further increases in doses may with some drugs produce effects opposite to their lower-dose effect, *e.g.*

(i) in myasthenia gravis, neostigmine enhances muscle power in therapeutic doses, but in high doses it causes muscle paralysis

(ii) physiological doses of vitamin D promotes calcification while hypervitaminosis D leads to decalcification.

9. **Diseases**

   Presence of certain diseases can influence drug responses, *e.g.*

   - **Malabsorption** Drugs are poorly absorbed.

   - **Liver diseases** Rate of drug metabolism is reduced due to dysfunction of hepatocytes. Also protein binding is reduced due to low serum albumin.

   - **Cardiac diseases** In CCF, there is edema of the gut mucosa and decreased perfusion of liver and kidneys. These may result in cumulation and toxicity of drugs like propranolol and lignocaine.

   - **Renal dysfunction** Drugs mainly excreted through kidneys are likely to accumulate and cause toxicity, *e.g.* Streptomycin, amphotericin B - doses of such drugs need to be reduced.

10. **Repeated dosing**

   Repeated dosing can result in
   - Cumulation
   - Tolerance
   - Tachyphylaxis.

   Cumulation: Drugs like digoxin which are slowly eliminated may cumulate resulting in toxicity.

   Tolerance: Tolerance is the requirement of higher doses of a drug to produce a given response. Tolerance may be natural or acquired.

   - *Natural tolerance:* The species/race shows less sensitivity to the drug, *e.g.* rabbits show tolerance to atropine; Black race are tolerant to mydriatics.

   - *Acquired tolerance* develops on repeated administration of a drug. The patient who was initially responsive becomes tolerant, *e.g.* barbiturates, opioids, nitrites produce tolerance.

   Tolerance may develop to some actions of the drug and not to others, *e.g.* morphine - tolerance develops to analgesic and euphoric effects of morphine but not to its constipating and miotic effects. Barbiturates - tolerance develops to sedative but not antiepileptic effects of barbiturates.

Mechanisms

The mechanisms of development of tolerance could be:

Pharmacokinetic Changes in absorption, distribution, metabolism and excretion of drugs may result in reduced concentration of the drug at the site of action and is also known as dispositional tolerance, *e.g.* barbiturates induce microsomal enzymes and enhance their own metabolism.

Pharmacodynamic Changes in the target tissue, may make it less responsive to the drug. It is also called functional tolerance. It could be due to down regulation of receptors as in opioids or due to compensatory mechanisms of the body, *e.g.* blunting of response to some antihypertensives due to salt and water retention.

Cross tolerance is the development of tolerance to pharmacologically related drugs, *i.e.* to drugs belonging to a particular group. Thus chronic alcoholics also show tolerance to barbiturates and general anaesthetics.

Tachyphylaxis is the rapid development of tolerance. When some drugs are administered repeatedly at short intervals, tolerance develops rapidly and is known as tachyphylaxis or acute tolerance, *e.g.* ephedrine, amphetamine, tyramine and 5-hydroxytryptamine. This is thought to be due to depletion of noradrenaline stores as the above drugs act by displacing noradrenaline from the sympathetic nerve endings. Other mechanisms involved may be slow dissociation of the drug from the receptor thereby blocking the receptor. Thus ephedrine given repeatedly in bronchial asthma may not give the desired response.

11. Psychological factor

The doctor patient relationship influences the response to a drug often to a large extent by acting on the patient's psychology. The patient's confidence in the doctor may itself be sufficient to relieve a suffering, particularly the psychosomatic disorders. This can be substantiated by the fact that a large number of patients respond to placebo. **Placebo** is the inert dosage form with no specific biological activity but only resembles the actual preparation in appearance (dummy medication) *Placebo* = 'I shall be pleasing' (in Latin).

Placebo medicines are used in -

1. Clinical trials as a control to compare and assess whether the new compound is significantly better than the placebo.

2. To benefit or please a patient psychologically when he does not actually require an active drug as in mild psychosomatic disorders and in chronic incurable diseases.

In fact all forms of treatment including physiotherapy and surgery have some placebo effect. Substances used as placebo include lactose, some vitamins, minerals and distilled water injections.

12. Presence of other drugs

The concurrent use of two or more drugs can influence the response of each other (See Drug Interactions page 51, 547).

5

Adverse Drug Reactions and Drug Interactions

- **Adverse drug reactions**
  - Side effects
  - Toxic effects
  - Intolerance
  - Iatrogenic diseases
  - Drug dependence
  - Teratogenicity
  - Carcinogenicity
  - Other adverse drug reactions
- **Drug interactions**
  - Definition
  - Site
  - Pharmacological basis of drug interactions

ADVERSE DRUG REACTIONS

All drugs can produce unwanted effects. WHO has defined an adverse drug reaction as "any response to a drug that is noxious and unintended and that occurs at doses used in man for prophylaxis, diagnosis or therapy."

All drugs can cause adverse effects. Some patients are more likely to exhibit adverse effects to drugs. **Pharmacovigilance** deals with the epidemiologic study of adverse drug effects.

1. **Side Effects:** Side effects are unwanted effects of a drug that are extension of pharmacological effects and are seen with the therapeutic dose of the drug. They are predictable, common and can occur in all people, *e.g.* hypoglycaemia due to insulin; hypokalaemia following frusemide.

2. **Toxic Effects:** Toxic effects are seen with higher doses of the drug and can be serious, *e.g.* morphine causes respiratory depression in overdosage.

3. **Intolerance:** Drug intolerance is the inability of a person to tolerate a drug and is unpredictable. Patients show exaggerated response to even small doses of the drug, *e.g.* vestibular dysfunction after a single dose

of streptomycin may be seen in some patients. Intolerance could also be qualitative, *e.g.* idiosyncrasy and allergic reactions.

- *Idiosyncrasy* is a genetically determined abnormal reaction to a drug, *e.g.* primaquine and sulfonamides induce haemolysis in patients with G_6PD deficiency; some patients show excitement with barbiturates. In addition, some responses like chloramphenicol-induced agranulocytosis, where no definite genetic background is known, are also included under idiosyncrasy. In some cases the person may be highly sensitive even to low doses of a drug (*e.g.* a single dose of quinine can produce cinchonism in some) or highly insensitive even to high doses of the drug.

- *Allergic reactions* to drugs are immunologically-mediated reactions which are not related to the therapeutic effects of the drug. The drug or its metabolite acts as an antigen to induce antibody formation. Subsequent exposure to the drug may result in allergic reactions. The manifestations of allergy are seen mainly on the target organs *viz.* skin, respiratory tract, gastrointestinal tract, blood and blood vessels.

Types of Allergic Reactions and their Mechanisms

Drugs can induce both types of allergic reactions *viz.* Humoral and cell-mediated immunity. Mechanisms involved in type I, II and III are humoral while type IV is by cell-mediated immunity.

Type I (Anaphylactic) reaction: The drug induces the synthesis of IgE antibodies which are fixed to the mast cells. On subsequent exposure, the antigen-antibody complexes cause degranulation of mast cells releasing the mediators of inflammation like histamine, leukotrienes, prostaglandins and platelet-activating factor. These are responsible for the characteristic signs and symptoms of anaphylaxis like bronchospasm, laryngeal edema and hypotension which could be fatal. Allergy develops within minutes and is called immediate hypersensitivity reaction, *e.g.* penicillins. Skin tests may predict this type of reactions. Penicillins, cephalosporins, lignocaine, procaine, iron dextran and streptomycin are some drugs known to cause anaphylaxis.

Type II (Cytolytic) reactions: The drug binds to a protein and together they act as antigen and induce the formation of antibodies. The antigen antibody complexes activate the complement system resulting in cytolysis causing thrombocytopenia, agranulocytosis and aplastic anaemia. Examples are carbamazepine, phenytoin, sulphonamides and phenylbutazone. Mismatched blood transfusion reactions are also cytolytic reactions.

Type III (Arthus) reactions: The antigen binds to circulating antibodies and the complexes are deposited on the vessel wall where it initiates the inflammatory response resulting in vasculitis. Rashes, fever, arthralgia, lymphadenopathy, serum sickness and Steven-Johnson's syndrome are some of the manifestations of arthus type reaction. Serum sickness is characterized by fever, arthritis, nephritis, edema and skin rashes. Penicillins, sulfonamides, phenytoin, streptomycin and heparin can cause serum sickness. Steven Johnson's Syndrome (SJS) is characterized by severe bullous erythema multiformae particularly in the mucous membranes with fever and malaise. Toxic Epidermal Necrolysis (TEN) is the most serious form of drug allergy with cutaneous reactions that can be fatal. Aminopenicillins, sulphonamides, sulfones, phenytoin, barbiturates, carbamazepine and phenylbutazone, quinolones are the drugs associated with SJS and TEN.

Type IV (delayed hypersensitivity) reactions: This type of reactions are mediated by T-lymphocytes and macrophages. The antigen reacts with receptors on T-lymphocytes which produce lymphokines leading to a local allergic reaction, *e.g.* contact dermatitis in nurses and doctors handling penicillins and local anaesthetics.

4. **Iatrogenic Diseases (Physician Induced):** These are drug induced diseases. Even after the drug is withdrawn toxic effects can persist, *e.g.* isoniazid induced hepatitis; chloroquine induced retinopathy. Drugs that can induce parkinsonism are chlorpromazine, haloperidol and other phenothiazines, metoclopramide, reserpine.

5. **Drug Dependence:** Drugs that influence the behaviour and mood are often misused to obtain pleasurable effects. Repeated use of such drugs result in dependence. Several words like drug abuse, addiction and dependence are used confusingly. Drug dependence is a state of compulsive use of drugs in spite of the knowledge of the risks associated with its use. It is also referred to as drug addiction. Dependence could be 'psychologic' or 'physical' dependence. Psychologic dependence is compulsive drug-seeking behaviour to obtain its pleasurable effects, *e.g.* cigarette smoking.

Physical dependence is said to be present when withdrawal of the drug produces adverse symptoms. The body undergoes physiological changes to adapt itself to the continued presence of the drug in the body. Stopping the drug results in 'withdrawal syndrome.' The symptoms of withdrawal syndrome are disturbing and the person then craves for the drug, *e.g.* alcohol, opioids and barbiturates.

Mild degree of physical dependence is seen in people who drink too much of coffee.

6. **Teratogenicity:** Teratogenicity is the ability of a drug to cause foetal abnormalities when administered to a pregnant woman. *Teratos* in Greek means monster. The sedative thalidomide taken during early pregnancy for relief from morning sickness resulted in thousands of babies being born with phocomelia (seal limbs). This thalidomide disaster (1958-61) opened the eyes of drug licensing authorities and various nations made it mandatory to conduct strict teratogenicity tests before a new drug is approved for use.

Depending on the stage of pregnancy during which the teratogen is administered, it can produce various abnormalities.

* Conception to 16 days - Usually resistant to teratogenic effects. If affected, abortion occurs.

* Period of organogenesis - (17 to 55 days of gestation) Most vulnerable period; major physical abnormalities occur.

* Foetal period - 56 days onwards - Period of growth and development-hence developmental and functional abnormalities result.

Therefore, in general, drugs should be avoided during pregnancy specially in the first trimester. The type of malformation also depends on the drug, *e.g.* thalidomide causes phocomelia; tetracyclines cause deformed teeth; sodium valproate causes spina bifida.

7. **Carcinogenicity and Mutagenicity:** Some drugs can cause cancers and genetic abnormalities. For example anticancer drugs can themselves be carcinogenic; other examples are radioactive isotopes and some hormones.

8. **Other Adverse Drug Reactions:** Drugs can also damage various organ systems.

Treatment of drug overdosage - see chapter 76

DRUG INTERACTIONS

Definition

Drug interaction is the alteration in the duration or magnitude of the pharmacological effects of one drug by another drug.

When two or more drugs are given concurrently, the response may be greater or lesser than the sum of their individual effects. Such responses may be beneficial or harmful. For example a combination of drugs is used in hypertension - hydralazine + propranolol for their beneficial interaction. But unwanted drug interactions may result in severe toxicity. Such interactions can be avoided by adequate knowledge of their mechanisms and by judicious use of drugs. Some important drug interactions are mentioned in Appendix-1.

Site

Drug interactions can occur:

1. *In vitro* in the syringe before administration - mixing of drugs in syringes can cause chemical or physical interactions - such drug combinations are incompatible in solution, *e.g.* penicillin and gentamicin should never be mixed in the same syringe.
2. *In vivo, i.e.* in the body after administration.

Pharmacological basis of drug interactions

The two major mechanisms of drug interactions include pharmacokinetic and pharmacodynamic interactions.

Pharmacokinetic mechanisms

Alteration in the extent or duration of response may be produced by influencing absorption,

	Organ system affected	Examples
	Table 5.1 Examples of drugs affecting various organ systems	
1.	Hepatotoxicity	Isoniazid, pyrazinamide, paracetamol, chlorpromazine, 6-Mercaptopurine, halothane, ethanol, phenylbutazone
2.	Nephrotoxicity	Analgesics, aminoglycosides, cyclosporine, cisplatin, cephexin, penicillamine, gold salts
3.	Ototoxicity	Aminoglycosides, frusemide
4.	Ocular toxicity	Chloroquine, ethambutol
5.	Gastrointestinal system	Opioids, broad spectrum antibiotics
6.	Cardiovascular system	Digoxin, doxorubicin
7.	Respiratory system	Aspirin, bleomycin, busulfan, amiodarone, methotrexate
8.	Musculoskeletal system	Corticosteroids, heparin
9.	Behavioural toxicity	Corticosteroids, reserpine
10.	Neurological system	INH, haloperidol, ethambutol, quinine, doxorubicin vincristine
11.	Dermatological toxicity	Doxycycline, sulfonamides, gold, d-penicillamine
12.	Electrolyte disturbances	Diuretics, mineralocorticoids
13.	Haematological toxicity	Chloramphenicol, sulfonamides
14.	Endocrine disorders	Methyldopa, oral contraceptives
15.	Sexual dysfunctions	Prazosin, reserpine, anticholinergics, barbiturates, methyl dopa, tricyclic, antidepressants

distribution, metabolism or excretion of one drug by another.

Absorption

Absorption of drugs from the gut may be affected by:

1. Binding –Tetracyclines chelate iron and antacids resulting in reduced absorption. Cholestyramine is a bile acid binding resin which also binds many drugs.

2. Altering gastric pH – Antacids raise gastric pH and interfere with the absorption of drugs like iron and anticoagulants

3. Altering GI motility. Atropine and morphine slow gastric emptying and delay the absorption of drugs. Purgatives reduce the absorption of riboflavin.

Distribution

Competition for plasma protein or tissue binding results in displacement interactions, e.g. warfarin is displaced by phenylbutazone from protein binding sites.

Metabolism

Enzyme induction and inhibition of metabolism can both result in drug interactions (page 23), e.g. phenytoin, phenobarbitone, carbamazepine and rifampicin are enzyme inducers while chloramphenicol and cimetidine are some enzyme inhibitors.

Excretion

When drugs compete for the same renal tubular transport system, they prolong each other's duration of action, e.g. penicillin and probenecid.

Pharmacodynamic mechanisms

Drugs acting on the same receptors or physiological systems result in additive, synergistic or antagonistic effects. Many clinically important drug interactions have this basis. Examples are-

• Atropine opposes the effects of physostigmine

• Naloxone antagonises morphine

• Antihypertensive effects of β blockers are reduced by ephedrine or other vasoconstrictors present in cold remedies

• Many diuretics produce hypokalemia which potentiate digitalis toxicity

• Organic nitrates (used in angina) act by increasing cGMP activity. Sildenafil inhibits phosphodiesterase which inactivates cGMP and thereby potentiates the effects of nitrates. Hence the combination can cause severe hypotension and even deaths have been reported.

• Aspirin inhibits platelet aggregation and enhances the risk of bleeding due to oral anticoagulants like warfarin.

• Many antihistamines produce sedation which may be enhanced by alcohol intake.

6

Drug Development, Drug Assay, Nomenclature and Essential Drugs Concept

- **Drug Development**
  - **- Preclinical evaluation**
  - **- Clinical trials**
  - **- Metaanalysis**
- **Drug assay**
  - **- Bioassay**
  - **- Chemical assay**
- **Drug Nomenclature**
- **Essential Drugs Concept**
- **Rational Drug Use**

DRUG DEVELOPMENT

The last few decades have seen the development of several new drugs which have revolutionised the practice of medicine. The discovery and development of a new drug is a time-consuming and expensive procedure.

A new drug may be identified by the following processes:

1. Chemical modification of a known drug.

2. Random screening of natural and synthetic chemicals to detect useful activity.

3. Rational drug designing based on the chemical structure.

After identification, the structure of the new compound and its purity are determined by the analytical chemist. The compound is screened for the presence of any useful biologic activity by a series of tests like bioassays, molecular and cellular studies, followed by tests in whole animals. If the compound is found to be promising, then it is subjected to preclinical evaluation in animals and clinical trials in humans.

Preclinical evaluation

The compound is evaluated in animals for the following:

1. Toxicity screening - includes acute, subacute and chronic toxicity studies.

2. Safety and efficacy evaluation; determination of therapeutic index.

3. Pharmacokinetic studies.

Clinical trials

When the drug is found to be reasonably safe in animals, it is subjected to clinical trials in human beings after obtaining permission from the regulatory agency. Clinical trials are conducted to compare the therapeutic efficacy of a new drug with an existing drug or a placebo.

Clinical trials include 4 phases (Table 6.1)

Phase I

Less than 50 normal healthy volunteers are given the drug to establish safety, to know the actions, determine pharmacokinetic profile and to design a safe dose for further use.

Phase II

If phase I is successful, the compound undergoes phase II evaluation in order to establish efficacy, to detect any adverse effects, appropriate dose and detailed pharmacology of the chemical in 100-300 patients suffering from diseases for which the drug under trial has therapeutic prospects.

Phase III

If the phase II establishes that the drug is useful and generally safe, phase III clinical trials are undertaken. A large number of selected patients are given the drug to establish the benefits of the drug in the target disease, to identify the latent side effects, susceptibility to tolerance and to design ideal dosage regimen for different groups of patients.

Phase IV

Postmarketing surveillance. If phase III studies are satisfactory, the new drug is marketed. Since the earlier phases involve a relatively smaller number of patients (3000) for short periods (<1 year), they cannot be expected to provide full safety information. Thus postmarketing surveillance is done for systematic detection and evaluation of long-term safety of the drug. It is done by collection and evaluation of data based on information sent by medical practitioners prescribing the drug. Phase IV trials are conducted by medical practitioners.

Meta-analysis

Data from several clinical trials or studies are combined and the results are analysed (each

TABLE 6.1 Phases of clinical trials			
Phases	**Number of subjects**	**Objectives**	**Conducted by**
Phase I	20-50 normal volunteers	To establish safety, to know biological effects, pharmacokinetic profile and to design a safe dose	Clinical pharmaco-logist
Phase II	100-300 patients	To establish efficacy, detect adverse effects and pharmacokinetics	Clinical pharmaco-logists and clinical investigators
Phase III	250 to > 1000 selected patients	To establish efficacy, safety, to identify latent side effects, tolerance, design ideal dose-range, and to compare with existing drugs	Clinical investigators
Phase IV (Post-marketing surveillance)	2000 to > 10,000 patients	Long-term safety and efficacy; to identify other possible therapeutic uses	Medical practitioners

study should have followed the same procedure). This is known as meta-analysis and helps to obtain more accurate results as a larger number of subjects are considered.

Orphan drugs are drugs to be used for prevention and treatment of rare diseases. Such drugs are not developed and marketed because they are not profitable for the manufacturer. Such rare diseases are called orphan diseases.

DRUG ASSAY

Assay is defined as the quantitative or qualitative evaluation of a substance for purity and potency.

Assay may be bioassay or chemical assay.

BIOASSAY

Bioassay is the estimation of concentration of a substance by measuring the biological activity of the substance. It is a quantitative estimation where the 'amount' of biological activity of a substance is determined by the magnitude of its effect on animals or living tissues.

We now have other more accurate and easier methods like chemical assays, but biological methods are still useful to measure the potency of drugs in some situations.

For example

- When the substance cannot be isolated.
- When chemical methods are more complex than biological methods.

In bioassay, the amount of biological activity in the 'test' sample is compared with the 'standard' preparation *i.e.* a known concentration of the given drug is the standard and the concentration of the test sample is estimated by comparing it with the response of the standard.

Biostandardisation is the procedure by which the potency of a new product is established against an existing standard.

Some examples of bioassays and the tissues/animals used are –

- Compound tissues/animals used.
- Insulin - Hypoglycaemic convulsions in mice
- Acetylcholine - contraction of frog's rectus abdominis muscle
- Tubocurarine - rabbit head drop due to paralysis of neck muscles
- Adrenaline - Blood pressure raising effect in the dog

Methods of bioassay

1. **Matching method:** A particular dose of the test sample is used to produce the response and the procedure is repeated till the response matches with a known dose of the standard.

2. **Interpolation:** Different concentrations of the standard are used and the responses are plotted on a graph. The concentration of the test is read from this graph.

3. **Four point assay:** Here matching as well as interpolation are used to obtain more accurate results.

Bioassay in man

Human beings may be used as subjects in bioassays as in clinical pharmacology studies and in clinical trials.

CHEMICAL ASSAY

Chemical methods are used to estimate the concentration of the drug. Some important chemical assay methods include spectrophotometry, fluorimetry, chromatographic techniques like gas chromatography and High Pressure Liquid Chromatography (HPLC) ; immunoassays like Radio ImmunoAssay (RIA) and Enzyme Linked Immuno Sorbant Assay (ELISA).

DRUG NOMENCLATURE

A drug can have three names.

1. Chemical name
2. Nonproprietary (generic) name
3. Proprietary (brand) name.

The chemical name gives the chemical description of the drug, *e.g.* 3, (10, 11-dihydro-5H-dibenz (b,f) -azepin-5-yl) propyldimethyla-mine. This is lengthy, complex and unsuitable for prescribing.

The nonproprietary name is given by an official agency like WHO and is internationally accepted, *i.e.* the drug has the same generic name all over the world. It gives a clue to the class of the drug, because they sound similar as they end with the same letters. *e.g.* propranolol, atenolol, esmolol, metoprolol - all are β-blockers and cimetidine, ranitidine, famotidine,and roxatidine are all H_2 receptor blockers. It is convenient and the drug is sometimes cheaper when prescribed by generic name. The nonproprietary name of the above example given under chemical name is imipramine.

Proprietary name is the brand name given by the manufacturer. Hence each drug may have many brand names, *e.g.* Crocin, Metacin, Pacemol, Calpol are different brand names of paracetamol. The main advantage in using brand name is the consistency of the product especially bioavailability. Hence, for drugs with low therapeutic index like digoxin and antiepileptics, prescribing the same brand name is beneficial.

ESSENTIAL DRUGS CONCEPT

WHO has compiled a list of drugs that are required to meet the primary health care needs of majority of the population and are called **essential drugs.** Essential drugs have been defined by WHO as those that satisfy the health care needs of majority of the population and should therefore be available at all times in adequate amounts and in the appropriate dosage forms. The original list has undergone revisions and updating from time to time to meet the changing requirements. Based on the WHO guidelines for selection of essential drugs and by referring its model list, each country puts forth its national list of essential drugs.

* Adoption of the list has resulted in greater coordination in health care development.

* The list serves as a guideline for indenting and stocking essential drugs.

* The concept has also helped in the development of national formularies.

* A short list is compiled for community health workers to aid in providing primary health care.

* The use of Essential Drug List has also emphasised the need for drug research and development, *e.g.* safety and efficacy of a new drug should be established for it to be included in the essential drugs list.

India's first National Essential Drugs List consisting of about 300 drugs was formulated in 1996. The revised tenth model list brought out by WHO is given in Appendix-2.

RATIONAL DRUG USE

Once a patient is diagnosed to have a particular disease and needs to be treated with drugs, the specific therapeutic objective should be defined. For example, in hypertension the objective is to bring down the BP to a particular level in order to prevent complications of prolonged hypertension. Once the objective is clear, the choice of drugs should be made. Various aspects should be considered while choosing the drug. When many drugs are available for the treatment of the particular condition, the right choice should be carefully made. For example hyperacidity and mild gastritis may be managed with antacids. When not controlled, a H_2 receptor blocker like ranitidine helps. Only more severe cases require to be treated with omeprazole. Patient factors including age, presence of other diseases, renal and liver function, other drugs being administered and cost of therapy should be considered. Newer drugs are all expensive. When less expensive older drugs are available, they should be preferred to the newer ones. Though human insulin is the rational choice for all diabetics who need insulin, majority of patients in the developing countries like India cannot afford such an expensive medication for the rest of their lives. Hence conventional insulins are still preferable in them - unless contraindicated.

The dose and the duration of treatment should be determined. When long term treatment is required, the regular review and monitoring of treatment should be planned. The therapeutic end point should be defined.

When a combination of drugs is to be administered, the guidelines like better therapeutic benefit , avoiding drugs with overlapping adverse effects and cost of therapy should be borne in mind. Equally important is to avoid irrational combination of drugs. The flourishing drug industry often comes out with absurd combinations of drugs. They serve no useful purpose, are more expensive and unnecessary, but are vigourously promoted and unfortunately often prescribed by doctors. Some such examples are:

1. Amoxicillin (250mg) with cloxacillin (250mg) - Combined with the view that cloxacillin can destroy the penicillinase producing *Staphylococcus Aureus* (PPSA) while amoxicillin can help if the infection is with other bacteria. But, in fact, if the infecting organism is PPSA, 250mg cloxacillin is an underdosage. If it is not PPSA, 250mg of amoxicillin is an underdosage. It should be noted that cloxacillin is not an efficient antibiotic in infections other than PPSA while amoxicillin is of no use in PPSA. Therefore the combination is totally irrational.

2. Ibuprofen with paracetamol - Either of them can be given based on the requirement. Combination serves no useful purpose.

3. Diclofenac + nimesulide - Either of them can be given based on the requirement. Combination serves no useful purpose. Nimesulide is now banned in most of the countries.

4. Ciprofloxacin + tinidazole - The combination is used in diarrhoea. It is claimed that it helps in diarrhoea due to both gram negative bacteria and amoeba. In reality the diarrhoea is due to either of the organisms and not both. Using the combination only exposes the patient to the risk of toxicity from the other antimicrobial agent and also adds to the cost of therapy.

SOME EXAMPLES

Drugs that are almost completely absorbed – on oral ingestion

- Diazepam
- Digitoxin
- Phenylbutazone
- Minocycline
- Doxycycline
- Valproic acid
- Chlordiazepoxide
- Indomethacin
- Lithium
- Phenobarbitone
- Salicylic acid

Drugs that undergo extensive first pass metabolism

- Propranolol
- Metoprolol
- Lignocaine
- Chlorpromazine
- Verapamil
- Morphine
- Pentazocine
- Pethidine
- Nitroglycerin
- Insulin
- Testosterone
- Isoprenaline
- Hydrocortisone
- Levodopa

Drugs that are highly bound to plasma proteins

- Warfarin
- Phenytoin
- Diazepam
- Sulfonamides
- Phenylbutazone
- Salicylates
- Indomethacin
- Tolbutamide
- Clofibrate
- Frusemide

Apparent volume of distribution (V_d)

Low V_d drugs	High V_d drugs
• Heparin	• Pethidine
• Warfarin	• Digoxin
• Aminoglycosides	• Chloroquine
• Aspirin	• Nortriptyline
• Furosemide	• Fluoxetine
• Ampicillin	• Haloperidol
• Amoxicillin	• Amiodarone

Hit and run drugs

- Reserpine
- Omeprazole

Some microsomal enzyme inducers

- Phenobarbitone
- Phenytoin
- Rifampicin
- Griseofulvin
- Tolbutamide
- Metronidazole
- Phenylbutazone
- Cigarette smoke
- DDT
- Alcohol
- Carbamazepine

Some microsomal enzyme inhibitors

- Cimetidine
- Fluoxetine
- Erythromycin
- Quinidine
- Omeprazole
- Ketoconazole
- Grape fruit juice
- Chloramphenicol
- Allopurinol

Prodrugs

Drug		Active metabolite
• Levodopa	→	Dopamine
• Prednisone	→	Prednisolone
• Enalapril	→	Enalaprilat
• Bacampicillin	→	Ampicillin
• Cortisone	→	Hydrocortisone
• Azathioprine	→	Mercaptopurine
• Cyclophosphamide	→	Aldophosphamide
• Zidovudine	→	Zidovudine triphosphate

Drugs metabolised by zero-order kinetics

- Alcohol
- Phenytoin
- Salicylates
- Heparin
- Phenylbutazone

Drugs that undergo enterohepatic recycling

- Tetracyclines
- Amphetamine
- Doxorubicin
- Metronidazole
- Mefloquine
- Morphine
- Indomethacin
- Phenytoin
- Estradiol

Drugs available as transdermal patches

- Nitroglycerin
- Hyoscine
- Fentanyl
- Estrogen
- Testosterone

Drugs to which tolerance develops easily

- Nitrates
- Hydralazine
- Barbiturates
- Opioids

Agents which exhibit tachyphylaxis

- Ephedrine
- Amphetamine
- 5–HT
- Tyramine

Drugs which need tapering (after long term use)

- β blockers
- Glucocorticoids
- Antiepileptics
- Clonidine
- Sedatives
- Antidepressants
- Antipsychotics

Drugs with very short t ½ (2-10 min)

- Dobutamine
- Sodium nitroprusside
- Dopamine
- Alteplase
- Esmolol
- 5–Fluorouracil
- Adenosine

Some haemodialysable drugs

- Isoniazid
- Ethyl and methyl alcohol
- Barbiturates
- Amphetamines
- Methaqualone
- Lithium
- Phenytoin
- Salicylates
- Theophylline

Nitric oxide donors

- Sodium nitroprusside
- Nitrites
- Nitrates

Drugs with long t½

Drug	t½ in days
Chloroquine	10-24
Etanercept	3-4
Phenylbutazone	3-4
Mefloquine	16-24
Gold salts	7

Drugs with low therapeutic index

- Digoxin
- Lithium
- Theophylline
- Quinidine

Drugs which need plasma concentration monitoring

- Lithium
- Carbamazepine
- Digoxin
- Theophylline
- Aminoglycosides

Teratogenic drugs

- Thalidomide
- Tetracylines
- Sodium valproate
- Phenytoin
- Carbamazepine
- Phenobarbitone
- Lithium
- Glucocorticoids
- Androgens
- Oestrogens
- Progestins
- Antithyroid drugs
- Anticancer drugs

Drugs to be used with caution in renal failure

- Aminoglycosides
- Amphotericin
- Cyclosporine
- Acyclovir
- Foscarnet
- Pentamidine
- Ifosphamide
- NSAIDs
- ACE inhibitors
- Sulphonamides
- Penicillamine
- Anticancer drugs like Cisplatin Methotrexate

Drugs that can produce gingival hyperplasia

- Phenytoin
- Cyclosporin
- Calcium channel blockers

Drugs that can induce haemolysis in G 6PD deficient patients

- Sulfonamides
- Nitrofurans
- Vitamin K analogs
- Some vegetablEs
- Primaquine
- NSAIDs
- Dapsone

Drugs excerted in saliva

- Clarithromycin
- Metronidazole
- Phenytoin
- Disulfiram
- Metoclopramide

GENERAL PHARMACOLOGY

7 Introduction to Autonomic Pharmacology

CHAPTER

- Autonomic innervation
- Neurotransmitters

The nervous system is divided into central and peripheral nervous systems (Fig. 7.1). The peripheral nervous system consists of autonomic and somatic nervous systems. The autonomic nervous system (ANS) is **not under voluntary control** and therefore was so named by Langley (*Autos* = self, *nomos* = governing—in Greek). The ANS innervates the heart, the smooth muscles, the glands and the viscera and controls the functions of these organs.(Fig 7.2)

The centres for autonomic reflexes are present in the hypothalamus, medulla and spinal cord.

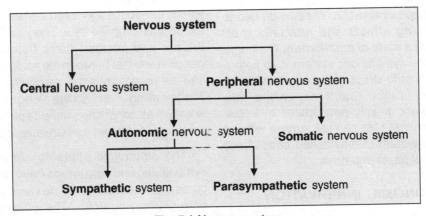

Fig. 7.1 Nervous system

63

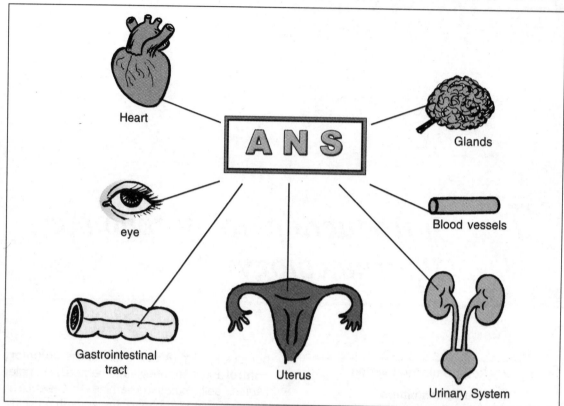

Fig. 7.2 Structures under the control of autonomic nervous system

Hypothalamus coordinates the autonomic activity.

The ANS consists of two major divisions - the **sympathetic** and the **parasympathetic** (Fig. 7.4). Most of the viscera have both sympathetic and parasympathetic innervation. *The two divisions have opposing effects and normally their effects are in a state of equilibrium.* The prime function of the sympathetic system is to help a person to adjust to stress and prepare the body for fight or flight reactions, while the parasympathetic mainly participates in tissue building reactions. Man can still survive without sympathetic system (if maintained stress-free) but not without parasympathetic.

AUTONOMIC INNERVATION

The autonomic afferents (Fig 7.3) are carried in visceral nerves through nonmyelinated fibres. For example, the parasympathetic afferents are carried by the 9th and 10th cranial nerves. The autonomic efferent innervation consists of a myelinated preganglionic fibre which synapses with the postganglionic fibre. The postganglionic fibre in turn forms a junction with the receptors of the organs supplied by it. The junction between the pre and postganglionic fibres is called a *ganglion* and that between the postganglionic fibre and the receptors is the *neuroeffector junction*. The travelling of an impulse along the nerve fibre is known as *conduction* while its passage across a synapse is known as *transmission*.

The autonomic efferents are divided into sympathetic and parasympathetic divisions. The parasympathetic efferents are carried through the craniosacral outflow. The parasympathetic ganglia are located close to the innervated structures and therefore their postganglionic fibres are short. The sympathetic efferents extend from

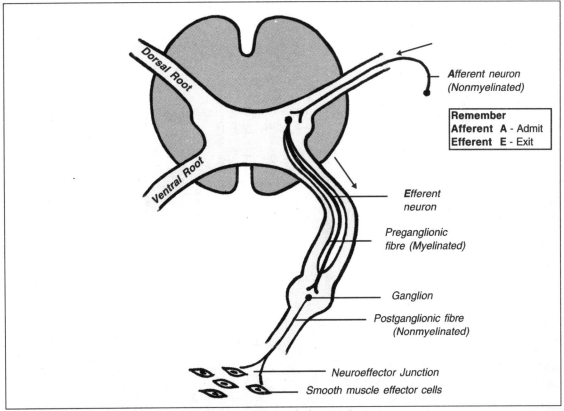

Fig. 7.3 Autonomic innervation

1st thoracic to 2nd or 3rd lumbar segments (T_1-L_3) of the spinal cord. The sympathetic ganglia are found at three sites - paravertebral, prevertebral and terminal. Postganglionic fibres arising from sympathetic ganglia are long and they innervate the head, neck and the viscera of the thorax and abdomen. Adrenal medulla is also considered as a sympathetic ganglion and differs from other sympathetic ganglia in that the principal catecholamine that is released is adrenaline.

NEUROTRANSMITTERS

For the transmission of an impulse across a synapse, a neurohumoral transmitter substance is released into the synaptic cleft. In the ANS, the neurotransmitters released are acetylcholine, noradrenaline, dopamine and in adrenal medulla, it is adrenaline and noradrenaline.

Cotransmission It has been noted that there are certain other substances apart from the principle neurotransmitter in the vesicles of the autonomic nerve terminals of some tissues. These include sustances like dopamine, nitric oxide, ATP, serotonin, vasoactive intestinal peptide (VIP), cholecystokinin (CCK) and GABA. These are called cotransmitters. Different set of neurons contain different neurotransmitters. For example: CCK, VIP and GABA are present in the excitatory neurons of the gut, while ATP and nitric oxide are cotransmitters at inhibitory neurons in the gut or enteric nervous system. The functions of these nonadrenergic and noncholinergic cotransmitters are not exactly known. They might modulate or influence the effects of the principle neurotransmitter.

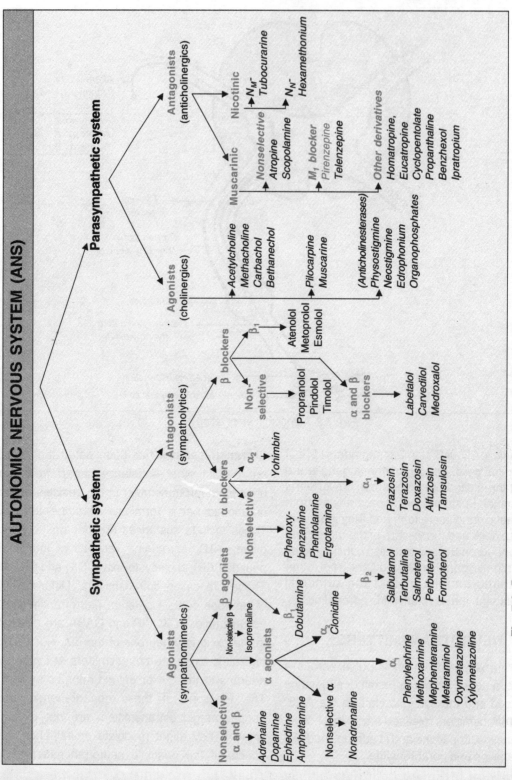

Fig. 7.4 Drugs acting on sympathetic and parasympathetic nervous system. Few examples.

8 *Cholinergic System*

- • **Synthesis of acetylcholine**
- • **Transmission of an impulse**
- • **Cholinergic receptors**
- • **Cholinergic Drugs**
  - **- Actions of acetylcholine**
  - **- Uses**
- • **Cholinomimetic alkaloids**
  - **- Pilocarpine**
- • **Anticholinesterases**
  - **- Reversible anticholinesterases**
  - **- Irreversible anticholinesterases**

Acetylcholine (ACh) an ester of choline, is the neurotransmitter of the parasympathetic system. The nerves that synthesize, store and release ACh are called *'cholinergic'*.

The **sites** of release of acetylcholine are (Fig. 8.1):

1. Ganglia - All the preganglionic fibres of ANS, i.e. at both the sympathetic and parasympathetic ganglia.

2. The postganglionic parasympathetic nerve endings.

3. Sweat glands - The sympathetic postganglionic nerve endings supplying the sweat glands.

4. Skeletal muscles - somatic nerve endings supplying skeletal muscles.

5. Adrenal medulla.

6. CNS - brain and spinal cord.

Synthesis of Acetylcholine

Acetylcholine is synthesized from acetyl-CoA and choline, catalysed by the enzyme choline acetyltransferase. This ACh is stored in small oval vesicles in the cholinergic nerve terminals.

Transmission of an impulse

When an action potential reaches the presynaptic membrane, ACh is released into the synaptic cleft

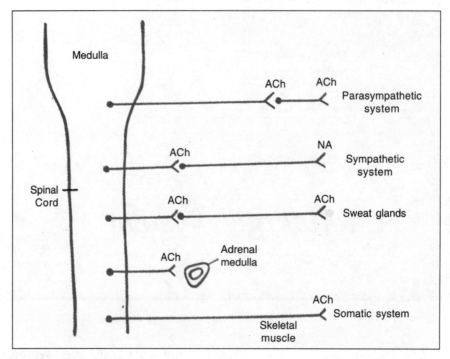

Fig. 8.1 Sites of release of neurotransmitters—acetylcholine and noradrenaline in the peripheral nervous system

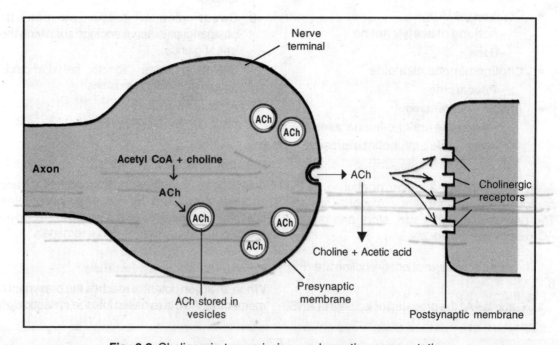

Fig. 8.2 Cholinergic transmission—schematic representation

TABLE 8.1: Subtypes and location of cholinergic receptors		
	Subtypes	**Location**
Muscarinic	M_1	Autonomic ganglia, gastric glands, CNS
	M_2	Heart, nerves, smooth muscles,
	M_3	Glands, smooth muscles
	M_4	CNS
	M_5	CNS
Nicotinic	N_M	Neuromuscular junction
	N_N	Autonomic ganglia Adrenal medulla, CNS

(Fig. 8.2). This ACh binds to and activates the cholinergic receptor on the postsynaptic membrane leading to the depolarisation of this membrane. Thus the impulse is transmitted across the synapse.

ACh released into the synaptic cleft is rapidly destroyed by the enzyme acetylcholinesterase (AChE). Then the postsynaptic membrane is repolarised.

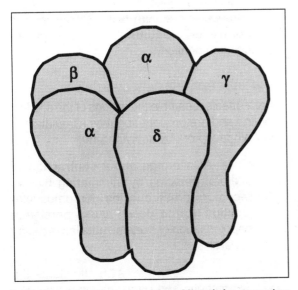

Fig 8.3 Nicotinic receptor. Nicotinic receptor contains 5 subunits - $2\alpha+\beta+\gamma+\delta$. Acetylcholine binds to the sites on a subunits resulting in opening of the channel

Cholinesterases

Acetylcholine is hydrolysed to choline and acetic acid by the enzymes cholinesterases. Two types of AChE are present:

1. True cholinesterase - at neurons, ganglia and neuromuscular junction.

2. Pseudocholinesterase (butyryl cholinesterase) - in plasma, liver and other organs.

Cholinergic receptors

There are two classes of cholinergic receptors - **muscarinic** and **nicotinic**. Muscarinic receptors are present in the heart, smooth muscles, glands, eyes and CNS. Muscarinic receptors are G protein coupled receptors. Five subtypes of muscarinic receptors, M_1-M_5 are recognised (Table 8.1).

Nicotinic receptors are present in the neuromuscular junction, autonomic ganglia and adrenal medulla. Nicotinic receptors are ion channels - five subunits ($2\alpha+1\beta+1\gamma+1\delta$) enclose the channel (Fig 8.3). Binding of acetylcholine to α subunits opens the channel allowing the entry of Na^+ into the cell. Two subtypes of nicotinic receptors are identified (Table 8.1). N_M receptors are present at the skeletal muscle end plate and N_N receptors at the autonomic ganglia and adrenal medulla.

CHOLINERGIC DRUGS

Cholinergic drugs are chemicals that act at the same site as acetylcholine and thereby mimic its actions. They are therefore called parasympathomimetics or cholinomimetics.

Cholinergic drugs may be classified as

1. Esters of choline
   Acetylcholine
   Methacholine
   Carbachol
   Bethanechol

2. Cholinomimetic alkaloids
   Pilocarpine
   Muscarine

3. Anticholinesterases

   Reversible - Neostigmine
   Physostigmine
   Pyridostigmine
   Ambenonium
   Edrophonium.

   Irreversible - Organophosphorus
   compounds.

Actions of Acetylcholine

Acetylcholine is taken as the prototype of parasympathomimetic drugs.

Muscarinic Actions

Muscarinic actions resemble the actions of the alkaloid muscarine found in some mushrooms. These actions result from the stimulation of the muscarinic receptors by acetylcholine.

1. Heart: The action of ACh is similar to that of vagal stimulation. It depresses the SA node and thereby reduces the heart rate and force of contraction. In larger doses, AV conduction is depressed.

2. Blood vessels: ACh relaxes the vascular smooth muscles and dilates the blood vessels of the skin and mucous membrane. The BP falls due to a fall in total peripheral resistance

3. Smooth muscle: ACh increases the tone of all other (nonvascular) smooth muscles.

   • *Gastrointestinal tract* - tone and peristalsis is enhanced, sphincters are relaxed, resulting in rapid forward propulsion of intestinal contents.

   • *Urinary bladder* - detrusor contracts and trigonal sphincter relaxes - promotes voiding of urine.

   • *Bronchial smooth muscle* - contracts resulting in bronchospasm.

4. Secretory glands: Acetylcholine enhances the secretions of all glands; salivary, lacrimal, nasopharyngeal, tracheobronchial, gastric and intestinal secretions are increased. Sweating is also increased. Enhanced bronchial secretions and bronchospasm result in severe dyspnoea.

5. Eye: Constriction of pupil (miosis) by contracting the circular muscles of the iris. Stimulation of muscarinic receptors present in the sphincter pupillae results in miosis. Drainage of aqueous humor is facilitated and intraocular pressure falls. Ciliary muscle contracts resulting in spasm of accommodation.

Nicotinic Actions

These effects resemble the actions of the alkaloid nicotine and are brought about by stimulation of nicotinic receptors by acetylcholine.

1. NMJ: ACh brings about contraction of skeletal muscles by stimulating the N_M receptors present in the neuromuscular junction. Large doses cause persistent depolarisation of skeletal muscles resulting in paralysis.

2. Autonomic ganglia: ACh stimulates the sympathetic and parasympathetic ganglia and the adrenal medulla.

3. CNS: ACh is a neurotransmitter at several sites in the CNS.

TABLE 8.2 Actions of acetylcholine

CVS	—	↓HR ↓BP
Non-vascular smooth muscle	—	contraction, ↑gut peristalsis, promotes urine voiding, bronchospasm
Glands	—	↑secretion
Eye	—	miosis, spasm of accommodation, ↓IOP
NMJ	—	muscle contraction
Ganglia	—	stimulation

The important actions of acetylcholine are summarised in Table 8.2.

Uses

Acetylcholine is destroyed in the gut when given orally. On intravenous administration, it is rapidly metabolised by pseudocholinesterases in the plasma and by true cholinesterase at the site of action. Therefore it is not used therapeutically except occasionally as 1% eye drops to produce miosis that is required during some eye surgeries.

Esters of choline are effective orally; carbachol and bethanechol are resistant to both cholinesterases and have a longer duration of action. Their muscarinic actions are prominent with a sustained effect on g.i. smooth muscles and urinary bladder. Methacholine is rarely used. Carbachol is used in glaucoma. Bethanechol may be used in hypotonia of bladder and g.i. smooth muscles and in some cases of postoperative paralytic ileus and urinary retention; in xerostomia as an alternative to pilocarpine.

Adverse effects include diarrhoea, flushing, salivation, sweating, bradycardia, hypotension, syncope and bronchospasm.

CHOLINOMIMETIC ALKALOIDS

Pilocarpine is an alkaloid obtained from the leaves of *Pilocarpus microphyllus*. Like ACh it stimulates cholinergic receptors, but its muscarinic actions are prominent.

Its actions on the eye are important - when applied to the eye it causes miosis, spasm of accommodation and a fall in intraocular tension. It also increases sweat (diaphoretic) and salivary secretions (sialogogue).

Adverse effects

When used as eye drops, burning sensation and painful spasm of accommodation, browache and corneal edema can occur. Long term use can cause retinal detachment.

Uses

1. Pilocarpine is used in glaucoma (see below). Pilocarpine ocusert is available and can deliver pilocarpine constantly for 7 days.

2. Pilocarpine is also used alternately with mydriatics like homatropine to break the adhesions between the iris and the lens.

3. It is used to counter dryness of mouth that is seen following radiation of head and neck.

Glaucoma is an eye disease characterised by increased intraocular pressure. Aqueous humor is secreted by the ciliary body and it drains through the canal of Schlemn. Rise in IOP (above 30mm of Hg) can damage the optic nerve. If untreated, irreversible damage can occur - optic nerve degenerates leading to permanent blindness. Glaucoma is one of the common causes of blindness. Hypertension, myopia and

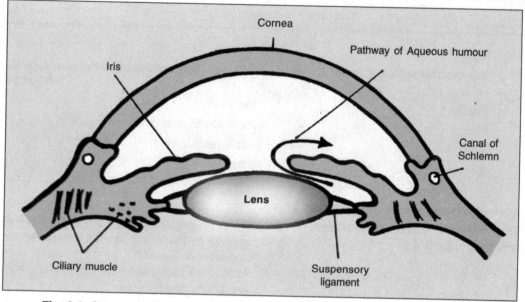

Fig. 8.4: Schematic diagram showing pathway for the drainage of aqueous humour

family history of glaucoma are risk factors. Glaucoma is of two types :

1. Acute congestive/narrow angle/closed angle glaucoma - in this, iris blocks the drainage of aqueous humor at the canal of Schlemn leading to increased intraocular pressure (Fig 8.4). It needs immediate treatment.

2. Chronic simple/wide angle/open angle glaucoma - onset is slow; needs long term treatment. Surgery is the preferred option.

Two categories of drugs may be used in the treatment of glaucoma. They are -

1. Drugs that decrease the formation of aqueous humor -

   Timolol, betaxolol, levobunolol, Carteolol, apraclonidine, brimonidine dipivefrine, adrenaline, acetazolamide & dorzolamide

2. Drugs that increase the drainage of aqueous humor -

   Carbachol, pilocarpine, physostigmine echothiophate & latanoprost.

Drugs used in glaucoma are summarised in Table 8.3.

- β blockers are the first line drugs. They reduce aqueous humor formation by blocking the β receptors in the ciliary body. Since they do not cause miosis, there is no associated headache or browache which are due to spasm of the iris and the ciliary muscles. The reduction in IOP is smoother and constant. However, even when used as eye drops, β blockers may be absorbed systemically. Hence β_1 selective agents are preferred particularly in asthmatics - even these should be used carefully. Use of β blockers may result in heart block and CCF particularly in the elderly.

- Epinephrine, dipivefrine and apraclonidine may act on the ciliary body to reduce aqueous humor formation or act by reducing ciliary blood flow (α_1). Apraclonidine is an analog of clonidine which has higher topical than systemic activity.

- Production of aqueous humor requires active

TABLE 8.3 Drugs used in Glaucoma

Drugs	Adverse effects	Comments
1. β blockers		
Timolol, betaxolol carteolol, levobunolol	Conjunctival irritation, redness and discomfort	• First line drugs • No miosis-hence no headache or browache
2. Cholinergics		
• Pilocarpine, carbachol	Corneal edema, spasm of accommodation, browache, myopia	Used with β blockers
• Physostigmine, echothiophate	Browache, cataract, retinal detachment	
3. Adrenergic agonists		
• Dipivefrine, adrenaline	Conjunctival redness, photosensitivity allergic reactions	II line drugs -may be combined with β blockers
• α_2 adrenergic agonists		
Apraclonidine Brimonidine	Conjunctival redness, photosensitivity clonidine	Higher topical activity than
4. Carbonic anhydrase inhibitors		
Acetazolamide, Methazolamide, Dorzolamide	Hypokalaemia, anorexia, drowsiness	II line drugs-given orally; slow release aceta-zolamide is better tolerated; topical dorzolamide is now available - has fewer side effects
5. PG Analogs		
Latanoprost, Bimatoprost		Used as adjuvant

transport of bicarbonate ions. Inhibition of carbonic anhydrase decreases aqueous humor formation by enhancing bicarbonate loss. Acetazolamide and methazolamide are given orally but are poorly tolerated. Topical agents are now available like dorzolamide eye drops. These can also be combined with β blockers and miotics.

• Miotics improve drainage of aqueous humor by constricting the pupil and opening the iridocorneal angle.

• Latanoprost is a prostaglandin analog - a prodrug of $PGF_{2\alpha}$. It increases the outflow of aqueous humor probably by relaxing the ciliary muscle. It can be used as an adjuvant to other drugs. Bimatoprost is similar to latanoprost.

ANTICHOLINESTERASES

Anticholinesterases (antiChEs) or cholinesterase inhibitors are drugs which inhibit the enzyme cholinesterase. As their structure resembles that of ACh, they bind to AChEs and inactivate them.

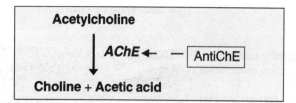

Thus ACh is not hydrolysed and it accumulates. The actions of all these drugs are due to this accumulated ACh. Hence the actions are similar to cholinergic agonists. The structure of AchE contains an anionic site and an esteratic site (Fig-8.5). Reversible anticholinesterases except edrophonium bind to both anionic and esteratic sites. Edrophonium binds only to anionic site and the binding is quickly reversible - hence it is very short acting. Organophosphates (OP) bind only to the esteratic site but the enzyme is phos phorylated (by covalent bonds) and the binding is stable. With some OPs the binding takes many days to be reversed while with others it is not fully reversible at all.

Anticholinesterases are either esters of carbamic acid (carbamates) or derivatives of phosphoric acid. They may be:

1. Reversible

  • *Carbamates* -

      Physostigmine
      Neostigmine
      Pyridostigmine
      Rivastigmine
      Donepezil
      Edrophonium

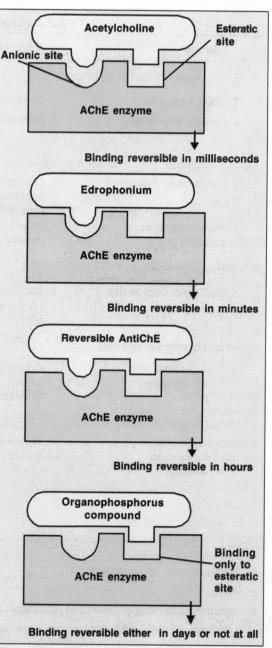

Fig 8.5: Acetycholine and reversible anticholinesterases bind to both anionic and esteratic sites of the acetylcholinesterase (AChE) enzyme. Edrophonium binds only the anionic site and is short acting because the binding is rapidly reversible. OP compounds bind only esteratic site but exception is echothiophate which binds both anionic and esteratic sites.

• *Carbamate insectisides* -

Carbaryl (SEVIN)
Propoxure (BAYGON)
Aldicarb (TEMIK)

2. Irreversible

• *Organophosphates* -

Echothiophate
Malathion
Sumithion
Toxic nerve gases - Sarin
Tabun

Physostigmine

Physostigmine is an alkaloid obtained from the plant *Physostigma venenosum*. It is a tertiary ammonium compound - hence has better penetration into tissues and also crosses the BBB. It is available as IV injection, as 0.1-1% eye drops and in combination with pilocarpine nitrate 2%. It is used in glaucoma and in atropine poisoning. Its use as eye drops can cause browache and on long term use, retinal detachment and cataract. (Table 8.4)

Neostigmine

Neostigmine is a synthetic quaternary ammonium com pound - poorly absorbed from the gut; it does not cross the BBB. It is used in myasthenia gravis, (see below) post-operative paralytic ileus and atony of the urinary bladder.

Edrophonium

Edrophonium is rapid and short-acting. It is used in myasthenia gravis, and intravenously in snake bite and in curare poisoning.

Uses of reversible anticholinesterases

1. As a miotic Physostigmine causes miosis, spasm of accommodation and a decrease in IOP. It is used:

   a. In glaucoma - can be used with pilocarpine for better effect.

b. Alternatively with a mydriatic to break adhesions between the iris and the lens.

2. Myasthenia gravis is a chronic autoimmune disease characterised by progressive weakness with rapid and easy fatiguability of skeletal muscles. Antibodies to nicotinic receptors are formed, resulting in a decrease in the number of these receptors at NMJ. Neostigmine (15 mg tab 6 hrly) or pyridostigmine or a combination of these may be given. Edrophonium is used IV for the diagnosis. In addition to its antiChE activity, neostigmine directly stimulates the nicotinic receptors and increases the amount of ACh released during each nerve impulse. AntiChEs enhance ACh levels at NMJ by preventing its destruction. They thus increase the force of contraction and improve muscle power by more frequent activation of the existing nicotinic receptors. In advanced disease antiChEs are not effective because the available nicotinic receptors are very few.

Factors like infection, surgery and stress can result in severe muscle weakness called - *myasthenic crisis.* But severe weakness may also result from an excess dose of an anticholinesterase drug (flaccid paralysis due to more of acetylcholine) called - *cholinergic crisis.* These two crises can be differentiated by 2 mg. IV edrophonium - the patient immediately improves if it is myasthenic crisis but the weakness worsens if it is cholinergic crisis. Treatment of cholinergic crisis is with atropine while myasthenic crisis requires a higher dose of or an alternate anticholinergic drug.

Other drugs used in myasthenia gravis are - glucocorticoids - inhibit the production of antibodies to the nicotinic receptors. These are used when anticholinesterases alone are not adequate.

Immunosuppressants - Azathioprine and cyclosporine can be used as alternatives to prednisolone in advanced myasthenia gravis. They inhibit the production of antinicotinic receptor antibodies.

3. Poisoning due to anticholinergic drugs Physostigmine is used in atropine poisoning and in toxicity due to other drugs with anticholinergic activity like phenothiazines, tricyclic antidepressants and antihistamines. Since physostigmine crosses the BBB, it reverses all the symptoms of atropine poisoning including CNS effects.

4. Curare poisoning Skeletal muscle paralysis caused by curare can be antagonised by AntiChEs. Neostigmine and pyridostigmine can be used. Though edrophonium is faster acting, it is less effective than neostigmine specially in severe poisoning.

5. Postoperative paralytic ileus and urinary retention Neostigmine may be useful.

6. Cobra bite Cobra venom, a neurotoxin causes skeletal muscle paralysis. Specific treatment is antivenom. Intravenous edrophonium prevents respiratory paralysis.

7. Alzheimer's disease: To overcome the deficient cholinergic neurotransmission, rivastigmine and donepezil are tried in Alzheimer's disease. Tacrine is another reversible anticholinesterase tried in this disease - but tacrine causes hepatotoxicity because of which it is not preferred (See chapter 28).

Irreversible Anticholinesterases

Organophosphorus (OP) compounds are powerful inhibitors of AChE enzyme; binding with the enzyme is stable - by covalent bonds. They bind only the esteratic site (Fig. 8.5) and the enzyme is phosphorylated. Effects are similar to that of cholinergic stimulation as ACh accumulates in the tissues. All organophosphates except echothiophate are highly lipid soluble and hence are absorbed from all routes including intact skin. This makes OP poisoning possible even while insecticides are used for spraying.

Uses

Glaucoma - echothiophate eye drops are sometimes used in glaucoma.

Organophosphorus Poisoning

Acute toxicity

As organophosphates are used as agricultural and domestic insecticides, poisoning by them is quite common. Poisoning may be occupational - as while spraying insecticides, accidental or suicidal. Symptoms result from muscarinic, nicotinic and central effects; vomiting, abdominal cramps, diarrhoea, miosis, sweating, increased salivary, tracheobronchial and gastric secretions and bronchospasm; hypotension, muscular twitchings, weakness, convulsions and coma. Death is due to respiratory paralysis.

Treatment

1. If poisoning is through skin - remove clothing and wash the skin with soap and water; if consumed by oral route - gastric lavage is given.

2. Maintain BP and patent airway.

3. Drug of choice is **atropine** IV 2 mg every 10 minutes till pupil dilates. Maximum dose can be anything from 50 to 100 mg or more depending on the severity of the poisoning. Treatment should be carefully monitored because of the risk of reappearance of symptoms due to delayed absorption of the OP compounds.

4. Cholinesterase reactivators - **pralidoxime, obidoxime, diacetylmonoxime.** These oxime compounds combine with cholinesterase organophosphate complex, release the binding and set free AChE enzyme. Thus they reactivate the cholinesterase enzyme. They should be

TABLE 8.4 Differences between Physostigmine and Neostigmine

	Physostigmine	Neostigmine
Source	Natural (*Physostigma venenosum*)	Synthetic
Chemistry	Tertiary ammonium compound	Quaternary ammonium compound
Absorption	Absorbed orally	Not absorbed
Tissue penetration	Good	Poor
BBB	Crosses BBB - has CNS effects	Does not cross BBB - no CNS effects
Primary use	In glaucoma	Myasthenia gravis
Use in poisoning	Used in atropine poisoning	Used in curare poisoning

given within minutes after poisoning preferably immediately, because the complex undergoes 'ageing' and the enzyme cannot be released. The complex becomes more stable by loss of a chemical group and this is responsible for 'ageing'. Cholinesterase reactivators are not useful in poisoning due to carbamate compounds because these compounds do not have a free site (anionic site) for the binding of oximes. Moreover pralidoxime itself has weak anticholinesterase activity particularly at higher doses.

In severe poisoning 1-2g of IV pralidoxime given within five minutes of poisoning gives best results. But in practice it is rather uncommon for a patient to get such quick treatment within minutes particularly in the rural setup and cholinesterase reactivators are tried upto a few hours (maximum 6 hours) after poisoning.

Diacetylmonoxime (DAM) is lipid soluble and therefore crosses the BBB and regenerates the cholinesterase in the brain.

Chronic organophosphate toxicity

Some OP compounds can produce neurotoxicity (polyneuropathy) several days after exposure to the compound. This toxicity came to light when thousands of people developed paralysis in America after consuming "Jamaica ginger" which contained small amounts of TOCP (triorthocresylphosphate). The symptoms include weakness, fatigue, ataxia, sensory disturbances, muscle twitching and in severe cases flaccid paralysis- which may last for several years.

9

Anticholinergic Drugs

- Classification
- Actions
- Pharmacokinetics
- Adverse effects
- Uses of Belladonna Alkaloids
- Atropine substitutes

Anticholinergic drugs are agents which block the effects of ACh on cholinergic receptors but conventionally antimuscarinic drugs are referred to as anticholinergic drugs. They are also called cholinergic blocking or parasympatholytic drugs. Drugs that block the nicotinic receptors are ganglion blockers and neuromuscular blockers.

Anticholinergic drugs include atropine and related drugs - atropine is the prototype.

Atropine is obtained from the plant *Atropa belladonna*. Atropine and scopolamine (hyo scine) are the belladonna alkaloids. They compete with acetylcholine for muscarinic

receptors and block these receptors - they are muscarinic antagonists.

Classification

1. Natural alkaloids

   Atropine, hyoscine (scopolamine)

2. Semisynthetic derivatives

   Homatropine, ipratropium bromide, tiotroprium bromide

3. Synthetic substitutes -

   - Mydriatics
     - *Eucatropine, cyclopentolate tropicamide*

   - Antispasmodic-antisecretory agents
     - *Propantheline, dicyclomine, oxyphenonium, glycopyrrolate, telenzepine, tolterodine, propiverine*

   - Antiparkinsonian agents
     - *Benzhexol, benztropine, trihexyphenidyl*

Actions

The actions of atropine and scopolamine are similar except that atropine is a CNS stimulant while scopolamine is a CNS depressant and causes sedation.

1. CVS - Atropine increases heart rate. In large doses, vasodilation and hypotension occurs.

2. Secretions - Atropine reduces all secretions except milk. Lacrimal, salivary, nasopharyngeal and tracheobronchial secretions are decreased. Decreased salivation results in dry mouth and difficulty in swallowing. Sweating is also reduced. In higher doses this results in increased body temperature.

   Atropine reduces gastric secretion - it decreases the volume as well as the quantity of acid, pepsin and mucous secretions. Atropine reduces gastric secretions - it decreases the volume as well as the quantity of acid, pepsin and mucous secretion.

3. Smooth muscle

   - *GIT* - reduces tone and motility and relieves spasm → these effects together with decreased secretions may result in constipation.

   - *Biliary tract* - smooth muscles are relaxed; biliary spasm is relieved.

   - *Bronchi* - atropine causes bronchodilatation. As the secretions are also reduced, it affords symptomatic relief in COPD patients.

   - *Genitourinary tract* - atropine relaxes ureters and the urinary bladder may cause urinary retention particularly in the elderly men since they may already have prostatic hypertrophy.

4. Eye - On local instillation, atropine produces mydriasis by blocking the muscarinic receptors in the sphincter pupillae. The ciliary muscle is paralysed resulting in cycloplegia or paralysis of accommodation. Because of mydriasis, the iris may block the drainage of aqueous humor - IOP increases and may precipitate glaucoma in some patients.

5. CNS - In higher doses atropine stimulates the CNS resulting in restlessness, disorientation, hallucinations and delirium. In contrast, scopolamine produces sedation and drowsiness.

Pharmacokinetics

Atropine and hyoscine are well-absorbed, cross the BBB and are metabolised in the liver.

Adverse effects

Adverse effects are common but not serious and include blurring of vision, dry mouth, dysphagia, dry skin, fever, constipation and urinary retention. Skin rashes may appear. High doses cause palpitation, flushing, restlessness, delirium, hallucinations, psychosis, convulsions and coma. Poisoning is treated with IV physostigmine.

Uses of Belladonna Alkaloids

1. *As antispasmodic*

   - In diarrhoea and dysentery, atropine relieves colic and abdominal pain. It is generally combined with loperamide.

   - In renal and biliary colic - atropine is used with morphine. Atropine partly overcomes the spasm of the sphinter of oddi.

   - Nocturnal enuresis in children and in paraplegia - atropine reduces urinary frequency.

2. *As mydriatric and cycloplegic*

   - *Diagnostic* for testing error of refraction and fundoscopic examination of the eye.

   - *Therapeutic* To provide rest to the iris in iritis, iridocyclitis and keratitis and after iridectomy

Mydriatics are used alternately with miotics to break the adhesions between the iris and the lens - both for the treatment and prevention of adhesion formation.

3. *As pre-anaesthetic medication* - When administered 30 min before anaesthesia, atropine reduces salivary and respiratory secretions. This will prevent the development of laryngospasm. It also prevents bradycardia during surgery. Its bronchodilator action is of additional value. *Glycopyrrolate* an atropine substitute, is most commonly used for this purpose.

4. *In organophosphorus poisoning* - Atropine is life saving in OP poisoning and is also useful in mushroom poisoning. (See page 76)

5. *In bronchial asthma, peptic ulcer and parkinsonism* Atropine derivatives are preferred over atropine - see next page.

6. *Motion sickness* - Hyoscine given 30 minutes before the journey prevents travelling sickness. Transdermal hyoscine patches are available to be applied behind the ear for a prolonged action.

7. *Labour* - Hyoscine can also be used during labour to produce sedation and amnesia.

Drug interactions

When anticholinergics are given with other drugs that also have anticholinergic property like antihistaminics, phenothiazines, tricyclic antidepressants - side effects get added up.

ATROPINE SUBSTITUTES

Belladonna alkaloids produce a wide range of effects, most of which are of therapeutic value. But these can also result in various side effects since they lack selectivity. Hence several semisynthetic and synthetic derivatives have been introduced some of which have selective actions (Table 9.1)

- Mydriasis and cycloplegia produced by atropine last for 7 - 10 days. The derivatives have shorter action (6 - 24 hrs), tropicamide being the shortest acting. Some can selectively produce either prominent mydriasis or cycloplegia.

- Antispasmodics or spasmolytics are used to relieve spasms of the gastrointestinal tract, biliary tract, ureter and uterus. They are also found to be useful in irritable bowel syndrome. Some of them in addition, reduce gastrointestinal motility.

- Pirenzepine and telenzepine are selective M_1 blockers which inhibit gastric secretion

TABLE 9.1 Atropine substitutes

Indications	Derivatives used
1. On the eye - mydriatics and cycloplegics	Homatropine, eucatropine cyclopentolate, tropicamide Propantheline, methantheline dicyclomine, flavoxate hydrochloride, oxybutynin chloride, oxyphenonium, glycopyrrolate, clidinium
2. As antispasmodics	Propantheline, methantheline, dicyclomine, flavoxate hydrochloride, oxybutynin chloride, oxyphenonium, glycopyrrolate, clidinium
3. Peptic ulcer	Pirenzepine, telenzepine
4. Bronchial asthma	Ipratropium, tiotropium
5. Preanaesthetic medication	Glycopyrrolate
6. Urinary disorders	Oxybutynin, tolterodine, propiverine, dicyclomine
7. Antiparkinonism drugs	Benzhexol, benztropine, trihexyphenidyl

at doses that do not affect other functions. Pirenzepine also does not cross the BBB - hence has no CNS effects. They are tried in peptic ulcer

- When used in bronchial asthma, atropine thickens the bronchial secretions and interferes with the movement of cilia, thus favouring formation of mucous plugs. Ipratropium bromide is a bronchodilator that does not affect mucociliary activity. When given as inhalation it acts only on the airways and does not produce any significant systemic effects because it is poorly absorbed.

- Glycopyrrolate is an antisialogogue (reduces salivary secretions). It is a quaternary ammonium compound - does not cross the BBB – therefore no effects on the CNS. It is given IM as preanaesthetic medication (See page 173).

- Benztropine, benzhexol, and trihexyphenidyl are the derivatives used in drug induced parkinsonism (See page 205).

- Urinary disorders – atropine substitutes are used to reduce urinary urgency and frequency to relieve bladder spasm and improve bladder capacity in urinary disorders and following urologic surgeries. They are also tried in nocturnal enuresis in children.

- Classification
- Peripherally acting skeletal muscle relaxants
  - Competitive blockers
  - Depolarising blockers
- Centrally acting muscle relaxants
- Directly acting muscle relaxants

Skeletal muscle relaxants (SMR) are drugs that reduce the muscle tone either by acting peripherally at the neuromuscular junction (neuromuscular blockers) or centrally in the cerebrospinal axis or directly on the contractile mechanism. They reduce the spasticity in a variety of neurological conditions and are also useful in surgeries.

Skeletal muscle relaxants may be classified as follows:

CLASSIFICATION
1. Drugs acting peripherally at the NMJ
• *Competitive blockers:-* (*Nondepolarising agents*)   d-Tubocurarine, pancuronium, alcuronium, atracurium, mivacurium, rocuronium, doxacurium, pipecuronium, vecuronium, rapacuronium, gallamine
• *Depolarising blockers:-*   Succinylcholine, decamethonium
2. Drugs acting centrally   Diazepam, baclofen, mephenesin, tizanidine.
3. Drugs acting directly on the muscle   Dantrolene.

PERIPHERALLY ACTING SKELETAL MUSCLE RELAXANTS

Neuromuscular Blockers (NMB)

Competitive Blockers

d-Tubocurarine

Curare was used by the South American Indians as arrow poison for hunting wild animals because curare paralysed the animals. On extensive research, the active principle from curare, **tubocurarine** was identified.

d-tubocurarine (d-Tc) is the dextrorotatory quaternery ammonium alkaloid obtained from the plant *Chondrodendron tomentosum* and plants of the Strychnos species. (l-tubocurarine is less potent) Several synthetic agents have been developed. All these are quaternary ammonium compounds because of which they are not well absorbed and are quickly excreted.

Mechanism of action

Non-depolarising blockers bind to nicotinic receptors on the motor end plate and block the actions of acetylcholine by competitive blockade (Fig. 10.1). These compounds slowly dissociate from the receptors and transmission is gradually restored. Thus the action of d-Tc is reversible.

Pharmacological actions

Skeletal muscle On parenteral administration, tubocurarine initially causes muscular weakness followed by flaccid paralysis. Small muscles of the eyes and fingers are the first to be affected, followed by those of the limbs, neck and trunk. Later the intercostal muscles and finally the diaphragm are paralysed and respiration stops. Consciousness is not affected throughout. Recovery occurs in the reverse order, i.e. the diaphragm is the first to recover. The effect lasts for 30-60 minutes (Table 10.1).

Autonomic ganglia In high doses tubocurarine can block autonomic ganglia and adrenal medulla resulting in hypotension.

Histamine release Tubocurarine can cause histamine release from the mast cells leading to bronchospasm, increased tracheobronchial and

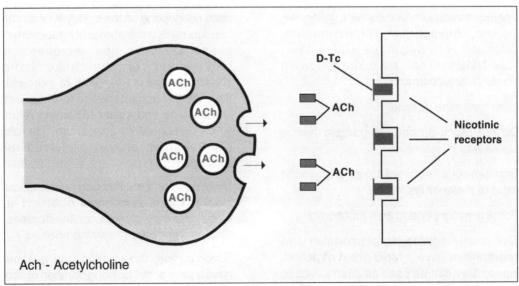

Ach - Acetylcholine

Fig. 10.1 d-Tc molecules bind to nicotinic receptors and prevent the binding of ACh on these receptors

gastric secretions. Histamine release also contributes to hypotension.

Pharmacokinetics

d-Tc is a quaternary ammonium compound - hence not absorbed orally. It is given either IM or IV.

Adverse reactions

1. Respiratory paralysis and prolonged apnoea - patient should be given artificial ventilation. Neostigmine may be used to reverse the skeletal muscle paralysis.

2. Hypotension is due to ganglion blockade and histamine release.

3. Flushing and bronchospasm due to histamine release by tubocurarine; this is not seen with newer agents.

Treatment of toxicity - Neostigmine reverses the skeletal muscle paralysis and it is the antidote in curare poisoning. Antihistamines should be given to counter the effects of histamine.

Synthetic Competitive Blockers

Pancuronium, atracurium, vecuronium, gallamine, doxacurium, mivacurium, pipecuronium, rapacuronium, rocuronium are (Table 10.1) synthetic NMBs. They have the following advantages over tubocurarine -

- Less histamine release

- Do not block autonomic ganglia hence cause less hypotension

- Spontaneous recovery takes place with most of these drugs

- Some are more potent than tubocurarine

- The newer agents *rapacuronium* and *rocuronium* have a rapid onset of action. Hence they can be used as alternatives to succinylcholine for muscle relaxation. When so used, rapacuronium can cause severe

TABLE 10.1 Duration of action of competitive neuromuscular blockers

Drug	Onset (min) of action	Duration (min)
Tubocurarine	5	35-60
Gallamine	5	35-60
Pancuronium	2-4	35-80
Doxacurium	5	90-120
Atracurium	2-4	20-35
Vecuronium	2-4	20-35
Mivacurium	2-4	12-18
Pipecuronium	2-4	80-100
Rapacuronium	1-2	15-30
Rocuronium	1-2	30-60

bronchospasm before endotracheal intubation.

- *Rocuronium* does not cause hypotension, tachycardia and is fast acting.

- *Atracurium* can be safely used in patients with renal impairment because it is degraded spontaneously by plasma esterases by *Hoffmann elimination* and does not depend on the kidney for excretion. Laudanosine, a metabolite of atracurium can cause seizures and increases the requirement of the anaesthetics. *Cisatracurium* is an isomer of atracurium, that has the advantages of forming lesser laudanosine and lesser histamine release when compared to atracurium. Therefore cisatracurium is now preferred over atracurium.

- Mivacurium is a short acting neuromuscular blocker with a slow onset of action. It is metabolised by plasma cholinesterases. It causes significant histamine release.

- Tubocurarine, doxacurium and gallamine have a slow onset but long duration of action (about 5 minutes). Pancuronium, vecuronium and atracurium have

Table 10.2 Comparision between Tubocurarine and Succinylcholine

	Tubocurarine	Succinylcholine
Mechanism	Compititive blockade	Persistant depolarization
Type of blockade	Nondepolarising	Depolarising
Phases of blockade	Single	Dual block
Anticholinesterases	Reverse blockade	Do not reverse
Initial fasciculations	Nil	Present
Metabolism	only partly metabolized in the liver	By pseudocholinesterase
Onset of action	Slow	Fast
Duration of action	Long (1 - 2hrs)	Short (10 min)

intermediate onset (2-4 minutes) while rapacuronium and rocuronium have fast onset of action(1-2 minutes)

Tubocurarine causes histamine release, ganglion blockade (resulting in hypotension) and its muscle relaxant effect needs to be reversed with drugs. Hence it is not used now. The synthetic compounds are preferred.

Depolarising blockers

Succinylcholine (SCh, Suxamethonium) is a quaternary ammonium compound with the structure resembling two molecules of acety lcholine joined together.

Mechanism of action

The neuromuscular effects of SCh are like those of ACh. SCh reacts with nicotinic receptors and depolarises the skeletal muscle membrane. But, unlike ACh which gets metabolised in a fraction of a second, SCh is destroyed very slowly by pseudocholinesterase (in about 5 minutes). Thus continued presence of the drug causes persistent depolarisation resulting in flaccid paralysis. This is phase I block. In high doses SCh produces a

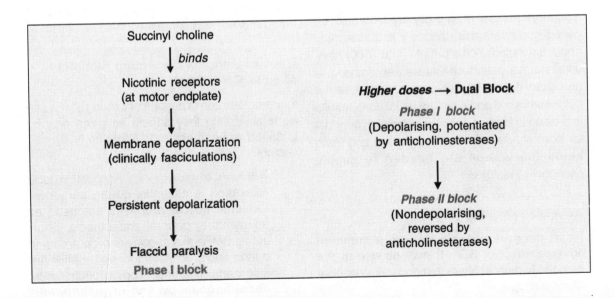

Succinyl choline
↓ *binds*
Nicotinic receptors
(at motor endplate)
↓
Membrane depolarization
(clinically fasciculations)
↓
Persistent depolarization
↓
Flaccid paralysis
Phase I block

Higher doses → **Dual Block**

Phase I block
(Depolarising, potentiated by anticholinesterases)
↓
Phase II block
(Nondepolarising, reversed by anticholinesterases)

dual block - initial depolarising block followed by non-depolarising block. The membrane gets slowly repolarised but cannot be depolarised again. The mechanism is not clearly known.

Pharmacological actions

Skeletal muscle On intravenous administration, onset of action is very rapid - within 1 minute. Initial transient muscular fasciculations and twitchings, mostly in the chest and abdominal regions, are followed by skeletal muscle paralysis. The fasciculations are maximum in 2 minutes and subside in 5 minutes. It is due to stimulation of the muscle fibres by the discharge of action potentials in them. SCh is a short acting muscle relaxant and the effect lasts for 5-10 minutes. Hence it has to be given continuously as an infusion for longer effect.

CVS: Initially hypotension and bradycardia may result from stimulation of vagal ganglia. This is followed by hypertension and tachycardia due to stimulation of sympathetic ganglia. Higher doses can cause cardiac arrhythmias. SCh can also cause histamine release if injected rapidly.

Pharmacokinetics

Succinylcholine is rapidly hydrolysed by pseudocholinesterase - hence it is short-acting about 5 minutes. Some people (1 in 2000) have an abnormal pseudocholinesterase enzyme, a hereditary defect. In such people, SCh does not get metabolised and even the usual dose results in prolonged apnoea and paralysis which may last for several hours. Artificial ventilation and fresh blood transfusion are needed to supply pseudocholinesterase.

Adverse reactions

Postoperative muscle pain is a common adverse effect of SCh. It may be due to the damage to muscle fibers that occur during initial fasciculations.

Hyperkalemia

Depolarising blockers can cause hyperkalemia due to sudden release of K^+ from the intracellular sites. This can be dangerous particularly in patients with CCF. It may result in cardiac arrest in patients with burns and nerve injuries.

Cardiac arrhythmias - SCh can cause cardiac arrhythmias.

Malignant hyperthermia - is a rare genetically determined condition where there is a sudden increase in the body temperature and severe muscle spasm due to release of intracellular Ca^{++} from the sarcoplasmic reticulum. Certain drugs like halothane, isoflurane and succinyl choline can trigger the process which can be fatal. Combination of halothane and SCh is the most common triggering factor. Intravenous dantrolene is life-saving in malignant hyperthermia. Oxygen inhalation and immediate cooling of the body also help.

Drug interactions

1. General anaesthetics augment the action of SMRs.

2. Anticholinesterases like neostigmine - reverse the action of competitive blockers.

3. Aminoglycosides and calcium channel blockers potentiate the action of SMRs.

Uses of Peripherally Acting Skeletal Muscle Relaxants

Inappropriate use of peripherally acting SMRs can be fatal. Hence they should be given only by qualified anaesthetists or adequately trained doctors.

1. **Adjuvant to anaesthesia** Adequate muscle relaxation is essential during surgeries. Skeletal muscle relaxants are used as adjuvants to general anaesthesia. Short acting SMRs like succinylcholine are used during endotracheal intubation. SMRs are also useful in laryngoscopy, bronchoscopy, oesophagoscopy and in orthopaedic

SUCCINYLCHOLINE! - NOT AN ANALGESIC

A young lady doctor in the pink of her health underwent a minor cosmetic surgery. She was recovering from anaesthesia in the post operative room. The nurse came smiling, wish the patient and loaded the syringe. She was supposed to give an analgesic injection. She instead administered succinylcholine. Within minutes the patient went into total muscular paralysis and cerebral anoxia resulting in brain death. The lady survived on ventilator for a few weeks and finally succumbed to it.

procedures like reduction of fractures and dislocations.

2. **In electroconvulsive therapy** SMRs protect the patient from convulsions and trauma during ECT.

3. **In spastic disorders** SMRs are used to overcome the spasm of tetanus, athetosis and status epilepticus.

CENTRALLY ACTING MUSCLE RELAXANTS

These drugs act on higher centres and cause muscle relaxation without loss of consciousness. They also have sedative properties.

Mechanism of Action

Centrally acting muscle relaxants depress the spinal polysynaptic reflexes. These reflexes maintain the muscle tone. By depressing these spinal reflexes, centrally acting muscle relaxants reduce the muscle tone.

Diazepam has useful antispastic activity. It can be used in relieving muscle spasm of almost any origin including local muscle trauma (See chapter 25).

Baclofen is an analog of the inhibitory neurotransmitter GABA. It is a $GABA_B$ agonist. It depresses the monosynaptic and polysynaptic reflexes in the spinal cord. It relieves painful spasms including flexor and extensor spasms and may also improve bladder and bowel functions in patients with spinal lesions. Normal tendon reflexes are not affected.

Baclofen is generally given orally. It should be gradually withdrawn after prolonged use because abrupt withdrawal can cause anxiety, palpitations and hallucinations.

Side effects are drowsiness, weakness and ataxia.

Mephenesin is not preferred due to its side effects. A number of related drugs like **carisoprodol, methocarbamol, chlorzoxazone** are used in acute muscle spasm caused by local trauma. All of them also cause sedation.

Tizanidine is a congener of clonidine. It is a central α_2 agonist like clonidine. It increases presynaptic inhibition of motor neurons and reduces muscle spasms. Adverse effects include drowsiness, weakness, hypotension and dry mouth. Tizanidine is used in the treatment of spasticity due to stroke, multiple sclerosis and amyotropic lateral sclerosis.

Other centrally acting spasmolytic agents include **riluzole, gabapentin** and **progabide**. Riluzole has both presynaptic and postsynaptic effects. It inhibits glutamate release in the CNS. It is well tolerated with minor adverse effects like nausea and diarrhoea. It is used to reduce spasticity in amyotropic lateral sclerosis.

Uses of Centrally Acting Muscle Relaxants

1. *Musculoskeletal disorders* like muscle strains, sprains, myalgias, cervical root syndromes, herniated disc syndromes, low backache, dislocations, arthritis, fibrositis and bursitis all cause painful muscle spasms. Muscle relaxants are used with analgesics in these.

2. *Spastic neurological disorders* like cerebral palsy, multiple sclerosis, poliomyelitis, hemiplegia and quadriplegia are treated with diazepam or baclofen.

3. *Tetanus* Diazepam is given IV.

4. *ECT* Diazepam is given along with peripherally acting SMRs.

5. *Orthopedic procedures* like fracture reduction may be done after administering diazepam.

DIRECTLY ACTING MUSCLE RELAXANTS

Dantrolene directly affects the skeletal muscle contractile mechanism. It inhibits the muscle contraction by preventing the calcium release from the sarcoplasmic reticulum.

Adverse effects include drowsiness, dizziness, fatigue, diarrhoea, muscle weakness and rarely, hepatotoxicity. Liver function tests should be done to look for hepatotoxicity.

Uses

Dantrolene is used in spastic disorders like hemiplegia and paraplegia. Dantrolene is the drug of choice in malignant hyperthermia. Dantrolene prevents the release of Ca^{++} from the sarcoplasmic reticulum and relieves muscle spasm in malignant hyperthermia.

DRUGS USED IN THE TREATMENT OF LOCAL MUSCLE SPASM

Several agents are used for the treatment of local muscle spasms which may result from injury or strain. Cyclobenzaprine, metaxalone, carisoprodol, chlorzoxazone, meprobamate and methocarbamol are some of them. They have the following common features-

• All these drugs act by depressing spinal polysynaptic reflexes.

• Common adverse reactions include drowsiness and dizziness.

• Cyclobenzaprine has anticholinergic effects and can therefore cause dryness of mouth, drowsiness and dizziness.

• Many of them are available in combination with NSAIDs.

• NSAIDs are equally or more effective in relieving muscle spasms.

Botulinum toxin is produced by the anaerobic bacterium *Clostridium botulinum.* The toxin inhibits the release of acetylcholine at the cholinergic synapses resulting in flaccid paralysis of skeletal muscles.

Botulinum toxin is useful (local injection) in the treatment of dystonias, including sports or writer's cramps, muscle spasms, tremors, cerebral palsy and in rigidity seen in extrapyramidal disorders. It is commonly used to relieve blepharospasm. Botulinum toxin is also gaining popularity in cosmetic therapy to remove facial lines by local injection.

11 *Adrenergic System*

- Distribution of the sympathetic system
- Neurotransmitters
- Synthesis of catecholamines
- Adrenergic receptors
- Mechanism of action

The prime function of the adrenergic or sympathetic nervous system is to help the human being to adjust to stress and prepare the body for fight or flight reactions. When exposed to stress, the heart rate and stroke volume increase with the resultant increase in cardiac output. The blood is shifted from the skin, gut, kidney and glands to the heart, skeletal muscles, brain and lungs, as these organs need more blood during stress. Pupils and bronchi are dilated and sweating is increased. Blood glucose increases by glycogenolysis.

Distribution of the sympathetic system

The sympathetic division consists of the thoracolumbar outflow extending from 1st thoracic to 2nd or 3rd lumbar segments. The sympathetic ganglia are paravertebral, prevertebral and terminal ganglia and adrenal medulla.

Tyrosine
  Tyrosine hydroxylase
DOPA
  DOPA decarboxylase
Dopamine
  DA β-hydroxylase
Noradrenaline
  N-methyl transferase
Adrenaline

Fig 11.1 Biosynthesis of catecholamines

Neurotransmitters

Neurotransmitters of the sympathetic system are noradrenaline (NA, norepinephrine) and dopamine (DA). Adrenaline (epinephrine) is the major hormone secreted by the adrenal medulla.

Synthesis of catecholamines

The three endogenous catecholamines - NA, adrenaline and DA are synthesized from the amino acid tyrosine (Fig. 11.2).

The sympathetic postganglionic nerve fibres that synthesize, store and release NA are called **adrenergic.** Noradrenaline is stored in small vesicles in the adrenergic nerve terminals (Fig 11.2). In response to nerve impulse, NA is released into the synaptic cleft by a process called **exocytosis**. This NA binds to adrenergic receptors located on the postsynaptic membrane to produce the response. A small portion of NA is metabolised by the enzyme COMT. But a large portion (nearly 80%) is taken back into the nerve terminals by an energy dependent active transport process termed **uptake 1**, which is responsible for termination of action of NA. Of

this, a fraction is metabolised by MAO and the remaining NA is then transferred to the storage vesicles. Some part of NA released into the synaptic cleft penetrates into the effector cells and is known as **uptake 2**.

Adrenergic receptors

Ahlquist classified adrenergic receptors into 2 types - α and β. With the availability of newer, synthetic, selective drugs, these are further classified into subdivisions. We now know α_1 α_2, β_1, β_2 and β_3 adrenergic receptors.

The stimulation of α receptors mainly produces excitatory effects (exception-GIT); β stimulation causes mainly inhibitory effects (exception-heart). The characteristics of these receptors are given in Table 11.1. α_2 receptors are located on the presynaptic membrane (Fig 11.3). Stimulation of presynaptic α_2 receptors inhibits the further release of NA. Thus α_2 receptors exert a negative feed back on NA release. α_2 receptors are also present postsynaptically in the pancreatic islets, platelets and brain.

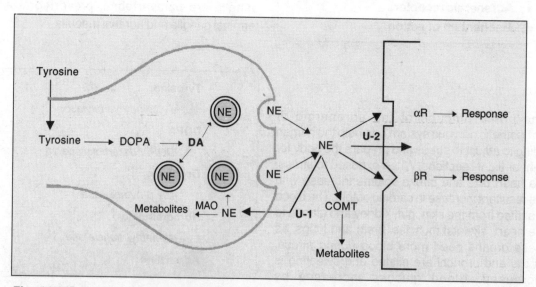

Fig. 11.2 Synthesis, storage, release and metabolism of noradrenaline. DA- Dopamine, NE-Norepinephrine, U-1- Uptake 1, U-2 - Uptake 2, MAO- Monoamine oxidase, COMT- Catechol -O-methyltransferase, α R - α receptor, βR - β receptor.

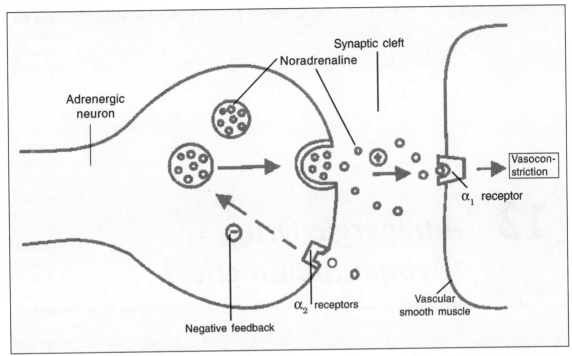

Fig 11.3 α_1 and α_2 receptor stimulation: NA binds to α_1 receptors and stimulates it to produce response like vasoconstriction. Presynaptic α_2 receptor stimulation inhibits the further release of NA from the storage vesicles

TABLE 11.1 Adrenergic receptor agonists and antagonists		
Receptor type	*Selective agonist*	*Selective antagonist*
α_1	Phenylephrine Mephenteramine Methoxamine	Prazosin Terazosin
α_2	Clonidine	Yohimbine
β_1	Dobutamine	Metoprolol Atenolol
β_2	Salbutamol	Butoxamine
β_3	-	-

Mechanism of action

Both α and β adrenergic receptors are G-protein coupled receptors (See page 38 - 40). Stimulation of alpha receptors activates phospholipase C in the cell membrane which acts through generation of second messengers inositol triphosphate (IP$_3$) and diacylglycerol (DAG) and increase intracellular calcium.

Stimulation of beta receptors activates an enzyme adenylyl cyclase resulting in increased intracellular cyclic AMP levels. This second messenger acts through various intracellular proteins to bring about the response.

12 | *Adrenergic Drugs (Sympathomimetics)*

- Classification
- Actions
- Pharmacokinetics
- Noradrenaline
- Isoprenaline
- Dopamine
- Epinine
- Dopexamine
- Dobutamine
- Fenoldopam
- Non-catecholamines
  - Ephedrine
  - Amphetamine
- Vasopressors
- Nasal decongestants
- Selective β₂ stimulants
- Anorectic agents

Sympathomimetics are drugs whose actions mimic that of sympathetic stimulation. Catecholamines and sympathomimetics or adrenergic drugs may be classified in various ways depending on the presence/absence of catechol nucleus, mode of action and therapeutic indications as follows:

CLASSIFICATION

I. **Chemical classification - based on the presence/absence of catechol nucleus**

1. Catecholamines
   Noradrenaline (NA), adrenaline, dopamine (DA), isoprenaline (Synthetic)
2. Non-catecholamines
   Ephedrine, amphetamine

II. Depending on the mode of action

1. Directly acting sympathomimetics
   (by interacting with adrenergic receptors)
   Noradrenaline, adrenaline, dopamine, isoprenaline
2. Indirectly acting sympathomimetics
   (by releasing NA from nerve terminals)
   Amphetamine, tyramine
3. Mixed action amines
   (both direct and indirect actions)
   Ephedrine, methoxamine

III. Therapeutic or clinical classification

1. **Vasopressors**

   Noradrenaline, dopamine, methoxamine, metaraminol

2. **Cardiac stimulants**

   Adrenaline, dopamine, dobutamine, isoprenaline, ephedrine

3. **CNS stimulants**

   Amphetamine, ephedrine

4. **Bronchodilators**

   Adrenaline, isoprenaline, salbutamol, terbutaline, salmeterol, perbuterol, fenoterol, formoterol

5. **Nasal decongestants**

   Ephedrine, pseudoephedrine, phenyl-propanolamine, phenylephrine, oxymeta-zoline, xylometazoline

6. **Appetite suppressants (anorectics)**

   Fenfluramine, dexfenfluramine

7. **Uterine relaxants**

   Salbutamol, terbutaline, isosuxprine, ritodrine

ADRENALINE

ACTIONS

1.Cardiovascular System

- **Heart** Adrenaline is a powerful cardiac stimulant. Acting through β_1 receptors, it increases the heart rate, force of contraction cardiac output and conduction velocity. The work done by the heart and the resultant O_2 consumption are increased.

- **Blood vessels and BP** Blood vessels of the skin and mucous membrane are constricted (α_1) and that of the skeletal muscles are dilated (β_2) by adrenaline. Since adrenaline causes cutaneous vasoconstriction, it is used to prolong the duration of action of local anaesthetics.

Small doses of (0.1 mg/kg) adrenaline produce a fall in blood pressure because of vasodilation of the blood vessels in skeletal muscles. This is because β_2 receptors are sensitive even to this small dose of adrenaline.

Moderate doses of adrenaline given IV produce a rapid increase in BP followed by a fall - a biphasic response.The systolic rises due to α_1 mediated vasoconstriction. Action on β receptors is more persistent and as the action on a receptors wears off, the action on β_2 receptors gets unmasked resulting in decreased BP due to the fall in the diastolic. Sir Henry Dale demonstrated that when α receptors are blocked (with - ergot alkaloids), adrenaline produces only a fall in BP and this is named after him as **Dale's vasomotor reversal** (or Dale's phenomenon).

Noradrenaline is mainly an alpha agonist and therefore brings about a rise in BP. This is associated with bradycardia due to baroreceptor stimulation.

- **Other vascular beds**

Adrenaline causes renal vasoconstriction resulting in a fall in renal blood flow; it also causes pulmonary and mesenteric vasoconstriction.

Cerebral and coronary blood flow is enhanced.

2. Smooth Muscles

- **Bronchi:** Adrenaline is a powerful broncho dilator and a weak respiratory stimulant. Pulmonary vasoconstriction relieves bronchial congestion. All these result in an increase in vital capacity.

- **Uterus**
  Nonpregnant uterus - contracts
  Last month of pregnancy - relaxes.

- **Gut** Smooth muscle is relaxed - but weak and transient action.

- **Splenic capsule**

  Contracts resulting in the release of RBCs into the circulation.

- **Pilomotor** muscles of the hair follicle contract.

- **Bladder** Detrusor is relaxed (β receptors) while trigone is contracted thereby increasing the holding capacity of the bladder.

3. Eye

Adrenaline causes mydriasis due to contraction of the radial muscles of the iris (α_1); it also reduces intraocular pressure. The exact mechanism is not known, but it is thought that adrenaline reduces both the production of aqueous humor (β) and improves its drainage (α receptor).

4. Metabolic Effects

Adrenaline increases the blood sugar level by enhancing hepatic glycogenolysis. It also inhibits insulin release. By enhancing breakdown of triglycerides in the adipose tissue, more free fatty acids are made available in the plasma by action on β_3 receptors in adipocytes.

5. Skeletal Muscles

Catecholamines facilitate neuromuscular transmission by action on both α and β receptors - they enhance the amount of ACh released.

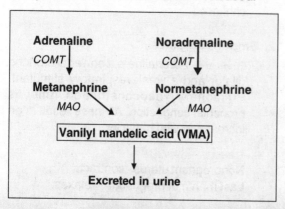

Pharmacokinetics

As catecholamines are rapidly inactivated in the gut and the liver, they are not given orally. Adrenaline and NA are metabolised by COMT and MAO.

Adverse reactions

Anxiety, palpitation, weakness, tremors, pallor, dizziness, restlessness and throbbing headache may follow adrenaline/NA administration. In patients with ischaemic heart disease, both adrenaline and NA can precipitate anginal pain. Rapid IV injection can cause sudden sharp rise in BP which may precipitate arrthythmias, subarachnoid haemorrhage or hemiplegia.

Preparations

Adrenaline 1:1000, 1: 10,000 and 1:1,00,000 solutions are available for injection. Adrenaline is given SC/IM; intracardiac in emergencies. Adrenaline aerosol for inhalation and 2% ophthalmic solution are also available.

Uses of adrenaline

1. **Anaphylactic shock:** Adrenaline is the drug of choice (0.3-0.5 ml of 1:1000 solution). It promptly reverses hypotension, laryngeal oedema and bronchospasm and is life saving in anaphylactic shock. IM route is preferred as absorption by SC route is not reliable in shock.

2. **Cardiac arrest:** Sudden cardiac arrest due to drowning, electrocution, etc. are treated with intracardiac adrenaline (into 4th or 5th intercostal space, 2-3 inches from the sternum); before injecting, ensure that the tip of the needle is in the heart. If the piston of the syringe is withdrawn, blood should enter the syringe.

3. **Control of haemorrhage:** Adrenaline in 1: 10,000 to 1 : 20,000 concentration is used as a topical hemostatic to control bleeding.

Bleeding stops due to vasoconstriction. Adrenaline packs are used for bleeding after tooth extraction and in epistaxis.

4. With local anaesthetics (See page 176, 179): Injected with LA, adrenaline produces vasoconstriction and reduces the rate of absorption of LA. By this it prolongs the action and reduces systemic toxicity of LA. 1: 10,000 to 1: 2,00,000 adrenaline is used.

5. Acute bronchial asthma: SC/inhalation adrenaline produces bronchodilation. But is not preferred as more selective drugs are available (See Chap. 38).

6. Glaucoma (See page 72) Adrenaline ↑IOP and can be used in glaucoma. But it has the disadvantages of being

   i. Poorly absorbed.

   ii. Short acting as it is quickly metabolised in the eye. **Dipivefrin** is a prodrug which gets converted to adrenaline in the eye by the action of corneal esterases. Dipivefrin has good penetrability due to high lipid solubility and it is used in glaucoma.

Contraindications

Adrenaline is contraindicated in patients with angina pectoris, hypertension and in patients on β blockers.

Noradrenaline can be used in shock to increase BP - but it is very rarely used.

Isoprenaline (Isoproterenol, Isopropyl arterenol) is a synthetic catecholamine with predominantly β receptor stimulant action and negligible ＼ actions. It has cardiac stimulant and smooth muscle relaxant properties. Due to vasodilation BP falls; it is a potent bronchodilator. Adverse effects include palpitation, angina, headache and flushing.

Isoprenaline is used in heart block and shock for its cardiac stimulant actions. It can be used in bronchial asthma (page 283).

Dopamine

Dopamine is the precursor of NA. It acts on dopaminergic and adrenergic receptors. It is a central neurotransmitter. Low doses stimulate vascular D_1 receptors in renal, mesenteric and coronary beds causing vasodilatation in these vessels. D_2 receptors stimulation in the sympathetic nerve terminals and in cardiovascular centres also results in renal vasodilation. Hence renal blood flow and GFR increase. Higher doses cause cardiac stimulation through β_1 receptors resulting in an increase in the force of contraction with a relatively minor increase in the heart rate. In high doses α_1 receptors are activated resulting in vasoconstriction and ↑BP. Dopamine does not cross the BBB - hence it has no CNS effects. It is given IV (2-5 µg/Kg/min). It is short acting and the infusion rate can be adjusted to get the appropriate effect by monitoring BP. Dopamine is metabolised by COMT & MAO. **Epinine** (Ibopamine) is an ester of methyldopamine which acts like dopamine.

Adverse effects Nausea, vomiting, palpitation, headache, angina, sudden rise in BP may occur.

Uses

Dopamine is used in the treatment of shock - cardiogenic, hypovolaemic and septic shock. It is specially useful when there is renal dysfunction and low cardiac output.

Dopexamine is a synthetic analog of dopamine acting on D_1 D_2 and β_2 receptors. It is found to have beneficial effects in CCF.

Dobutamine a derivative of dopamine is a relatively selective β_1 agonist. Though it also activates α_1 receptors, in therapeutic doses the only dominant action is an increase in the force of contraction of the heart without a significant increase in the heart rate. Hence the increase in myocardial demand is milder when compared to dopamine and is therefore more useful than dopamine in cardiogenic shock. Dobutamine is used in patients with CCF or acute myocardial infarction or following cardiac surgery when there may be pump failure.

Fenoldopam is a selective D_1 agonist which dilates coronary, renal and mesentric arteries. It is used as an i.v. infusion in severe hypertension to rapidly reduce the BP.

NONCATECHOLAMINES

Noncatecholamines are devoid of catechol nucleus, they act both by direct stimulation of the adrenergic receptors and indirectly by releasing NA. In contrast to catecholamines, they are effective orally, relatively resistant to MAO and therefore are longer-acting; they cross the blood-brain barrier and have CNS effects.

Ephedrine is an alkaloid obtained from the plants of the genus *Ephedra*. Ephedrine acts by direct stimulation of α and β receptors and indirectly through release of NA. Repeated administration at short intervals result in tachyphylaxis. Ephedrine raises BP by peripheral vasoconstriction and by increasing the cardiac output. Like adrenaline it relaxes smooth muscles; it is a CNS stimulant and produces insomnia, restlessness, anxiety, tremors and increased mental activity.

Adverse effects include gastric upset, insomnia, tremors and difficulty in micturition.

Uses

1. Bronchial asthma: Ephedrine is useful in mild chronic bronchial asthma (See page 283) but it is not preferred.

2. Nasal decongestion: Ephedrine nasal drops are used. *Pseudoephedrine* - an isomer of ephedrine is used orally for decongestion. It causes vasoconstriction in the skin and mucous membrane but its effects on the CNS and the heart are milder.

3. Mydriasis Ephedrine eye drops are used to produce mydriasis without cycloplegia.

4. Hypotension For prevention and treatment of hypotension during spinal anaesthesia - IM ephedrine is used.

5. Narcolepsy is a condition with an irresistible desire and tendency to sleep. As ephedrine is a CNS stimulant, it is useful in narcolepsy.

6. Nocturnal enuresis (Bed wetting) in children may be treated with ephedrine as it increases the holding capacity of the bladder. Drugs should be used only when non-pharmacological measures have failed.

7. Stokes Adam's syndrome As an alternative to isoprenaline.

Amphetamine is a synthetic compound with actions similar to ephedrine; tachyphylaxis can occur on repeated use. Amphetamine readily crosses the BBB to reach the CNS. Amphetamine is a potent CNS stimulant; it produces increased mental and physical activity, alertness, increased concentration and attention span, elation, euphoria and increased capacity to work.

It also increases initiative and self confidence, postpones fatigue and improves physical performance (temporarily) as seen in athletes. All these properties make amphetamine a drug of dependence and abuse. Higher doses produce confusion, delirium and hallucinations.

Respiration: Amphetamine stimulates respiration - it is an analeptic.

Depression of appetite acting on the feeding centre in the hypothalamus, amphetamine reduces hunger and suppresses appetite.

Amphetamine also has weak anticonvulsant property.

Adverse effects include restlessness, tremors, insomnia, palpitation, anxiety, confusion and hallucinations. Prolonged use may precipitate psychosis.

High doses ca use angina, delirium, arrhy thmias, hypertension, acute psychosis, coma and death due to convulsions.

Dependence: Amphetamine causes psycho logic dependence.

Uses

1. **Attention deficit hyperactivity disorder (ADHD)** in children is characterised by decreased ability to concentrate and hold attention, aggressive behaviour and hyperactivity; Amphetamine increases attention span in such children and improves performance in school.

2. **Narcolepsy:** Amphetamine is preferred over ephedrine. Other drugs used in narcolepsy include **methylphenidate** and **modafinil**. Methylphenidate is an indirectly acting sympathomimetic like amphetamine. Modafinil is a centrally acting CNS stimulant which may act by stimulating α_1 adrenoceptors. In addition it also influences GABA and serotonin receptors. It is better tolerated with fewer adverse effects.

3. **Obesity:** Though appetite is suppressed, due to risk of dependence and other side effects, amphetamine should not be used for this purpose.

4. **Epilepsy:** Amphetamine can be used as adjuvant and to counter the sedation due to antiepileptics.

Methamphetamine has more prominent central than peripheral actions. Methylphenidate, phenmetrazin and pemoline are other amphetamine - like drugs with actions and abuse potential similar to amphe tamine.

VASOPRESSORS

These are a_1 agonists and include noradrenaline, dopamine, metaraminol, mephenteramine, phenylephrine and methoxamine. They increase the BP by increasing total peripheral resistance (TPR) or cardiac output (CO) or both. The rise in BP is associated with reflex bradycardia. They are given parenterally with constant monitoring of BP. Tachyphylaxis may develop.

Uses

Vasopressors are used to raise the BP in hypotension as seen in cardiogenic or neurogenic shock and during spinal anaesthesia.

Metaraminol is an alpha stimulant and also acts indirectly by NA release. CO is increased. It is also a nasal decongestant.

Mephenteramine acts on both α and β receptors to ↑TPR and ↑CO and thereby raises BP. It is orally effective. Pressor effect is accompanied by bradycardia.

Phenylephrine is a selective α_1 stimulant; it is also a nasal decongestant. Reflex bradycardia is prominent. It produces mydriasis without cycloplegia.

Methoxamine has actions similar to phenylephrine.

NASAL DECONGESTANTS

Nasal decongestants are α_1 agonists.

Mechanism of action

Nasal decongestants act by stimulating the α_1 receptors present in the blood vessels of the nasal mucosa.

They bring about vasoconstriction of the nasal mucosa, resulting in its shrinkage and decreased volume of the mucosa. Thus they relieve nasal congestion and decrease resistance to airflow through the nose.They also reduce nasal secretion. The nasal decongestants thus provide symptomatic relief in rhinitis due to allergy and upper respiratory infections.

Table 12.1 Uses of adrenergic agonists	
Indication	**Sympathomimetic used**
1. Cardiac arrest	- Adrenaline
2. Hypotension	- Methoxamine, mephenteramine
3. Hypertension	- Clonidine (α_2 agonist)
4. Anaphylactic shock	- Adrenaline IM
5. Severe allergic reactions (bee sting, food & drug allergy)	- Adrenaline IM
6. To arrest local bleeding	- Adrenaline
7. To prolong local anaesthesia	- Adrenaline
8. Bronchial asthma	- Salbutamol, terbutaline, salmeterol, ibuterol
9. Narcolepsy	- Amphetamine, ephedrine
10. Glaucoma	- Adrenaline, dipivefrine
11. Weight reduction	- Fenfluramine, dexfenfluramine, mazindol, amphetamine,
12. Nasal decongestion	- Oxymetazoline, xylometazoline,
13. Mydriasis for fundoscopy	- Phenylephrine
14. Attention deficit hyperactivity disorder	- Amphetamine, methylphenidate

They may be used

1. *Orally*   Ephedrine
                 Pseudoephedrine

2. *Topically (as nasal drops)*

      Oxymetazoline, xylometazoline
      Naphazoline, phenylephrine
      Mephenteramine
      Metaraminol
      Phenylpropanolamine

Adverse effects

1. When orally used, ephedrine and pseudoephedrine can cause insomnia, tremors and irritability

2. Topical agents - can cause nasal irritation. Most disadvantages result from long term use.

3. Prolonged use can cause

   - Atrophy of the nasal mucosa due to intense vasoconstriction.
   - Recongestion or 'after congestion' may result when the drug is stopped (due to vasodilatation).

- Loss of efficacy or tolerence due to desensitization of the receptors.
- Nasal decongestants should be used carefully in patients with hypertension.
- Phenylpropanolamine has been widely used in cold remedies and as an anorexiant. Its use is associated with an increased risk of haemorrhagic stroke and is therefore banned.

Uses

- Rhinitis in upper respiratory infections.
- Allergic and vasomotor rhinitis, sinusitis.
- Blocked eustachian tubes.

Nasal decongestants afford symptomatic relief in the above conditions.

SELECTIVE β_2 STIMULANTS

Selective β_2 stimulants include orciprenaline, salbutamol, terbutaline and the newer ones include salmeterol, perbuterol, bitolterol, fenoterol and formoterol. These are smooth muscle relaxants which produce bronchodilatation, vasodilation and uterine relaxation without significant cardiac stimulation.

Selective β_2 agonists are used in:

i. Bronchial asthma (chap 38) - they can be given by inhalation.
ii. As uterine relaxants to delay premature labour.

Side effects include muscle tremors, palpitation and arrhythmias.

Isoxsuprine is a selective β receptor stimulant used as uterine relaxant in premature labour, threatened abortion and dysmenorrhoea.

ANORECTIC AGENTS (ANOREXIANTS)

Though **amphetamine** suppresses appetite, it is not recommended for the treatment of obesity due to its central stimulant effects. Many amphetamine like drugs which suppress appetite but lack significant CNS stimulant effects are now available. They are **fenfluramine, dexfen fluramine, mazindol, phenylpropanolamine, phenmetrazine** and others.

Adverse effects include risk of abuse, drowsiness and depression because of which they are only used for short periods as adjuncts to other measures. Phenylpropanolamine is now banned because of the risk of stroke.

Sibutramine suppresses appetite and has been tried in obesity. It inhibits the uptake of NA and 5-HT but causes many serious adverse effects including insomnia, anxiety, mood changes, hypertension and cardiovascular deaths.

13 *Adrenergic Antagonists*

- **Alpha adrenergic blocking agents**
    - **Actions**
    - **Phenoxybenzamine**
    - **Ergot alkaloids**
    - **Selective α_1 blockers**
    - **Yohimbine**
- **Beta adrenergic blocking agents**
    - **Classification**
    - **Pharmacological actions**
    - **Pharmacokinetics**
    - **Adverse reactions**
    - **Some important drug interactions**
    - **Cardioselective β blockers**
    - **Partial agonists**
    - **Some individual β antagonists**
    - **Uses of β-blockers**
- **Alpha and Beta adrenergic blockers**

Adrenergic blockers bind to the adrenergic receptors and prevent the action of adrenergic drugs. They may block alpha or beta receptors or both.

ALPHA ADRENERGIC BLOCKING AGENTS

Alpha receptor antagonists block the adrenergic responses mediated through alpha adrenergic receptors. Some of them have selectivity for α_1 or α_2 receptors.

Actions

The important effects of α receptor stimulation are α_1 mediated vasoconstriction and α_2-(presynaptic) receptor mediated inhibition of NA release. The result of alpha blockade by α-antagonists (Fig. 11.3 Page 91) are:

α_1-blockade - inhibits vasoconstriction leading to vasodilation and thereby $\downarrow$ BP. This fall in BP is opposed by the baroreceptor reflexes which tend to ↑ heart rate and cardiac output.

α_2-blockade - enhances release of NA which stimulates β receptors (α are already blocked) β_1 stimulation in heart results in tachycardia and - cardiac output.

Thus the predominant effects of nonselective α–blockade is hypotension with tachycardia.

Selective α_1-blockade - results in hypotension without significant tachycardia. This is because α_2 receptors are not blocked which means there is no increase in NA release.

Selective α_2 - blockade - ↑NA release resulting in hypertension.

α - blockade also results in miosis and nasal stuffiness. α - blockade in the bladder and prostate leads to decreased resistance to the flow of urine.

Adverse effects of α-blockers - Postural hypotension, palpitation, nasal stuffiness, miosis, impaired ejaculation and impotence.

α blockers are classified as follows-

1. Non-selective
   a. *Non-competitive blocker*
      Phenoxybenzamine

   b. *Competitive blockers*
      Ergot alkaloids (ergotamine), tolazoline, phentolamine, chlorpromazine

2. Selective
   a. *α_1-blockers*
      Prazosin, terazosin, trimazosin doxazosin, tamsulosin, alfuzosin, indoramin

   b. *α_2-blocker*
      Yohimbine

Phenoxybenzamine

Phenoxybenzamine binds covalently to alpha receptors causing irreversible blockade or non equilibrium type of blockade. Given IV, blood pressure gradually falls over 1-2 hours and is associated with tachycardia and ↑ CO. The BP reduction is more in patients with increased sympathetic tone. The action lasts for 3-4 days. It also blocks histamine, 5-HT and cholinergic receptors. Phenoxybenzamine can be given orally - started with a low dose which is gradually increased. It is used in the treatment of pheochromocytoma.

Ergot alkaloids

Ergotamine (See page 270), ergotoxine and their derivatives are competitive antagonists and the blockade is of short duration. Some of them have a direct stimulant effect on smooth muscles - cause contraction of the uterus and ↑ BP due to vasoconstriction. Prolonged use of these can cause gangrene of the toes and fingers.

Phentolamine and tolazoline

Phentolamine and tolazoline are imidazoline derivatives. They are competitive α–blockers. In addition they also block 5-HT receptors, stimulate gut motility and ↑ gastric secretion. Hence they can cause vomiting and diarrhoea in addition to the effects of α–blockade.

SELECTIVE α_1 BLOCKERS

Prazosin

Prazosin is a potent, highly selective, α_1-blocker with 1000 times greater affinity for α_1 receptors. Arterioles and venules are dilated resulting in decreased peripheral vascular resistance and cardiac output. (CO falls because of reduced preload which is due to venodilation. There is no significant tachycardia (as α_2 receptors are spared, there is no ↑ in NA release). In addition it may decrease central sympathetic outflow. Prazosin also inhibits phosphodiesterase, the enzyme that degrades cAMP resulting in ↑ cAMP which also contributes to vasodilation.

Other actions

- Prazosin and its congeners are found to ↓ LDL and triglycerides and ↑ HDL cholesterol.
- They also relax the urinary bladder neck and the prostatic capsule because of which they are useful in prostatic hypertophy.

Prazosin is orally effective, extensively bound to plasma proteins (about 97%) and is metabolised in the liver. Its duration of action is 8-10 hrs.

Adverse effects

First dose phenomenon - one hour after the initial dose, marked postural hypotension occurs which may lead to fainting. To avoid this, prazosin should be started with a low dose and taken at bed time. Other side effects include headache and dizziness. Tamsulosin can cause abnormal ejaculation.

Congeners of prazosin include terazosin, doxazosin, alfuzosin and tamsulosin. Others are indoramin and urapidil.

- These congeners are longer acting and can be given once daily
- Highly selective for α_1 receptors.
- Postural hypotension is milder than with prazosin.
- No significant effect on cardiac function.
- ↓LDL and ↑HDL cholesterol
- Tamsulosin has selective activity on α_{1A} receptors which are dominant in the bladder

and prostate while hypotension mediated by α_{1B} receptors is milder. Therefore tamsulosin relieves the symptoms of benign prostatic hypertrophy (BPH) with milder fall in BP. Hence it is preferred in BPH.

- Alfuzosin is also useful in BPH.
- Terazosin and doxazosin are used in hypertension.
- Urapidil has α_1 and β_1 (weak) blocking properties. It is used in hypertension and BPH.
- Indoramin is a selective α_1 blocker. It is used in the treatment of benign prostatic hypertrophy.

α_2 BLOCKER

Yohimbine

Yohimbine is a relatively selective α_2-blocker which increases BP and heart rate due to ↑ NA release. It causes congestion of genitals because of which it is used to treat psychogenic impotence. It is also claimed to be an aphrodisiac though the effect is only psychological.

Uses of α-blockers

1. Hypertension   Selective α_1-blockers like prazosin are used in the treatment of hypertension (See page 149). Phenoxy-benzamine or phentolamine can be used in hypertensive crisis.

2. Pheochromocytoma is an adrenal medullary tumor which secretes large amounts of catecholamines resulting in hypertension. The tumor has to be removed surgically. Phenoxybenzamine and phentolamine are used for the preoperative management of the patient and during the operation. Inoperable cases are put on long-term treatment with phenoxybenzamine.

3. Peripheral vascular diseases like

Raynaud's phenomenon may be be .efited by α - blockers which afford symptomatic relief.

4. Congestive cardiac failure Because of its vasodilator action, prazosin is useful in CCF. But ACE inhibitors are preferred.

5. Benign prostatic hypertrophy (BPH) Blockade of α_1 receptors in the bladder, prostate and urethra reduces resistance to urine outflow. Prazosin, tamsulosin and alfuzosin are useful in patients who cannot be operated upon. Of these, tamsulosin is preferred because of its selective activity on α_{1A} receptors.

BETA ADRENERGIC BLOCKING AGENTS

β–blockers are drugs that block the actions of catecholamines mediated through the β receptors.

Classification

1. Non-selective

Propranolol, nadolol

timolol, sotalol

2. Cardioselective (β_1)

Metoprolol, atenolol,

acebutolol, esmolol, betaxolol

3. Partial agonists

Pindolol, oxprenolol,

carteolol, bopindolol, penbutotol

4. With additional alpha blocking property

Labetalol, carvedilol

5. β_1 blocker β_2 agonist

Celiprolol

Pharmacological Actions

1. *CVS* β - blockers decrease heart rate, force of contraction and cardiac output. Blood pressure falls. The effect is more pronounced in presence of increased sympathetic tone than in a normal situation.

AV conduction is delayed. Myocardial oxygen requirement is reduced due to reduced cardiac work. They also improve exercise tolerance in angina patients. β - blockers prevent the exercise - induced increase in heart rate and force of contraction.

High doses produce membrane-stabilising activity like quinidine causing direct depression of the heart.

2. *Respiratory tract* Blockade of β_2 receptors in the bronchial smooth muscle causes increase in airway resistance - may precipitate acute attack in asthmatics.

3. *Eye* Many β - blockers reduce intraocular pressure by decreased secretion of aqueous humour.

4. *Metabolic* β - antagonists block lipolysis and glycogenolysis (β_2 mediated) induced by sympathetic stimulation. Hence nonselective β blockers may interfere with recovery from hypoglycaemia in diabetics. Plasma triglycerides may increase and HDL levels decrease in some patients.

Pharmacokinetics

Though well absorbed on oral administration, some β–blockers like propranolol undergo extensive first pass metabolism. Most of them have short t½ and are metabolised in the liver.

Adverse Reactions

1. Bradycardia is common. Patients with AV conduction defects may develop arrhythmias and heart block with β - blockers.

2. CCF In patients with impaired myocardial function, sympathetic activity supports the heart. β - blockade eliminates this and may precipitate CCF and acute pulmonary edema.

3. Cold extremities especially in patients with

peripheral vascular disease may occur.

4. β - blockers can precipitate acute asthmatic attack in asthmatics and is contraindicated in them.

5. CNS Insomnia, depression and rarely hallucinations can follow the use of β - blockers.

6. Fatigue due to decreased blood flow to the muscles during exercise and reduced cardiac output.

7. Metabolic effects Weakness, ↓ exercise capacity may be seen due to its metabolic effects.

8. Abrupt withdrawal of β - blockers after prolonged use can cause rebound hypertension and precipitate anginal attacks. This is due to up-regulation of β receptors. Hence β - blockers should be gradually tapered.

9. β blockers can also cause dizziness.

10. Topical - Timolol eye drops can sometimes cause burning and dryness of the eyes.

Some important drug interactions

1. Propranolol + insulin - when diabetics on insulin also receive propranolol:

    i. β - blockade masks tachycardia which is the first warning signal of hypoglycaemia.

    ii. β–blockade delays the recovery from hypoglycaemia by preventing glycogenolysis induced by sympathetic stimulation (acting through β2 receptors). This may be avoided by using a β1-selective blocker.

2. Propranolol + verapamil - since both cause myocardiac depression, profound depression may result when both are used together. Hence the combination should be avoided.

3. β - blockers + catecholamines - in patients

on nonselective β - blockers, blockade of vascular β receptors could predispose peripheral vessels to intense vasoconstriction (receptor up regulation) from even small doses of adrenaline used with LAs. Hence it is safer to use plain local anaesthesia in such patients.

Cardioselective β - blockers e.g. Atenolol, metoprolol, esmolol.

These drugs:
- Selectively block β1 receptors, β2 - blockade is weak
- Bronchospasm is less/negligible
- Inhibition of glycogenolysis is lower - hence safer in diabetics
- Exercise performance is impaired to a lesser degree
- Lesser chances of peripheral vascular disease.

Partial agonists - Pindolol, oxprenolol.

These have intrinsic sympathomimetic activity due to their partial β - agonistic property. As a result, bradycardia and myocardiac depression are less marked. They are therefore preferred in patients with low cardiac reserve or those who are likely to have severe bradycardia.

Some individual β - antagonists

Atenolol
- Selective β1-blocker
- Longer acting - given once daily
- Less lipid soluble - does not cross BBB - hence no CNS side effects
- No side effects on lipid profile.

Hence very commonly used (25 - 100mg daily).

Esmolol
- Selective β1 - blocker
- Ultra short-acting - t½ - 8 minutes.
- Used IV

TABLE 13.1 Doses of some β-blockers

Drug (Trade name)	Total daily dose (mg)	Frequency
Propranolol (INDERAL)	40-240	6-12 hr
Metoprolol (MEFOCARD)	50-200	12-24 hr
Atenolol (ATEN)	25-100	once daily
Pindolol (PINADOL)	10-45	6 hr
Acebutolol (SECTRAL)	200-400	12-24 hr

- Safer in critically ill patients and in emergencies when immediate β - blockade is needed.

Nadolol

- Nonselective β - blocker
- Long acting

Metoprolol

- Selective, β_1 blocker
- Well absorbed but undergoes significant first - pass metabolism
- Given twice daily (50 - 200 mg)
- Used in hypertension and angina pactoris

Acebutolol

- β_1 selective with some partial agonistic effects
- May be used in hypertension and arrhythmias

Celiprolol

- β_1 blocker, β_2 agonist effects
- Safer in asthmatics
- Used in hypertension

Timolol

- Nonselective, short-acting
- Used in glaucoma - as eye drops.

Uses of β-blockers

1. **Hypertension** β - blockers are useful in the treatment of mild to moderate hypertension. β - blocker can be used alone or with other antihypertensives (page 149).

2. **Angina pectoris** β - blockers are useful in the prophylaxis of exertional angina. Both the severity and frequency are reduced (page 138). They ↓ both cardiac work and O_2 demand.

3. **Cardiac arrhythmias** β - blockers are useful in the treatment of both ventricular and supraventricular arrhythmias. Sotalol has additional antiarrhythmic effects (page 133).

4. **Myocardial infarction** IV β - blockers in acute MI may limit the size of the infarct. In patients who have recovered from MI, long-term treatment with β - blockers prolongs survival (See page 141).

5. **Congestive cardiac failure** Earlier experience has shown that β - blockers can worsen CCF because of their negative inotropic effect (See page 125). But several recent studies have shown that when judiciously used in selected patients, β blockers can be beneficial in CCF. They reduce the risk of sudden death and prolong survival on long term use. The exact mechanism is not known. Sympathetic system is stimulated in CCF which may infact be deleterious to the heart in many ways and even contribute to cardiac remodelling. Blocking the β receptors may help to improve cardiac function and

prevent cardiac remodelling.

6. **Obstructive cardiomyopathy** β - blockers are found to be beneficial.

7. **Pheochromocytoma** Propranolol is given with α - blockers before surgery to control hypertension.

8. **Thyrotoxicosis** Propranolol controls symptoms like palpitation, tremors and affords symptomatic relief in thyrotoxicosis; it is used as an adjuvant. Propranolol can also be used in thyrotoxic crisis or thyroid storm as it quickly affords symptomatic relief. It also impairs conversion of T_4 to T_3. (See chapter 63)

9. **Glaucoma** Timolol is used topically in open angle glaucoma and narrow angle glaucoma. It is the first line treatment in glaucoma. Newer β - blockers are now developed.

10. **Prophylaxis of migraine** Propranolol reduces the frequency and severity of migraine headache; used for prophylaxis.

11. **Anxiety** Propranolol prevents the acute panic symptoms seen in public speaking, examination and other such anxiety-provoking situations. Performance in musicians can be improved. Tremors, tachycardia and other symptoms of sympathetic overactivity are alleviated.

ALPHA AND BETA-ADRENERGIC BLOCKERS

Labetalol

Labetalol blocks both α_1 and β (β_1 and β_2) receptors. It is a competitive antagonist. Heart rate, contractility, AV conduction and BP fall. Vasodilation (α_1 and β blockade) and ↓ CO contribute to antihypertensive effect. Blood flow to the limbs increases.

Side effects include postural hypotension, gastrointestinal disturbances and other effects of alpha and β - blockade.

Uses Labetalol is used in hypertensive emergencies and pheochromocytoma.

Carvedilol and **medroxalol** also are alpha and β–antagonists. Carvedilol blocks α_1, β_1 and β_2 receptors. In addition it has antioxidant property. It is used in the treatment of hypertension and CCF.

Contraindications to β blockers

- β blockers prevent an increase in heart rate and cardiac output. These effects may be dangerous in patients with CCF. They should be used cautiously and only in selected patients with CCF.
- β blockers should be avoided in patients with bradycardia.
- β blockers are contraindicated in patients with heart block because they depress AV conduction.
- They are to be avoided in patients with bronchial asthma and COPD. If needed, a cardioselective β blocker may be used with caution in them.
- β blockers should be avoided in diabetics because they mask the initial symptoms of hypoglycaemia as discussed under durg interactions.

DRUGS ACTING ON THE KIDNEY

◆ Diuretics and Antidiuretics

14 Diuretics and Antidiuretics

- Physiology of urine formation
- Classification
- High efficacy diuretics
- Thiazides
- Potassium sparing diuretics
- Carbonic anhydrase inhibitors
- Osmotic Diuretics
- Antidiuretics
  - Vasopressin analogs
  - Miscellaneous
    - Thiazide diuretics
    - Chlorpropamide
    - Carbamazepine

DIURETICS

Kidney, the excretory organ of our body serves the important functions of excretion of waste products, regulation of fluid volume and electrolyte content of the extracellular fluid.

PHYSIOLOGY OF URINE FORMATION

Normally about 180 litres of fluid is filtered everyday, of which 99% gets reabsorbed and about 1.5 litres of urine is formed. For simplification, the nephron can be divided into four sites (Fig. 14.1).

Proximal tubule

Sodium bicarbonate, sodium chloride, amino acids and glucose are reabsorbed in the proximal tubule along with water by specific transport mechanisms. Osmotic diuretics act here.

Henle's loop

In the thin descending limb of the loop of Henle, water is reabsorbed by osmotic forces. Hence osmotic diuretics are acting here too. The thick ascending limb actively reabsorbs sodium chloride from the lumen (but is impermeable to water) by $Na^+/K^+/2Cl^-$ co-transporter. 'Loop diuretics' selectively block this transporter.

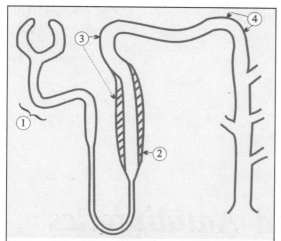

Fig. 14.1: Simplified diagram of a nephron showing sites of action of diuretics (1) Proximal tubule - osmotic diuretics, mannitol, (2) Ascending limb of Henle's loop - loop diuretics, (3) Early distal tubule - thiazides, (4) Distal tubule and collecting duct - K^+ sparing diuretics

Distal convoluted tubule

In the early distal tubule, sodium chloride is reabsorbed by an electrically neutral Na^+ and Cl^- transporter. This transporter is blocked by thiazide diuretics.

Collecting tubule

In the late distal tubule and collecting duct, $NaCl^-$ is actively reabsorbed, in exchange for K^+ and H^+ to maintain the ionic balance regulated by aldosterone. Absorption of water is under the control of antidiuretic hormone (ADH).

Diuretic is an agent which increases urine and solute excretion. Diuretics may be classified as follows-

CLASSIFICATION

1. **High efficacy diuretics**

   Furosemide, bumetanide, piretanide, ethacrynic acid, torsemide, azosemide

2. **Moderate efficacy diuretics**

   - *Thiazides*

     Benzothiadiazines - Chlorothiazide, hydrochlorothiazide, polythiazide, bendroflumethiazide

   - *Thiazide related agents*

     Chlorthalidone, clopamide, indapamide, metolazone, xipamide

3. **Low efficacy diuretics**

   - *Potassium sparing diuretics*

     Triamterene, amiloride, spironolactone

   - *Carbonic anhydrase inhibitors*

     Acetazolamide, methazolamide, dorzolamide

   - *Osmotic diuretics*

     Mannitol, urea, glycerol

   - *Methylxanthines*

     Theophylline

HIGH EFFICACY, HIGH CEILING OR LOOP DIURETICS

Frusemide (Furosemide)

Frusemide is a sulfonamide derivative. It is the most popular loop diuretic. Frusemide is a powerful diuretic.

Mechanism of action

Frusemide acts by inhibiting $NaCl^-$ reabsorption in the thick ascending limb of the Henle's loop (Fig 14.2). It blocks the Na^+, K^+, $2Cl^-$ symporter in the thick ascending limb of the Henle's loop because of which it is called is a loop diuretic. It greatly increases the excretion of Na^+ and Cl^- in the urine. As a large amount of $NaCl^-$ is absorbed in this segment, loop diuretics are highly efficacious. Diuretic response increases with dose and over-enthusiastic treatment can cause

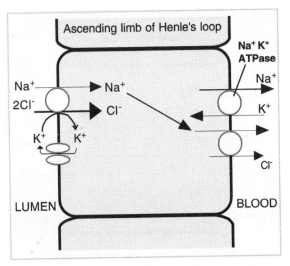

Ascending limb of Henle's loop

Na⁺ K⁺ ATPase

Na^+
$2Cl^-$
Na^+
Cl^-
K^+
K^+
Na^+
K^+
Cl^-

LUMEN   BLOOD

Fig 14.2: Mechanism of action of loop diuretics

and duration of action is 4 to 6 hours. Loop diuretics reach the ascending limb of Henle's loop as they are secreted by the organic acid transport system.

Bumetanide is a sulfonamide like frusemide but is 40 times more potent. Bioavailability is 80% and is better tolerated.

Ethacrynic acid is more likely to cause adverse effects and hence is not commonly used.

Torsemide Is a recently introduced loop diuretic. It is longer acting and therefore can be given once a day.

Adverse Effects of Loop Diuretics

1. *Hypokalaemia and metabolic alkalosis* (due to loss of H⁺) is dose dependent and can be corrected by K⁺ replacement and correction of hypovolaemia.

2. *Hyponatraemia, dehydration hypovolaemia* and *hypotension* should be treated with saline infusion.

3. *Hyperuricaemia* may precipitate acute attacks of gout.

4. *Hypocalcaemia and hypomagnesaemia* - After prolonged use this may result in osteoporosis.

5. *Ototoxicity* Loop diuretics cause hearing loss by a toxic effect on the hair cells in the internal ear. Associated tinnitus and vertigo may also occur. Ototoxicity is more common with ethacrynic acid. It is dose-related, more common on IV administration and generally reversible. Concurrent use of other ototoxic drugs should be avoided.

6. *Hyperglycaemia and hyperlipidaemia* are mild in therapeutic doses.

7. *GIT disturbances* like nausea, vomiting and diarrhoea are common with ethacrynic acid.

dehydration (high ceiling of effect).

Other actions

Loop diuretics also enhance the excretion of K⁺, Ca⁺⁺ and Mg⁺⁺ (but Ca⁺⁺ is reabsorbed in the distal tubule - hence no hypocalcaemia). They increase reabsorption of uric acid in the proximal tubule. On long term use, they also alter renal haemodynamics to reduce fluid and electrolyte reabsorption in the proximal tubule. Frusemide is also a weak carbonic enhydrase inhibitor hence it increases the excretion of HCO_3^- and phosphate. Loop diuretics enhance renin release.

Given intravenously frusemide acts in 2-5 minutes, while following oral use, it takes 20-40 minutes; duration of action is 3-6 hours.

Intravenous frusemide causes venodialation and reduces left ventricular filling pressure. It thus relieves pulmonary congestion in congesti. heart failure and in pulmonary edema even before the onset of diuresis.

Pharmacokinetics

Fúrosemide is rapidly absorbed orally, highly bound to plasma proteins, metabolised in the liver and excreted by kidneys. Plasma t½ is 1½ hours

8. *Allergic reactions* like skin rashes are more common with sulfonamide derivatives.

Uses

1. *Oedema* Loop diuretics are highly effective for the relief of oedema of all origins like cardiac, hepatic or renal oedema. In chronic congestive cardiac failure loop diuretics reduce venous and pulmonary congestion.

2. *Acute pulmonary oedema* is quickly relieved by IV frusemide due to its immediate vasodilator effect and then by diuretic action.

3. *Cerebral oedema* - frusemide is used as an alternative to osmotic diuretics.

4. *Forced diuresis* In poisoning due to drugs like barbiturates and salicylates, frusemide is used with IV fluids.

5. *Hypertension* with renal impairment may be treated with loop diuretics.

6. *Hypercalcaemia and hyperkalaemia* Loop diuretics enhance excretion of Ca^{++} and K^+. But Na^+ and Cl^- should be replaced to avoid hyponatraemia and hypo chloraemia.

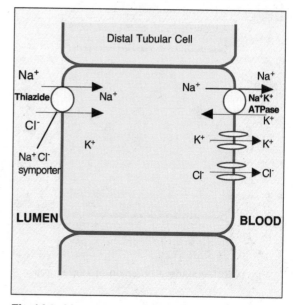

Fig 14.3: Mechanism of action of thiazide diuretics

and hyperuricaemia.

Pharmacokinetics

Thiazides are well-absorbed orally and are rapid acting- acts within 60 minutes. Duration varies from 6-48 hr (Table 14.1). They are excreted by the kidney.

Adverse Effects

Hypokalaemia, metabolic alkalosis, hyper uricaemia, hypovolaemia, hypotension, dehy dration, hyponatraemia, hypomagnesemia, hypochloremia hypercalcaemia, and hyper lipidaemia are similar to that seen with loop diuretics. Hyperglycaemia induced by thiazides may precipitate diabetes mellitus probably by inhibition of insulin secretion. The exact mechanism is not known but correction of hypokalemia also reduces hyperglycaemia. It is more common when long-acting thiazides are used for a long time. Thiazides can cause impotence in male. Weakness, fatigue, anorexia, gastrointestinal disturbances and allergic reactions like rashes and photosensitivity can be seen.

THIAZIDES AND THIAZIDE-LIKE DIURETICS

Chlorothiazide was the first thiazide to be synthesized. All thiazides have a sulfonamide group.

Actions and mechanism of action

Thiazides have a moderate efficacy because 90% of the filtered sodium is already reabsorbed before reaching the distal tubule. This group of drugs block Na^+/Cl^- co-transport system (Fig 14.3).in the early distal tubule (Fig 14.1). They also inhibit carbonic anhydrase activity and increase bicarbonate loss. Thiazides also enhance excretion of Mg^+ and K^+ (in distal segments, Na^+ in the lumen is exchanged for K^+ which is then excreted). But they inhibit urinary excretion of Ca^{++} and uric acid resulting in hypercalcaemia

Uses

1. *Hypertension* Thiazides are the first line drugs (see page 143).

2. *Congestive heart failure* Thiazides are useful in the management of oedema due to mild to moderate CHF.

3. *Oedema* Thiazides may be tried in hepatic (cirrhosis) or renal oedema. Renal oedema may be due to nephrotic syndrome, acute glomerulonephritis or chronic renal failure. Metolazone may be combined with loop diuretics in severe refractory oedema.

4. *Renal stones* Hypercalciuria with renal stones can be treated with thiazides which reduce calcium excretion.

5. *Diabetes insipidus* Thiazides reduce plasma volume and GFR - a paradoxical effect - and benefit such patients.

Indapamide

Indapamide is particularly suitable in hypertension because it is claimed to lower blood pressure in subdiuretic doses and in such doses adverse effects are milder. It is well absorbed orally and has a long duration of action to permit once a day dosing.

POTASSIUM SPARING DIURETICS

Aldosterone enhances the Na+ reabsorption through Na^+ channels in the collecting tubule and enhances K^+ secretion. Aldosterone enters the cells of the collecting duct and binds to the mineralocorticoids receptor in the cell. The agonist - receptor complex moves to the nucleus and directs the synthesis of aldosterone induced protiens (AIP) which are responsible for the actions of aldosterone.

Spironolactone is a synthetic steroid which is structurally similar to aldosterone. It is an aldosterone antagonist. Spironolactone binds mineralocorticoid receptors on the distal tubule

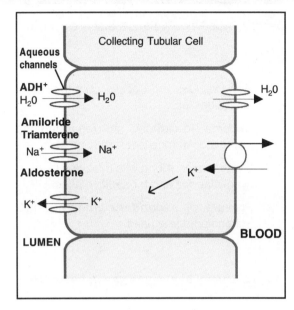

Fig 14.4: Mechanism of action of potassium sparing diuretics. Spironolactone antagonises the action of aldosterone while amiloride and triamnctere directly inhibit the Na^+ channels. (ADH promotes reabsorption of water through aqueous channels - it also increases the number of these channels).

and collecting duct and competitively inhibits the action of aldosterone. Spironolactone is an aldosterone antagonist. As major amount of Na^+ is already reabsorbed in the proximal parts, spironolactone has low efficacy. Spironolactone also reduces K^+ loss due to other diuretics.

It enhances the excretion of calcium by a direct action on the renal tubules.

Adverse effects include gynaecomastia, drowsiness, hyperkalaemia especially in presence of renal insufficiency; metabolic acidosis and skin rashes.

Amiloride and triamterene are directly acting agents which enhance Na^+ excretion and reduce K^+ loss by acting on ion channels in the distal tubule and collecting duct. They block the Na^+ transport through ion-channels in the luminal membrane. Since K^+ secretion is dependent on Na^+ entry, these drugs reduce K^+ excretion.

Adverse effects are gastrointestinal disturbances, hyperkalaemia and metabolic acidosis.

Uses

1. *With thiazides and loop diuretics* to prevent potassium loss.

2. *Oedema* In cirrhosis and renal oedema where aldosterone levels may be high.

3. *Hypertension* Along with thiazides to avoid hypokalaemia and for additive effect.

4. *Primary or secondary aldosteronism* Spironolactone is used.

CARBONIC ANHYDRASE INHIBITORS

Carbonic anhydrase is an enzyme that catalyses the formation of carbonic acid which spontaneously ionises to H^+ and HCO_3^-. This HCO_3^- combines with Na^+ and is reabsorbed.

$$H_2O + CO_2 \rightleftharpoons H_2CO_3$$

$$H_2CO_3 \rightleftharpoons H^+ + HCO_3^-$$

Carbonic anhydrase inhibitors block sodium bicarbonate reabsorption and cause HCO_3^- diuresis. Carbonic anhydrase is present in the nephron, eyes, gastric mucosa, pancreas and other sites.

Acetazolamide, a sulfonamide derivative is a carbonic anhydrase inhibitor and enhances excretion of sodium, potassium, bicarbonate and water. The loss of bicarbonate leads to metabolic acidosis.

Other Actions

1. *Eye* The ciliary body of the eye secretes bicarbonate into the aqueous humour. Carbonic anhydrase inhibition results in decreased formation of aqueous humour and thereby reduces intraocular pressure.

2. *Brain* Bicarbonate is secreted into CSF and carbonic anhydrase inhibition reduces the formation of CSF.

Adverse Effects

1. Metabolic acidosis due to HCO_3^- loss.

2. Renal stones - Ca^{++} is lost with HCO_3^- resulting in hypercalciuria. This excess Ca^{++} may precipitate resulting in the formation of renal stones.

3. Hypokalaemia, drowsiness and allergic reactions can occur.

Uses

1. Glaucoma - (see page 71) IOP is decreased by acetazolamide; it is given orally. Newer ones - **methazolamide** and **dorzolamide** are better tolerated and are available as eye drops.

2. Alkalinization of urine - as required in overdosage of acidic drugs. Also, uric acid and cysteine excretion can be enhanced as these are soluble in alkaline urine.

3. Metabolic alkalosis - acetazolamide enhances HCO_3^- excretion.

4. Mountain sickness - In mountain climbers who rapidly ascend great heights, severe pulmonary oedema or cerebral oedema may occur. Acetazolamide may relieve symptoms by reducing the formation and pH of CSF - it can also be used for prophylaxis.

5. Epilepsy - acetazolamide is used as an adjuvant as it increases the seizure threshold.

OSMOTIC DIURETICS

Mannitol is a pharmacologically inert substance. When given IV (orally not absorbed), mannitol gets filtered by the glomerulus but is not reabsorbed. It causes water to be retained in the proximal tubule and descending limb of Henle's loop by osmotic effect resulting in water diuresis. There is also some loss of Na^+.

Adverse effects are dehydration, ECF volume expansion, headache and allergic reactions.

Uses

1. To maintain urine volume and prevent oliguria in conditions like massive haemolysis and shock.

2. To reduce intracranial and intraocular pressure - following head injury and glaucoma respectively.

Glycerol is effective orally - reduces intraocular and intracranial pressure.

Methylxanthines like theophylline have mild diuretic effect.

Drug Interactions with Diuretics

1. Frusemide and ethacrynic acid are highly protein bound and may compete with drugs like warfarin and clofibrate for protein binding sites.

2. Other ototoxic drugs like aminoglycosides should not be used with loop diuretics to avoid enhanced toxicity.

3. Hypokalaemia induced by diuretics enhance digitalis toxicity.

4. NSAIDs blunt the effect of diuretics as they cause salt and water retention to avoid enhanced toxicity.

5. Diuretics enhance lithium toxicity by reducing renal excretion of lithium.

6. Other drugs that cause hyperkalaemia (ACE inhibitors) and oral K^+ supplements should be avoided with K^+ sparing diuretics because, given together they can cause severe hyperkalaemia.

ANTIDIURETICS

Antidiuretics are drugs that reduce urine volume. These include

1. Antidiuretic hormone (Vasopressin)
2. Thiazide diuretics
3. Miscellaneous
   - Chlorpropamide
   - Carbamazepine.

TABLE 14.1: Dose and duration of action of commonly used diuretics

Diuretic	Daily dose (mg)	Duration (hrs)	Brand name
Furosemide	20-80 mg	3-6	LASIX
Bumetanide	0.5-2 mg	3-6	BUMET
Hydrochlorothiazide	25-100	8-12	ESIDREX
Polythiazide	1-3	24-48	NEPHRIL
Chlorthalidone	50-100	48-72	HYTHALTON
Xipamide	20-60	24-36	XIPAMID
Metolazone	5-10	18-24	ZAROXYLIN
Spironolactone	50-100	6-12	ALDACTONE
Triamterene	50-100	4-6	DYTIDE (with benzthiazide)
Amiloride	5-10	20-24	LASIRIDE (with frusemide)

Antidiuretic hormone (ADH)

Antidiuretic hormone is secreted by the anterior pituitary along with oxytocin. It is synthesized in the supraoptic and paraventricular nuclei of the hypothalamus, transported along the hypothalamo-hypophyseal tract to the posterior pituitary and is stored there.

ADH is released in response to two stimuli - dehydration and rise in plasma osmolarity.

Vasopressin receptors

ADH acts on V_1 and V_2 receptors. V_1 receptors are present in vascular and other smooth muscles, kidneys and anterior pituitary; V_2 receptors in collecting duct in the kidneys. (See fig 14.4).

Actions

ADH enhances water reabsorption by acting on the collecting duct. ADH activates the V_2 receptors present on the cell membrane of the collecting duct and increases the water permeability of these cells. ADH causes vasoconstriction and raises BP mediated by V_1 receptors. It also acts on other smooth muscles to increase peristalsis in the gut and contracts the uterus.

Vasopressin is given parenterally as injection - SC/IM/IV.

Adverse Effects

When used intranasally ADH can cause nasal irritation, allergy, rhinitis and atrophy of nasal mucosa. Other effects include nausea, abdominal cramps and backache (due to contractions of the uterus).

Uses

1. Diabetes insipidus of pituitary origin - Desmopressin is the preparation used. It should be used life long.

2. Bleeding oesophageal varices - ADH constricts mesenteric blood vessels (V_1 receptors) and may help. Analogs like desmopressin, terlipressin and lypressin can be used.

3. Before abdominal radiography - expels gases from the bowel.

4. Haemophilia and Von Willebrand's disease - ADH may release factor VIII and prevent bleeding.

Vasopressin analogs

Desmopressin is selective for V_2 receptors and is longer acting. It is given as nasal spray. *Terlipressin* is longer acting while felypressin is short acting. *Felypressin* is used with local anaesthetics to prolong the duration of action because of its vasoconstrictor properties. *Lypressin* is another analog used in place of ADH.

Miscellaneous

Thiazides Paradoxically thiazides reduce urine volume in diabetes insipidus of both pituitary and renal origin by an unknown mechanism.

Chlorpropamide an oral hypoglycaemic, sensitizes the kidney to ADH action.

Carbamazepine an antiepileptic, stimulates ADH secretion.

15   *Cardiac Glycosides and Treatment of Cardiac Failure*

- **Cardiac action potential**
- **Congestive cardiac failure**
- **Cardiac Glycosides**
    - Pharmacological actions
    - Mechanism of action
    - Pharmacokinetics
    - Adverse Effects
- **Other Positive - inotropic Drugs**
- **Drugs used in Congestive cardiac failure**
    - Diuretics
    - Vasodilators
    - Angiotensin converting enzyme inhibitors
    - Sodium nitroprusside
    - Prazosin
    - Calcium channel blockers
    - Positive inotropic agents
- **Digitalis**
- **β adrenergic agonists**
- **PDE inhibitors**

The cardiac muscle is a specialised tissue with unique properties like excitability, contractility and automaticity. The myocardium has two types of cells - the contracting cells and the conducting cells. The contracting cells participate in the pumping action of the heart. Parts of the conducting tissue have the characteristic property of automaticity. **Automaticity** is the ability of the cell to generate electrical impulses spontaneously. SA node, AV node and His-Purkinje system comprise the conducting tissue of the heart. Normally the SA node acts as the pace maker. **Excitability** is the ability of the cell to undergo depolarization in response to a stimulus. **Contractility** is the ability of the myocardium to adequately contract and pump the blood out of the heart.

Cardiac action potential

When a stimulus reaches the cardiac cell, specific ions move into and out of the cell eliciting an action potential. Such movement of ions across

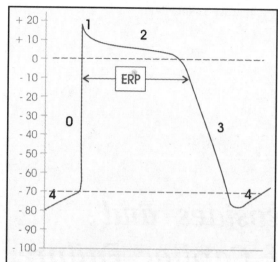

Fig. 15.1 Cardiac action potential phases 0-4: Phase 0 - indicates rapid depolarisation, Phases 1-3 - indicate repolarisation, Phase 4 - gradual depolarisation during diastole

the cardiac cell may be divided into phases (Fig. 15.1).

Phase 0 is rapid depolarisation of the cell membrane during which there is fast entry of sodium ions into the cell through the sodium channels. This is followed by repolarisation.

Phase 1 is a short, initial, rapid repolarisation due to efflux of potassium ions.

Phase 2 is a prolonged plateau phase due to slow entry of calcium ions into the cell through the calcium channels. Cardiac cell differs from other cells in having this phase of action potential.

Phase 3 is a second period of rapid repolarisation with potassium ions moving out of the cell.

Phase 4 is the resting phase during which potassium ions return into the cell while sodium and calcium ions move out of it and the resting membrane potential is restored.

During phases 1 and 2, the cell does not depolarise in response to another impulse, i.e. it is in absolute refractory period. But during phases 3 and 4, the cell is in relative refractory period

and may depolarise in response to a powerful impulse.

The cardiac output is determined by heart rate and stroke volume. The stroke volume in turn depends on the preload, afterload and contractility. **Preload** is the load on the heart due to the volume of blood reaching the left ventricle. It depends on the venous return. **Afterload** is the resistance to the left ventricular ejection, i.e. the total peripheral resistance.

Congestive cardiac failure (CCF)

CCF is one of the common causes of morbidity and mortality. In congestive cardiac failure, the heart is unable to provide adequate blood supply to meet the body's oxygen demand. The pumping ability of the heart is reduced and the cardiac output decreases. The ventricles are not completely emptied resulting in increased venous pressure in the pulmonary and systemic circulation. This causes pulmonary oedema, dyspnoea, liver enlargement and peripheral oedema. As a compensatory mechanism, there is stimulation of the sympathetic system, renin angiotensin system and release of atrial natriuretic peptides which help in maintaining the cardiac output. Atria, ventricles and vascular endothelium store natriuritic peptides and release them in volume overload. These peptides increase renal excretion of salt and water and dilate vascular smooth muscles. The myocardium also undergoes structural alterations like ventricular hypertrophy and remodelling to adapt itself to the stressful situation. These compensatory changes maintain the cardiac output for sometime.

Low output failure could result from ischaemic heart disease, hypertension, valvular and congenital heart diseases. High output failure results from anaemia, thyrotoxicosis, beriberi and certain congenital heart diseases.

The drugs used in CCF include **diuretics, vasodilators** and **cardiac glycosides**. The pharmacology of cardiac glycosides has been discussed first, followed by the role of other drugs in CCF.

CARDIAC GLYCOSIDES

Cardiac glycosides are obtained from the plants of the foxglove family. Though these plants were known to Egyptians 3000 years ago, they were irrationally used. William Withering, an English physician first described the clinical effects of digitalis in CCF in 1785.

Source

Digitoxin is obtained from the leaves of *Digitalis purpurea*. From the leaves of *Digitalis lanata*, digitoxin and digoxin are derived and the seeds of *Strophanthus gratus* contain ouabain. They are all called cardiac glycosides but digoxin is the most commonly used of them because of its favourable pharmacokinetic properties. The word digitalis is used to mean cardiac glycosides.

Chemistry

The glycosides consist of an aglycon attached to sugars. The aglycon has pharmacodynamic activity while sugars influence pharmacokinetic properties.

Pharmacological Actions

1.Cardiac actions

- Digoxin is a cardiotonic drug.
- Positive inotropic effect

Cardiac glycosides increase the force of contraction of the heart - the stroke volume increases and thereby the cardiac output. The systole is shortened and the diastole is prolonged which allows more rest to the heart. The ventricles are more completely emptied because of more forceful contractions.

The *heart rate* is reduced due to -

- Increased vagal tone
- Decreased sympathetic overactivity due to

improved circulation

- By a direct action on SA and AV nodes.

The effects on *electrophysiological properties* of the heart varies with dose and in different parts of the heart. Digitalis shortens ventricular refractory period, depresses AV conduction and enhances automaticity of the ventricles and the Purkinje cells. Digitalis also produces the characteristic ECG changes like T wave inversion, changes in P wave, increased PR interval, (in AV node) shortened QT interval and ST segment depression.

Blood pressure

No significant effects on BP in CCF patients. Pulse pressure may increase.

Coronary circulation

Coronary circulation improves due to increased cardiac output and prolonged diastole during which the coronaries get filled better.

2. Extracardiac actions

- Kidney - Diuresis occurs which relieves oedema in CCF patients.
- CNS - High doses stimulate CTZ resulting in nausea and vomiting.

Mechanism of action

Cardiac glycosides inhibit the enzyme Na^+/K^+ ATPase - also called *'sodium pump'* present on the cardiac myocytes (Fig 15.2). This results in an increase in intracellular Na^+ and Ca^{++}. Thus more calcium is available for contraction, resulting in increased force and velocity of contraction.

Inhibition of the 'sodium pump' increases intracellular sodium. This prevents Ca^{++} extrusion and also drives more calcium into the cell during depolarisation through voltage-sensitive calcium channels. Excess calcium is stored in the sarcoplasmic reticulum and thus increases the amount of calcium released during each action potential.

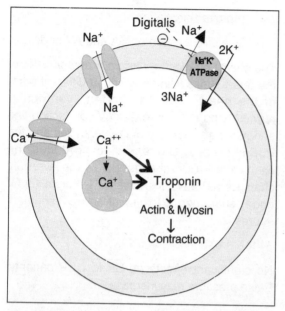

Fig. 15.2 Mechanism of action of cardiac glycosides. Cardiac glycosides inhibit the Na⁺ K⁺ ATPase pump and -intracellular Na⁺ which in turn prevents Ca⁺⁺ extrusion. Thus more calcium is available for contraction.

Pharmacokinetics

Digoxin is well-absorbed (Table 15.1). Presence of food in the stomach delays absorption. Bioavailability varies with different manufacturers and because the safety margin is low, in any given patient, the preparations from the same manufacturer should be used. Glycosides are cumulative drugs.

Digitalization

Response to digitalis develops over 5-7 days with the maintenance dose as given in mild to moderate cases of CCF. But when rapid response is required, rapid digitalization can be done by more frequent dosing with constant monitoring.

Adverse effects

Cardiac glycosides have a low safety margin and adverse effects are common. They inhibit Na⁺/K⁺ - ATPase in all excitable tissues - including neurons and smooth muscle cells where spontaneous activity is increased and this activity is responsible for toxicity. It can be cardiac and extracardiac.

Extracardiac

- GI toxicity - anorexia, nausea, vomiting and diarrhoea are the first symptoms to appear. Cardiac glycosides directly stimulate the CTZ which is responsible for nausea and vomiting.

- Neurotoxicity - digitalis can cause vertigo, blurred vision, disturbances of colour vision, headache, confusion, neuralgia, disorientation, delirium, hallucinations and

Properties	Digoxin	Digitoxin
Absorption	40-60%	90-100%
Plasma protein binding	25%	95%
Onset of action	15-30 min	30-120 min
t½	24-48 hr	5-7 days
Route of elimination	Renal excretion	Hepatic metabolism
Time for digitalization (without loading dose)	5-7 days	25-30 days
Daily dose (slow loading or maintenance)	0.125-0.5 mg	0.05-0.2 mg
Rapid digitalising dose	0.5-0.75 mg every 8 hours 3 doses	0.2-0.4 mg every 12 hours 3 doses

TABLE 15.1: Pharmacokinetic properties of digoxin and digitoxin

rarely convulsions.

- Others - cardiac glycosides can also cause allergic skin rashes and long term use can cause gynaecomastia. The cause for gynaecomastia is not exactly known.

Cardiac toxicity

Arrhythmias of any type including extrasystoles, bradycardia, pulses bigeminy and AV block can be caused by cardiac glycosides (ventricular tachycardia or fibrillation) and paroxysmal atrial tachycardia can also occur but rare.

Several factors influence digitalis induced cardiotoxicity like -

- Hypokalemia enhances digoxin toxicity. Un fortunately plasma K^+ is not an indicator of myocardial K^+ status. Vomiting, diarrhoea and diuretic therapy may all result in hypokalemia and potentiate digoxin toxicity.

- Hypercalcaemia can enhance cardiac toxicity due to digitalis.

- Rapid digitalization and IV administration of cardiac glycosides are likely to precipitate toxicity.

- Patients with poor cardiac status especially elderly are more prone to digoxin toxicity than young adults with normal heart.

Treatment of toxicity

- Stop digitalis

- Oral or parenteral K^+ supplements are given (but K^+ is contraindicated in presence of hyperkalemia or AV block) depending on the severity. Mild cases respond to oral potassium chloride (5g daily in divided doses). When parentral K^+ is required, it should be given slowly as a drip with constant ECG monitoring.

- Ventricular arrhythmias are treated with IV phenytoin

- Bradycardia is treated with atropine and

TABLE 15.2: Drug interactions

Drugs that enhance digoxin toxicity
- Diuretics (due to hypokalaemia), calcium
- Quinidine, verapamil, methyldopa - ↑digoxin levels

Drugs that reduce digoxin levels
- Antacids, neomycin, metoclopramide - ↓ absorption
- Rifampicin, phenobarbitone - hasten metabolism due to enzyme induction

---

supraventricular arrhythmias with propranolol

- Antidigoxin immunotherapy (Digibind) is now available. Antidigoxin antibodies bind cardiac glycosides and reverse their effects. These antibodies are life saving in severe toxicity due to cardiac glycosides.

Uses

1. Congestive cardiac failure (see below)

2. Cardiac arrhythmias

   - Atrial fibrillation and atrial flutter - digoxin reduces the ventricular rate

   - Paroxysmal supraventricular tachycardia (PSVT) - digoxin is an alternative to verapamil.

Precautions and contraindications to digitalis therapy

- Hypokalaemia - enhances toxicity

- MI, thyrotoxicosis patients - more prone to arrhythmias

- Acid base imbalance - prone to toxicity

OTHER POSITIVE INOTROPIC DRUGS

Phosphodiesterase inhibitors

Amrinone (inamrinone) and milrinone inhibit the enzyme phosphodiesterase (which degrades cAMP) resulting in an increased cAMP levels. They increase the force of contraction and also cause vasodilatation. But because of the adverse effects and increased mortality seen with the use of these drugs, they are generally not preferred. However, they may be used for short periods in severe heart failure. Milrinone has shorter t½ and fewer side effects.

DRUGS USED IN CONGESTIVE CARDIAC FAILURE

In congestive cardiac failure, the heart is unable to provide adequate blood supply to meet the demand. The aim of treatment is to reduce morbidity and mortality by restoring cardiac output and relieving congestion.

The drugs used in CCF include

1. Diuretics

2. Vasodilators

3. Positive inotropic agents -

   - Digitalis
   - β adrenergic agonists
   - Phosphodiesterase (PDE) inhibitors
   - Others

1. Diuretics: High ceiling diuretics like frusemide are used. They increase salt and water excretion and reduce blood volume. By this they *reduce preload* and venous pressure, improve cardiac performance and relieve oedema.

2. Vasodilators: Vasodilators reduce the mortality in patients with cardiac failure. Vasodilators may be arteriolar or venular dilators or both.

- Arteriolar dilators (↓after load) - hydralazine - relax arterial smooth muscles, thus reducing peripheral vascular resistance (↓ afterload). As a result, the work load on the heart is reduced.

- Venodilators (↓ preload) - nitrates - reduce the venous return to the heart (↓ preload) thus reducing the stretching of the ventricular walls and myocardial

oxygen requirements.

Organic Nitrates

Nitroglycerine and isosorbide dinitrate are good vasodilators with a rapid and short action. They can be used for short periods to decrease the ventricular filling pressure in acute heart failure. Nitroglycerine can be used IV in acute CCF. Nitrates may be given in combination with hydralazine.

- Both arteriolar and venular dilators - ACE inhibitors, sodium nitroprusside, prazosin, calcium channel blockers - these reduce both preload and afterload.

Angiotensin converting enzyme inhibitors (ACE-I)

ACE inhibitors (See page 144) like captopril, enalapril, lisinopril and ramipril act by -

- Reduction of afterload Angiotensin II is a powerful vasoconstrictor present in the plasma in high concentrations in cardiac failure. ACE - I prevent the conversion of angiotensin I to angiotensin II and thereby reduce the after load.

- Reduction of preload Aldosterone causes salt and water retention and increases plasma volume. ACE-I prevent the formation of aldosterone (by reducing Ang-II) and thereby reduce the preload. They also prevent bradykinin degradation and increase bradykinin levels which also causes vasodilatation.

- Reversing compensatory changes Angiotensin II formed locally in the myocardium is responsible for various undesirable compensatory changes like ventricular hypertrophy and ventricular remodelling seen in CCF. ACE-I reverse these changes.

ACE inhibitors are the most preferred drugs in chronic congestive cardiac failure.

Sodium nitroprusside

Sodium nitroprusside is a powerful vasodilator. Since it dilates both arterioles and venules, it reduces both ventricular filling pressure and peripheral arterial resistance. It is given IV, has a rapid (30-60sec) and short action (3 minutes). Hence it is useful in acute severe heart failure.

Prazosin

Prazosin an α_1 antagonist, is a vasodilator. It can be used in acute heart failure for longer periods than nitrates.

Calcium channel blockers

These are not routinely used. Amlodipine or felodipine may be tried in patients in whom other vasodilators are contraindicated.

3.Positive inotropic agents

Digitalis: Mild to moderate cases of low output failure are treated with diuretics and vasodilators (ACE-inhibitors preferred). When the patients do not respond to these, digoxin may be given. Digoxin improves cardiac performance in the dilated, failing heart. If there is associated atrial fibrillation, digoxin is the preferred drug in such patients.

β Adrenergic agonists Dobutamine is a positive inotropic agent. It stimulates the cardiac β_1 receptors and enhances the force of contraction of the cardiac muscle. It increases the cardiac output without significant tachycardia. It also produces some vasodilation by stimulating the β_2 receptors. Dopamine may be used in patients with associated renal impairment because dopamine increases renal perfusion in addition to increased cardiac output.

PDE Inhibitors Amrinone or milrinone may be used for short periods to enhance the cardiac output in severe heart failure.

4.Others

β Adrenergic blockers Though β blockers are negative inotropic agents, several recent studies have shown that when used carefully along with other drugs, β blockers can improve long term survival (See page 105).

16 *Calcium Channel Blockers*

- Mechanism of action
- Actions
- Drug interactions
- Verapamil
- Diltiazem
- Bepridil
- Dihydropyridine CCBs

The discovery of the calcium channels in the cardiac myocyte helped in understanding the mechanisms involved in smooth muscle contraction. Verapamil was the first agent found to have calcium channel blocking properties and many more soon followed.

Calcium channel blockers (CCB)

Dihydropyridines

Nifedipine	Nicardipine
Nimodipine	Nitrendipine
Nisoldipine	Felodipine
Amlodipine	Isradipine

Others

Verapamil	Diltiazem
	Bepridil

Mechanism of Action

The depolarisation of the cardiac and vascular smooth muscle cells depend on the entry of extracellular calcium into the cell through the calcium channels. Intracellular calcium is also increased by receptor - mediated action - *i.e.,* agonist induced calcium release - mediated by the second messenger IP_3. This calcium triggers the release of intracellular calcium from the sarcoplasmic reticulum. All these calcium ions bring about contraction of the cardiac and vascular smooth muscle cells.

Calcium channel antagonists inhibit the entry of calcium by blocking the L-type of calcium channels. (There are 3 types of calcium channels - L, N and T types) This decreases calcium current and calcium entry into cardiac and vascular smooth muscle cells resulting in the following effects.

Actions

1. **Vascular smooth muscle**

   Relaxation of the arteriolar smooth muscles results in reduced peripheral vascular resistance and blood pressure. The effect on venous beds is not significant. Reflex tachycardia may occur with some CCBs like nifedipine. Dihydropyridine CCBs have prominent effects on the blood vessels i.e. they are vascular selective.

2. **Heart**

   CCBs depress myocardial contractility, reduce heart rate and in higher doses they slow AV conduction. They reduce cardiac work and thereby myocardial oxygen consumption. Verapamil, bepridil and diltiazem have prominent cardiac effects.

3. **Coronary circulation**

   CCBs dilate the coronary vessels, increasing the coronary blood flow. Hence they are useful in variant angina.

4. **Other effects**

   - Nimodipine is highly lipid soluble, crosses the BBB and relaxes the cerebral blood vessels.
   - CCBs relax the uterus and may be useful in premature labour.

Pharmacokinetics

CCBs are well-absorbed but undergo extensive first pass metabolism. They are all highly plasma protein bound and are metabolized in the liver. Dose - Table 16.1.

Therapeutic uses

1. **Angina Pectoris**

   CCBs are useful in the the prophylaxis of patients with exertional angina as they decrease myocardial oxygen demand and bring about coronary vasodilatation. CCBs are also useful in variant angina as they bring about coronary vasodilation.

2. **Hypertension**

   Long acting CCBs or sustained release preparations may be used in chronic hypertension. In hypertensive crisis nifedipine is used sublingually or the capsule is bitten and swallowed.

3. **Arrhythmias**

   Verapamil, diltiazem and bepridil have

Table 16.1 Therapeutic doses of some calcium channel blockers		
CCB	*Dose*	*Route*
Nifedipine	5-20 mg	oral 8 hrly
	10 mg	SL or capsule bitten & swallowed
Amlodipine	5-10 mg	orally once daily
Felodipine	5-10 mg	orally once daily
Nicardipine	20-40 mg	orally 8 hourly
Isradipine	2.5-10 mg	orally 12 hourly
Nitrendipine	5-20 mg	orally once daily
Nisoldipine	20-40mg	orally once daily
Nimodipine	30-60 mg	orally 4 hourly
Verapamil	40-120mg	orally 8 hourly
	2.5 - 10mg	slow IV
Diltiazem	30-60 mg	orally 6 hourly
	20 mg	slow IV

Isoptin - what are you doing?

Leela a 40 year old lady was admitted for cardiac arrhythmias. She was prescribed Isoptin (verapamil). The intern reported to the doctor that the patient's heart rate was not coming down and instead had severe tachycardia. When the medication was checked, it was found that the patient was receiving Isoprin (Isoprenaline) and not isoptin. This was the reason for her tachycardia which was however brought to light before any mishap.

antiarrhythmic properties. Verapamil is used in PSVT and to control ventricular rate in atrial flutter or fibrillatrion.

4. **Peripheral vascular disease**

Nifedipine, felodipine and diltiazem can be used in Raynaud's disease for their vasodilator effects.

5. **Other uses**

- *Hypertrophic cardiomyopathy* - verapamil produces beneficial effects

- *Migraine* – Verapamil is useful in the prophylaxis of migraine

- *Subarachnoid haemorrhage* – vasospasm that follows subarachnoid haemorrhage is believed to be responsible for neurological defects. As nimodipine brings about cerebral vasodilatation, it is used to treat neurological deficits in patients with cerebral vasospasm.

- *Atherosclerosis* – There are claims that dihydropyridines slow the progress of atherosclerosis

- *Preterm labour* – Nifedipine inhibits uterine contractions and is found to be useful in delaying labour in premature uterine contractions.

Drug interactions

- Verapamil and diltiazem should be avoided in patients receiving beta-adrenergic blockers because the myocardiac depressant effects get added up.

- Verapamil can precipitate digoxin toxicity by increasing digoxin levels (verapamil reduces digoxin excretion).

Verapamil has prominent myocardiac depressant

actions. AV conduction is depressed and usually bradycardia is seen. Hence it should not be combined with b-blockers. Fall in BP is mild as the vasodilator effect of verapamil is less potent.

Diltiazem has less potent vasodilator effects but is a myocardiac depressant.

Bepridil can cause serious arrhythmias and agranulocytosis – hence not preferred.

Adverse effects

Verapamil and diltiazem produce constipation, bradycardia, heart block, hypotension and skin rashes. They may precipitate CCF in patients with diseased heart. Long term use of CCBs can cause gum hyperplasia.

Dihydropyridine CCBs

Nifedipine is a potent vasodilator and causes a significant fall in BP and evokes reflex tachycardia. Myocardiac depressant effect is weak. It can be given sublingually.

Adverse effects of nifedipine are headache, flushing, palpitation, dizziness, fatigue, hypotension, leg cramps and ankle oedema.

Other dihydropyridines

- Amlodipine, felodipine, nitrendipine and nicardipine are similar to nifedipine with some pharmacokinetic variations. They have higher vascular selectivity.

- Amlodipine, felodipine, nitrendipine and nisoldepine are longer acting and can be given once daily.

- Nimodipine selectively relaxes cerebral vasculature as it crosses the BBB owing to its high lipophilicity.

17 *Antiarrhythmic Drugs*

- **Classification**
- **Sodium Channel Blockers**
  - **- Class IA drugs**
  - **- Class IB drugs**
  - **- Class IC drugs**
- **Class II drugs**
- **Class III drugs**
- **Class IV drugs**
- **Other antiarrhythmics**

Mechanisms of arrhythmogenesis

Abnormal impulse generation
- altered normal automaticity
- abnormal automaticity
- after depolarization $\Big\langle$ early / delayed

Abnormal impulse conduction
- Reentry
- Conduction Block - I, II or III degree

An arrhythmia is an abnormality of the rate, rhythm or site of origin of the cardiac impulse or an abnormality in the impulse conduction. The word dysrhythmia is also used by some. Cardiac arrhythmias may be due to abnormal generation or conduction of impulses. Factors like myocardial hypoxia, myocardial ischaemia, electrolyte disturbances, trauma, drugs and autonomic influences can cause arrhythmias.

Clinical features include palpitation, syncope, fatigue, breathlessness, cardiac failure and in more severe cases - cardiac arrest.

Disturbances of impulse generation may be due to altered normal and abnormal automaticity or after - depolarisations. In disturbances of impulse conduction, an impulse may recirculate in the heart and cause repeated activation (re-entry - Fig.17.2) or there could be conduction blocks. Arrhythmias may be tachyarrhythmias, brady-arrhythmias or digitalis-induced arrhythmias. Based on the site of impulse origin, they may be supraventricular (SA node, AV node,

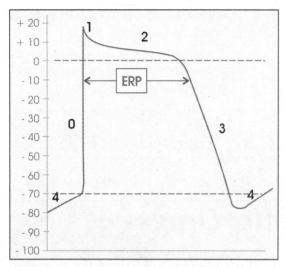

Fig. 17.1 Cardiac action potential: **Phase 0** - rapid depolarisation, **phase 1** - initial rapid repolarisation, **phase 2** - prolonged plateau phase, **phase 3** - second rapid repolarisation, **phase 4** - resting phase

atria) or ventricular arrhythmias (in ventricles). Ventricular arrhythmias are a common cause of death, particularly sudden death.

CLASSIFICATION

Based on the cardiac cycle, Vaughan Williams classified antiarrhythmics as follows:

Class I. Sodium channel blockers

1. Prolong repolarization
   - Quinidine, procainamide, disopyramide, moricizine

2. Shorten repolarization
   - Lignocaine, mexiletine, phenytoin

3. Little effect on repolarization
   - Encainide, flecainide, propafenone

Class II. β-adrenergic blockers
(reduce sympathetic tone)
   - Propranolol, acebutolol, esmolol, etc.

Class III. K⁺ channel blockers
(Prolong repolarization)
   - Amiodarone, bretylium, sotalol, dofetilide, ibutilide

Class IV. Ca⁺⁺ channel blockers
(Prolong conduction and refractoriness specially in SA and AV nodes)
   - Verapamil, diltiazem

SODIUM CHANNEL BLOCKERS

CLASS IA DRUGS

Mechanism of action

All drugs in class I block the sodium channels and prevent the inward movement of Na^+ ions. The sodium channels exist in three states- resting, open and inactivated (refractory) state. Sodium channel blockers preferentially bind Na^+ channels in the open and inactivated state.

Class IA drugs block Na^+ channels and depress phase-0 depolarization. They also prolong repolarization by blocking K^+ channels.

Quinidine

Quinidine is the D-isomer of quinine obtained from the cinchona bark. By blocking Na^+ channels, it depresses all cardiac properties - automaticity, excitability, conduction velocity and prolongs repolarization - quinidine thus has membrane-stabilizing activity, i.e. it inhibits propagation of the action potential.

Quinidine also has vagolytic and α-blocking properties. It is also a skeletal muscle relaxant.

Pharmacokinetics Given orally quinidine is rapidly absorbed, 90% bound to plasma proteins, metabolised in the liver and excreted in the urine.

Adverse effects Quinidine is not well - tolerated due to adverse effects and may need to be stopped.

● *Cardiac*

Quinidine itself can cause arrhythmias and heart block. It can also cause hypotension, prolongation of QT interval and *torsades de pointes*. *Torsades de pointes* refers to polymorphic ventricular tachycardia and is so called because of the pattern of EEG changes - in French, it means twisting of points. All drugs which prolong QT interval can also cause this. Hence treatment should be monitored.

● *Non-cardiac*

Diarrhoea, nausea, vomiting and hypersensitivity reactions including thrombocyto - penia and rarely bone marrow depression, hepatitis and idiosyncratic reactions can occur. Higher doses can cause cinchonism like quinine.

Drug interactions

● Quinidine is a microsomal enzyme inhibitor. It raises the plasma levels of propafenone and reduces the conversion of codeine to morphine thereby decreasing its analgesic efficacy.

● Microsomal enzyme inducers like phenytoin and phenobarbitone enhance metabolism of quinidine resulting in therapeutic failure.

● Quinidine reduces the clearance of digoxin thereby precipitating digoxin toxicity.

Procainamide

Procainamide, a derivative of the local anaesthetic procaine has the advantages over quinidine that it has weak vagolytic properties and is not an a-blocker. It is better tolerated than quinidine. But it can cause nausea, vomiting and hypersensitivity reactions including lupus syndrome. Higher doses can cause hypotension, heart block and *Torsades de pointes*.

Disopyramide

Disopyramide has significant anticholinergic properties which is responsible for adverse effects like dry mouth, blurred vision, constipation and

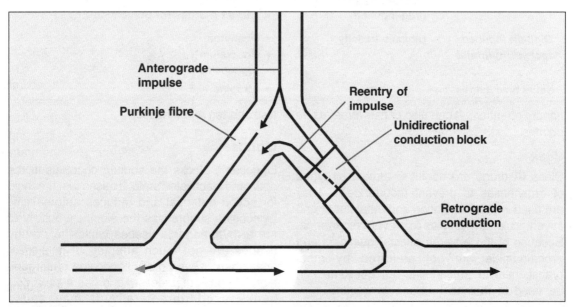

Fig 17.2 Reentry circuit in the ventricle. The impulse from the SA node generally passes to the AV node, purkinje fibres and then to the ventricle. But when there is a conduction block, an impulse may recirculate in the heart and cause reentry arrhythmias.

TABLE 17.1 Choice of drugs in cardiac arrhythmias		
Arrhythmia	*Cause*	*Treatment*
Sinus tachycardia	↑ **sympathetic tone, fever, thyrotoxicosis**	• **Treat the cause** • **If severe →propranolol**
Atrial extrasystoles	**Excess caffeine, nicotine, alcohol**	• **Treat the cause** • **Reassurance** • **If severe→propranolol / disopyramide**
Atrial flutter/fibrillation	**Rheumatic heart disease, cardiomyopathy, hypertension**	• **Cardioversion** • **Propranolol / quinidine/ disopyramide / digitalis**
PSVT		• **Vagal manouvers like carotid massage** • **Verapamil/adenosine** • **β-blockers**
Ventricular ectopics	**Normal heart—benign; also in cardiomyopathy, ischaemia, digitalis induced**	• **β-blockers** • **Lignocaine**
Ventricular tachycardia	**Organic heart disease, ventricular dysfunction, drug-induced**	• **Cardioversion** • **Lignocaine**
Ventricular fibrillation	**Acute MI, organic heart disease, surgical trauma, drug-induced**	• **Cardioversion** • **Lignocaine** • **Class I A drugs for prevention**
Digitalis induced tachyarrhythmias	**Digitalis toxicity**	• **Phenytoin** • **Potassium** • **Lignocaine**
Sinus bradycardia		• **Atropine**

urinary retention. It can also cause *torsades de pointes.*

Uses

Class IA drugs are useful in almost all types of arrhythmias to prevent recurrences. They are used in atrial fibrillation and atrial flutter and in ventricular arrhythmias to prevent recurrence. Because of the adverse effects, quinidine and procainamide are not preferred by most practitioners in arrhythmias but quinidine can be used in malaria in place of quinine.

CLASS IB DRUGS

Class IB drugs block the sodium channels and also shorten repolarization.

Lignocaine

Lignocaine blocks the sodium channels in the open and inactivated state. It raises the threshold for action potential and reduces automaticity. Lignocaine suppresses the electrical activity of the arrhythmogenic tissues while the normal tissues are not much affected. It is a local anaesthetic. Given orally lignocaine undergoes high first pass metabolism and has a short t½ - hence used parenterally. It may cause drowsiness, hypotension, blurred vision, confusion and convulsions. Lignocaine is used in the treatment of ventricular arrhythmias, especially that caused by acute myocardial infarction or open heart surgery and in digitalis induced arrhythmias. Lignocaine is **not** useful in atrial arrhythmias because atrial action potentials are so short that sodium channel is in the inactivated state only for a very short period.

Phenytoin

Phenytoin is an antiepileptic also useful in ventricular arrhythmias (not preferred due to toxicity) and digitalis induced arrhythmias.

Mexiletine

Mexiletine can be used orally; causes dose related neurologic adverse effects including tremors and blurred vision. Nausea is common. It is used as an alternative to lignocaine in ventricular arrhythmias.

CLASS IC DRUGS

Class IC drugs are the most potent sodium channel blockers. Because of the risk of cardiac arrest, sudden death and other adverse effects, they are not commonly used. They may be used in severe ventricular arhythmias and to maintain sinus rhythm in atrial fibrillation.

CLASS II DRUGS

β - blockers

β - blockers like propranolol (Chapter 13) exert antiarrhythmic effect due to blockade of cardiac β receptors. They depress myocardial contractility, automaticity and conduction velocity. In higher doses they also have membrane stabilising activity like class I drugs.

Propranolol and cardioselective β blockers like atenolol and metoprolol are used in the treatment and prevention of supraventricular arrhythmias especially those associated with exercise, emotion or hyperthyroidism.

Esmolol given intravenously is rapid and short-acting and can be used to treat arrhythmias during surgeries, following myocardial infarction and other emergencies.

CLASS III DRUGS

These drugs prolong the action potential duration and refractory period by blocking the potassium channels.

Amiodarone

Amidarone an analog of the thyroid hormone is a powerful antiarrhythmic. It acts by multiple mechanisms.

- Prolongs APD by blocking K^+ channels.
- ERP is prolonged.
- Blocks sodium channels.
- Blocks β adrenergic receptors.

Pharmacokinetics Amiodarone has complex pharmacokinetic properties. Following oral administration bioavailability is variable (35-65%), onset of action is slow - may vary from 2- 3 days to several weeks, duration of action and $t_{1/2}$ may range from weeks to months. It is metabolised in the liver by microsomal enzymes. Hence drugs that induce or inhibit microsomal enzyme can alter plasma levels of amiodarone - resulting in many drug interactions. Amiodarone itself inhibits certain microsomal enzymes thereby increasing plasma levels of drugs like digoxin and warfarin.

Adverse effects

Amiodarone can cause various adverse effects including cardiac and extracardiac effects like heart block, QT prolongation, bradycardia, cardiac failure, hypotension particularly on IV injection; Bluish discolouration of the skin, gastrointestinal disturbances and hepatotoxicity can occur. Amiodarone can interfere with thyroid function. It blocks the peripheral convertion of T_4 to T_3. It can cause hypothyroidism - or hyperthyroidism. Thyroid function should be monitored. It can cause pulmonary fibrosis that can be fatal.

Uses Amiodarone is a toxic drug and requires constant monitoring. Hence it is used only in resistant cases of chronic ventricular arrhythmias and to prevent recurrence of atrial fibrillation and flutter.

Bretylium

Bretylium is an adrenergic neurone blocker used in resistant ventricular arrhythmias.

Sotalol

Sotalol a β-blocker, also prolongs the action potential duration and is classified under class III antiarrhythmic drugs and is often preferred when a β-blocker is needed.

CLASS IV DRUGS

Calcium channel blockers (see page 126) inhibit the inward movement of calcium resulting in reduced contractility, automaticity and AV nodal conduction. Verapamil, diltiazem, and bepridil have prominent cardiac effects, because they block the Ca^{++} channels in the cardiac cells in therapeutic doses.

Verapamil

Verapamil is used to terminate paroxysmal supraventricular tachycardia (PSVT). It is also used to control ventricular rate in atrial flutter or fibrillation because it depresses the AV nodal conduction. Diltiazam can be used in place of verapamil.

Drug Interactions Verapamil displaces digoxin from tissue binding sites and also reduces its renal clearance resulting in digoxin toxicity- dose of digoxin should be reduced.

Dofetilide

Defetilide is a newly introduced and selective K^+ channel blocker. It has no other actions as it is a pure K^+ channel blocker and prolongs APD. It is used orally in atrial fibrillation to convert and to maintain sinus rhythm. The only adverse effect known is *torsades de pointes* in 1% patients.

Ibutilide

Ibutilide is a K^+ channel blocker used as intravenous infusion to quickly convert atrial flutter/fibrillation to sinus rhythm. It can cause *torsades de pointes.*

Other antiarrhythmics

Adenosine, atropine, digoxin, potassium and magnesium sulphate also have antiarrhythmic properties but are not included in Vaughan Williams classification.

Adenosine is a purine nucleotide having rapid and short antiarrhythmic action. Given IV it suppresses automaticity, AV conduction and dilates the coronaries. Adenosine is the drug of choice for acute termination of paroxysmal supraventricular tachycardias (PSVT).

Adverse effects are nausea, dyspnoea, flushing, dizziness and headache but are of short duration. Theophylline blocks adenosine receptors and inhibits the action of adenosine.

Atropine is used in sinus bradycardia. It acts by blocking M_2 muscarinic receptors.

Digitalis Depresses AV conduction, reduces heart rate and increases the force of contraction of the myocardium. Digoxin is used in atrial fibrillation to control the ventricular rate.

Magnesium sulphate is used IV to treat digitalis induced arrhythmias and *torsades de pointes.*

Potassium is a myocardiac depressant. It brings about a decrease in conduction velocity, automaticity and prolongs the refractory period. Higher doses produce defects in AV conduction. (Digitalis toxicity is potentiated by hypokalemia).

18 Drugs used in the treatment of Angina Pectoris and Myocardial infarction

- Angina pectoris
- Antianginal drugs
- Nitrates
- Calcium channel blockers
- β -blockers
- Potassium channel openers
- Miscellaneous
- Pharmacotherapy of Angina
- Combination of drugs in angina
- Unstable angina
- Drugs used in myocardial infarction
    - Immediate treatment
    - Long-term treatment
    - Risk factor management

Angina pectoris

Angina Pectoris is the chief symptom of ischaemic heart disease (IHD) characterised by sudden, severe, substernal discomfort or pain which may radiate to the left shoulder and along the flexor surface of the left arm. Myocardial oxygen consumption is mainly determined by preload (venous return and stretching of the heart), afterload (peripheral arterial resistance) and heart rate. When the oxygen supply to the myocardium is insufficient for its needs, myocardial ischaemia develops. Pain is due to accumulation of metabolites in the cardiac muscle.

Two forms of angina are

1. **Classical angina** (stable angina, angina of effort, exertional angina) Pain is induced by exercise or emotion, both of which increase myocardial oxygen demand (even a heavy meal can precipitate angina). In such patients there is narrowing of the coronary arteries due to atherosclerosis and therefore the coronaries cannot dilate to increase the blood supply during exercise. Hence there is an imbalance between oxygen supply and demand.

2. **Variant or Prinzmetal's angina**

    It occurs at rest and is caused by spasm of the coronary artery. Drugs are used to improve the balance between oxygen supply and demand either by increasing oxygen supply to the myocardium (coronary dilation) or by reducing the oxygen demand (reducing preload/afterload/heart rate or all of these).

ANTIANGINAL DRUGS

1. Nitrates

Nitroglycerin, isosorbide dinitrate, isosorbide mononitrate, pentaerythritol tetranitrate.

2. Calcium channel blockers

Verapamil, diltiazem, amlodipine, nifedipine.

3. β-blockers

Propranolol, atenolol, etc.

4. Potassium channel openers

Nicorandil, Pinacidil.

5. Miscellaneous

Dipyridamole, aspirin, trimetazidine

NITRATES

Nitroglycerin was introduced for the treatment of angina in 1879.

Mechanism of action

Nitrates are vasodilators (Fig 18.1). They are converted to nitric oxide which activates vascular guanylyl cyclase which in turn increases the synthesis of cGMP. This cGMP brings about de phosphorylation of protein kinases (prevents interaction of actin with myosin). It also reduces free cytosolic calcium by preventing Calcium release from sarcoplasmic reticulum or increasing Ca^{++} efflux. These effects result in relaxation of smooth muscles. Thus it causes vasodilation and also relaxation of other smooth muscles.

Pharmacological actions

Nitrates are predominantly venodilators. Venodilation reduces venous return to the heart thereby reducing preload. Arteriolar dilation reduces vascular resistance thus decreasing afterload. As both preload and afterload are reduced, work load of the heart is decreased thereby reducing oxygen requirement of the heart.

Nitrates also bring about some coronary vasodilation. But, the beneficial effect in stable angina is due to its vasodilator properties. However in variant angina, nitrates relieve vasospasm due to coronary vasodilation.

Nitrates also cause dilation of blood vessels

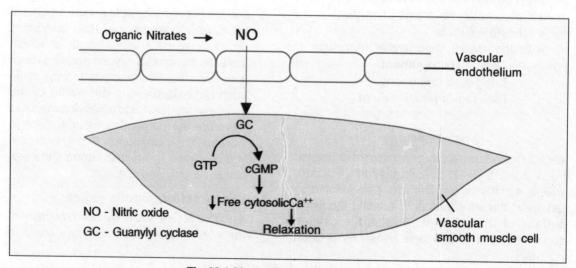

Fig 18.1 Mechanism of action of nitrates

in the skin - resulting in flushing; dilatation of the meningeal vessels result in headache. Bronchial smooth muscles are also relaxed.

Nitrates also inhibit platelet aggregation but the therapeutic benefit from this is yet to be established.

Pharmacokinetics

Nitrates are well absorbed orally but they undergo extensive first pass metabolism. All nitrates have good lipid solubility.

Nitroglycerin, isosorbide dinitrate, isosorbide mononitrate (Table 18.1) and pentaerythritol tetranitrate are the nitrates used in angina. Isosorbide mononitrate is longer acting (needs to be given twice daily) and has 100% bioavailability. Amyl nitrite is used in cyanide poisoning.

Nitrates are available for oral, sublingual, parenteral use and as ointment and transdermal patches for topical use . Topical preparations are used for the prevention of nocturnal episodes of angina. But there is an increased risk of development of tolerance with topical and slow release preparations.

Adverse effects

Headache is common; flushing, sweating, palpitation, weakness, postural hypotension and rashes can occur. Tolerance to vascular effects of nitrates develops on repeated long term use particularly when continuous high plasma nitrate levels are present. By adopting proper dosing schedule, tolerance can be avoided. The patient must be free of nitrates for atleast 8 hours of the day to prevent the development of tolerance. Tolerance can also be minimized by twice/thrice daily dosing schedule.

Drug interactions

Nitrates should not be abruptly withdrawn after long term use because it can precipitate acute angina and spasm of the vascular and other smooth muscles. Thus nitrates are said to cause a sort of dependence.

Nitrates and sildenafil - Sildenafil (Viagra), a drug used in erectile dysfunction - is a phosphodiesterase inhibitor. It thus increases cGMP activity resulting in relaxation of cavernosal as well as vascular smooth muscles. Vasodilation results in hypotension. Sildenafil potentiates the action of nitrates and together can cause severe hypotension. Deaths have been reported due to myocardial infarction.

Uses

1. *Exertional Angina* Sublingual nitroglycerin is the drug of choice for acute anginal attacks and for acute prophylaxis of angina. It relieves pain in 3 minutes. If the pain is not relieved, the dose may be repeated (up to 3 tablets in 15 minutes).

Nitrates are also used orally for the prophylaxis of angina. Longer acting nitrates are preferred for this but patients can develop

TABLE 18.1: Some nitrates used in angina pectoris		
Drug	*Dose and route*	*Duration of action*
Nitroglycerin (GTN) (ANGISED)	0.5 mg SL	15-40 min
	5 mg oral	4-8 hr
	2% Skin ointment applied 1-2 inches on the precardial region	4-6 hr
Isosorbide dinitrate (SORBITRATE)	5-10 mg SL	20-40 min
	10-20 mg oral	2-3 hr
Isosorbide mononitrate (ISMO)	10-20 mg oral	6-8 hr

tolerance to nitrates. Nitroglycerin ointment may be applied over the chest specially to control angina at night. Transdermal patch delivers nitroglycerin constantly for 24 hours.

2. *Vasospastic angina* Nitroglycerin relieves pain by relieving coronary vasospasm.

3. *Unstable angina* Intravenous nitroglycerin helps to relieve pain but the exact reason for the benefit is not understood. Both a reduction in cardiac work load and coronary vasodilation may be of value in such patients.

4. *Cardiac failure* Nitrates are useful due to their vasodilator property (See page 124)

5. *Myocardial infarction* IV nitroglycerin is used by many physicians to reduce cardiac work. The dose should be carefully adjusted to avoid tachycardia.

6. *Cyanide poisoning* Cyanide rapidly binds to cytochrome oxidase and other vital enzymes resulting in inhibition of cellular respiration and blocks the utilization of oxygen. It requires immediate treatment. Amylnitrite is given by inhalation and sodium nitrite by IV injection (10ml of 3% solution). Sodium thiosulphate is given IV (50ml of 25% solution). Nitrates convert haemoglobin to methemoglobin which has a high affinity for cyanide and binds to cyanide forming cyanmethaemoglobin. Sodium thiosulphate reacts with cyanmetheamoglobin to form thiocyanate which is easily excreted by the kidneys. It thus protects the important enzymes from binding to cyanide. Early treatment is very important.

CALCIUM CHANNEL BLOCKERS

CCBs (Chapter - 16) relax the arterioles leading to a decrease in the peripheral vascular resistance and a reduction in the afterload. Some reflex tachycardia can occur particularly with dihydropyridines. But CCBs, particularly

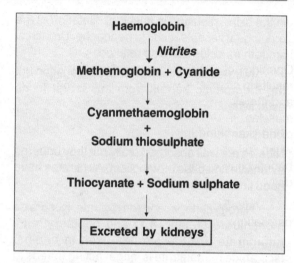

verapamil and diltiazem also depress the myocardial contractility thereby reducing the heart rate and force of contraction. This results in reduced cardiac work load and oxygen consumption. CCBs also dilate the coronaries thereby increasing the coronary blood flow.

CCBs are used for the prophylaxis of exertional angina. They can be combined (except verapamil) with beta blockers like propranolol. CCBs are also useful in vasospastic angina since they dilate the coronaries and relieve vasospasm. Infact they are preferred over nitrates in vasospastic angina.

β-BLOCKERS

β-blockers reduce the frequency and severity of attacks of exertional angina and are useful in the prevention of angina. Exercise, emotion and similar situations increase sympathetic activity leading to increased heart-rate, force of contraction and BP, thereby increasing O_2 consumption by the heart. β-blockers prevent angina by blocking all these actions (Chap. 13) and thereby prevent an increase in myocardial oxygen demand. They are used for the long-term prophylaxis of classical angina and may be combined with nitrates. β - blockers should always be tapered after prolonged use. They are not useful in variant angina.

POTASSIUM CHANNEL OPENERS

Nicorandil is an arterial and venous dilator. Opening of the ATP-sensitive K^+ channels results in efflux of K^+ leading to hyperpolarization and therefore relaxation of the vascular smooth muscles. In addition it also acts through nitric oxide like nitrates. Nicorandil is tried in angina when other drugs do not afford significant benefit. It is expensive. Dose 10 - 20mg twice daily.

Adverse effects are headache, flushing, palpitation, dizziness and hypotension.

Pinacidil is similar to nicorandil. It is also useful in hypertension.

MISCELLANEOUS

Dipyridamole is a coronary vasodilator but it diverts the blood from ischaemic zone and is therefore not beneficial. It inhibits platelet aggregation for which it is used in post MI and post-stroke patients for prevention of coronary and cerebral thrombosis.

Aspirin Long term administration of low dose aspirin is recommended to prevent myocardial infarction. Aspirin inhibits platelet aggregation and thereby prevents MI in patients with angina.

Trimetazidine is a calcium channel blocker claimed to have a protective effect on the ischemic myocardium and to maintain left ventricular function. It is tried in exertional angina - 20 mg t.d.s.(Flavedon 20mg MR).

PHARMACOTHERAPY OF ANGINA

Exertional angina

Acute attack Sublingual nitroglycerin is the drug of choice. If the pain does not subside in 5 minutes, repeat the dose. After the relief of pain, the tablet should be discarded.

Acute prophylaxis Sublingual nitroglycerin given 15 minutes before an exertion (e.g. walking uphill) can prevent the attack. The prophylactic effect lasts for 30 minutes.

Chronic prophylaxis Long-acting nitrates or β-blockers (preferred) or calcium channel blockers can be used. All are given orally. If one drug is not effective, a combination of drugs may be used.

Vasospastic angina

Nitroglycerin and nifedipine given sublingually are effective in preventing and treating vasospastic episodes.

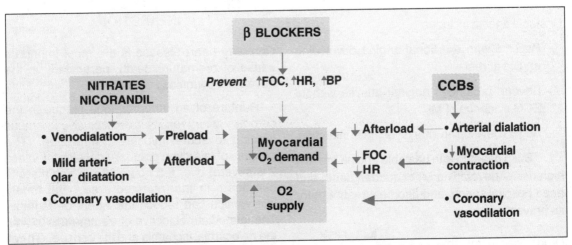

Fig. 18.2 Cardiovascular effects of antianginal drugs

Unstable angina not gastritis!

A 53 year old obese but otherwise healthy man at the peak of his career complained of discomfort in the retrosternal region. It was passed off as gastritis and self treated with antacids. The discomfort recurred on and off and on the third day the patient died a sudden death while he was travelling in his car. The patient had a massive MI and the discomfort he had earlier was retrospectively diagnosed as unstable angina.

Combination of drugs in angina

1. Nitrates + β-blockers - very effective in exertional angina. Reflex tachycardia due to nitrates is countered by β - blockers. Ventricular dilatation due to β - blockers is opposed by nitrates.

2. Nifedipine + β - blockers. The antianginal effects are additive. Reflex tachycardia due to nifedipine is countered by β-blockers.

3. Nitrates + CCBs - nitrates decrease preload, CCBs reduce afterload and the combination reduces cardiac work load.

4. CCBs + β -blockers + Nitrates - if the angina is not controlled by 2 drug combinations, 3 drugs can be used. Nitrates reduce preload, CCBs reduce afterload while β-blockers decrease heart rate. This combination is useful in severe angina.

UNSTABLE ANGINA

Unstable angina includes:

- Patients with exertional angina developing angina at rest

- Severe, prolonged anginal attacks without ECG evidence of MI

- Angina developing after myocardial infarction.

Such patients with unstable angina are at a high risk of developing MI or sudden death and need hospitalisation and rigorous treatment for its prevention.

Drugs used in unstable angina are

1. Aspirin - Platelet aggregation can occlude narrowed coronary arteries and can also release potent vasoconstrictors. Aspirin (75- 300mg daily) prevents platelet aggregation and thereby could prevent myocardial infarction.

2. Heparin - In high risk patients IV/SC heparin reduces pain.

3. Nitrates - Intravenous nitroglycerin reduces the cardiac workload and relieves pain.

4. Other drugs - β adrenergic blockers like atenolol (50-100mg daily) may be given; if they are contraindicated, calcium channel blockers like verapamil may be given. Glycoprotein receptor antagonists (abciximab, integrilin and tirofiban) inhibit the final steps of platelet aggregation and are being tried in unstable angina.

DRUGS USED IN MYOCARDIAL INFARCTION

Coronary heart disease is the most important cause of premature death, particularly in the developed countries.

Rupture of an atheromatous plaque in the coronary artery results in an occlusive thrombus leading to acute myocardial infarction. The process of infarction gradually develops (unless it is severe) over 6-8 hours after which there is cell death in the infarcted area. But timely intervention can reduce the extent of damage. The immediate objective of treatment is to limit the myocardial ischemia and the consequent cell death.

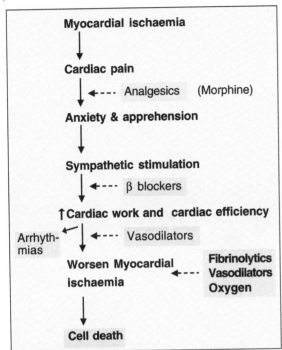

Fig. 18.3 Pathophysiology and sites of drug action in Myocardial infarction.

Immediate treatment

1. **Analgesia** Morphine 10 mg or pethidine 50mg is given intravenously through an IV cannula. They relieve pain and thereby reduce anxiety. Hence the demerits of sympathetic overactivity are reduced. Diazepam may also be given to reduce anxiety and produce sedation.

2. **Thrombolytics** Streptokinase 1.5 million units infusion is given over 1 hour. Urokinase or alteplase may be given as alternatives as 15 mg bolus and 0.5 mg/kg over the next 90 minutes. It is very expensive and hence is mostly reserved for patients in whom streptokinase cannot be used (See page 306)

Thrombolytics should be **started at the earliest possible** (within 6 - 12 hours) because they can limit the extent of damage and reduce mortality. Anistreplase is a form of streptokinase which is convenient to use because it is long acting and therefore can be used as a single IV injection.

3. **Aspirin** 300 mg of soluble aspirin given orally reduces mortality and improves the effect of thrombolysis. It should be continued (75-150 mg/day) even after the patient recovers.

4. **Oxygen** High flow oxygen should be given by inhalation.

5. **Other drugs**

   i. *ß - adrenergic antagonists* - IV atenolol (5 - 10 mg over 5 minutes) reduces short-term mortality and lowers the incidence of arrhythmias.

   ii. *Antiemetics* - an antiemetic may be given intravenously.

   iii. *Antiarrhythmics* - Arrhythmias are common in patients in acute MI; suitable antiarrhythmics should be used depending on the arrhythmia.

Long term treatment

Once the patient is stabilized, certain drugs are recommended for prevention of further ischemic events. Long term administration of low dose aspirin, a ß - adrenergic blocker and an ACE inhibitor are useful in reducing long term mortality.

ACE inhibitors prevent ventricular remodeling and cardiac failure.

Risk factor management

- Smoking should be stopped.
- Hyperlipidemia if any should be controlled.
- Body weight should be reduced.
- Regular moderate exercises should be advised
- Adequate control of diabetes and hypertension if any.

19 *Antihypertensive Drugs*

- • **Classification**
- • **Diuretics**
- • **Angiotensin Converting Enzyme inhibitors**
- • **Angiotensin II receptor blockers**
- • **Sympatholytics**
- • **Calcium Channel Blockers**
- • **Vasodilators**
- • **Treatment of hypertension**

Hypertension is an elevation of systolic and/or diastolic BP above 140/90 mm of Hg. It is a common cardiovascular entity. Hypertension may be *primary* (essential) hypertension - where the cause is not known or *secondary* - when it is secondary to other conditions like renal, endocrine or vascular disorders.

Based on the diastole, the degree of severity of hypertension can be graded as:

- • Mild - diastole upto 104
- • Moderate - 105 - 114
- • Severe - more than 115.

Blood pressure is determined by cardiac output (CO) and total peripheral vascular resistance (PVR). Blood pressure is controlled by baroreceptor reflexes acting through autonomic nervous system along with the renin-angiotensin-aldosterone system.

Prolonged hypertension damages the blood vessels of the heart, brain and the kidneys and may result in several complications like stroke, coronary artery disease or renal failure. Hence hypertension needs to be treated even though as such it does not generally produce obvious troublesome symptoms.

Antihypertensives act by influencing the BP regulatory systems *viz.* the autonomic system, renin - angiotensin system, calcium channels or sodium and water balance (plasma volume).

Antihypertensives may be classified as follows :

CLASSIFICATION	
1. **Diuretics**	
• *Thiazides*	Hydrochlorothiazide, chlorthalidone, indapamide
• *Loop diuretics*	Frusemide, bumetanide, torsemide
• *K+ Sparing diuretics*	Spironolactone, amiloride, triamterene
2. **Angiotensin converting enzyme inhibitors**	
	Captopril, enalapril, lisinopril, ramipril. perindopril, fosinopril, trandolapril, quinapril, benazepril
3. **Angiotensin II receptor antagonists**	
	Losartan, candesartan, valsartan, eprosartan, irbesartan, olmesartan
4. **Sympatholytics**	
• *Centrally acting drugs*	Clonidine, methyldopa, guanabenz, guanfacine
• *Ganglion blockers*	Trimethaphan
• *Adrenergic neuron blockers*	Guanethidine, reserpine
• *Adrenergic receptor blockers:*	
α-blockers	Prazosin, terazosin, doxazosin phenoxybenzamine, phentolamine
β -blockers	Propranolol, atenolol, esmolol, metoprolol
• *Mixed α and β blockers*	Labetalol, carvedilol
5. **Ca++ channel blockers**	Verapamil, nifedipine, nicardipine nimodipine, amlodipine, felodipine
6. **Vasodilators**	
• *Arteriolar dilators*	Hydralazine, minoxidil, diazoxide
• *Arteriolar & venular dilators*	Sodium nitroprusside

DIURETICS

The antihypertensive effect of diuretics (see Chap. 14) is mild - BP falls by 15-20 mm of Hg over 2-4 weeks. Diuretics act as antihypertensives as follows.

Diuretics enhance the excretion of sodium and water resulting in

1. ↓ Plasma volume → ↓ cardiac output → ↓ BP

2. ↓ Body sodium → relaxation of vascular smooth muscles (due to Na+ depletion in the vascular smooth muscle - ↓ PVR → ↓ BP.

Restriction of dietary salt intake will reduce the dose of the diuretic needed. Thiazides are the first-line antihypertensives and are inexpensive.

An initial dose of 12.5 mg daily hydrochlorothiazide/chlorthalidone is given. If the response is not adequate the dose may be increased to a maximum of 25 mg daily. They may be combined with a K+ sparing diuretic which is the best way to avoid hypokalaemia -1.25 mg amiloride with 12.5 mg hydrochlorothiazide. Thiazides may be used in combination with other antihypertensives particularly with those that cause salt and water retention as a side effect.

Indapamide is particularly useful in hypertension because it lowers BP in subdiuretic doses. Moreover it causes milder electrolyte disturbances.

Loop diuretics Although loop diuretics like frusemide are powerful diuretics, their antihypertensive efficacy is low. They are used only in hypertension with chronic renal failure or congestive heart failure.

Angiotensin Converting Enzyme (ACE) Inhibitors

Angiotensin II is a powerful vasoconstrictor. Aldosterone also raises the BP by increasing the plasma volume (Fig 19.2). ACE inhibitors prevent the formation of angiotensin II and (indirectly) aldosterone. There is vasodilation and decrease in PVR resulting in a fall in ↓ BP. As ACE also degrades bradykinin, ACE inhibitors raise the bradykinin levels which is a potent vasodilator. This also contributes to the fall in BP.

The blood flow to the kidneys, brain and heart increases due to selective vasodilation and thus maintains adequate blood supply to these vital organs.

Pharmacokinetics

ACE inhibitors are generally well-absorbed. Except captopril and lisinopril all others are prodrugs. They differ in their potency and pharmacokinetic properties like bioavailability, distribution, plasma $t\frac{1}{2}$ and excretion. Most ACE inhibitors are excreted through the kidney. Hence their dose should be reduced in renal dysfunction.

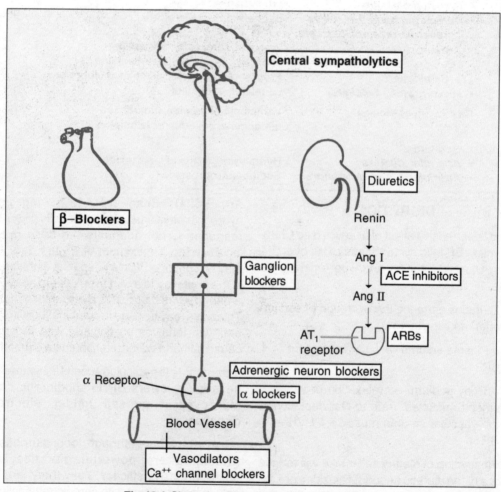

Fig 19.1 Sites of action of antihypertensive drugs

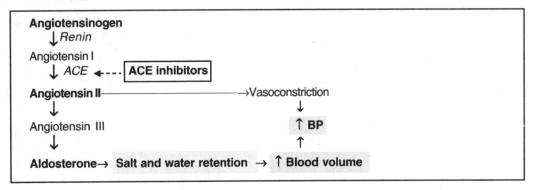

Fig 19.2 Renin-angiotensin system

Adverse effects

ACE inhibitors are well-tolerated. Adverse effects include -

1. **Persistent dry cough:** Due to ↑ bradykinin levels is more common in women. It may require withdrawal of the ACE inhibitors. An angiotension II receptor antagonist may be used in such patients. (See below)

2. **Hypotension:** On initiation of therapy, ACE inhibitors may cause significant hypotension - first dose phenomenon. Hence, treatment should be started with small doses and if patients are already on diuretics - temporarily diuretics should be stopped.

3. **Hyperkalemia:** ACE inhibitors may cause hyperkalemia particularly in patients on K^+ sparing diuretics or on K^+ supplements.

4. **Dysguisia:** An altered taste sensation is more common with captopril - it is however reversible.

5. **Angioneurotic edema:** ACE inhibitors can rarely cause (0.1% incidence) angio oedema with swelling in the lips, nose, larynx and airway obstruction. It may be due to increased bradykinin levels and can be fatal. ACE inhibitors should be immediately withdrawn at the first sign of angio oedema. Severe cases may need adrenaline and glucocorticoids.

6. **Skin rashes:** ACE inhibitors can occasionally cause skin rashes which are self-limiting.

7. **Teratogenicity:** Given during second and third trimester of pregnancy, ACE inhibitors can cause various foetal malformations including foetal growth retardation, malformed lungs and even death. ACE inhibitors are therfore contraindicated in pregnancy.

8. **Other effects:** They can cause headache, nausea, abdominal pain, proteinuria and rarely, neutropenia.

Neutropenia is more common in patients with collagen diseases and should be watched for. ACE inhibitors can precipitate acute renal failure in patients with renal artery stenosis.

Uses

1. **Hypertension**

- ACE inhibitors are presently the first line antihypertensives.
- ACE inhibitors are useful in the treatment of hypertension of all grades due to all causes.
- Addition of a diuretic potentiates their antihypertensive efficacy. They are generally combined with thiazides without a K^+ sparing diuretic because there can be significant hyperkalemia.
- ACE inhibitors are well tolerated.

- They are specially indicated as antihypertensives in :

    a. Hypertension with left ventricular hypertrophy - hypertrophy is gradually reversed by ACE inhibitors.

    b. Patients with diabetes mellitus because ACE-I slow the development of nephropathy.

    c. Renal diseases with HT - ACE inhibitors slow the progression of chronic renal diseases like glomerulosclerosis.

    d. Patients with co-existing IHD including post-MI patients.

    e. In severe hypertension, they may be combined with other antihypertensives like β blockers, CCBs or diuretics.

2. CCF : ACE inhibitors are the first line drugs (see page 124).

3. Myocardial infarction : ACE inhibitors started within 24 hours and given for several weeks prevent the development of CCF and reduce mortality.

4. Coronary artery disease : In patients who are at a high risk of ischaemic cardiovascular conditions like MI and stroke, ACE inhibitors afford significant benefit by reducing the risk of MI, stroke and sudden death.

5. Chronic renal failure : In patients with diabetic nephropathy and chronic renal failure, ACE inhibitors delay the progression of renal disease.

6. Scleroderma renal crisis: ACE inhibitors may be life saving in these patients.

Precautions and contraindications

- ACE inhibitors are contraindicated in pregnancy

- ACE inhibitors should not be combined with K^+ sparing diuretics.

- At the first sign of angio-oedema, ACE inhibitors should be stopped.

- ACE inhibitors are contraindicated in patients with renal artery stenosis as they can cause renal failure in them.

- ACE inhibitors may enhance plasma levels of digoxin.

ANGIOTENSIN II RECEPTOR BLOCKERS (ARBS)

Losartan was the first orally effective AT_1 receptor antagonist to be developed. There are 2 subtypes of angiotensin II receptors - AT_1 and AT_2. AT_1 receptors are present in vascular and myocardial tissue, brain, kidney and adrenal glomerular cells. Losartan is the first AT_1 receptor blocker to be available. It has high affinity for AT_1 receptors when compared to AT_2 receptors. By blocking AT_1 receptors, losartan blocks the effect of angiotensin II. It thus relaxes vascular smooth muscles, promotes salt and water excretion and reduces plasma volume.

TABLE 19.1: Dose and duration of action of some commonly used ACE inhibitors

Drug	Duration of action (in hrs)	Daily dose in hypertension (mg)
Captopril	6-12	12.5-50 mg BD
Enalapril	24	2.5-20 mg OD
Lisinopril	>24	5-40 mg OD
Ramipril	8-48	1.25-10 mg OD
Fosinopril	12-24	10-60 mg OD
Benazepril	12-24	10-40 mg OD
Perindopril	24	2-8 mg OD

TABLE 19.2 Dose and route of administration of some commonly used antihypertensives

Antihypertensives	Daily doses	Routes
Hydrochlorothiazide +	12.5-25 mg +	Oral
amiloride	1.25-2.5 mg daily	
Losartan	50 mg OD	Oral
Clonidine	100-300 µg	Oral
Methyldopa	250-500 mg q 6-12 hr	Oral
Atenolol	25-100 mg OD	Oral
Prazosin	2-20 mg daily	Oral
Hydralazine	25-50 mg q 8-24 hr	Oral
Diazoxide	50-100 mg every 5-10 min	IV
Sodium nitroprusside	0.2-0.3 mg/min	IV
Nifedipine	10 mg	SL
	5-20 mg q 8-12 hr	Oral

For ACE inhibitors see Table 19.1

The main **advantage of ARBs over ACE inhibitors** is that there is no increase in bradykinin levels and its associated adverse effects like dry cough and angiooedema.

Many other ARBs have now been synthesized including candesartan, irbesartan, valsartan, telmisartan and eprosartan.

ARBs are all given orally. Their bioavailability is generally <50%. They are all extensively protein bound and excreted by kidneys.

Adverse effects

ARBs are well tolerated. They can cause hypotension and hyperkalaemia like ACE inhibitors. Angiooedema is rare. ARBs are contraindicated in pregnancy because of their teratogenic potential.

Uses

1. Hypertension

   ARBs are used in the treatment of hypertension in similar indications as that of ACE inhibitors as alternatives to ACE inhibitors. They can be considered as first line drugs in hypertension. Losartan, candesartan and irbesartan are available in India. ARBs can be usefully combined with diuretics (Dose - Table 19.2)

2. Cardiac failure

   ARBs may be used as alternatives to ACE inhibitors in cardiac failure. *i.e.,* in patients who poorly tolerate ACE inhibitors.

SYMPATHOLYTICS

Drugs Acting Centrally

Clonidine

Clonidine, an imidazoline derivative, is a selective α_2 agonist. Stimulation of α_2 receptors in the CNS (in the vasomotor centre and hypothalamus), decreases central sympathetic outflow, blocks the release of noradrenaline from the nerve terminals leading to a fall in BP and bradycardia.

Adverse effects include drowsiness, dryness of mouth, nose and eyes; parotid gland swelling and pain, fluid retention, constipation and impotence. Sudden withdrawal of clonidine will lead to rebound hypertension, headache, tremors, sweating and tachycardia. Hence the dose should be tapered.

Uses

1. Mild to moderate hypertension.

Other uses

2. In Opioid withdrawal Most withdrawal symptoms in opioid addicts are of sympathetic overactivity and can be benefited by treatment with clonidine.

3. Diabetic neuropathy Clonidine controls diarrhoea by improving absorption of NaCl and water in the gut by stimulation of α_2 receptors in the intestines.

4. With anaesthetics Clonidine given preoperatively reduces the dose of the general anaesthetic needed due to its analgesic effects.

Guanfacine and guanabenz are α_2 agonists similar to clonidine and can be used as antihypertensives

α-methyl dopa

Alpha methyldopa, an analog of dopa, is a prodrug. It is metabolised in the body to α- methyl norepinephrine which is an α_2 agonist and acts like clonidine. Renin levels also fall. Left ventricular hypertrophy is reversed in about 12 weeks of treatment.

Adverse effects are sedation, dryness of mouth and nose, headache, postural hypotension, fluid retention and impotence.

Uses

Methyldopa is used in mild to moderate hypertension along with a diuretic. It is safe in hypertension during pregnancy and is the preferred antihypertensive in such patients. Started with 250 mg twice daily, the dose may be increased to a maximum of 750 mg BD.

GANGLION BLOCKERS

These drugs block both sympathetic and parasympathetic ganglia resulting in decreased sympathetic tone and a fall in BP. But they produce several side effects as they block both sympathetic and parasympathetic ganglia and except trimethaphan, ganglion blockers are not used now.

Trimethaphan

Trimethaphan is the only ganglion blocker that is in use now. It is given intravenously to produce controlled hypotension during certain surgical procedures due to its rapid and short action (15 minutes).

ADRENERGIC NEURON BLOCKERS

Guanethidine

Guanethidine depletes the stores of noradrenaline in the adrenergic neurons and also blocks its release. Because of the adverse effects like postural hypotension, diarrhoea and sexual dysfunction, guanethidine is not used.

Reserpine

Reserpine is an alkaloid obtained from *Rauwolfia serpentina* (Sarpagandhi) that grows in India. In the adrenergic neurons, it binds to the vesicles that store monoamines like noradrenaline, dopamine and 5-HT and destroys these vesicles. The monoamines then leak into the nerve terminals where they are destroyed by monoamine oxidase. Reserpine thus depletes the stores of these monoamines and reduces BP. Depletion of monoamines particularly dopamine is thought to be responsible for antipsychotic effects of reserpine (See page 247).

Reserpine causes various side effects like drowsiness, depression, parkinsonism, postural hypotension, oedema, weight gain, gynaecomastia and sexual dysfunction. Though it is generally not preferred, it has the advantages of being inexpensive, effective, long acting (once daily dose) and generally well tolerated when given with a diuretic.

α - blockers

Nonselective α blockers (see Chapter 13) like phenoxybenzamine and phentolamine are used in the treatment of hyper-tension due to pheochromocytoma. Selective α_1 blockers like prazosin, terazosin and doxazosin dilate both arterioles and venules. Peripheral vascular resistance is decreased leading to a fall in BP with only mild tachycardia.

30-60 minutes after the first dose of prazosin, the patient could experience postural hypotension which may lead to fainting particulary if the patient suddenly gets up from lying down position. This 'First dose phenomenon' can be avoided by starting with a low dose prazosin (0.5 mg) given at bed time. Dose is gradually increased. α_1 blockers are used in mild to moderate hypertension; they may be combined with diuretics and β-blockers.

β-blockers

β-blockers (see Chapter 13) are mild antihypertensives. Blockade of cardiac β_1 receptors results in decreased myocardial contractility and cardiac output. Thus they reduce the BP due to a fall in the cardiac output. They also lower plasma renin activity and have an additional central antihypertensive action.

β blockers are effective and well-tolerated and are of special value in patients who also have arrhythmias or angina. They may be used alone but are also suitable for combination with other antihypertensives, particularly with drugs that cause tachycardia as their side effect (*eg.* vasodilators). They are thus the first line antihypertensive drugs in mild to moderate

hypertension. Atenolol is the preferred β-blocker because of the advantages like once a day dosing, absence of CNS side effects and β_1 selectivity. β-blockers should always be tapered while withdrawing.

α and β-blockers

Labetalol and carvedilol block α_1 and β receptors. They are used IV in the treatment of hypertension in pheochromocytoma and in hypertensive emergencies.

CALCIUM CHANNEL BLOCKERS

Calcium channel blockers (CCBs) (see chap 16) are another important group of antihypertensives. They dilate the arterioles resulting in reduced peripheral vascular resistance. Nifedipine produces some reflex tachycardia while this is not seen with verapamil and diltiazem as they are cardiac depressants. Fluid retention is negligible unlike other arteriolar dilators. CCBs were earlier considered first line antihypertensives and were extensively used. But several recent large scale studies have shown them to have many disadvantages. They are not preferred in patients who also have left ventricular hypertrophy and previous myocardial infarction. Short acting DHPs produce frequent changes in BP and sympathetic activity and hence should be avoided in hypertension.

Use in hypertension

- CCBs are well-tolerated, and effective.

- CCBs are particularly effective in elderly patients.

- CCBs may be used as monotherapy or in moderate to severe HT along with other antihypertensives.

- It has now been shown that sublingual nifedipine does not actually achieve plasma concentration quicker than oral formulation. Thus in HT emergencies, short acting DHPs can be used parenterally.

- There is a growing concern that use of CCBs, especially short acting ones, is associated with increased mortality and risk of sudden death.

- Sustained release preparations or long acting dihydropyridine CCBs may be used for smoother control of BP.

VASODILATORS

Vasodilators relax the vascular smooth muscles thus reducing BP due to decreased peripheral vascular resistance. Salt and water retention and reflex tachycardia are common with vasodilators.

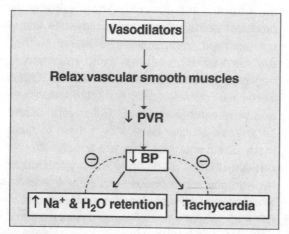

Hydralazine

Hydralazine is a directly acting arteriolar dilator. The fall in BP is associated with tachycardia, renin release and fluid retention. Coronary, cerebral and renal blood flow are increased.

Hydralazine is metabolised by acetylation in the liver (like INH) and the rate of acetylation is genetically determined - people may be fast or slow acetylalors.

Adverse effects are headache, dizziness, flushing, palpitation, nausea, hypotension and salt and water retention. It may precipitate angina in some patients because of increased O_2 demand due to reflex tachycardia and decreased

myocardial blood supply due to peripheral vasodilatation. Hypersensitivity reactions like serum sickness and lupus erythematosus (arthralgia, fever, pleuritis, pericarditis) may occur and is more common in slow acetylators.

Uses Hydralazine is used with a β-blocker and/or a diuretic in moderate to severe hypertension not controlled by the first line drugs. It can be given in hypertension during pregnancy (2nd and 3rd trimester).

Minoxidil

Minoxidil is a directly acting arteriolar dilator used in severe hypertension not responding to other drugs. It acts by opening K^+ channels in the smooth muscles. Opening of the K^+ channels causes efflux of K^+ resulting in hyperpolarisation and smooth muscle relaxation.

Uses: Minoxidil is used with a diuretic - as a reserve drug - in patients with severe hypertension who do not respond to other drugs. Minoxidil directly stimulates the growth of hair on prolonged use (hypertrichosis). It appears to activate the gene that controls the protein of hair shaft - by this it stimulates the maturation and growth of cells of the hair shaft. Hence it is used topically (2% solution) in *alopecia*. Young men with relative alopecia are more likely to respond.

Minoxidil can cause fluid retention, tachycardia and anginal episodes. Hypertrichosis on the face, arms, legs and back make it unacceptable in women.

Diazoxide

Diazoxide is related to thiazide diuretics and is a potent arteriolar dilator. Its mechanism of action is like that of minoxidil. Diazoxide can cause hyperglycaemia because it inhibits the insulin secretion from pancreas. Other side effects include salt and water retention, palpitation and myocardial ischaemia. It is used intravenously in hypertensive emergencies where monitoring of infusion is not possible. Diazoxide has a long duration of action (24 hours) and is suitable in such situations.

Sodium nitroprusside

It is a rapidly acting vasodilator and it relaxes both arterioles and venules. Both peripheral resistance and cardiac output are reduced resulting in lower myocardial oxygen consumption.

Nitroprusside acts through the release of nitric oxide which activates guanylyl cyclase, resulting in the formation of cGMP which relaxes the vascular smooth muscles. On IV administration, it is rapid (acts within 30 seconds) and short-acting (duration 3 minutes) allowing titration of the dose. This makes it suitable for use in hypertensive emergencies with close monitoring. It decomposes on exposure to light; *the infusion bottle and tubing should be covered with opaque foil.*

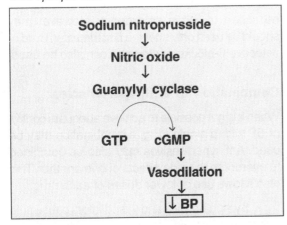

Adverse reactions are palpitation, sweating, weakness, nausea, vomiting and hypotension. In higher doses nitroprusside gets converted to cyanide and thiocyanate which can result in toxicity. Symptoms of toxicity include nausea, anorexia, weakness, disorientation and psychosis. Administration of sodium thiosulphate along with nitroprusside prevents the accumulation of cyanide.

Uses

1. Nitroprusside is the drug of choice in hypertensive emergencies. Started with 0.5 mcg/kg/min infusion and may be gradually increased upto 10 mcg/kg/min. The BP should be constantly monitored.

2. It is used in situations where short-term reduction of myocardial work load is required as in myocardial infarction.

Drug Interactions of antihypertensives

1. Sympathomimetics and tricyclic antidepressants can antagonise the effects of sympatholytics.

2. Antihistamines add to sedation produced by clonidine and methyldopa.

3. NSAIDs tend to cause salt and water retention and may blunt the effect of antihypertensives.

TREATMENT OF HYPERTENSION

Mild hypertension

Treatment is started with low dose of a single drug - a thiazide diuretic or a β-blocker. If the patient does not adequately respond in 3-4 weeks, an ACE inhibitor or a calcium channel blocker should be tried. If BP is not controlled by one drug, another should be added.

Moderate hypertension

A combination of a diuretic with a sympatholytic may be given. If response is inadequate add a third drug.

Severe hypertension

It may be associated with cardiac or renal disorder. A vasodilator with a diuretic and a β-blocker is useful.

Hypertensive Crises

Hypertensive crises include hypertensive emergencies and urgencies.

Hypertensive emergencies are situations with very high BP (210/120 mm of Hg) associated with target organ damage. They may be life threatening. Conditions like malignant hypertension, hypertensive encephalopathy, acute myocardial infarction, dissecting aneurysm of aorta, acute LVF with pulmonary edema,

Table 19.3 Drugs in hypertensive emergencies

Drug	Dose	Duration
Sodium nitroprusside	0.5 to 10 mcg/kg/min IV infusion	1 - 2 min
Nifedipine	10mg sub lingual	2 - 3 hours
Nitroglycerin	5 to 100 mcg/min IV infusion	3 - 5 min
Fenoldopam	0.1 to 1.6 mcg/kg/min IV infusion	15 - 30 min
Hydralazine	10 to 20 mg IV bolus or 10-50mg IM	4 - 8 hours
Esmolol	50 to 300 mcg/kg/min IV infusion	10 - 15 min
Labetalol	20 to 80 mg IV every 10 min (Max 300mg)	3 - 6 hours

eclampsia and hypertensive crisis in pheochromocytoma are some hypertensive emergencies, *Malignant hypertension* is severe hypertension associated with vascular damage due to arteriolopathy. It is a medical emergency manifested by papilloedema, retinal haemorrhages and hypertensive encephalopathy.

Hypertensive emergencies require treatment in an ICU with constant monitoring of BP. Blood pressure should be lowered gradually. This is because, in patients with chronic hypertension, autoregulatory changes take place in the blood vessels of vital organs.

Hypertensive urgencies are conditions with highly elevated BP but no target organ damage. They require gradual reduction of BP over about 24 hours - the diastole is brought down to about 100 mm of Hg.

Parenteral drugs are preferred in the treatment of hypertensive crises. IV sodium nitroprusside under close monitoring is the drug of choice (See Table 19.3). IV esmolol, diazoxide, fenoldopam, nitroglycerine, labetatol, hydralazine and sublingual nifedipine are alternatives. BP should be constantly monitored because drugs like sodium nitroprusside can bring down BP suddenly which results in hypoperfusion of vital organs. As soon as possible switching over to oral drugs is desirable because the control of BP is smoother with oral antihypertensives.

Hypertension in pregnancy

The drugs found safe are - methyldopa orally for maintenance and hydralazine (parenteral) for reduction of BP in emergency. However they should be used only after the first trimester. Cardio-selective β-blockers (atenolol) can also be used.

Combination of antihypertensives

When it is not possible to achieve adequate control of BP with a single drug, a combination may be used. Antihypertensives may also be combined to overcome the side effects of one another. This also allows use of lower doses of each drug.

Sympatholytics and vasodilators cause fluid retention which can be overcome by adding a diuretic.

Vasodilators like nifedipine and hydralazine evoke reflex tachycardia. This can be countered by β-blockers, while propranolol may cause initial rise in PVR which is countered by vasodilators.

Combination of ACE inhibitors and diuretics is synergistic.

Non-pharmacological measures

Low salt diet, weight reduction and transcendental meditation - all go a long way in controlling the blood pressure. Smoking and alcohol should be given up. These measures also help in reducing the dose of the antihypertensive needed.

20 *Pharmacotherapy of Shock*

- **Hypovolaemic shock**
- **Septic shock**
- **Cardiogenic shock**
- **Anaphylactic shock**
- **Neurogenic shock**

SHOCK

Shock is acute circulatory failure with underperfusion of tissues. In shock, symptoms of sympathetic overactivity are generally seen - like pallor, sweating, cold extremities and tachycardia. Shock may be -

1.Hypovolaemic shock

Decreased fluid volume due to sudden loss of plasma or blood as in haemorrhage, burns or dehydration - results in hypovolaemic shock.Fluid and electrolytes (see Chapter 21) should be replaced and BP monitored.

2.Septic shock

Septic shock is precipitated by severe bacterial infection. It may be due to release of bacterial toxins - should be treated with appropriate antibiotics apart from general measures.

Drotrecogin alpha - is activated human protein C obtained by recombinant DNA technology. In septic shock, the bacterial toxins evoke an inflammatory response which is associated with an impairment of coagulation and fibrinolysis. Protein C inhibits coagulation, improves fibrinolysis and may also inhibit TNF synthesis. It has been tried in severe sepsis with multiorgan failure. It is very expensive.

Preparation: XIGRIS - 24 mcg/hour IV infusion for 96 hours.

3.Cardiogenic shock

Cardiogenic shock is due to failure of heart as a

pump as in myocardial infarction. IV morphine is the drug of choice to relieve pain and anxiety. (see page 219)

4. Anaphylactic shock

Anaphylactic shock is a Type I hypersensitivity reaction causing release of massive amounts of histamine which is triggered by antigen-antibody reaction.Adrenaline (IM) is the drug of choice (see page 94)

5. Neurogenic shock

Neurogenic shock is due to venous pooling as following spinal anaesthesia, abdominal or testicular trauma (vagal inhibition).

Shock of all types needs immediate treatment

General measures

- The cause should be identified and treated

- Maintain BP and plasma volume - Appropriate intravenous fluids should be administered based on the requirement. Vasopressors like dopamine may be given intravenously when the BP cannot be brought up by IV fluids. Plasma expanders (see chapter 21) may help in maintaining the plasma volume when there is severe hypovolemia.

- Correct the acid base and electrolyte disturbances

- Ensure adequate urine output.

21 | *Plasma Expanders & Intravenous Fluids*

- **Plasma Expanders**
  - **- Dextrans**
  - **- Gelatin products**
  - **- Hydroxyethyl starch**
  - **- Polyvinyl pyrrolidine**
  - **- Human albumin**
  - **- Uses of plasma expanders**
- **Intravenous Fluids**
  - **- Types of IV solutions**

PLASMA EXPANDERS

To restore the intravascular volume, the component that is lost should ideally be replaced like plasma in burns and blood after haemorrhage. But in emergency, immediate volume replacement is important. In such situations plasma expanders are used. These are high molecular weight substances which when infused IV exert osmotic pressure and remain in the body for a long time to increase the volume of circulating fluid.

An ideal plasma expander should exert oncotic pressure comparable to plasma, be long-acting, non - antigenic and pharmacologically inert.

The plasma expanders used are dextrans, gelatin polymer, hydroxyethyl starches and polyvinyl pyrrolidone - all colloidal compounds. Human albumin obtained from pooled human plasma is also useful.

Dextrans

Dextrans (Dextran 70 - mol. wt. 70,000 and dextran 40 - mol. wt. 40,000) are polysaccharides obtained from sugar beet. Their osmotic pressure is similar to that of plasma proteins. Dextran 70 effectively expands the plasma volume and remains so for 24 hours. It interferes with coagulation, blood grouping and cross matching.

Dextran 40 is faster but shorter acting. It can improve microcirculation in shock by preventing rouleax formation of RBCs and have an antisludging effect. It can clog renal tubules resulting in renal failure - though rare should be watched for. Allergic reactions are common as dextrans are antigenic.

Dextrans have a long shelf-life (10 years) and can be easily sterilized. Dextrans are the commonly used plasma expanders.

Gelatin products

Gelatin prodeucts have a mol. wt. of 30,000 and a duration of action of 12 hours. Gelatin polymers can remain stable for almost 3 years at a pH of 7.2-7.3. They do not interfere with coagulation, blood grouping and cross matching. They can rarely cause urticaria, allergic reactions and bronchospasm.

Hydroxyethyl starch (Hetastarch)

Hydroxyethyl maintains blood volume for a long period. Allergic reactions are rare and it does not interfere with coagulation.

Polyvinyl pyrrolidone (PVP)

PVP is a synthetic polymer. It is not preferred due to various disadvantages like - it provokes histamine release and interferes with blood grouping.

Human albumin

Human albumin is obtained from pooled human blood. It is given as 5% or 20% solution. It is nonantigenic, does not interfere with coagulation, blood grouping or cross matching.

Human albumin is used in edema, burns, hypovolemic shock, hypoproteinaemia, acute liver failure and in dialysis.

Allergic reactions and fever can occur though rarely.

Uses of plasma expanders

These are used as plasma substitutes in hypovolaemic shock, burns and in extensive fluid loss - as an emergency measure to restore plasma volume.

INTRAVENOUS FLUIDS

Intravenous fluids are sterile solutions meant for intravenous administration. The content and quantity of solute varies. Intravenous fluids are used for replacement of fluid, electrolytes and nutrition. There are different types of IV fluids to be given depending on the patient's requirements.

Types of I.V solutions

Intravenous solutions are of 3 types depending on osmolality - *isotonic, hypotonic or hypertonic.* Fluids having an osmolality nearly equal to that of extracellular fluid (ECF) or if the electrolyte content (cations + anions) is nearly equal to 310 mEq/L – they are considered isotonic.

Isotonic electrolyte content = 310 mEq/L

Hypotonic electrolyte content < 250 mEq/L

Hypertonic electrolyte content > 375 mEqL

(Plasma osmolality is nearly equal to 300 m mol / L. Osmolality of 10% dextrose is 505 m mol / L)

Isotonic fluids

As isotonic fluids have an osmolality nearly equal to that of ECF, they do not alter the size of RBCs (neither shrink not swell). 1 litre of isotonic solution expands ECF by 1 litre. But it quickly diffuses into the ECF compartment and therefore the plasma volume is increased only by ¼ litre (250 ml). Hence around 3 litres of isotonic fluid is needed to replenish volume of one litre of lost blood. However patients with hypertension and cardiac failure need careful monitoring to avoid fluid overload. Isotonic solutions include normal saline and lactated ringer solution.

Normal saline solution – (0.9 % sodium chloride) remains in the ECF because the electrolytes make up its osmolality. It is used in hyponatraemia. It should be avoided in heart failure, pulmonary edema and renal impairment.

Lactated ringer solution contains potassium, calcium and sodium chloride. It is used to correct dehydration, hyponatraemia and to replace gastrointestinal fluids. Many other similar solutions are available with minor changes in the electrolyte content.

Hypotonic fluids

Hypotonic fluids replace cellular fluid because they are hypotonic as compared to plasma. Half normal saline (0.45% sodium chloride solution) is the commonly used hypotonic solution but other electrolyte solutions are also available. Hypotonic sodium solution is used in hypernatraemia and other hyperosmolar conditions. Overdosage can result in intravascular fluid depletion, hypotension, cellular odema and later cell damage.

Hypertonic fluids

Fiver percent dextrose in normal saline or lactated ringer's solution or in hypotonic solution has osmolality more than ECF. Once thedextrose is metabolized, the normal saline becomes isotonic and lactated Ringer becomes hypotonic. 45% to 50% dextrose solution may be administered in hypoglycemia or to supplement calories. Since these solutions are strongly hypertonic, they should be injected into central veins for rapid dilution. Hypertonic saline solutions draw water from the cells and the cells shrink. They should be injected slowly and carefully to avoid ECF volume overload.

CENTRAL NERVOUS SYSTEM

22 *Introduction*

- Excitatory neurotransmitters
- Inhibitory neurotransmitters
- Other transmitters

The central nervous system is the most complex of all the systems in the body. Several drugs act on the CNS including drugs used therapeutically and those used for pleasurable effects. Drugs may stimulate or depress the CNS. To understand the effects of drugs, a basic idea of the important neurotransmitters acting on the CNS and their receptors is very much essential.

The central neurotransmitters include

- Excitatory transmitter
  Glutamate
- Inhibitory transmitters
  GABA, glycine
- Other transmitters
  Noradrenaline, dopamine, 5-HT, acetylcholine, histamine, adenosine

EXCITATORY NEUROTRANSMITTERS

Glutamate is the chief excitatory neurotransmitter present throughout the CNS. It is stored in synaptic vesicles and is released into the synapse by exocytosis. It acts on specific glutamate receptors for excitatory amino acid receptors

Excitatory amino acid (EAA) receptors are of 4 subtypes -
- NMDA
- AMPA
- Kainate
- Metabotropic receptor

NMDA, AMPA and Kainate receptors are ionotropic receptors.

NMDA is N-methyl-D-Aspartate. Activation of NMDA receptors is by glycine and glutamate - each at different sites (Fig 22.1).

The NMDA receptors mediate slow excitatory responses and also play a role in long term adaptive changes in the brain. Drugs like ketamine

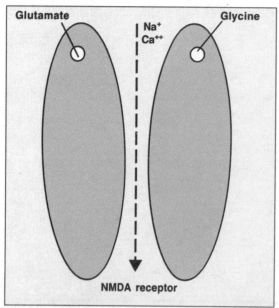

Fig 22.1 NMDA receptor is a ligand gated ion channel. Binding of glutamate and glycine opens the channel resulting in entry of Ca^{++} and some Na^{+}.

(See page 170), phencyclidine, memantine and magnesium block the NMDA receptor channels. Ketamine produces dissociative anaesthesia.

AMPA and Kainate receptors are involved in fast excitatory transmission. They are both activated

Table 22.1: Central neurotransmitters and their receptors	
Transmitter	**Receptor**
Excitatory	
Glutamate	NMDA
	AMPA
	Kainate
	Metabotropic
Inhibitory	
GABA	GABA$_A$
	GABA$_B$
Glycine	Glycine
Others	
Noradrenaline	α_{1-2}, β_{1-3}
Dopamine	D$_{1-5}$
Acetylcholine	Muscarinic (M$_{1-5}$)
5-Hydroxytryptamine	5HT$_{1-7}$
Histamine	H$_{1-3}$

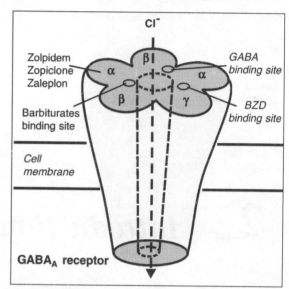

Fig 22.2: GABA$_A$ receptor is a ligand gated chloride channel. Binding of the agonist opens the channel resulting in entry of Cl^{-}.

by glutamate while the AMPA receptor activity is modulated by cyclothiazide and aniracetam. (AMPA=α-amino-3-hydroxy-5-methylisoxazole, AP-5, 2-amino-5-phos phonopentanoic acid).

Metabotropic receptors are G-protein coupled receptors and are involved in long-term adaptive changes in the brain.

INHIBITORY NEUROTRANSMITTERS

GABA

GABA is the principal inhibitory neurotransmitter in the brain. Agonists may bind to different sites on the GABA receptor. There are two subtypes of GABA receptors. GABA$_A$ and GABA$_B$ receptors. GABA$_A$ receptor is a ligand - gated chloride channel (Fig 22.2) while GABA$_B$ receptors are G -protein coupled receptors. Drugs like benzodiazepines and barbiturates bring about their effects by acting on the GABA$_A$ receptors. Flumazenil is a GABA$_A$ antagonist.

Baclofen is a GABA$_B$ receptor agonist which

brings about skeletal muscle relaxation.

Glycine

Glycine is an inhibitory transmitter in the brain stem and spinal cord. It acts on glycine receptor which is a ligand - gated chloride channel. Tetanus toxin inhibits the release of glycine in the spinal cord resulting in powerful muscle spasms.

Other transmitters in the CNS include noradrenaline, dopamine, acetylcholine serotonin, histamine, purines and nitric oxide.

DRUGS ACTING ON CNS

GENERAL ANAESTHETICS

Inhalational: N$_2$O, Ether, Halothane, Enflurane, Isoflurane, Desflurane, Sevoflurane

Intravenous: Thiopentone sodium, BZDs, Ketamine, Neuroleptanalgesic (Droperidol + Fentanyl)

SEDATIVE HYPNOTICS

BZDs: Diazepam, Flurazepam, lorazepam, alprazolam

Newer agents: Zolpidem, Zopiclone, Zaleplon

Barbiturates: Phenobarbitone, Pentobarbitone, Thiopentone

Misc: Paraldehyde, Chloral hydrate, Glutethimide

DRUGS USED IN PSYCHIATRY

Antipsychotics: Chlorpromazine, Trifluoperazine, Fluphenazine, Haloperidol, Trifluperidol, Thiothixene, Clozapine, Olanzepine, Risperidone, Quetiapine

Antidepressants:
- *TCAs*: Imipramine, Amitriptyline, Doxepin
- *SSRIs*: Fluoxetine, Fluvoxamine, Citalopram, Sertraline, Venlafaxine
- *MAOI*: Phenelzine, Tranylcypromine
- *Atypical*: Trazodone, Nefazodone, Bupropion, Mianserin, Mirtazapine

Mood Stabilizers: Lithium, Carbamazepine, Valproic and

Antianxiety drugs
- *BZDs*: Diazepam, alprazolam
- *5-HT agonist-antagonist*: Buspirone, Gepirone, Ipsapirone
- *β blockers*: Propranolol

ANTIEPILEPTICS

Phenytoin, Phenobarbitone, Primidone, Carbamazepine, Ethosuximide, Valproic acid, BZDs,

Newer agents: Gabapentine, Lamotrigine, Vigabatrin, Felbamate, Tiagabine, Topiramate, Zonisamide, Levetiracetam.

ANALGESICS

Opioids

Agoinsts: Morphine, Codiene, Pethidine, Methadone

Antagonists: Naloxone, Naltrexone, Nalmefene

Mixed agonist-antagonists: Pentazocine, Nalbuphine, Butorphanol, Buprenorphine, Nalorphine

NSAIDs

Non-selective COX inhibitors: Aspirin, Paracetamol, Phenylbutazone, Azapropazone, Indomethacin, Diclofenac, Ibuprofen, Ketoprofen, Flufenamic acid, Piroxicam, Tenoxicam, Nabumetone,

Selective COX-2 inhibitors: Nimesulide, Celecoxib, Rofecoxib.

DRUGS IN PARKINSONISM

Levodopa, Amantadine, Bromocryptine, lisuride, Ropinirole, Selegiline, Tolcapone, Entacapone

Anticholinergics: Benztropine, Benzhexol, Trihexyphenidyl

ALCOHOLS

Ethanol, Methanol

CNS STIMULANTS

Resp. Stimulants: Doxapram, Nikethamide

Psychomotor Stimulants: Amphetamine, Cocaine, Methylxanthine

Convulsants: Leptazol, Strychnine

23 *General Anaesthetics*

- Stages of general anaesthesia
- Mechanism of action
- Pharmacokinetics
- Inhalational anaesthetics
- Intravenous anaesthetics
  - Inducing agents
  - Dissociative anaesthesia
  - Neuroleptanalgesia
  - Benzodiazepines
- Preanaesthetic medication

GENERAL ANAESTHETICS

General Anaesthetics are agents that bring about reversible loss of sensation and consciousness. Before 1846, alcohol, opium, packing a limb with ice and concussion, i.e. making the patient unconscious by a blow on the headwere used to relieve surgical pain. Dr Horace Wells a dentist, tried to demonstrate the effect of nitrous oxide as

an anesthetic in 1844 but was unsuccessful as he removed the gas bag too early. Dr William Morton who was present at the demonstration, worked on it and in 1846 demonstrated ether anaesthesia successfully. Chloroform was introduced by James.Y. Simpson in 1847. Since then several anaesthetics have been synthesized over the decades. Halothane was introduced into anaesthetic practice by Johnstone in 1956 .

Stages of General Anaesthesia

1. **Stage of analgesia** is from the beginning of inhalation of the anaesthetic to loss of consciousness.

2. **Stage of delirium** This stage is from loss of consciousness to beginning of surgical anaesthesia. It may be associated with excitement - shouting, crying and violent behaviour.

3. **Stage of surgical anaesthesia** This has 4 planes. As anaesthesia passes to deeper

planes, respiratory depression is seen. There is gradual loss of reflexes and relaxation of skeletal muscles.

4. **Stage of medullary paralysis** is seen only with overdose. It is the stage of medullary depression. Cessation of breathing, circulatory failure and death may follow.

Ideal anaesthetic

An ideal anaesthetic should be pleasant, non-irritating, provide adequate analgesia, immobility and muscle relaxation; should be non-inflammable and administration should be easy and controllable and have a wide margin of safety. Induction and recovery should be smooth and should not affect cardiovascular functions. It should be inexpensive.

Mechanism of action of general anae sthetics.

The exact mechanism of action of general anaesthetics is not known. The most accepted mechanisms of action are as follows.

1. Inhaled and some intravenous anaesthetics bind to specific sites on GABA receptor chloride channels and activate these receptors. By this they increase the inhibitory neurotransmission and depress the CNS.

2. Inhalational anaesthetics also enhance the sensitivity of glycine - gated chloride channels to glycine. These glycine receptors bring about inhibitory neurotransmission in the brain stem.

3. Some anaesthetics like ketamine and nitrous oxide bind to and inhibit the N-methyl D - aspartate (NMDA) receptors.

4. Inhalational and intravenous agents act at multiple sites in the nervous system and depress the neuronal activity at many sites in the brain.

General anaesthetics are as follows-

CLASSIFICATION

I. Inhalational

A. *Gases*
  - Nitrous oxide, cyclopropane

B. *Liquids*
  - Ether, halothane, enflurane, isoflurane, methoxyflurane, desflurane, sevoflurane

II. Intravenous

A. *Inducing agents*
  - Thiopentone sodium, methohexitone, propofol, etomidate

B. *Dissociative anaesthesia*
  - Ketamine

C. *Neuroleptanalgesia*
  - Fentanyl + droperidol

D. *Benzodiazepines*
  - Diazepam, lorazepam, midazolam

INHALATIONAL ANAESTHETICS

Pharmacokinetics

Inhalational anaesthetics are administered at a specific concentration. Since the brain is a highly perfused organ, steady state can be achieved quickly. When the steady state is reached, the partial pressure of the anaesthetic in the lung and the brain are equal and this makes it possible to monitor the anaesthesia. But, for anaesthetics with high solubility in blood and tissues, rise in alveolar partial pressure (and thereby induction) is slower. Such anaesthetics need to be administered at higher pressures.

Factors which influence the partial pressure (PP) of the anaesthetic attained in the brain are:

1. *Partial pressure of the anaesthetic in the inspired gas* - Higher the partial pressure of the anaesthetic in the inspired air, greater is its quantity moving into the blood.

2. *Pulmonary ventilation* - Delivery of the anaesthetic into the alveoli is directly proportional to pulmonary ventilation.

3. *Alveolar exchange* - When ventilation perfusion is appropriate, volatile anaesthetics freely diffuse across the alveoli.

4. *Solubility of the anaesthetic in the blood* - Lower the solubility of the anaesthetic in the blood, faster is the rise of its PP in the blood and faster is the induction.

5. *Solubility of the anaesthetic in the tissue* Anaestheics which are more soluble in tissues like the adipose tissue, require a longer time to attain equilibrium.

6. *Cerebral blood flow* Since the blood flow to the brain is high, GAs reach it rapidly and if other factors are favourable, anaesthesia can be rapidly attained.

Minimum Alveolar Concentration (MAC) is the concentration that immobilizes 50% of subjects in response to a surgical skin incision. MAC is used to describe the potencies of different volatile anaesthetics.

Second Gas Effect - When certain anaesthetics like nitrous oxide are administered in high conc entrations, the other anaesthetic gases are also pulled in and their alveolar tension rises more rapidly. This is known as second gas effect.

Concentration Effect - When an anaesthetic is administered in high concentration, its alveolar tension rises more rapidly than when the same gas is inhaled in lower concentration. For example if 75% nitrous oxide is administered, its alveolar tension rises faster than 50% nitrous oxide administration.

Elimination

Once the administration of the anaesthetic is discontinued, recovery from anaesthesia depends on the rate of elimination of anaesthetics from the brain. The same factors which influence induction also influence recovery. Most anaesthetics are eliminated unchanged. Inhalation anaesthetics are eliminated from the lungs. Agents which are soluble in fat and tissues require longer time for elimination and therefore recovery is slower.

NITROUS OXIDE

Priestly discovered nitrous oxide in 1776 and was used by Horace Wells in 1944 for its anaesthetic properties. Nitrous oxide is a gas with a slightly sweetish odour. It produces light anaesthesia without significant depression of respiration or vasomotor centre.

Advantages

1. Strong analgesic

2. Induction is rapid and smooth

3. It is non-irritating and non-inflammable

4. Recovery is rapid

5. Postoperative nausea is not significant

6. Has little effect on respiration and cardiovascular functions, hence ideal for combination

7. It is non-toxic to liver, kidney and brain and is quickly removed from lungs.

Disadvantages

1. It is less potent and should be used with other agents.

2. Poor muscle relaxant.

3. N_2O displaces nitrogen in the air-filled cavities and while doing so, it enters the cavities faster *i.e.* even before nitrogen escapes. This results in expansion of such cavities like pneumothorax and air embolus. Hence N_2O should be avoided in such patients.

4. Repeated use can depress the bone marrow.

5. Long term exposure (like in staff of operation theatre) to low doses can impair DNA synthesis which may result in foetal abnormalities on conception.

Status in anaesthesia Nitrous oxide is used as an adjuvant to other anaesthetics. It is used along with oxygen (30%).

ETHER

Ether is a colourless volatile liquid. It is highly inflammable; vapours are irritating.

Advantages

1. Potent and reliable anaesthetic.
2. Good analgesic.
3. Effect on cardiovascular and respiratory functions are not significant in therapeutic doses; reflexes are well-maintained.
4. It is a bronchodilator.
5. Provides full muscle relaxation in deep anaesthesia.
6. Does not sensitize the heart to adrenaline.
7. Easy to administer as complicated equipment is not necessary.
8. Inexpensive.

Disadvantages

1. It is inflammable - hence diathermy is contraindicated.
2. Highly soluble in body tissues - induction is slow and unpleasant.
3. It is irritating and therefore enhances respiratory secretions. Premedication with atropine is essential - laryngeal spasm may occur during induction.
4. Postoperative nausea and vomiting are frequent.
5. Recovery is slow.

Status in anaesthesia Ether is not preferred now because of its flammability and irritant

property. But it is still used in developing countries like India because it is inexpensive, potent, easy to administer (by open drop method) and relatively safe.

HALOTHANE

Halothane is a colourless volatile liquid with a sweet odour. It is non-irritant and non-inflammable.

Advantages

1. Potent, non-inflammable anaesthetic.
2. Induction is smooth and rapid - in 2-5 min surgical anaesthesia can be produced
3. Non-irritant - therefore does not augment salivary or bronchial secretions.
4. Recovery is rapid.
5. Postoperative nausea and vomiting are of low incidence.

Disadvantages

1. Neither a good analgesic nor a muscle relaxant.
2. Halothane is a direct myocardiac depressant. Cardiac output and BP start falling and heart rate may decrease. It sensitizes the heart to the arrhythmogenic action of adrenaline.
3. It also causes some respiratory depression.
4. Severe hepatitis which may be fatal occurs in 1: 50,000 patients. A metabolite may be responsible for this toxicity.
5. Malignant hyperthermia - a genetically determined reaction occurs rarely. Succinylcholine accentuates this effect of halothane. It is due to intracellular release of calcium from the sarcoplasmic reticulum which causes muscle contraction and increased heat production. It is treated with dantrolene.

Status in anaesthesia

Halothane is one of the most popular anaesthetics.

Analgesics and muscle relaxants are used as adjuvants. Properties such as non-flammability, non-irritancy, bringing about rapid induction and recovery have made it an important and preferred anaesthetic - most widely used.

ENFLURANE

Enflurane is similar to halothane except that:

1. it is metabolised to a lesser extent than halothane - therefore safer regarding the liver toxicity.

2. does not sensitize the heart to adrenaline. But enflurane may precipitate seizures in epileptics and should be avoided in them.

ISOFLURANE

Isoflurane is an isomer of enflurane and is similar to halothane. It differs as follows:

1. more potent than halothane

2. does not sensitize the heart to adrenaline

3. metabolism is negligible - therefore safer regarding the liver toxicity

4. it does not provoke seizures

Isoflurane is extensively used now. It is expensive and can cause hypotension.

DESFLURANE

Desflurane is a congener of isoflurane. It has all the advantages of isoflurane. In addition desflurane has low solubility in blood and tissues. because of which it rapidly attains therapeutic concentration in the alveoli. Therefore induction and recovery are very rapid and smooth.

Desflurane also has some disadvantages:

- It is pungent - may induce coughing and sometimes laryngspasm. It is therefore used for maintenance of anaesthesia and is not preferred for induction.

- Because of low volatility a special vaporizer is required for administration.

- It can cause transient sympathetic stimulation and tachycardia.

SEVOFLURANE

Sevoflurane is the latest introduction to inhalation anaesthetics. It has the advantages of desflurane but is not pungent. It has the advantages of rapid and smooth induction and recovery because of low solubility in blood and tissues. This also makes it suitable for day-case surgeries and for anaesthesia for children.

Disadvantages:

1. Sevoflurane is chemically unstable and is degraded by carbondioxide absorbants (sodalime) to a metabolite that can cause nephrotoxicity.

2. Sevoflurane undergoes biotransformation (about 3%) in the liver to release fluoride ions which can cause nephrotoxicity.

If the above disadvantages of sevoflurane are overcome, we would have found an ideal anaesthetic.

Oxygen in anaesthesia

Oxygen should be added routinely to inhalational agents to protect against hypoxia (especially when halothane or nitrous noxide is used). When O_2 is not available, ether is the safest agent for maintenance of anaesthesia.

INTRAVENOUS ANAESTHETICS

Intravenous anaesthetics allow an extremely rapid induction because the blood concentration can be raised rapidly - in one arm - brain circulation (~11 sec) there is loss of consciousness. But when we administer anaesthetics intravenously, there is no channel for quick elimination like the lungs. Moreover, elimination of inhaled anaesthetics can be hastened by inducing hyperventilation, while this is not possible with intravenous anaesthetics.

Hence IV anaesthetics are used for induction because of the rapid onset of action and anaesthesia is maintained by an inhalational agent.

INDUCING AGENTS

Thiopentone sodium is an ultrashort - acting barbiturate which when administered IV, rapidly induces hypnosis and anaesthesia without analgesia. It is highly water soluble. Extravasation of the solution produces intense pain, necrosis and gangrene.

On IV inj (3 - 5 mg/kg as a 2.5% solution) thiopentone sodium produces unconsciousness in 20-30 sec. Duration of action is 4 - 7 minutes. It is highly lipid soluble and gets rapidly redistributed in the body tissues.

Advantages

Quick onset of action; induction is smooth, rapid and pleasant.

Disadvantages

*   Not a good analgesic nor muscle relaxant.

*   It cannot be used alone as the dose required results in delayed recovery, respiratory and circulatory depression.

*   A short period of apnoea occurs. Overdosage results in profound respiratory depression. Artificial ventilation has to be given.

*   Severe hypotension, hiccoughs may occur. Hypotension should be treated with plasma expanders, head low position and pressor agents.

*   Should not be mixed with acidic drugs because barbiturates may be precipitated.

Uses

Thiopentone sodium is used for induction of anaesthesia before to administration of inhalational anaesthetics

Precautions Equipment for resuscitation should be ready.

Methohexitone is similar to thiopentone but is more potent. It is not preferred due to toxicity.

Propofol is an oily liquid; quick induction (30 sec) and recovery (4 min) are possible from a single dose. It is used for induction and maintenance for short procedures of up to 1 hour duration. The effect of a single dose is terminated by distribution. Propofol can be used for total IV anaesthesia as continuous infusion or intermittent injection. It has antiemetic property which is an added advantage. Because of rapid recovery, it is particularly preferred for 'day - cases' when the patient has to be discharged the same day. Propofol can be safely used in pregnant women.

Etomidate is similar to thiopental but it differs in that -

*   it is rapidly metabolised - as a result recovery is fast.
*   less cardiovascular and respiratory depression.

But etomidate may cause -

*   involuntary movements and excitatory effects during induction.
*   pain at the injection site.
*   adrenocortical suppression on long term use.

Etomidate is preferred for induction in patients with cardiovascular problems.

DISSOCIATIVE ANAESTHESIA

Ketamine is a phencyclidine derivative. In anaesthetic doses it produces a trans - like state known as *dissociative anaesthesia* characterised by intense analgesia, immobility, amnesia and a feeling of dissociation from ones own body and surroundings with or without actual loss of consciousness.

Mechanism of action Ketamine acts by blocking the NMDA receptor which is an excitatory aminoacid receptor. (Fig 22.1, Page 160)

Ketamine is highly lipid soluble and gets rapidly distributed into highly perfused organs and then redistributed to less vascular structures. Ketamine hydrochloride given 1 - 2 mg/kg slow IV or 10 mg/kg IM produces dissociative anaesthesia within 3 - 5 min which lasts for 10 - 15 min after a single injection. Amnesia lasts for 1-2 hr. Premedication with atropine is needed. Return to 'consciousness' is gradual. Delirium with vivid dreams may be accompanied. If diazepam is administered pre and postoperatively, delirium can be avoided. Heart rate, CO and BP are increased due to sympathetic stimulation.

Advantages

- Provides profound analgesia and amnesia; can be used as the sole agent for minor procedures

- Respiration is not depressed, does not induce hypotension

- Less likely to induce vomiting

- Pharyngeal and laryngeal reflexes are only slightly affected

- It is of particular value in children and poor-risk patients and also in asthmatic patients since it does not induce bronchospasm.

Disadvantages

- Hallucinations, delirium, involuntary movements and nystagmus may occur during recovery if used as a sole agent. Diazepam may be used as preanaesthetic medication

Drug	Main features	uses
Thiopental	• Fast onset of action • CV*and respiratory depression	For induction
Propofol	• Fast onset and recovery • Pain at injection site • CV and respiratory depression	Short procedures
Etomidate	• Fast onset and recovery • Less CV and respiratory depression • Involuntary movements during induction • Suppresses adrenal steroidogenesis • Pain at injection site	For induction particularly in patients with low cardiovascular reserve
Ketamine	• Slow onset • Good analgesia and amnesia • No respiratory depression, no hypotension • ↑ BP • Hallucinations and involuntary movements during recovery	Short procedures particularly in children.
Midazolam	• Slow onset and recovery • Less CV and respiratory depression	Short procedures like endoscopy, fracture reduction.
Fentanyl + Droperidol	• Slow onset and recovery • Profound analgesia	Short procedures

Table 23.1: Intravenous anaesthetics

CV= Cardiovascular

to prevent these symptoms.

- May be dangerous in hypertensives as it raises the BP.
- Ketamine increases cerebral blood flow and intracranial pressure.

Contraindications

Hypertension, CCF, cerebral haemorrhage, increased intracranial tension, psychiatric disorders and pregnancy before term.

Precautions

Pulse and BP should be closely monitored; during recovery patients must be undisturbed and under observation.

NEUROLEPTANALGESIA

A combination of a neuroleptic (droperidol) with an analgesic (fentanyl) is used.

Fentanyl is a short-acting (30-50 min) and potent opioid analgesic. (See page 216)

Droperidol is a rapidly acting, potent neuroleptic related to haloperidol.

When the combination is given IV, a state of neuroleptanalgesia is produced. This is characterised by quiescence, psychic indifference and intense analgesia without loss of consciousness. It lasts for 30-40 min. Fentanyl 0.05 mg + droperidol 2.5 mg/ml - 4 to 6 ml of the solution is infused IV over 10 min. Patient is drowsy but cooperative. Respiratory depression is present. There is a slight fall in BP and HR (vagal stimulation). During recovery EPS may be seen - due to droperidol. It is employed for endoscopies, burn dressing, angiographies and other diagnostic and minor surgical procedures.

Neuroleptanaesthesia

Addition of 65% N_2O + 35% O_2 to the above combination produces neuroleptanaesthesia.

BENZODIAZEPINES

Benzodiazepines like diazepam, lorazepam and midazolam are used to induce or supplement anaesthesia. They cause sedation, amnesia and reduce anxiety which are beneficial in such patients. BZDs may be employed alone in procedures like endoscopies, reduction of fractures, cardiac catheterisation and cardioversion. IV midazolam is particularly preferred as it is faster and shorter - acting, more potent, does not cause significant respiratory and cardiovascular depression and does not cause pain or irritation at the injection sites. BZDs are also used as preanaesthetic medication.

PREANAESTHETIC MEDICATION

Prior to anaesthesia, certain drugs are administered in order to make anaesthesia safer and more pleasant and is known as preanaesthetic medication. It is given in order to:

1. decrease anxiety
2. provide amnesia for the preoperative period
3. relieve preoperative pain if present
4. make anaesthesia safer
5. reduce side effects of anaesthetics
6. reduce gastric acidity.

To achieve the above purpose, more than one drug is required. An informative, supportive, preoperative visit by the anaesthesiologist is very much essential.

Sedative hypnotics

Antianxiety agents like benzodiazepines are used extensively as preanaesthetic medication. They reduce anxiety and produce sedation. Diazepam

5-10 mg is given orally. It also produces amnesia. Barbiturates are not preferred due to the disadvantages like respiratory depression.

Antihistamines

have sedative, antiemetic and anticholinergic properties and are useful, e.g. promethazine.

Antiemetics

Metoclopromide, domperidone or ondansetron may be used. Antihistamines with antiemetic properties may also be used.

Anticholinergic drugs

Some irritant anaesthetics like ether increase the salivary and respiratory secretions. The secretions from the oral cavity and trachea may creep into the larynx inducing laryngospasm. They may enter into the lungs causing aspiration pneumonia. This indicated the need for drugs that reduce secretions. Fortunately we now have less irritant anaesthetics and secretions are less of a problem. Atropine 0.6 mg IM or scopolamine 0.6 mg IM or glycopyrrolate 0.2mg IM can be used. Scopolamine produces more sedation.

Anticholinergics -

- reduce the secretions
- prevent bradycardia due to vagal stimulation
- prevent laryngospasm which is due to excessive secretions.

Glycopyrrolate

As compared to atropine, glycopyrrolate is longer acting, is a better antisialogogue and is less likely to cause significant tachycardia. It also produces less sedation than scopolamine.

Drugs that reduce acidity

General anaesthetics may induce vomiting. This is associated with an increased risk of aspiration into the respiratory tract because normal protective airway reflexes are blunted by anaesthetics. Aspiration of the acidic gastric contents into the lungs cause damage to the lungs. H_2 blockers like ranitidine decrease gastric acid secretion (See page 321) and are given on the night before surgery. Decrease in gastric secretions reduces the damage to lungs if aspiration occurs while on anaesthesia.

Gastrokinetic agents

Metoclopramide is a dopamine antagonist that promotes gastrointestinal motility and increases the tone of oesophageal end of the stomach. This speeds up gastric emptying. The combination of H_2 blocker + metoclopramide provides best protection against aspiration.

Opioids like morphine and pethidine reduce anxiety and apprehension, provide analgesia and reduce the dose of the anaesthetic required. But they depress respiration and may cause hypotension, postoperative constipation, and urinary retention; precipitateasthma and delay recovery.

Balanced anaesthesia

Since it is not possible to achieve ideal anaesthesia with a single drug, multiple drugs are employed to attain this - preanaesthetic medication, IV anaesthetics for induction, inhalational agents for maintenance, oxygen, skeletal muscle relaxants and analgesics. This is termed *balanced anaesthesia.*

24 | *Local Anaesthetics*

- Classification
- Chemistry
- Mechanism of action
- Actions
- Pharmacokinetics
- Adverse effects
- Individual compounds
- Uses of local anaesthetics

Local anaesthetics are drugs that block nerve conduction when applied locally to nerve tissue in appropriate concentrations. Their action is completely reversible. They act on every type of nerve fibre and can cause both sensory and motor paralysis in the innervated area. They act on axons, cell body, dendrites, synapses and other excitable membranes that utilize sodium channels as the primary means of action potential generation.

Cocaine was the first agent to be isolated by Niemann in 1860. Inspite of its addiction potential, cocaine was used for 30 years as a surface anaesthetic. In an effort made to improve the properties of cocaine, procaine was synthesized in 1905. It ruled the field for the next 50 years. In 1943, lignocaine was synthesized and it continues to dominate the field till today.

Classification of local anaesthetics (LAs) based on the route of administration and duration of action is as follows.

CLASSIFICATION

I. Injectable

1. *Short-acting*
   Procaine, chloroprocaine

2. *Intermediate-acting*
   Lignocaine, prilocaine

3. *Long-acting*
   Tetracaine (amethocaine), bupivacaine, dibucaine, ropivacaine, etidocaine.

174

II. Surface anaesthetics

Lignocaine, cocaine, tetracaine, benzocaine, oxethazaine.

Chemistry

Local anaesthetics are bases and consist of a hydrophilic amino group on one side and a lipophilic aromatic residue on the other, joined by an intermediate chain through an ester or amide linkage. Since ester links are more prone to hydrolysis than amide links, generally esters have a shorter duration of action. Depending on the linkage, LAs can be classified as:

Ester linked

Cocaine, procaine, tetracaine, benzocaine, chloroprocaine.

Amide linked

Lignocaine (Lidocaine), mepivacaine, bupivacaine, ropivacaine, etidocaine, prilocaine.

Since local anaesthetics are weak bases and the infected tissues have a low extracellular pH, LA ionise in such medium and a very low fraction of non-ionised LA is available for diffusion into the cell. Therefore, LAs are much less effective in infected tissues.

Mechanism of Action

Local anaesthetics prevent the generation and the conduction of nerve impulses (Fig 24.1). The primary mechanism of action is blockade of voltage-gated sodium channels.

Local anaesthetics diffuse through the cell membrane and bind to the voltage-sensitive sodium channels from the inner side of the cell membrane. They prevent the increase in permeability to Na^+ and gradually raise the threshold for excitation. With increasing concentration, impulse conduction slows, rate of rise of action potential (AP) declines, AP amplitude decreases and finally the ability to generate an AP is abolished. These result from binding of LA to more and more sodium channels. Thus it prevents the generation of an AP and its conduction.

Small nerve fibres are more susceptible as they present a greater surface area per unit volume. Thus smaller fibres are blocked first - autonomic fibres are blocked first followed by sensory fibres conducting pain, temperature sense, then touch, pressure and vibration sensations in the same order. This is called **'differential blockade'**. Sensory and motor fibres are equally sensitive. Non-myelinated fibres are blocked more readily than the myelinated.

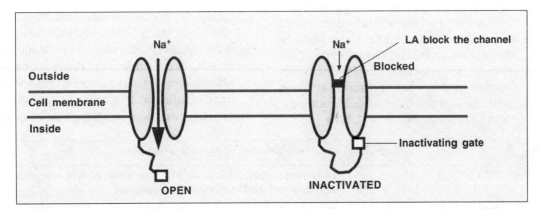

Fig 24.1: Mechanism of action of local anaesthetics. In the open state the Na^+ moves in and within milliseconds the channel is inactivated due to closure of the inactivating gate. LA block the sodium channels.

Addition of a vasoconstrictor like adrenaline (1:1,00,000 to 1: 2,00,000) or phenylephrine (1:20,000) :

1. prolongs the duration of action of LAs by slowing the rate of absorption from the site of administration.

2. reduces systemic toxicity of LAs since the absorption rate is reduced and as it gets absorbed, it gets metabolised.

ACTIONS

Systemic Actions

Depending on the concentration attained in the plasma, any LA can produce systemic effects. LAs interfere with the functions of all organs in which conduction or transmission of impulses occur. Thus CNS, autonomic ganglia, NMJ and all muscles are affected.

- **CNS** Local anaesthetics depress the cortical inhibitory pathway thereby allowing unopposed activity of excitatory components. This loss of inhibition is manifested as restlessness, tremors and may proceed to convulsions. This central stimulation is followed by generalised CNS depression and death may result from respiratory failure.

- **CVS** The primary site of action is the myocardium - lignocaine decreases excitability, conduction rate and force of contraction (quinidine like effects). They also cause arteriolar dilatation. Since procaine is short-acting, procainamide is used as an antiarrhythmic. Bupivacaine is more cardiotoxic than other LAs.

- **Smooth muscle** LAs depress contractions in the intact bowel. They also relax vascular and bronchial smooth muscles.

Pharmacokinetics

Local anaesthetics are rapidly absorbed from the mucous membranes and abraded skin. Rate of absorption is dependent on the vascularity of the area. Thus vasoconstriction decreases the absorption. Toxicity depends on the balance between absorption and metabolism, i.e. if it gets metabolised as it gets absorbed, then toxicity is less. Binding to tissues decreases the concentration in systemic circulation and thereby toxicity. Ester - linked LAs are rapidly hydrolysed by plasma pseudocholinesterase and in the liver. Amide linked LAs are metabolised by the liver microsomes by dealkylation and hydrolysis and are not effective orally (as antiarrhythmics). They undergo extensive first pass metabolism.

Adverse Effects (Table 24.1)

1. **Hypersensitivity reactions** - include skin rashes, dermatitis, asthma or rarely anaphylaxis. These reactions are more common with ester type of drugs. Ester type LA are metabolised to PABA derivatives. These are responsible for allergic reactions while with amides, allergy is rare. Intradermal sensitivity test should be done before using these drugs. Drugs including to manage such reactions should be kept ready. Moreover, allergy is most often due to the preservative methylparaben. Preparations that do not contain this preservative are now available.

TABLE 24.1: Adverse effects of local anaesthetics	
CNS	: Dizziness, confusion, anxiety, tremors, occasionally convulsions and respiratory depression
CVS	: Hypotension, bradycardia, arrhythmias
Hypersensitivity reactions	: Rashes, dermatitis, asthma, rarely anaphylaxis

2. **CNS** - Dizziness, auditory and visual disturbances, mental confusion, disorientation, anxiety, muscle tremors, convulsions and respiratory failure can result from large doses. Intravenous diazepam controls convulsions. In fact, these can be prevented by preanaesthetic administration of diazepam (1-2 mg/kg), especially if large doses are to be used.

3. **CVS** - Hypotension, bradycardia and arrhythmias may be encountered. Rarely cardiac arrest can occur.

4. **Local irritation** - can be seen with bupivacaine. Wound healing may be delayed.

INDIVIDUAL COMPOUNDS

A. Injectable (Table 24.2)

1. **Lignocaine** - is the most widely used LA. It is fast and long -acting. It is useful for all types of blocks. Maximum anaesthetic effect is seen in 2-5 minutes and lasts for 30-45 minutes. In contrast to other LAs, lignocaine causes drowsiness and mental clouding. Though it is a good corneal anaesthetic, it is not generally preferred because it causes irritation.

Lignocaine (XYCOCAINE) is available as 4% topical solution, 2% Jelly, 5% ointment, 1% and 2% injection, 5% for spinal anaesthesia, 10% lignocaine spray. Though lignocaine can be used on the eye for surface anasthesia, it is not preferred because it causes some irritation.

2. **Bupivacaine HCl** - is more potent and longer acting than lignocaine - it is widely used. But it can cause more cardiotoxicity than others. Injection 0.25-0.5% with or without adrenaline. **Levobupivacaine** HCl is a derivative of bupivacaine that seems to be less neurotoxic and less cardiotoxic than bupivacaine.

3. **Ropivacaine** - is similar to bupivacaine except that it is less cardiotoxic.

Drug	Preparation	Uses
TABLE 24.2: Preparations and uses of some local anaesthetics		
1. Tetracaine	1-2% ointment, eye drops, cream, powder 0.25, 0.5% inj	Topical, spinal anaesthesia
2. Lignocaine	2-4% drops, spray, jelly, ointment, cream, 1-10% Inj	Topical, infiltration, nerve block, spinal, epidural and IV regional anaesthesia
3. Benzocaine	1-2% dusting powder, 5% suppository, cream, gels, ointments, 20% spray	Topical anaesthesia
4. Oxethazaine	0.2% suspension	Topical anaesthesia (used in peptic ulcer)
5. Prilocaine	5% Cream, 4% Inj	Topical, nerve block anaesthesia
6. Dibucaine	0.5-1% Cream	Topical anaesthesia
7. Mepivacaine	1-3% Inj	Nerve block, epidural anaesthesia
8. Bupivacaine	0.25-0.75% Inj	Infiltration, nerve block, spinal, epidural anaesthesia
9. Ropivacaine	2-10% Inj	Infiltration, nerve block, spinal, epidural anaesthesia
10. Etidocaine	1% Inj	Epidural anaesthesia

4. Chloroprocaine HCl - potency is twice that of procaine and its toxicity is lower because of its more rapid metabolism.

5. Etidocaine HCl - its analgesic action lasts 2-3 times longer. It is used for epidural and all types of infiltration and regional anaesthesia.

6. Mepivacaine - action is more rapid in onset and more prolonged than that of lignocaine.

7. Prilocaine HCl - onset of action and duration are longer. Because of its toxicity, its use is restricted to dental procedures.

8. Cocaine - produces euphoria and is a drug of dependence and abuse. It is a surface anaesthetic. It is a protoplasmic poison and hence cannot be injected. Cocaine was used for ocular anaesthesia earlier. But it causes constriction of conjunctival vessels, clouding and sometimes corneal sloughing and is therefore not used to produce corneal anaesthesia. Cocaine is used topically for anaesthesia of upper respiratory tract. It has the advantage of being a vasoconstrictor and a local anaesthetic - both in one.

9. Procaine - was widely used once. But is now replaced by other agents. It is hydrolysed to PABA which interferes with the action of sulfonamides. It is rapidly absorbed following parenteral administration. It is ineffective when applied topically because it is poorly absorbed from the

mucous membranes - thus not useful as a surface anaesthetic.

10. Tetracaine (amethocaine) - is a PABA derivative and is 10 times more toxic and more active than procaine. It is used on the eye as 0.5% drops, ointments 0.5% and cream 1% for topical use. 0.25 to 0.5% injection is used for spinal anaesthesia.

B. Local anaesthetics used only on the eye

Benoxinate HCl - within 60 seconds of administration it produces corneal anaesthesia enough to perform tonometry.

Proparacaine HCl - produces little or no initial irritation - 0.5% ophthalmic solution is used.

C. Local anaesthetics used on the skin and mucous membranes

LAs used on the skin and mucous membranes are dibucaine, dyclonine hydrochloride and pramoxine hydrochloride. These drugs are effective when used topically in the symptomatic relief of anal and genital pruritus, poison ivy rashes, acute and chronic dermatoses. Dibucaine is the most potent, most toxic and longest-acting LA. It is available as cream and ointment.

D. Poorly Soluble Anaesthetic

These are too slowly absorbed to be toxic. They can be applied to wounds directly and ulcerated surfaces as they produce sustained anaesthetic effect, e.g. benzocaine. Benzocaine is a PABA derivative. It is poorly soluble in water because of which it remains at the site for a longer time and toxicity is low as absorption is poor. It is used topically to anaesthetise the skin and mucous membrane.

Corneal anaesthetics used clinically

Proparacaine	Benoxinate
Tetracaine	Lignocaine

USES OF LOCAL ANAESTHETICS

Local anaesthesia is the loss of sensation without the loss of consciousness or impairment of central control of vital functions. Depending on the site and technique of administration, LA can be:

Surface anaesthesia

Anaesthesia of mucous membrane of the eye, nose, mouth, tracheobronchial tree, oesophagus and genitourinary tract can be produced by direct application of the anaesthetic solution. Tetracaine 2%, lignocaine 2-10% are most often used. Phenylephrine (but not adrenaline as its penetration is poor) produces vasoconstriction on topical application and prolongs duration of action.

Anaesthesia is entirely superficial and does not extend to submucosal structures. But LAs are absorbed from mucous membranes and may result in systemic toxicity. Patient should be cautioned to expectorate the excess solution to avoid excess absorption. Local anaesthetics can also be used on abraded skin. Surface anaes thesia is useful -

1. On the eye
   a. for tonometry, surgery
   b. to remove foreign bodies from the cornea and conjunctiva
   c. for preoperative preparation.

2. Others
   Nasal lesions, stomatitis, sore throat, tonsillectomy, endoscopies, intubation, gastric ulcer, burns and proctoscopy.

An eutectic mixture containing 2.5% each of lignocaine and prilocaine at room temperature has a lower melting point than either of the drugs. This is emulsified and applied as a cream to anaesthetise the intact skin. The cream should be applied on the skin under an occlusive dressing and can produce anaesthesia upto a depth of 5mm. It can be used for procedures like venipuncture and skin graft harvesting.

Infiltration anaesthesia

Injection of a local anaesthetic solution directly into the tissue can be (i) superficial - only into the skin, or (ii) into deeper structures including intra-abdominal organs. Duration can be doubled by adrenaline (1:2,00,000). Adrenaline should not be used (i) around end arteries to avoid necrosis, and (ii) intracutaneously to avoid sloughing. Drugs used are lignocaine, procaine, bupivacaine.

Advantage

By using infiltration anaesthesia, it is possible to provide anaesthesia without disruption of normal bodily functions.

Disadvantage

In major surgeries - systemic toxicity due to local anaesthetic is likely as large amounts of the anaesthetic are required for such procedures.

Uses

For minor procedures like incisions, drainage of an abscess, excision, etc.

Field block

Subcutaneous injection of a LA solution proximal to the site to be anaesthetised, interrupts nerve transmission in the region distal to the injection. Sites such as forearm, scalp, anterior abdominal wall and lower extremity are used for field block. Knowledge of the relevant neuroanatomy is essential.

Advantage

With a small dose anaesthesia could be provided to a greater area.

Nerve block

Injection of a solution of a LA about/around individual peripheral nerves or nerve plexuses produces larger areas of anaesthesia with a smaller amount of the drug than the above techniques. Anaesthesia starts a few centimeters distal to the injection.

Nerve block anaesthesia is useful for:

1. blocks of brachial plexus for procedures on the arm (distal to deltoid).

2. intercostal nerve blocks to anaesthetise anterior abdominal wall.

3. cervical plexus block for surgery of the neck.

4. sciatic and femoral nerve blocks for surgeries distal to the knee.

5. blocks of nerves at wrist and ankle.

6. radial and ulnar nerve block at the elbow.

7. sensory cranial nerves block.

8. facial and lingual nerves block.

9. inferior alveolar nerve block for extraction of lower jaw teeth.

Onset of action is within 3 minutes with lignocaine. Duration depends on lipid solubility and protein binding. Anaesthesia lasts longer than by field block or infiltration techniques. Nerve blocks are done for tooth extraction, operations on the eye, limbs and in neuralgias.

Spinal anaesthesia (SA)

Local anaesthetic solution is injected into the subarachnoid space between L2 - 3 or L3 - 4 below the lower end of the spinal cord. The drug acts on nerve roots. Lower abdomen and lower limbs are anaesthetised and paralysed. The level of anaesthesia can be altered by the volume of injection, specific gravity of the solution and posture of the patient. Generally a hyperbaric solution (in 10% glucose) is injected. Iso and hypobaric solutions can also be given. Level of sympathetic block produced is 2 segments higher and motor paralysis 2 segments lower than sensory or cutaneous anaesthesia. Duration depends on the concentration, dose and the drug itself. Lignocaine, tetracaine, bupivacaine and ropivacaine are used for spinal anaesthesia.

Advantages

Safe, affords good analgesia and muscle relaxation and there is no loss of consciousness.

Keybox 24.1
Other Drugs with local anaesthetic property
• **Chlorpromazine**
• **Propranolol**
• **Quinine**
• **H_1 antihistamines**

In cardiac, pulmonary and renal diseases, SA may be preferred over general anaesthesia whenever possible.

Uses

Surgical procedures on the lower limb, pelvis, lower abdomen, obstetric procedures, Caesarean section and other operations are done on spinal anaesthesia.

Complications of SA

1. *Hypotension and bradycardia* - Sympathetic blockade results in venous pooling of the blood leading to decreased venous return, decreased cardiac output and hypotension.

2. *Respiratory paralysis* - Hypotension and ischaemia of the respiratory centre results in respiratory failure. Due to paralysis of the abdominal muscles; cough reflex is less effective resulting in stasis of respiratory secretions, leading to respiratory infections.

3. *Headache* due to seepage of CSF can be treated with analgesics.

4. *Cauda equina syndrome* is uncommon - control over bladder and bowel sphincters is lost because of damage to nerve roots.

5. *Sepsis* - resulting in meningitis

6. *Nausea and vomiting* - premedication can be given to prevent this.

Epidural Anaesthesia

LA is injected into the spinal extradural space. It acts on nerve roots while small amounts diffuse into SA space. It is technically more difficult and comparatively larger volumes of the anaesthetic are needed. After repeated injections tachyphylaxis may develop.

Advantages

1. Sensory blockade is 4 - 5 segments higher than motor blockade. This difference is useful for obstetric analgesia, as the mother has painless labour and can still cooperate in the process of labour and is conscious throughout.

2. As there is no risk of injecting into SA space, there are no chances of infection.

Intravenous Regional Anaesthesia

This type of anaesthesia is useful for rapid anaesthetization of an extremity. A rubber bandage is used to force the blood out of the limb (veins) and a tourniquet is applied to prevent the re-entry of the blood. A dilute solution of the local anaesthetic is then injected intravenously. It diffuses into extravascular tissues. Onset of anaesthesia is in 2 minutes. Because of the pain produced by the tourniquet, this type of anaesthesia is used for procedures lasting less than one hour. About 25% of the drug enters into the systemic circulation. This type of anaesthesia is commonly used on the upper limbs though it can also be used on the legs and the thighs.

25 *Sedative Hypnotics*

- **Benzodiazepines (BZD)**
  - **Mechanism of action**
  - **Pharmacokinetics**
  - **Adverse effects**
  - **Uses of BZDs**
- **Barbiturates**
  - **Classification**
  - **Mechanism of action**
  - **Pharmacological actions**
  - **Adverse reactions**
  - **Uses**
- **Newer agents**
- **Miscellaneous**
  - **Chloral hydrate**
  - **Paraldehyde**

Sedative is a drug that produces a calming or quietening effect and reduces excitement. It may induce drowsiness. **Hypnotic** is a drug that induces sleep resembling natural sleep. Both sedation and hypnosis may be considered as different grades of CNS depression.

All human beings need sleep. Approximately 1/3 rd of our life is spent in sleep.

Sleep can be classified into two types depending on the physiological characteristics -

1. NREM (Non-rapid eye movement) sleep

2. REM (Rapid eye movement) sleep.

Throughout the night, NREM and REM sleep cycles repeat alternately for brief periods. NREM sleep is of 0 to 4 levels of depth.

Stages or levels of NREM sleep

Stage 0   - From lying down to falling asleep.

Stage 1   - Eye movements are less and the neck muscles relaxed.

Stage 2   - Eye movements are further reduced but the person is still easily arousable.

Stage 3   - Deeper sleep with minimum eye

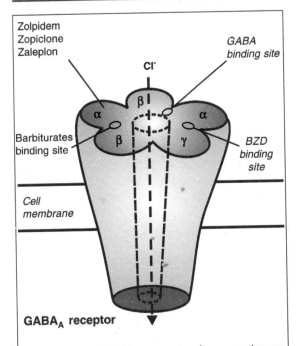

Zolpidem
Zopiclone
Zaleplon

GABA
binding site

Cl⁻

α

β

α

Barbiturates
binding site

β

γ

BZD
binding
site

Cell
membrane

GABA$_A$ receptor

Fig 25.1: GABA$_A$ receptor is a pentamer made of 5 subunits (2α, 2β and 1γ). BZDs, GABA, barbiturates and newer non-BZD agents bind to different sites on the GABA$_A$ receptor to facilitate the opening of the Cl⁻ channel. Binding of agonists opens the Cl⁻ ion channels. β carbolines bind to the BZD receptors and produce opposite effects (inverse agonists).

movement eye movement and not easily arousable.

Stage 4   - Slow wave sleep which is the deepest level of sleep. In this stage the metabolic rate is the lowest and growth hormone secretion is highest.

These stages of NREM alternate with REM sleep (which is associated with dreaming) throughout the night for brief periods.

Insomnia is sleeplessness. Since centuries man has sought the help of drugs and other remedies for insomnia.

CLASSIFICATION

1. **Benzodiazepines**

   Long-acting (24-48 hrs)

       Diazepam, Chlordiazepoxide

       Clonazepam, Flurazepam

       Chlorazepate, Clobazam

   Short-acting (12 - 24 hrs)

       Temazepam, Lorazepam

       Oxazepam, Nitrazepam

       Alprazolam, Halazepam.

   Ultra short acting (< 6 hrs)

       Triazolam, Midazolam

2. **Newer agents**

       Zolpidem, Zopiclone, Zaleplon

3. **Barbiturates**

       Phenobarbitone,

       Mephobarbitone

       Pentobarbitone, Secobarbitone

       Thiopentone, Hexobarbitone

4. **Miscellaneous**

       Paraldehyde, Chloral hydrate

       Glutethimide, Meprobamate

BENZODIAZEPINES (BZD)

Chlordiazepoxide was the first BZD to be introduced into clinical medicine in 1961 and since then about 2000 BZDs have been synthesized, of which 35 are now in clinical use.

Pharmacological actions

The most important actions of BZDs are on the CNS and include.

1. Sedation and hypnosis
2. Reduction in anxiety

3. Anaesthesia
4. Muscle relaxation
5. Anticonvulsant effects
6. Amnesia.

Sedation and hypnosis

BZDs produce a calming effect. They hasten the onset of sleep. At slightly higher doses they induce sleep (hypnosis) and increase the duration of sleep. The stage 2 NREM sleep is prolonged while the duration of REM sleep is decreased. But the suppression of REM sleep is very little with BZD when compared to other sedative hypnotics. The quality of sleep resembles natural sleep more closely when compared to other older hypnotics. Tolerance develops to this effect gradually after about 1-2 week of use.

Anxiolytic or antianxiety effects

BZDs reduce anxiety and aggression and produce a calming effect. Alprazolam has additional antidepressant properties.

Anaesthesia

BZDs produce CNS depression in a dose dependent manner. Sedation, hypnosis, stupor, anaesthesia and coma are the different grades of CNS depression. BZDs in higher doses than that used for sedation produce general anaesthesia. Midazolam is used as an IV anaesthetic. BZDs can be used as adjuvants to general anaesthetics.

But they carry the risk of prolonging respiratory depression.

Muscle relaxant action

BZDs reduce muscle tone by a central action. They depress the spinal polysynaptic reflexes which maintain the muscle tone. Generally anxiety is associated with an increased muscle tone and may be responsible for aches and pains in these patients. The muscle relaxation by BZDs adds to its beneficial effects in such patients.

Anticonvulsant effects

BZDs increase the seizure threshold and act as anticonvulsants. Diazepam is used intravenously for the treatment of status epilepticus. Other BZDs like clonazepam are used in the treatment of absence seizures and myoclonic seizures in children (See page 200).

Amnesia

BZDs produce anterograde amnesia i.e.loss of memory for the events happening after the administration of BZDs. This property is an advantage when BZDs are used in surgical procedures as the patient does not remember the unpleasant events.

Other actions

In higher doses BZDs decrease BP and increase heart rate and also depress respiration. Diazepam

Table 25.1	Effects of ligands on GABA$_A$ receptor BZD binding site (BZD receptor)		
	Agonist	Antagonist	Inverse agonist
• Ligand	BZD	Flumazenil	Beta carbolines
• Principle effects	Sedation, Hypnosis, Antianxiety, Anticonvulsant, Muscle relaxation	Blocks and reverses the BZD effects	Arousal, Anxiety, Increased muscle tone Convulsions

decreases nocturnal gastric acid secretion.

Mechanism of action

GABA is the principle inhibitory neurotransmittor of the central nervous system and it acts through GABA receptors. BZDs bring about their effects through GABA i.e they modulate the response to GABA by acting on $GABA_A$ receptors. Benzodiazepines bind to the $GABA_A$ receptor present in the neurons of the CNS. They bind (Fig. 25.1) at a site which is different from the GABA-binding site. They enhance the affinity of GABA for the receptor. GABA enhances chloride ion conductance through this receptor and this effect is potentiated or intensified by BZDs. BZDs bind to the receptor (BZ_1 subtype) and increase the frequency of chloride channel opening in response to GABA. This in turn leads to increased flow of chloride ions into the neurons, resulting in hyperpolarization of these neuronal membranes which, in turn, result in decreased synaptic transmission.

BZDs as hypnotics -

When compared to barbiturates:

1. BZDs induce sleep which more closely resembles natural sleep and has less hangover. The suppression of REM sleep is lesser when compared to barbiturates.

2. In hypnotic doses they do not affect respiration or cardiovascular functions.

3. BZDs have a higher safety margin and are safer than barbiturates even in overdoses. The respiratory depression in overdoses is milder.

4. In case of BZD overdosage, a specific BZD antagonist - flumazenil can be used to reverse the symptoms.

5. BZDs do not cause microsomal enzyme induction and therefore do not alter the blood levels of other drugs.

6. BZDs have lower abuse liability.

Because of the above advantages, BZDs are the most preferred sedative hypnotics.

Pharmacokinetics

There are significant pharmacokinetic diffe rences among BZDs due to their difference in lipid

Table 25.2: Dose and duration of action of some commonly used hypnotics.		
Hypnotic	**Hypnotic dose (mg.)**	**Duration of action (hrs.)**
Long acting		
Diazepam	5-10	24-48
Chlordiazepoxide	10-20	24-48
Nitrazepam	5-10	24
Alprazolam	0.25-0.5	24
Short acting		
Triazolam	0.125-0.25	<6
Midazolam	7.5-10	<6
Lorazepam	1-2	12-18
Temazepam	10-20	12-18
Newer agents		
Zolpidem	5-10	<4 <8
Zaleplon	5-20	<4
Zopiclone	7.5-10	<4

solubility. BZDs are completely absorbed on oral administration. Intramuscular absorption is slow - hence oral route is preferred. They are extensively bound to plasma proteins, metabolised in the liver by glucuronide conjugation. Many BZDs particularly long acting ones are converted to metabolites which are active-thereby prolonging their effects.

Adverse effects   *ADR*

BZDs are generally well tolerated. The common side effects include drowsiness, confusion, amnesia, lethargy, weakness, headache, blurred vision, ataxia, day time sedation and impaired motor coordination such as driving skills - therefore, while on BZDs driving should be avoided.

In some patients it may cause paradoxical irritability and anxiety.

Tolerance and dependence

Both tolerance and dependence liability are less with BZDs as compared to barbiturates. Patients develop tolerance to the sedative effects very slowly.

The withdrawal symptoms are mild and slow in onset because of the longer plasma half-life of most BZDs, but they may be abrupt and more intensive with short-acting agents. Withdrawal symptoms include anxiety, nervousness, tremor, dizziness and anorexia. When given to a pregnant mother during labour, BZDs cause hypotonia and respiratory depression in the neonate.

Acute overdosage

BZD overdosage induces sleep but the respi ratory depression is mild. Hence BZDs are safe and the availability of a specific antagonist-flumazenil- makes it safer to use BZDs because poisoning can be treated.

Uses of BZDs

1. **Insomnia** When drugs are to be used to treat insomnia, BZDs are the agents of choice. Lorazepam, oxazepam, temazepam, nitrazepam or triazolam may be used.

2. **In anxiety states** BZDs are the most commonly used anxiolytics for the treatment of anxiety states and anxiety neuroses (See page 247). Any of the BZDs except the ultra short acting ones may be used.

3. **As anticonvulsants** IV diazepam is the drug of choice in the treatment of status epilepticus. Clonazepam or clobazam are used as an adjuncts with other antiepileptic drugs (See page 200).

4. **Muscle relaxant** BZDs are centrally acting muscle relaxants used in chronic muscle spasm and spasticity.

5. **As preanaesthetic medication** - for their sedation, amnestic and anxiolytic effects BZDs are useful (See page 173).

6. **General anaesthesia** - IV midazolam is used as an intravenous anaesthetic. BZDs are also used to suppliment anaesthesia. (See page 172)

7. **During alcohol withdrawal** - BZDs are useful in patients during withdrawal of alcohol or other sedative-hypnotics and opioids.

BENZODIAZEPINE ANTAGONIST

Flumazenil is a BZD receptor antagonist which competes with BZDs for the receptor and blocks the effects of BZD. Given intravenously flumazenil is rapid and short acting. It may rarely induce seizures.

Uses

1. To reverse BZD sedation/anaesthesia

2. In BZD overdosage.

NEWER AGENTS

The Newer agents zolpidem, zopiclone and zaleplon are sedative hypnotics.

- They are not BZDs but produce their effects by binding to the $GABA_A$ receptors and facilitate the inhibitory actions of GABA. (Fig 25.1)

- The modification of sleep pattern is negligible in therapeutic doses.

- The risk of dependence and tolerance is lower than with BZDs.

- These newer agents are used for short periods to treat insomnia.

- They are all rapid and short acting agents and produce minimum hangover.

- Their actions are blocked by flumazenil.

Zolpidem

Zolpidem is a good hypnotic but has weak anticonvulsant, anxiolytic and muscle relaxant effects.

Zolpidem does not suppress deep sleep (stages 3 and 4 NREM sleep) and the suppression of REM sleep is negligible. It is short acting (t½-2 hrs.) but the effects on sleep continue for a longer time even after stopping zolpidem. The duration of sleep is 8 hrs after a single dose.

It is well absorbed from the gut and metabolized in the liver. Dose should be reduced in hepatic dysfunction.

Adverse effects include dizziness and diarrhoea.

Zaleplon

Zaleplon is rapidly absorbed from the gut and has a short t½ of about 1 hour. It is metabolised in the liver both by microsomal and non - microsomal enzymes. It has the advantages that withdrawal symptoms are very mild after stopping it and no tolerance develops. It has rapid onset but short duration of action. No significant side effects are reported in therapeutic doses.

Uses

Because zaleplon has a rapid onset of action, it is useful in patients who require a long time to fall asleep (long sleep latency). Duration of sleep is not much prolonged with zaleplon.

Zopiclone

Zopiclone is another new hypnotic. Its actions resemble those of BZDs. Zolpiclone binds to the $GABA_A$ receptor (Fig 25.1) and potentiate, the effects of GABA. It does not suppress REM sleep and prolongs deep sleep (stages 3 and 4 NREM)

Adverse effects include dryness of mouth, metallic taste; higher doses can cause impaired psychomotor performance.

BARBITURATES

Barbiturates are derivatives of barbituric acid and were the largest group of hypnotics in clinical use until the 1960s.

Classification

Barbiturates can be classified based on their duration of action as:

Long-acting
Phenobarbitone, Mephobarbitone

Short-acting
Pentobarbitone, Butobarbitone

Ultrashort-acting
Thiopentone, Hexobarbitone, Methohexitone

Mechanism of Action

Barbiturates bind to a specific site on the GABA receptor Cl⁻ channel complex (which is different from the BZD binding site). They facilitate inhibitory neurotransmission by prolonging the duration of opening of the chloride ion channels by GABA and hyperpolarise the neural membrane. At high concentrations barbiturates directly enhance the chloride conductance i.e - by a GABA - mimetic effect.

Table 25.3 Other drugs that can produce sedation	
• Most antipsychotics	• Alcohol
• Most antidepressants	• Reserpine
• Some antihistamines	• Opioids
• Clonidine	• Methyldopa
• Most antiepileptics	

Pharmacological Actions

CNS

Barbiturates cause depression of all excitable tissues of which CNS is the most sensitive.

Sedation and hypnosis: In hypnotic doses, barbiturates induce sleep and prolong the duration of sleep. The REM-NREM sleep cycle is altered with decreased duration of REM and prolonged NREM sleep. On waking up there is some hangover with headache and residual sedation.

Barbiturates reduce anxiety, impair short-term memory and judgement. They can produce euphoria and are drugs of addiction while some people may experience dysphoria. Barbiturates produce hyperalgesia (increased sensitivity to pain). Therefore barbiturates, when given as hypnotics for a patient in pain may be more troublesome than being of any benefit.

Anaesthesia: In higher doses barbiturates produce general anaesthesia. The ultra short-acting barbiturates are used intravenously for this effect.

Anticonvulsant effects: All barbiturates have anticonvulsant action. Phenobarbitone and mephobarbitone have specific anticonvulsant activity in subhypnotic doses and are used in the treatment of epilepsy.

Respiratory system

Barbiturates cause significant depression of respiration. High doses cause profound respiratory depression and also bring about a direct paralysis of the medullary respiratory centre.

Cardiovascular system

Hypnotic doses of barbiturates produce a slight reduction in blood pressure and heart rate as seen during natural sleep.

Toxic doses of barbiturates produce a significant fall in BP due to direct decrease in myocardial contractility and vasomotor centre depression.

Skeletal muscles

Higher doses of barbiturates depress the excitability of the neuromuscular junction.

Pharmacokinetics

Barbiturates are well-absorbed and widely distributed in the body. The highly lipid soluble barbiturates like thiopentone have a fast onset of action while duration of action is short due to redistribution into adipose tissues. Barbiturates are metabolised in the liver. They are hepatic microsomal enzyme inducers. The metabolites are excreted in urine.

Adverse reactions

Hangover - due to residual depression of the CNS may be accompanied by nausea, vomiting, vertigo and diarrhoea. Distortions of mood, impaired judgement and fine motor skills may be evident. Barbiturates may cause excitement and irritability in some patients particularly children.

Barbiturates cause respiratory depression and in the presence of respiratory disorders even the hypnotic doses of barbiturates can cause serious respiratory depression. Hypersensitivity reactions like skin rashes, swelling of the eyelids and lips and rarely exfoliative dermatitis may be seen.

Barbiturates are contraindicated in porphyrias because they increase porphyrin synthesis.

Tolerance and dependence On repeated administration, tolerance develops to the effects of barbiturates.

Development of both psychological and physical dependence to barbiturates make them one of the drugs with abuse liability. Withdrawal symptoms include anxiety, restlessness, abdominal cramps, hallucinations, delirium and convulsions.

Acute barbiturate poisoning

The fatal dose of phenobarbitone is 6-10 g. Manifestations include respiratory depression with slow and shallow breathing, hypotension, skin eruptions, cardiovascular collapse and renal failure.

Treatment There is no specific antidote. The measures include:

1. Gastric lavage followed by administration of activated charcoal to prevent further absorption of barbiturates.

2. Artificial ventilation and oxygen administration.

3. General supportive measures like maintenance of BP, patent airway, adequate ventilation and oxygen administration.

4. Forced alkaline diuresis with sodium bicarbonate, a diuretic and IV fluids will hasten the excretion of long-acting barbiturates through the kidneys since they are acidic drugs

5. Haemodialysis should be done especially if there is renal failure.

Uses

Because of respiratory depression and abuse liability, barbiturates are generally not preferred.

1. *Sedation and hypnosis* Benzodiazepines are preferred to barbiturates as sedative hypnotics.

2. *Anaesthesia* Thiopentone sodium is used IV for the induction of general anaesthesia.

3. *Preanesthetic medication* Barbiturates were used earlier for the sedative-hypnotic property, but are not preferred now.

4. *Antiepileptic* Phenobarbitone is used as an antiepileptic (See page 198).

5. *Neonatal jaundice* Phenobarbitone is a microsomal enzyme inducer because of which it enhances the production of glucuronyl transferase-the enzyme required for metabolism and excretion of bilirubin. It therefore helps in the clearance of jaundice in the neonates.

MISCELLANEOUS

Chloral hydrate is used as an alternative to BZD. It has a bad taste and is an irritant - causes nausea and vomiting. It produces hypnosis without affecting respiratory and cardiovascular functions.

Meprobamate has sedative and antianxiety properties but is now not recommended. It produces respiratory depression, ataxia and is a drug of abuse. Not preferred now.

Paraldehyde is a colourless, transparent, pungent, inflammable liquid. It is an irritant and can dissolve plastic - cannot be given by a plastic syringe. It is a good hypnotic causing little hangover. It can be given rectally, intramuscularly or orally.

Paraldehyde also has anticonvulsant properties.

Uses

1. As anticonvulsant in status epilepticus particularly in children; tetanus and eclampsia.

2. Hypnotic - rarely used.

26 Alcohols

- **Ethyl alcohol (Ethanol)**
  - Actions
  - Mechanism of action
  - Pharmacokinetics
  - Uses
  - Acute alcoholic intoxication

- **Disulfiram**

- **Methyl alcohol (Methanol)**

ETHYL ALCOHOL (Ethanol)

Ethyl alcohol is a monohydroxy alcohol manufactured by fermentation of sugars. It is a colourless, volatile, inflammable liquid. The ethanol content of various alcoholic beverages ranges from 4-55%.

Actions

1. Local

On topical application, ethanol evaporates quickly and has a cooling effect. It is an astringent - precipitates surface proteins and hardens the skin. 40-50% alcohol is rubefacient and counter irritant. Alcohol is also an antiseptic. At 70%, it has maximum antiseptic properties, which decrease above that. It is not effective against spores.

2. CNS

Alcohol is a CNS depressant. Small doses cause euphoria, relief of anxiety and loss of social inhibitions. Moderate doses impair muscular coordination and visual acuity making driving dangerous. With higher doses mental clouding, impaired judgement, drowsiness and loss of self control result. High doses cause stupor and coma. Death is due to respiratory depression.

Alcohol may precipitate convulsions in epileptics. Tolerance develops on long-term use.

3. CVS

The actions are dose dependent. Small doses cause cutaneous vasodilation resulting in flushing and feeling of warmth. Large doses cause hypotension due to depression of myocardium and vasomotor centre.

4. GIT and liver

Alcohol is an irritant - increases gastric secretion and produces vasodilation and warmth. It is an appetizer. Chronic alcoholism results in peptic ulcer.

Chronic consumption of moderate amounts of alcohol results in accumulation of fat in the liver, liver enlargement, followed by fatty degeneration and cirrhosis.

Alcohol induces microsomal enzymes.

5. Other effects

Though alcohol is called an aphrodisiac, this effect could be due to loss of inhibition. Low doses taken over a long time increases HDL and lowers LDL cholesterol. Alcohol is a diuretic ($^{-}$ADH secretion). It interferes with folate metabolism and may cause megaloblastic anaemia. Though alcohol causes a feeling of warmth, heat loss is increased due to vasodilation and should not be used for 'warming up' in cold surroundings. Food value is 7 calories/gram.

Mechanism of action

Ethanol acts by -

1. Inhibiting central neuronal nicotinic acetylcholine receptors

2. Inhibiting excitatory NMDA and kainate receptor functions.

3. Promoting the function of 5 HT_3 receptors.

4. Ethanol also influences many ion channels including K^+ channels.

Pharmacokinetics

Alcohol is rapidly absorbed from the stomach and is metabolised in the liver by dehydrogenases (See Fig. 26.1).

Metabolism follows zero order kinetics - a constant amount is metabolised per unit time, i.e. about 10 ml absolute alcohol is metabolised per hour. It is excreted through kidneys and lungs.

Drug interactions

1. Alcohol potentiates other CNS depressants including hypnotics, opioids and antipsychotics.

2. Sulfonylureas, metronidazole and griseofulvin have disulfiram like effects on alcohol consumption.

3. Alcohol is an enzyme inducer.

Uses

1. *Antiseptic* - 70% alcohol is applied topically.

2. *Bed sores* When rubbed onto the skin, alcohol hardens the skin and prevents bed sores.

3. Alcoholic sponges are used for reduction of body temperature *in fevers*.

4. *Appetite stimulant* About 50 ml of 6-10% alcohol given before meals is an appetite

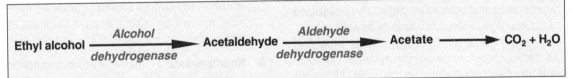

Fig. 26.1 Metabolism of ethanol

stimulant.

5. *Neuralgias* In severe neuralgias like trigeminal neuralgia, injection of alcohol around the nerve causes permanent loss of transmission and relieves pain.

6. *In methanol poisoning (See below)*

Acute alcoholic intoxication

Acute alcoholic intoxication causes severe gastritis, hypotension, hypo glycaemia, respiratory depression, coma and death.

Treatment measures include gastric lavage, airway maintenance, positive pressure ventilation and maintenance of fluid and electrolyte balance. Haemodialysis is needed in severe intoxication.

Chronic alcoholism

Chronic alcoholism causes dependence. Wernicke's encephalopa thy, Korsakoff's psychosis, tremors, cirrhosis of liver, hypertension and cardiomyopathy can occur. In addition, nutritional deficiencies such as polyneuritis, anaemia and pellagra can occur. In pregnant women, alcohol is teratogenic. Even moderate drinking during pregnancy can produce fetal alcohol syndrome with manifestations like low IQ, microcephaly, growth retardation and facial anomalies. It can also cause stillbirths and abortions.

DISULFIRAM

Disulfiram inhibits the enzyme aldehyde dehydrogenase. If alcohol is consumed after taking disulfiram, acetaldehyde accumulates and within a few minutes it can produce flushing, throbbing headache, nausea, vomiting, sweating, hypotension and confusion - called **the antabuse reaction,** due to accumulation of acetaldehyde. The effect lasts for 7-14 days after stopping disulfiram. Therefore the person develops aversion to alcohol and often gives up the habit. However the willingness on the part of the person to give

up the habit goes a long way in the success of this aversion therapy. The reactions can sometimes be very severe and therefore treatment should be given in a hospital.

Other drugs that cause antabuse reaction are metronidazole, chlorpropamide, tolbutamide, griseofulvin, cephalosporins and phenylbutazone.

Contraindications Patients with liver disease, patients physically dependent on alcohol.

Drugs used in alcohol dependence

Alcohol dependence is a common social evil which is difficult to treat.

Several drugs are tried in chronic alcoholism

1. **Disulfiram** is used to make alcohol consumption an unpleasant experience so that the person gives up drinking. (see above)

2. **Benzodiazepines** to reduce the symptoms of alcohol withdrawal - benzodiazepines relieve symptoms like anxiety and insomnia.

3. **Clonidine** an α_2 receptor agonist reduces the release of sympathetic neurotransmitters while propranolol blocks the effects of sympathetic overactivity like tremors and tachycardia.

4. **Naltrexone** is an orally effective opioid antagonist which has been thought to be useful in alcohol withdrawal. It is given in the dose of 50mg once daily. Some studies have shown naltrexone to reduce alcohol craving and 'relapse' of heavy drinking. Naltrexone and disulfiram should not be given concurrently as both can cause hepatotoxicity - moreover, chronic alcoholics are likely to have an already damaged liver. Nalmefene can also be used in place of naltrexone.

5. **Acamprosate** a NMDA receptor antagonist has been found to be useful in preventing relapse of heavy drinking and in achieving

alcohol abstinance.

6. **Ondansetron** a $5HT_3$ antagonist antiemetic has been shown to reduce alcohol consumption and is being evaluated for use in alcohol withdrawal.

METHYL ALCOHOL (METHANOL, WOOD ALCOHOL)

Methanol is used to denature ethyl alcohol. It has no therapeutic value. Ingestion results in methanol poisoning. Methanol is converted to formaldehyde - catalysed by alcohol dehydr ogenase; formaldehyde is converted to formic acid by the action of aldehyde dehydrogenase (Fig. 26.2). Toxic effects are due to formic acid.

Manifestations of toxicity are vomiting, headache, vertigo, severe abdominal pain, hypotension, delirium, acidosis and coma. Formic acid has affinity for optic nerve and causes retinal damage resulting in blindness. There are reports of even 15 ml of methanol causing blindness. Death is due to respiratory failure.

Treatment

1. *Correction of acidosis* As acidosis hastens retinal damage, immediate correction of acidosis with IV sodium bicarbonate infusion helps in preventing blindness.

2. *Protect eyes* Patient should be kept in a dark room to protect the eyes.

3. *Gastric lavage* should be given.

Keybox 26.1

Some drugs that can precipitate disulfiram like reaction

Metronidazole
Sulfonylureas
Griseofulvin
Some Cephalosporins
Phenylbutazone
Nitrofurantoin

---

4. *BP and ventilation* must be maintained.

5. *Ethyl alcohol* should be given immediately. It competes with methanol for alcohol dehydrogenase, because of its higher affinity for alcohol dehydrogenase. It thus slows the metabolism of methanol and prevents the formation of toxic metabolites. A loading dose of 0.6g/Kg is followed by an infusion of 10g/hour.

6. *Antidote* **Fomepizole** specifically inhibits the enzyme alcohol dehydrogenase and thereby prevents the formation of toxic metabolites - formaldehyde and formic acid. Fomepizole is considered the antidote in methanol poisoning. It has the advantage over alcohol that it does not cause any intoxication by itself.

7. *Haemodialysis* should be started at the earliest possible to enhance the removal of methanol.

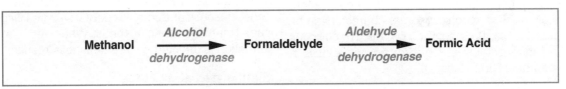

Fig. 26.2 Metabolism of methanol

27 *Antiepileptics*

- **Types of epilepsy**
- **Antiepileptics**
  - **Classification**
  - **Mechanism of action**
- **Phenytoin**
- **Phenobarbitone**
- **Carbamazepine**
- **Ethosuximide**
- **Valproic acid**
- **Benzodiazepines**
- **Newer antiepileptics**
- **Treatment of epilepsies**

Epilepsy is a common neurological abnormality that affects about 0.5-1% of the population. Epilepsy is a chronic disorder characterised by recurrent seizures often accompanied by episodes of unconsciousness and/or amnesia. It is a disorder of brain function.

Seizure indicates a transient alteration in behaviour because of disordered firing of groups of brain neurons. Such discharges may spread to other parts of the brain to different extents. In most of the cases, the cause is not known. It may be due to various reasons including trauma during birth process, head injury, childhood fevers, brain tumors, meningitis or drug induced.

TYPES OF EPILEPSY

Seizures have been classified into partial and generalised seizures.

Partial seizures
Partial seizures account for about 60% of all epilepsies and begin focally in the cortex.i.e.they involve focal brain regions. It is classified as simple partial in which there is no impairment of consciousness and complex partial seizures with impairment of consciousness. When reticular formation is affected unconsciousness results.

Simple partial seizures
There is no impairment of consciousness. The

194

manifestation depends on the site in the cortex that is activated by the seizure, e.g. if the motor cortex representing the right thumb is involved, there is recurrent contractions of the right thumb. If the sensory area representing the left palm is involved, there is numbness or paresthesia of the left palm. This type of seizures lasts for 20-60 seconds.

Complex partial seizures

Complex partial seizures are the most common types of epilepsy. This is characterised by purposeless movements like lipsmacking, hand wringing or swallowing that lasts for 30 sec to 2 minutes. Consciousness is impaired and may be preceded by an *aura.*

Partial with secondarily generalised seizures

Simple or complex partial seizure may evolve into a generalised seizure.

Generalised seizures

Generalised seizures account for 40% of all epilepsies and is usually of genetic aetiology. Generalised seizures affect the whole brain. It may be:

Absence seizures (Petitmal)

In this, there is a sudden onset of impaired consciousness associated with staring. The person stops all on-going activities and the episode lasts for a brief period usually less than 30 sec.

Myoclonic seizures involve a sudden, brief, shock like contraction of muscles. It may be limited to a part of the body or may affect the whole body.

Atonic seizures (Drop attacks)

Atonic seizures are characterised by sudden loss of postural tone and the head may drop for a few seconds or the person may drop to the ground for no obvious reasons.

Tonic-clonic seizures (Grand mal epilepsy)

Tonic-clonic seizures are characterised by sudden loss of consciousness followed by sustained contraction of muscles throughout the body (known as tonic phase), lasting for 1 minute and then, a series of jerks, i.e. periods of muscle contraction alternating with periods of relaxation (clonic phase) lasting for 2 - 4 minutes follow. CNS depression then occurs and the person goes into

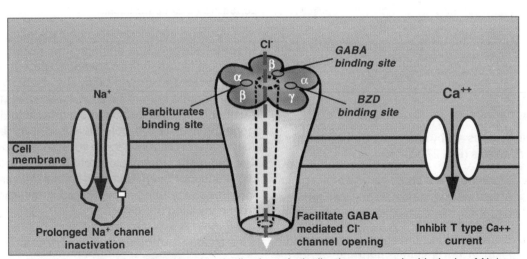

Fig 27.1: Mechanisms of action of antiepileptics. Antiepileptics may act by blockade of Na^+ channels, by facilitating GABA activity or by blockade of Ca^{++} current.

sleep. Injury may occur during the convulsive episode.

Status epilepticus

Status epilepticus is continuous or recurrent seizures of any variety without recovery of consciousness between the attacks.

ANTIEPILEPTICS

Antiepileptics can be classified as follows -

Classification

Hydantoins	Phenytoin, mephenytoin
Barbiturates	Phenobarbitone, mephobarbitone
Deoxybarbiturate	Primidone
Iminostilbene	Carbamazepine
Succinimide	Ethosuximide
GABA transaminase *inhibitors*	Valproic acid, vigabatrin
Benzodiazepines	Diazepam, clonazepam, lorazepam, clorazepate

Newer agents

GABA analogues	Gabapentin, vigabatrin, tiagabine.
Others	Lamotrigine, levetiracetam, felbamate, topiramate, zonisamide.

Mechanism of action of antiepileptics

Antiepileptics act by one or more of the following mechanisms (Fig. 27.1) -

- Blockade of Na^+ channels and prolongation of their inactive state delaying their recovery e.g. phenytoin, carbamazapine, lamotrigine.

- Blockade of low threshold Ca^{++} current (T-type) in the thalamic neurons - controls absence seizures e.g. ethosuximide.

- Enhancing GABA mediated inhibition
  - by acting on GABA receptors - e.g, Benzodiazepines
  - by inhibiting GABA metabolism - Valproic acid, Vigabatrin.
  - by blocking exitatory glutamate receptors
  - Topiramate and some drugs under investigation.

PHENYTOIN

Phenytoin (Diphenylhydantoin) was synthesized in 1908, but its anticonvulsant property was discovered only in 1938.

Pharmacological Actions

CNS Phenytoin has good antiseizure activity and is one of the most effective drugs against generalised tonic-clonic seizures and partial seizures. It brings about its effect without causing general depression of the CNS.

Mechanism of action

Phenytoin causes blockade of the voltage dependent sodium channels and stabilizes the neuronal membrane. It inhibits the generation of repetitive action potentials.

Voltage dependent Na^+channels enter an inactive stage after each action potential. Phenytoin blocks the Na^+ channels which are in an inactivated state and delay the recovery of these channels from inactivation. It decreases the number of channels which are available for the generation of action potentials and it inhibits membrane excitability of these voltage-dependent Na^+ channels. Phenytoin preferentially blocks high frequency firing (neurons in normal state have low frequency firing while in seizures, high-frequency firing occurs).

Pharmacokinetics

Phenytoin is poorly water-soluble - hence absorption is slow. Phenytoin is 90% bound to plasma proteins. Valproic acid competes with phenytoin for plasma protein binding sites and may result in phenytoin toxicity. It is metabolised in the liver initially by first order and later by zero order kinetics as the dose increases. Therefore monitoring of plasma concentration is useful. Phenytoin is an enzyme inducer. Dose - Table 27.1.

Adverse effects

Adverse effects depend on the dose, duration and route of administration.

1. Nausea, vomiting, epigastric pain, anorexia.
2. Nystagmus, diplopia, ataxia are common.
3. Gingival hyperplasia is more common in children on prolonged use.
4. Peripheral neuropathy.
5. Endocrine
   - Hirsutism, acne, coarsening of facial features.
   - Hyperglycaemia - as phenytoin inhibits insulin release.
   - ↓ release of ADH.
   - Osteomalacia, hypocalcaemia due to altered metabolism of vitamin D and inhibition of intestinal absorption of Ca^{++}
   - Phenytoin also reduces target tissue sensitivity to vitamin D.
6. Hypersensitivity - rashes, SLE, hepatic necrosis, lymphadenopathy and neutropenia. Idiosyncratic reactions including hepatic necrosis and SLE have been reported.
7. Megaloblastic anaemia - as phenytoin decreases absorption and increases excretion of folates.
8. Teratogenicity - when taken by the pregnant lady, phenytoin produces foetal hydantoin syndrome characterised by hypoplastic phalanges, cleft palate, harelip and microcephaly in the offspring.

Toxic doses - cerebellar and vestibular effects are prominent; drowsiness, delirium, confusion, hallucinations, altered behaviour and coma follow.

Drug	Dose	Trade name
Table 27.1: Therapeutic dose of antiepileptic drugs		
Phenytoin	100mg BD Children 5-8 mg/kg/day	EPILEPTIN EPTOIN
Carbamazepine	200-400mg TDS Children 15-30 mg/kg/day	TEGRETOL, CARBATOL
Phenobarbitone	60mg OD - TDS Children 3-6 mg/kg/day	GARDINAL
Ethosuximide	20-30 mg/kg/day	ZARONTIN
Valproic acid	200-500 mg TDS Children 15-30 mg/kg/day	VALPARIN
Clonazepam	0.5 - 5 mg TDS Children 0.01 - 0.2 mg/kg/day	CLONOTRIL
Clobazam	10-20mg HS Max 60mg HS	FRISIUM
Lamotrigine	50-300mg/day	LAMITOR
Gabapentin	300mg OD - TDS	NEURONTIN

Keybox 27.1

PHENYTOIN

- Blocks voltage dependent Na^+ channels
- Preferrably blocks high frequency firing that is seen in seizures.
- Blocks Na^+ channels in an inactivated state and delays their recovery.
- Main adverse effects include vestibular effects, G.I.disturbances; long term use results in gum hyperplasia, hirsutism and megaloblastc anaemia.
- It is teratogenic.
- Used in partial and generalised tonic-clonic seizures.

Uses

1. Generalised tonic-clonic seizures and partial seizures (not useful in absence seizures).

2. Status epilepticus - phenytoin is used by slow IV injection.

3. Trigeminal neuralgia - as an alternative to carbamazepine.

4. Cardiac arrhythmias: Phenytoin is useful in digitalis induced arrhythmias (See page 133).

Drug Interactions

- Phenytoin is an enzyme inducer. Given with phenobarbitone, both increase each other's metabolism. Also phenobarbitone competitively inhibits phenytoin metabolism.
- Carbamazepine and phenytoin enhance each other's metabolism.
- Valproate displaces protein bound phenytoin and may result in phenytoin toxicity.
- Cimetidine and chloramphenicol inhibit the metabolism of phenytoin resulting in toxicity.

- Antacids ↓ absorption of phenytoin.

Mephenytoin, ethotoin and phenacemide are congeners of phenytoin. Ethatoin can be used as an alternative in patients allergic to phenytoin. Adverse effects of ethotoin are milder. Phena cemide is used in patients with refractory partial seizures when other drugs fail. It is a highly toxic drug.

PHENOBARBITONE

Phenobarbitone (Chap 25) was the first effective antiepileptic drug to be introduced in 1912. It still remains one of the widely used drugs.

Antiepileptic actions

Phenobarbitone has specific antiepileptic activity and raises the seizure threshold. Primidone which is rarely used now is metabolised to phenobarbitone. Phenobarbitone is effective in tonic-clonic seizures and is ineffective in absence seizure.Though other barbiturates also have anticonvulsant effects, the dose required produce significant sedation.

Mechanism of action

Barbiturates enhance the inhibitory neurotransmission in the CNS by enhancing the activation of $GABA_A$ receptors and thus facilitating the GABA - mediated opening of chloride ion channels.

Pharmacokinetics

Oral absorption of phenobarbitone is slow but complete. About 50%is bound to plasma proteins. It is a microsomal enzyme inducer and can result in many drug interactions.

Adverse effects

Sedation is the most common side effect. Tolerance develops to some extent to sedation after prolonged use. Phenobarbitone, like phenytoin can also cause nystagmus, ataxia, megaloblastic anaemia and osteomalacia .Skin rashes and other hypersensitivity reactions can occur.

Uses

Phenobarbitone is one of the widely used antiepileptic and because of its efficacy and low cost. It is used in:

1. Generalised tonic - clonic seizures.

2. Partial seizures.

CARBAMAZEPINE

Carbamazepine is a tricyclic compound closely related to imipramine. It is one of the most commonly used antiepileptic drugs.

Antiseizure activity

Carbamazepine has good anti-seizure activity. Its mechanism of action and antiepileptic actions are similar to phenytoin, i.e. it blocks sodium channels.

Carbamazepine is also useful in the treatment of trigeminal neuralgia (severe pain along the distribution of the trigeminal nerve) and glossopharyngeal neuralgia. It is also found to be beneficial in mood disorders. Carbamazepine has mild antidiuretic effects.

Keybox 27.2
Newer antiepileptics:
• Gabapentin, vigabatrin, tiagabine, lamotrigine, levetiracetam, topiramate, felbamate, zonisamide.
• All are generally well tolerated except that felbamate can rarely cause aplastic anaemia, hepatitis.
• Presently they are recommended as add-on drugs in refractory partial seizures.

Pharmacokinetics

Absorption is slow and erratic; has a $t^1/_2$ of 10-30 hours. But it is a powerful microsomal enzyme inducer. Therefore after repeated administration, its $t^1/_2$ reduces to 15 hours due to autoinduction.

Adverse effects

Drowsiness, vertigo, ataxia, diplopia, blurring of vision, nausea, vomiting and dizziness are common. Driving is dangerous for patients on carbamazepine. It also causes water retention due to antidiuretic effects. Hyper-sensitivity reactions - like skin rashes may occur. Haematological toxicity includes leukopenia, thrombocytopenia and rarely agranulocytosis and aplastic anaemia. It is a teratogen. Its t1/2 reduces to 15 hrs due to autoinduction.

Uses

1. Generalised tonic clonic seizures (grand mal epilepsy).

2. Simple and complex partial seizures - especially temporal lobe epilepsy.

3. Trigeminal neuralgia and glossopharyngeal neuralgia - carbamazepine is the drug of choice for these neuralgias and has to be given for several months.

4. Carbamazepine is also found to be useful in chronic neuropathic pain and in tabetic pain.

5. Bipolar mood disorder - carbamazepine is used as an alternative to lithium as a mood stabilizer (See page 254).

Oxcarbazepine

Oxcarbazepine is similar to carbamazepine in action and uses. It has the following advantages over carbama zepine-fewer hypersensitivity reactions, milder induction of microsomal enzymes - hence fewer drug interactions. It has been tried as an alternative to carbamazepine in partial seizures.

ETHOSUXIMIDE

Ethosuximide is a succinimide. It raises the seizure threshold.

Mechanism of action

Ethosuximide reduces the low threshold calcium currents (T-currents) in the thalamic neurons. These T currents are thought to be responsible for absence seizures.

Pharmacokinetics

Absorption is complete on administration of oral dosage forms. It is metabolised in the liver.

Adverse effects

The most common adverse effects are nausea, vomiting, epigastric pain, gastric irritation and anorexia. These can be avoided by starting with a low dose and gradually increasing it. CNS effects like drowsiness, fatigue, lethargy, euphoria, dizziness, headache and hiccough are dose-related effects. Hypersensitivity reactions like rashes, urticaria, leukopenia, thrombocytopenia or pancytopenia have been reported.

Uses

Ethosuximide is the drug of choice for absence seizures.

VALPROIC ACID

Valproic acid (salt-sodium valproate) is a very effective antiepileptic drug useful in many types of epilepsies including absence seizures, partial and generalised tonic-clonic seizures.

Divalproex sodium is a combination of valproic acid and sodium valproate. The combination is said to have a better bioavailability and is better tolerated.

Mechanism of action

Valproic acid acts by multiple mechanisms.

1. It enhances the level of GABA by:
   - increasing the synthesis of GABA - by increased activity of GABA synthetase enzyme.
   - decreasing the metabolism of GABA - by inhibiting GABA transaminase enzyme.
2. Like phenytoin, valproic acid blocks the sodium channels.
3. Like ethosuximide valproate decreases low threshold Ca^{++} (T-currents in the thalamus).

Adverse effects

Gastrointestinal symptoms like nausea, vomiting, epigastric distress occur initially. Tremors, sedation, ataxia, rashes and alopecia are rare. Sodium valporate can cause hepatotoxicity in children below 2 years of age which can be fatal. Hepatotoxity is thought to be an idiosyncratic response. Though it is more likely to occur in children below 2 years of age who are also on other antiepileptics, hepatotoxicity can occur in patients of all age groups. Hence careful monitoring of liver functions is mandatory. Valporic acid should be avoided in patients with hepatic dysfunction.

Valproic acid is teratogenic, it can cause neural tube defects including spina bifida.

Uses

Useful in partial and generalised seizures. Valproic acid is particularly useful in absence seizures. In patients with both absence seizures and generalised tonic-clonic attacks, valproate is the drug of choice.

Valproate is also useful as a mood stabilizer in bipolar mood disorder (See page 254).

BENZODIAZEPINES

Benzodiazepines have useful anticonvulsant properties. **Diazepam** is the drug of choice in status epilepticus. **Clonazepam** is a potent antiepileptic useful in absence and myoclonic seizures. But tolerance develops to its antiepileptic effects. **Clobazam** causes less sedation and is effective in most types of epilepsies - used as an adjuvant to other antiepileptic drugs.

NEWER ANTIEPILEPTICS

Gabapentin

Gabapentin is a highly lipid soluble analogue of GABA which was designed to cross the BBB. It is effective in tonic clonic seizures. Its exact mechanism of action is not known, but it does not act on GABA receptors.

Absorption of gabapentin depends on a carrier protein and does not increase with increase in dose hence it is safe. It is well tolerated. It does not influence the plasma concentrations of other antiepileptics.

Progabalin is a prodrug, which is more potent than gabapentin.

Adverse effects include ataxia, fatigue, drowsiness and dizziness. Tolerance develops to these effects in 1 - 2 weeks.

Gabapentin is used in combination with other antiepileptic drugs, as an add - on drug in partial seizures. It is also used in migraine, neuropathic pain and in bipolar mood disorder.

Lamotrigine

Lamotrigine has a broad spectrum of antiepileptic activity. It inhibits the sodium channels and also inhibits the release of the excitatory amino acids like glutamate. It is completely absorbed from the gut. Lamotrigine may cause skin rashes, nausea, ataxia and dizziness. It is used either alone or with other drugs in partial and generalized seizures.

Vigabatrin

Vigabatrin is a GABA analogue which acts by irreversibly inhibiting the enzyme GABA transaminase thereby raising brain GABA levels. It can cause depression in some patients. Vigabatrin is useful in patients not responding to other antie pileptics.

Levetiracetam

Levetiracetam a pyrrolidine, is effective against partial and secondarily generalized seizures. Its mechanism of action is not known. It is not an enzyme inducer - no related drug interactions. Levetiracetam can be used as an add-on drug in refractory partial seizures.

Tiagabine

Tiagabine a GABA analogue, inhibits the reuptake of GABA into neurons and thereby enhances extracellular GABA levels. It may cause drowsiness and dizziness. Tiagabine can be used as add-on drug for refractory partial seizures.

Topiramate

Topiramate a monosaccharide, acts by multiple mechanisms. It blocks the sodium channels, enhances $GABA_A$ receptor currents, blocks AMPA receptors (glutamate receptor). It is effective in partial and generalized seizures. Topiramate can be used as add-on therapy in refractory epilepsy.

Felbamate

Felbamate an analogue of meprobamate is found to have good antiepileptic action. It blocks the NMDA receptors in addition to weak sodium channel blocking effect. But felbamate can sometimes cause serious adverse effects like aplastic anaemia and hepatitis because of which it is employed only in refractory epilepsy.

Zonisamide

Zonisamide a sulfonamide derivative acts by

inhibiting T type Ca^{++} currents and also by blocking Na^+ channels. It is well tolerated and is indicated in refractory partial seizures.

TREATMENT OF EPILEPSIES

An attempt should be made to detect the cause. When drugs are found to be necessary, the goal of therapy is to keep the patient free of seizures (Table 27.2) without interfering with normal daily activity. Treatment should be started with a single drug at a low dose; dosage is increased gradually, preferably by monitoring the drug levels in plasma. If a single drug is not effective, another drug should be tried.

Good compliance is very important for success. Regarding the duration - decision should be made on an individual basis and dose should be very gradually reduced over months to avoid status epilepticus.

Almost all antiepileptics produce side effects related to the CNS. Drowsiness is the most common side effect of most of them.

The ratio of $\dfrac{ED50\ (Neurological\ impairment)}{ED50\ (Seizure\ protection)}$

is called protective index. Higher the protective index, safer is the drug.

Febrile convulsions

Two to four per cent of children experience convulsions during fever; of them 2 - 3 per cent become epileptics. Treatment is controversial. Children <18 months developing febrile convulsions, those with neurological abnormalities and those with seizures lasting for > 15 minutes, complex seizures - all these have greater risk of recurrence. Diazepam (0.5 mg/kg) given orally or rectally at the onset of fever prevents convulsions. Timely use of paracetamol and tepid sponging prevent high fever. If convulsions occur, diazepam rectally

TABLE 27.2 Choice of antiseizure drugs	
Types of seizures	*Preferred drugs*
1. Simple partial seizures	Carbamazepine, Phenytoin Valproic acid.
2. Complex partial seizures	Carbamazepine, Phenytoin, Valproic acid.
3. Partial with secondarily generalised tonic-clonic seizures	Carbamazepine, Phenytoin, Valproic acid
4. Absence seizures	Ethosuximide, Valproate.
5. Tonic-clonic seiw2qzures	Carbamazepine, Phenytoin Valproic acid.
6. Tonic-clonic + absence seizures	Valproic acid drug of choice
7. Myoclonic seizures	Diazepam, Valproic acid
8. Status epilepticus	Diazepam, Phenytoin, General anaesthesia
9. Febrile convulsions	Diazepam

or intravenously can be used.

Status epilepticus

Status epilepticus is a neurological emergency which may be fatal. Diazepam IV 5-10 mg every 10-15 minutes up to 30 mg is the drug of choice or phenytoin IV can be given. A loading dose 500-1000 mg phenytoin (max 1000 mg in 24 hr) takes 15-20 min to act. Some prefer to combine diazepam and phenytoin (60 mg/min). If seizures continue-general anaesthesia is the last resort Airway maintenance is important. After the cont. ol of seizures, long-term antiepileptic therapy is needed.

In pregnancy - antiepileptics should be continued because abrupt discontinuation increases the risk of status epilepticus which is hazardous to the foetus.

28 Drugs used in Parkinsonism

- • **Classification**
- • **Dopamine precursor**
- • **Drugs that release dopamine**
- • **Dopamine receptor agonists**
- • **Drugs that inhibit DA metabolism**
  - - MAO inhibitors
  - - COMT inhibitors
- • **Anticholinergics**
- • **Drug induced parkinsonism**
- • **Drugs used in Alzheimer's disease**

Parkinsonism is a chronic, progressive, motor disorder characterised by rigidity, tremors and bradykinesia. Other symptoms include excessive salivation, abnormalities of posture and gait, seborrhoea and mood changes. It was described by James Parkinson in 1817 and is therefore named after him.

The incidence is about 1 per cent of population above 65 years of age. It is usually idiopathic in origin but can also be drug induced. In idiopathic parkinsonism, there is degeneration of nigrostriatal neurons in the basal ganglia resulting in dopamine deficiency (Fig 28.1). The balance between inhibitory dopaminergic neurons and excitatory cholinergic neurons is disturbed.

Antiparkinsonian drugs can only help to alleviate the symptoms and improve the quality of life. The two strategies in the treatment are -

i. to enhance dopamine activity

ii. to depress cholinergic overactivity.

Often combination of drugs are used to influence both functions. Drugs used in parkinsonism can be classified as -

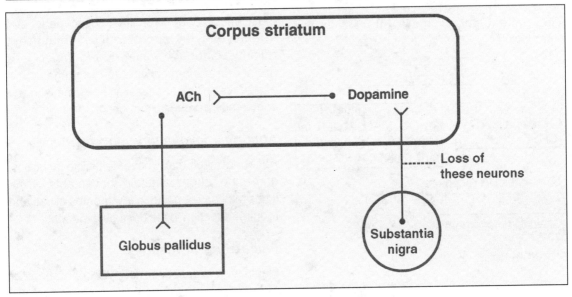

Fig 28.1 Pathophysiology of parkinsonism

CLASSIFICATION

1. Drugs that increase dopamine influence

  i. **DA precursor**
      Levodopa

  ii. **Drugs that release dopamine**
      Amantadine

  iii. **Dopaminergic agonists**
      Bromocryptine
      Lisuride
      Ropinirole
      Pramipexole

  iv. **Inhibit dopamine metabolism**
    • *MAO$_B$ inhibitors*
      Selegiline
    • *COMT inhibitors*
      Tolcapone
      Entacapone

2. Drugs influencing cholinergic system

  i. **Central anticholinergics**
      Benztropine
      Benzhexol
      Biperidine
      Trihexyphenidyl

  ii. **Antihistamines**
      Diphenhydramine
      Orphenadrine
      Promethazine

DOPAMINE PRECURSOR

Levodopa

Though parkinsonism is due to dopamine deficiency, dopamine is of no therapeutic value because it does not cross the blood-brain barrier. Levodopa is a prodrug which is converted to dopamine in the body. It crosses the BBB and is taken up by the surviving nigrostriatal neurons.

$$\text{Levodopa} \xrightarrow{\text{Dopa decarboxylase}} \text{Dopamine}$$

Antiparkinsonian effect On administration of levodopa, there is an overall improvement in the patient as all the symptoms subside.

Bradykinesia, rigidity and tremors respond. There is an improvement in sialorrhea, seborrhoea, mood changes and general motor performance.

The patient shows more interest in the surroundings.

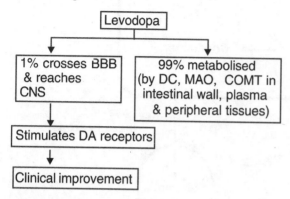

Other actions

Large amounts of levodopa are converted to dopamine in the periphery which brings about other actions.

- **CTZ** - Dopamine stimulates the CTZ to induce vomiting.

- **CVS** - It causes postural hypotension, tachycardia and arrhythmias. Dopamine is a catecholamine.

- **Endocrine** - Dopamine suppresses the prolactin secretion.

Pharmacokinetics

Levodopa is rapidly absorbed from the small intestine. An active transport process that is meant for amino acids is responsible for absorption and transport of levodopa into the brain across the BBB. Therefore some amino acids in food compete with levodopa for both absorption and transport into the brain. Presence of food delays its absorption. It undergoes first pass metabolism in the gut and the liver. Its t½ is 1-2 hours.

Adverse reactions

As 99% of levodopa is converted to dopamine in the periphery, several adverse effects are expected. Nausea, vomiting, anorexia, postural hypotension, palpitation and occasionally arrhythmias can occur. Tolerance develops to these effects after some time. These peripheral effects can be prevented by concurrent administration of domperidone which is a peripheral dopamine antagonist. Behavioural effects like anxiety, depression, hallucinations and sometimes psychosis can occur.

Abnormal involuntary movements

Abnormal involuntary movements like facial tics, grimacing, choreoathetoid movements of the limbs may develop after a few months of use and require reduction in the dose of levodopa.

Fluctuation in response

Fluctuation in response to levodopa can occur after 2-5 years of use - known as 'on-off' phenomenon - where the patient swings alternately from periods of good response to severe disabling disease.

Uses

Levodopa is the most effective drug in idiopathic parkinsonism but is not useful in drug induced parkinsonism.

Drug interactions

1. Pyridoxine enhances peripheral decarboxy-lation of levodopa and thus reduces its availability to the CNS.

2. Phenothiazines and metoclopramide are DA antagonists. They reverse the effects of levodopa.

CARBIDOPA AND BENSERAZIDE

These are peripheral dopa decarboxylase inhibitors. When carbidopa or benserazide are given with levodopa, they prevent the formation of dopamine in the periphery. They do not cross the BBB and hence allow levodopa to be converted to DA in the CNS. The combination is synergistic and therefore levodopa is always given with carbidopa/benserazide.

Levodopa

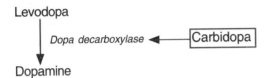

Dopamine

Advantages of the combination

1. Dose of L-dopa can be reduced by 75%.

2. Response to L-dopa appears earlier.

3. Side effects like vomiting and tachycardia are largely reduced.

4. Pyridoxine does not interfere with treatment.

Dose: Fixed dose combination of 1:10 or 1:4 i.e 10mg carbidopa with 100mg levodopa or 25mg carbidopa with 100/250mg levodopa is available.

DRUGS THAT RELEASE DOPAMINE

Amantadine

Amantadine is an antiviral drug. It enhances the release of DA in the brain and diminishes the re-uptake of DA. The response starts early and its adverse effects are minor. Large doses produce insomnia, dizziness, vomiting, postural hypotension, hallucinations and ankle oedema. Amantadine is used in mild cases of parkin sonism. It can also be used along with levodopa as an adjunct.

DOPAMINE RECEPTOR AGONISTS

Bromocriptine and pergolide

Bromocriptine and pergolide are ergot derivatives having dopamine agonistic activity at D_2 receptors. Bromocriptine is also a partial agonist while pergolide is an agonist at D_1 receptors. The newer agents ropinirole and pramipexole are selective D_2 agonists, are better tolerated and quickly attain therapeutic levels. Their adverse effects are milder except that they may cause some sleep disorders.

Dopamine agonists are all longer acting because of which they are useful in the treatment of 'on-off' phenomenon.

Adverse effects include nausea, vomiting, hallucinations and skin eruptions. Ergot derivatives can cause postural hypotension or hypertension initially and first dose phenomenon → sudden cardiovascular collapse.

DA agonists are used:

1. in the treatment of 'on-off' phenomenon

2. as alternatives in the initial treatment of par-kinsonism (particularly newer agents).

Lisuride is similar to bromocriptine.

DRUGS THAT INHIBIT DA METABOLISM

MAO$_B$ Inhibitor

Selegiline

Selegiline (Deprenyl) is a selective MAO-B inhibitor. MAO-B is present in DA containing regions of the CNS. Selegiline prolongs the action of levodopa by preventing its degradation. Selegiline may delay the progression of parkinsonism.

Adverse effects include nausea, postural hypotension, confusion and hallucinations.

Uses

Mild cases of parkinsonism are started on selegiline. It is also used as an adjunct to levodopa.

COMT inhibitors

Tolcapone and **entacapone** inhibit the peripheral metabolism of levodopa by inhibiting the enzyme COMT - thereby they increase the bioavailability of levodopa. Tolcapone crosses the BBB and enhances the availability of levodopa in the brain.

Adverse effects are nausea, orthostatic hypotension, confusion and hallucinations. Tolcapone can also cause hepatotoxicity.

COMT inhibitors are used as add-on drugs in parkinsonism.

ANTICHOLINERGICS

The cholinergic overactivity is overcome by anticholinergics. Tremors, seborrhoea and sialorrhoea are reduced more than rigidity. Atropine derivatives like benzhexol, benztropine, trihe xyphenidyl are used. Antihistamines owe their beneficial effects in parkinsonism to their anticholinergic properties. Atropine-like side effects such as dry mouth, constipation, urinary retention and blurred vision may be encountered.

Uses

Anticholinergics are used as (i) adjunct to levodopa, (ii) drugs of choice in drug-induced parkinsonism.

DRUG INDUCED PARKINSONISM

Drugs like reserpine, metoclopramide and phenothiazines can induce parkinsonism. Reserpine depletes catecholamine stores, while metoclopramide and phenothiazines are dopamine antagonists.

Treatment Withdrawal of the drug usually reverses the symptoms. When drugs are needed, one of the anticholinergics are effective. Levodopa or other dopamine agonists are not effective because DA receptors are blocked by drugs like meto clopramide and phenothiazines.

DRUGS USED IN ALZHEIMER'S DISEASE

Alzheimer's disease (AD) is a neurodegenerative disorder, characterized by progressive impairment of memory and cognitive functions. Other symptoms like depression, anxiety and disturbed sleep may also be seen. Pathological features include atrophy of the cerebral cortex and loss of neurons - mainly cholinergic neurons with multiple senile (amyloid) plaques and neurofibrillary tangles in the brain. Since there is loss of cholinergic neurons, drugs that enhance cholinergic function have been tried. Many other drugs have also been used to improve cognitive functions with variable results.

Drugs used in Alzheimer's disease are -

Cholinesterase inhibitors
Tacrine, rivastigmine, donepezil, galanthamine

Nootropic agents
Piracetam, aniracetam

Drugs under trial
Memantine, ibuprofen, indomethacin

Tacrine

Tacrine is a centrally acting cholinesterase inhibitor. It enhances cholinergic transmission in the brain. But it is short acting and also causes various side effects including nausea, vomiting abdominal cramps, diarrhoea and hepatotoxicity. The newer agents *rivastigmine* and *donepezil* are better tolerated with fewer side effects.

- Donepezil, rivastigmine and *galanthamine* are selective central ChE inhibitors - hence do not cause the g. i. side effects which are due to peripheral cholinergic activity.

- They are not hepatotoxic

- They are longer acting.

Nootropic agents have not shown consistent results in Alzheimer's Disease (See page 257).

Memantine, an NMDA receptor antagonist and NSAIDs - ibuprofen and indomethacin have been found to be useful in Alzheimer's Disease.

29 Opioid analgesics and Antagonists

CHAPTER

- Classification
- Mechanism of action
- Pharmacological actions
- Pharmacokinetics
- Adverse effects
- Management of addiction
- Acute morphine poisoning
- Precautions and contraindications
- Other opioids
- Derivatives of pethidine
- Uses of morphine and its congeners
- Mixed agonists and antagonists
- Opioid antagonists

Pain or analgesia is an unpleasant subjective sensation. It cannot be easily defined. Pain is a warning signal and indicates that there is an impairment of structural and functional integrity of the body. It is the most important symptom that brings the patient to the doctor and demands immediate relief. Prompt relief of pain instills enormous confidence in the patient regarding the

doctor's treating ability.

Pain arising from the skin and integumental structures, muscles, bones and joints is known as **somatic pain.** It is usually caused by inflammation and is well-defined or sharp pain.

Pain arising from the viscera is vague, dull-aching type, difficult to pinpoint to a site and is known as **visceral pain.** It may be accompanied by autonomic responses like sweating, nausea and hypotension. It may be due to spasm, ischaemia or inflammation.

When pain is referred to a cutaneous area which receives nerve supply from the same spinal segment as that of the affected viscera, it is known as **referred pain**, e.g. cardiac pain referred to the left arm.

Pain consists of 2 components - the original 'sensation' and the 'reaction' to it. The original sensation is carried by the afferent nerve fibres and is the same in all. The reaction component

209

differs widely from one person to another. Perception of pain is enhanced in presence of anxiety. A person who is already in stress can poorly tolerate pain.

Pain may be acute or chronic. Acute pain may result from wounds, irritants, burns or from ischemia. The cause is usually well defined. In chronic pain the origin may not be well defined. Example: Pain due to arthritis, cancers and neuroplasmic pain.

Analgesic

Analgesic is a drug which relieves pain without loss of consciousness. Analgesics only afford symptomatic relief from pain without affecting the cause.

Analgesics are of 2 classes.

- Opioid or morphine type of analgesics
- Non-opioid or aspirin type of analgesics.

Opium is the dark brown gummy exudate obtained from the poppy capsule *(Papaver somniferum)*. On incising the unripe seed capsule, a milky juice emerges which turns brown on drying and this is crude opium. The word opium is derived from Greek in which *'opos'* means juice. Opium has been in use since 4000 BC. It was used both for medicinal and recreational purposes. By 18th century, opium smoking had become quite popular in Europe. It was Serturner who isolated a pure opium alkaloid in 1806. He named it **Morphine** after Morpheus, the Greek God of dreams. As the research progressed, opium was found to contain 20 alkaloids. By around 19th century, the pure opium alkaloids were available for therapeutic use - but because they were equally abused, efforts were made to isolate the analgesic property, *i.e.* to obtain an opioid that is only an analgesic and has no euphoric effects. In the process, various agonists, antagonists and partial agonists were synthesized. **'Opioid'** is the term used for drugs with morphine-like actions. They were earlier called narcotic analgesics.

CLASSIFICATION

1. Agonists
   Natural opium alkaloids
   Morphine, codeine
   Synthetic opioids
   Pethidine, methadone

2. Antagonists
   Naloxone, naltrexone

3. Mixed agonist-antagonists
   Pentazocine, nalbuphine, butorphanol, buprenorphine, nalorphine

Chemically the opium alkaloids can be grouped into

1. The Phenanthrene group
   Morphine, codeine, thebaine

2. The Benzylisoquinoline group
   Papaverine, noscapine, narcine.

Opioids can also be classified depending on their source as

1. Natural opium alkaloids
   Morphine, codeine, noscapine

2. Semisynthetic derivatives
   Heroin, oxymorphone, pholcodeine

3. Synthetic opioids
   Pethidine, fentanyl, diphenoxylate, loperamide, dextropropoxyphene, methadone, tramadol, ethoheptazine.

Morphine

Morphine is the most important alkaloid of opium. Many new opioids with actions similar to morphine have been synthesized. But none of them are superior to morphine as an analgesic. Morphine is discussed as the prototype of the group.

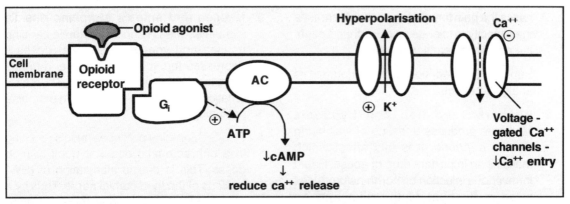

Fig 29.1: Mechanisms of action of opioids. Opioid receptors are G-Protein coupled receptors. Stimulation of these receptors ↓ cAMP formation, ↑ K⁺ efflux causing hyperpolarisation and also inhibit Ca⁺⁺ entry through voltage gated Ca⁺⁺ channels. AC=Adenylyl cyclase cAMP=cyclic AMP.

Mechanism of Action

Morphine and other opioids produce their effects by acting on specific opioid receptors. (Fig 29.1) These receptors are abundant in the CNS and other tissues. The opioid receptors are *mu* (μ) *kappa* (κ) and *delta* (δ). It is found that there are 3 families of endogenous opioid peptides released in the body is response to pain *viz* the *enkephalins,* the *endorphins* and the *dynorphins.* This indicates that we have a natural system in the body that releases various opioid peptides in response to pain. These opioid peptides act on opioid receptors and relieve pain. Most pharmacological effects of opioids including analgesia, sedation, euphoria, respiratory depression, miosis and constipation are mediated through μ receptors. 'Endomorphins' are endogenous ligands for μ receptors but other endegenous peptides also bind to μ receptors. Dynorphins are endogenous ligands for κ receptors while enkephalins bind δ receptors. Various subtypes of these receptors are now known. A fourth type of opioid receptor was recently identified. It is called nociceptin (N) / orphanin FQ receptor.

All opioid receptors are G-protein-coupled receptors. Stimulation of these receptors inhibit adenylate cyclase resulting in decreased intracellular cAMP formation. They also facilitate the opening of K⁺ channels leading to hyperpolarisation and inhibit the entry of calcium into the cell. In addition to this they inhibit the opening of calcium channels. All these result in a decrease in the intracellular calcium which, in turn, decrease the release of neurotransmitters. Various neurotransmitters including dopamine, glutamate, GABA, NA, 5HT and substance P are involved in transmission of pain impulses.

Opioids also directly inhibit the transmission in the dorsal horn ascending pathway. Opioids stimulate the descending pain control pathway - from the midbrain and brain stem to the dorsal horn of the spinal cord. Opioid receptors are abundant in these areas including the peri-aqueductal grey (PAG) area, substantia gelatinosa and the spinal cord.

Pharmacological Actions

Central nervous system

1. Analgesia Morphine is a potent analgesic and relieves pain without loss of consciousness. Dull aching visceral pain is relieved better than sharp pricking pain. But in higher doses it relieves even the severe pain as that of biliary colic. Morphine alters both the perception and reaction to pain. It

raises the pain threshold and thus increases the capacity to tolerate pain. Further, it alters the emotional reaction to pain.

Euphoria and sedation also contribute to its analgesic effects.

2. **Euphoria, sedation and hypnosis** Morphine produces a feeling of well-being termed *euphoria*. It is this effect which makes it an important drug of abuse. Rapid intravenous injection of morphine produces a warm flushing of the skin and an immensely pleasurable sensation in the lower abdomen lasting for about 45 seconds which is known as 'high', 'rush' or 'kick'. The person loses rational thinking and is lost in colourful day dreams. It also produces drowsiness, a calming effect, inability to concentrate, feeling of detachment and indifference to surroundings.

The effects of morphine may not be pleasurable in all. A person has to learn to perceive its pleasurable effects. It may produce dysphoria in some.

3. **Respiration** Morphine produces significant respiratory depression. It directly depresses the respiratory centre in the brain stem. This action is dose dependent. It depresses all phases of respiratory activity - rate and tidal volume. It may also alter the rhythm to produce irregular and periodic breathing. Death from morphine poisoning is almost always due to respiratory arrest.

Morphine suppresses neurogenic (originating in RAS), chemical (hypercapnoeic) and hypoxic drive in the order. The respiratory centre is insensitive to increased plasma CO_2 concentration. With toxic doses breathing is maintained by hypoxic drive.

Sedation and indifference to surroundings add to the depression.

4. **Cough centre** It directly depresses the cough centre and thereby suppresses cough.

5. **Nausea and emesis** Morphine directly stimulates the CTZ in the medulla causing nausea and vomiting. In higher doses it depresses the vomiting centre and hence there is no vomiting in poisoning. Therefore, emetics should not even be tried in morphine poisoning.

6. **Pupils** Morphine produces miosis resulting in a characteristic pinpoint pupil in high doses. This is due to stimulation of (EW) nucleus of the third cranial nerve. Thus by a central effect it produces miosis. Hence morphine used as eye drops does not produce miosis.

7. **Vagus** Morphine stimulates vagal centre causing bradycardia.

8. **Heat regulation** Opioids shift the equilibrium point of heat-regulating centre so that body temperature falls slightly.

9. **Excitatory effect** In high doses opioids produce convulsions. They may increase the excitability of the spinal cord.

Cardiovascular system

In therapeutic doses, morphine produces hypotension by:

* direct peripheral vasodilatation
* inhibition of baroreceptor reflexes

In higher doses it causes depression of vasomotor centre and histamine release both contributing to a fall in BP. Postural hypotension and fainting may occur.

GIT

Opioids decrease the motility of the gut.

• *Stomach* Gastric motility is decreased resulting in increased gastric emptying time. Oesophageal reflux may increase. Gastric acid secretion is reduced. Opioids increase the tone of the antrum and first part of the duodenum which also contribute to delayed emptying by almost 12 hrs and this can retard the absorption of orally given drugs.

• *Intestines* Morphine diminishes all intestinal secretions, delays digestion of food in the small intestine; resting tone is increased. There can be spasms of the intestine. The tone of the sphincters is increased leading to spasm. The intestinal motility (propulsive) is markedly diminished. The resulting delay in the passage of the intestinal contents in the large intestine, together with reduced secretions and inattention to the sensory stimuli for defecation reflex - all contribute to produce marked constipation. The effects of morphine on the gut are by stimulation of μ and δ receptors in the gut.

Other smooth muscles

• *Biliary tract* Morphine causes spasm of the sphincter of Oddi. Intrabiliary pressure rises and may cause biliary colic. Atropine partly antagonises this while opioid antagonists relieve it.

• *Urinary bladder and ureter* Tone and amplitude of contractions of the ureter is increased; tone of external sphincter and volume of the bladder are increased. Opioids inhibit urinary voiding reflex. All these result in urinary retention especially in the elderly male with prostatic hypertrophy.

• *Uterus* No significant effect. May prolong labour in high doses.

• *Bronchi* Morphine causes release of histamine from the mast cells leading to bronchoconstriction. This can be dangerous in asthmatics.

Neuroendocrine effects

Morphine acts in the hypothalamus to inhibit the release of gonadotrophin-releasing hormone and CRF, thus decreasing blood levels of FSH, LH, ACTH and b-endorphins. Tolerance develops after long-term use. These effects are reversible on cessation of therapy.

Pharmacokinetics

Given orally, absorption of morphine is slow and incomplete. Morphine undergoes extensive first pass metabolism. Bioavailability is 20 to 40%. Some opioids are also given as rectal suppositories while highly lipid soluble opioids are available as transdermal preparation. Dose - Table 29.2.

Given subcutaneously, onset of action is in 15-20 min, peak effect - in 1 hr, duration of action is - 3-5 hr. Morphine is metabolised in the liver by glucuronide conjugation. The active metabolite morphine-6-glucuronide, is more potent than morphine and is excreted through the kidneys. Morphine undergoes enterophepatic circulation.

Adverse Effects

Morphine can produce a wide range of adverse effects like nausea, vomiting, dizziness, mental clouding, respiratory depression, constipation, dysphoria, urinary retention and hypotension.

Allergic reactions including skin rashes, pruritus and wheal at the site of injection of morphine may be seen. Morphine is a histamine liberator and this action is responsible for the allergic effects. Rarely intravenous injection can cause anaphylaxis due to the same reason. It is a drug of dependence.

Tolerance and dependence

Repeated administration of morphine results in the development of tolerance to some of its effects including respiratory depression, analgesia, sedation and euphoriant effects and other CNS depressant effects. Constipation and miosis show no tolerance. Though lethal dose of morphine is about 250 mg, addicts can tolerate morphine in grams. Patients in pain can also tolerate a higher dose of morphine. Cross-tolerance is seen among different opioids.

Tolerance is mainly pharmacodynamic, where the cells adapt to the drugs action - at the receptor level, though pharmacokinetic mechanisms like increased metabolism also contribute. An addict needs progressively higher doses to get his 'kick' or 'rush'.

Dependence

Opium has been a drug of addiction for many centuries. Its ability to produce euphoria makes it a drug of addiction. Opioids produce both psychological and physical dependence. Sudden cessation of opioids or administration of opioid antagonists produce significant withdrawal symptoms in such dependent individuals. Manifestations are lacrimation, sweating, yawning, anxiety, apprehension, restlessness, rhinorrhoea and tremors - seen 8-12 hr after the last dose. The person craves for the drug. As the syndrome progresses, fever, insomnia, abdominal colic, severe sneezing, violent yawning, diarrhoea, blurring of vision due to mydriasis, hypertension, severe dehydration, gooseflesh, palpitation, prostration and cardiovascular collapse can occur. There is profound weakness, depression and irritability. Goose flesh is due to pilomotor activity; skin resembles that of a plucked turkey. Hence the word 'cold turkey' is used for abrupt withdrawal. Abdominal cramps, pain in the bones and muscles of the back and limbs are also characteristic.

Inspite of all these disturbing symptoms, withdrawal symptoms are generally not life-threatening. Administration of a suitable opioid, dramatically and completely reverses the symptoms of withdrawal. Without treatment, symptoms disappear in 7-10 days.

Withdrawal in the newborn

Babies born to mothers who were addicts prior to delivery - will also be dependent. Withdrawal symptoms seen are irritability, excessive crying, tremors, frantic suckling of fists, diarrhoea, sneezing, yawning, vomiting and fever. Tincture of opium 0.2 ml /kg/3-4 hr is started at birth and gradually withdrawn.

Management of Addiction

Morphine is slowly withdrawn over several days and substituted by oral methadone.

Advantages of methadone administration are:

1. Methadone is effective orally and by this route no 'kick' is experienced.

2. It is more potent, long - acting and prevents withdrawal symptoms because it is slowly released from the tissues.

The dose is adjusted as per the degree of dependence - 1 mg methadone for every 4 mg of morphine (once a day). Methadone is then gradually withdrawn.

Most addicts can be completely withdrawn from opioids in about 10 days though mild tolerable withdrawal symptoms persist. Symptoms like insomnia, malaise, restlessness, irritability, fatigue and GI hyperactivity may last up to several months.

Clonidine

Clonidine a central α_2 agonist can suppress some of the autonomic withdrawal symptoms like anxiety, nausea, vomiting and diarrhoea. It is given for 7 - 10 days and withdrawn over 3 - 4 days. Night time sedation with a hypnotic like diazepam is helpful.

Acute morphine poisoning may be accidental, suicidal or homicidal. Lethal dose in non - addicts is about 250 mg but addicts can tolerate grams of morphine. Signs and symptoms include respiratory depression with shallow breathing, pin point pupils, hypotension, shock, cyanosis, flaccidity, stupor, hypothermia, coma and death due to respiratory failure and pulmonary oedema.

Treatment

1. Positive pressure respiration.

2. Maintenance of BP.

3. Gastric lavage with potassium

permanganate to remove unabsorbed drug.

4. Specific antidote is naloxone - 0.4 - 0.8 mg IV repeated every 10-15 min.

Precautions and Contraindications

1. Avoid opioids in patients with respiratory insufficiency - COPD.

2. An attack of bronchial asthma can be precipitated by morphine.

3. In extremes of age - more susceptible to respiratory depression.

4. Head injury - morphine is contraindicated because:

    i. morphine increases CSF pressure by retaining CO_2 and thereby increases the intracranial tension.

    ii. causes marked respiratory depression.

    iii. vomiting, miosis and mental clouding seen with morphine interfere with diagnosis and assessment of progress in head injuries.

5. In hypovolaemic shock, morphine further decreases the BP.

6. Opioids potentiate CNS depressants.

7. Undiagnosed acute abdomen - morphine relieves pain and may interfere with the diagnosis. It induces vomiting and its spasmogenic effect may add to its drawbacks. Hence it can be administered only after the diagnosis is established - if necessary.

Other Opioids

Heroin or diamorphine or diacetyl morphine is converted to morphine in the body. It has higher lipid solubility because of which euphoric effects are faster and greater resulting in higher abuse potential. It has a strong smell of vinegar. Though it can be used as an analgesic it is banned in most countries.

Levorphanol is similar to morphine but it is longer acting.

Codeine is a naturally occurring opium alkaloid. Codeine depresses the cough centre in suban algesic doses. It is effective orally and is well-absorbed.

It is less potent (one-sixth) than morphine as an analgesic (60 mg codeine = 10 mg morphine).

It produces less respiratory depression and is less constipating. Codeine has less addiction liability and tolerance is uncommon.

Hence codeine is used as an antitussive. It is well-absorbed when given orally compared to morphine. Duration of action is 4-6 hr. 10 to 30 mg is the antitussive dose. About 10% of codeine is converted to morphine. Constipation is the most common side effect.

Uses

Codeine is a commonly used antitussive. It is also available in combination with paracetamol for analgesia. It is to be given at bed time (CODOPLUS - Codeine 30 mg + Paracetamol 500 mg).

Papaverine is devoid of opioid and analgesic activity.

Noscapine is a naturally occurring opium alkaloid. In therapeutic doses, it has no significant actions on the CNS except for antitussive effects. Hence it has no disadvantages of opioids. In large doses it may cause bronchoconstriction due to the release of histamine. Dose: 15-30 mg, 3-4 times a day. Noscapine is highly effective and safe. The only adverse effect is nausea. It is used as a cough suppressant.

Several other centrally acting antitussives have been synthesized including, pholcodeine, and dextromethorphan.

Pholcodeine though structurally related to opioids, has no other opioid-like actions. It is as effective as codeine as an antitussive; has a long half-life and therefore can be given once a day.

Dextromethorphan has no analgesic or addictive properties. It acts centrally to elevate the threshold for coughing for which it is as effective as codeine. Toxicity is very low; extremely high doses cause CNS depression. Antitussive dose: 10 - 30 mg, 3 - 4 times a day.

Tramadol is a recently developed synthetic codeine analog. It is an effective analgesic but its mechanism of action is not clear. It is a weak opioid agonist. In addition it inhibits the reuptake of noradrenaline and serotonin in the CNS.

Adverse effects include drowsiness, dryness of mouth, sedation and nausea. Respiratory depression is mild. It is a drug of dependence. It may precipitate seizures. It should be avoided in patients on MAO inhibitors because tramadol inhibits serotonin uptake.

Tramadol is used in acute and chronic pain, like postoperative pain and neuralgias.

Pethidine (Meperidine)

Pethidine is a phenylpiperidine derivative of morphine. Many of its actions resemble that of morphine. When compared to morphine:

- pethidine is $1/10$th as potent as morphine (100 mg pethidine = 10 mg morphine). However, efficacy as an analgesic is equal to morphine
- the onset of action is more rapid and duration of action is shorter
- it produces corneal anaesthesia
- it is not a good antitussive
- it is less constipating
- in some patients, it may cause dysphoria
- it also has anticholinergic effects which can cause dry mouth, and blurring of vision.
- in toxic doses, pethidine sometimes produces

CNS stimulation with tremors, restlessness and convulsions instead of sedation. This is

because of the toxic metabolite - norpethidine.

Adverse effects are similar to morphine except that constipation and urinary retention are less common.

Uses

Dose 25-100 mg IM/SC is the analgesic dose.

In pain Pethidine is used as an analgesic in visceral pain and also for other indications of morphine. Because of its better oral efficacy and less spasmogenic effect, pethidine is preferred to morphine.

During labour Given during labour, pethidine produces less respiratory depression in the newborn when compared to morphine. Moreover it does not interfere with uterine contractions and labour and is therefore preferred to morphine for obstetric analgesia.

Preanaesthetic medication - pethidine can also be used as preanaesthetic medication.

DERIVATIVES OF PETHIDINE

Fentanyl

Fentanyl is a pethidine congener.

Advantages

- It is about 100 times more potent than morphine as an analgesic.
- Fentanyl is highly lipid soluble and fast acting (maximum effect within 5 minutes.)
- Fentanyl has mild effects on the cardio vascular system. It slightly reduces HR and BP. Hence it is found to be safer than other opioids in cardiovascular surgeries.
- Transdermal patches of fentanyl are available which acts for 48 hours.
- Unlike morphine, fentanyl does not increase the intracranial pressure.
- Fentanyl is not a histamine liberator.

- It can be used in combination with droperidol, a neuroleptic agent to produce neuroleptanalgesia.

Because of the above advantages fentanyl is a commoly used opioid analgesic.

For neuroleptanalgesia the combination is given IV to produce sedation and intense analgesia without loss of consciousness. This state is maintained for 30-40 minutes as both have rapid and short-action (See page 172). A fixed dose combination is available with 0.05 mg fentanyl + 2.5 mg droperidol per ml. 5 ml is the dose used IV over 10 minutes. Patient is drowsy but responds to commands.

Uses

1. Neuroleptanalgesia is used for short surgical procedures especially in 'poor risk' patients.

2. Epidural fentanyl is used for postoperative and obstetric analgesia. For this morphine/fentanyl may be combined with local anaesthetics so that lower doses of both drugs are sufficient.

3. Fentanyl can also be used in chronic pain where opioid use is permissible.

Adverse effects

Bolus doses of fentanyl cause muscle rigidity. This can be reduced by avoiding bolus doses. Other adverse effects include nausea, vomiting and respiratory depression.

Congeners of fentanyl are sufentanil, alfentanil and remifentanil. Alfentanil and remifentanil are faster acting (act within one minute) and recovery is rapid. They are used for short surgical procedures.

Methadone

Methadone a synthetic opioid, has actions similar to morphine. Its outstanding features are:

- It is an effective analgesic
- It is effective by oral route
- It has a long duration of action ($t\frac{1}{2}$ 24 - 36 hours) and therefore effectively suppresses withdrawal symptoms in addicts.

Methadone is about 90% bound to plasma proteins; it is firmly bound to proteins in various tissues, including brain. After repeated administration, it gradually accumulates in tissues. When administration is discontinued, the drug is slowly released from these binding sites. This

Table 29.1: Difference between morphine and pethidine		
	Morphine	**Pethidine**
Source	Natural opium alkaloid	Synthetic
Potency	More potent	Less potent (1/10th of mophine)
Corneal anaesthesia	No effect	Corneal anaesthetic
Higher doses	Profound CNS depression	CNS stimulation (due to norpethidine)
Antitussive property	Good	Poor or nil
Constipation effect	Marked	Less
Analgesic dose	10 mg	100 mg
Anticholinergic effect	Absent	Present
Use during labour	Significant respiratory depression in the neonate	Less neonatal respiratory depression - hence preferred over morphine

probably accounts for its milder withdrawal symptoms. As euphoric effects are less intense, abuse potential is less. Tolerance develops more slowly. Even in addicts, withdrawal symptoms are gradual in onset, less intense, but prolonged.

Preparation 10 mg inj, (2 mg/5 ml syrup) Dose - 10 mg oral or IM.

Uses

1. *Substitution therapy* in opioid dependence. 1 mg oral methadone is given for every 4

mg morphine.

2. *Opioid maintenance:* Gradually increasing doses of methadone is given orally to produce a high degree of tolerance. Such subjects do not experience the pleasurable effects of IV morphine, i.e. opioids are not pleasurable in them and they give up the habit.

3. Methadone can also be used as an *analgesic.*

LAAM (L - alpha - acetyl - methadol) is a

Name	Dose (mg)	Duration of analgesia (hours)	Preparations*	Trade name
Morphine	20-40	4-5	10,30mg CR-Tabs	Morcontin Continus
Ethyl morphine	16-32	6-8	16mg tab	Dionindon
Methadone	10	4-6	------	------
Pethidine	50-100	2-4	50mg, 100mg inj.	Pethidine
Fentanyl	0.05-0.2	1-2	50mcg inj. TD Patch-release 25-75 mcg/hr.	Trofentyl
Sufentanil	0.02	1-2	-----	------
Codeine	30-60	3-5	Codeine 30mg+Paracetamol 500mg tab	Codoplus
Dextropropoxyphene	60 q	4-6	60mg caps	Parvodex
Pentazocine	30-60	3-4	30mg inj. IM/SC 30 IV q 4-6 hr	Pentawin
Nalbuphine	10-15	3-6	-----	-----
Buprenorphine	0.3-0.6 IM/Slow IV q 6 - 8 hr	4-8	0.3mg inj., 0.2mg SL tab	Pentorel
Butorphanol	2mg	3-4	1,2mg inj.	Butrum
Ethoheptazine	75mg	3-4	75mg tab with aspirin 325mg	Equagesic
Tramadol	50-100 IM q 4-6hr	4-6	50,100mg inj.	Urgendol

Table 29.2: Dose, duration of action and preparations of opioid analgesics

* Preparations available in India.

derivative of methadone. L- alpha- acetyl-methadol is found to have longer duration of action than methadone so that it can be given three times a week. It is used to prevent withdrawal symptoms in addicts.

Dextropropoxyphene

Dextropropoxyphene is a congener of methadone. It binds to the opioid receptors and produces effects similar to morphine. It is less constipating, longer acting and has good oral efficacy. But dextropropoxyphene is an irritant when given parenterally. Large doses cause CNS stimulation. It also has abuse potential.

Uses

Used in mild to moderate pain. It is marketed in combination with aspirin.

Dextropropoxyphene 32   mg+aspirin 600 mg.

Ethoheptazine

Ethoheptazine is related to pethidine and has mild analgesic effects with low addiction potential. It is used orally in combination with NSAIDs for relief of pain.

Uses of Morphine and its congeners

Dose Morphine 10 to 20 mg IM/SC; 20 mg tablet of ethylmorphine is now available for oral use.

1. **Analgesic** Morphine is one of the most potent analgesics available. It affords **symptomatic relief of pain** without affecting the underlying disease. It is an excellent analgesic for severely painful conditions such as acute myocardial infarction, fractures, burns, pulmonary embolism, terminal stages of cancer, acute pericarditis, spontaneous pneumothorax and postoperative pain. In excruciating pain, morphine can be given IV.

In **myocardial infarction,** morphine relieves

pain and thereby apprehension. As a result reflex sympathetic stimulation is reduced and shock is minimized.

- Morphine is given with atropine to relieve **renal and biliary colic.** Atropine relieves spasm of the sphincter of oddi. Morphine relieves pain but may cause spasm of the sphincter of oddi which in turn raises intrabiliary pressure. Hence atropine is given which relieves spasm of the sphincter of oddi.

- Since opiate receptors are present in the spinal cord, epidural morphine can be used to produce **epidural analgesia.** Such analgesia is segmental in distribution and there is no interference with motor function or autonomic changes and no systemic adverse effects. Small doses of morphine can produce profound analgesia for 12-24 hours.

- **Obstetric analgesia** Pethidine is preferred to morphine for this condition

- Opioids can be liberally given to control pain of **terminal illness** like cancers

- But opioids should *not be* freely used in case of other chronic pain due to their addiction liability.

Various alternative routes of administration are tried for opioids - in order to reduce their systemic effects and provide longer duration of analgesia particularly for patients with chronic pain. Morphine and other opioids are being tried as intraspinal infusion, rectal, transmucosal, transdermal administration and by inhalation. In Patient controlled analgesia (PCA) with opioids the patients decide their own need for the analgesic. A specific dose of the opioids is pushed through an intravenous device careful monitoring is needed to avoid overdosage.

2. **As preanaesthetic medication** Morphine and pethidine are commonly used as preanaesthetic medication. They reduce anxiety, provide analgesia, allow smoother

induction and reduce the dose of the anaesthetic required. But they have certain disadvantages:

- Opioids depress respiration
- Morphine precipitates bronchospasm and is dangerous in patients with poor respiratory reserve
- They cause vasomotor depression
- They may induce vomiting
- They may interfere with pupillary response to anaesthesia because they cause miosis.
- Postoperative urinary retention and constipation may be troublesome.

3. **Acute left ventricular failure** Morphine is used to alleviate the dyspnoea of LVF and pulmonary oedema in which the response to IV morphine may be dramatic. The mechanism is not clear. The relief may be due to:

i. alteration in the patient's reaction to impaired respiratory function.

ii. reduction in the work of the heart due to decreased fear and apprehension. Reduced anxiety decreases sympathetic stimulation which in turn decreases cardiac work.

iii. cardiovascular effects like decreased PVR leading to shifting of blood from pulmonary to peripheral circulation, thereby reducing cardiac work load.

Morphine is contraindicated in bronchial asthma and pulmonary oedema due to respiratory irritants.

4. **Diarrhoea** Opioids are effective for the symptomatic treatment of diarrhoea. Synthetic opioids - diphenoxylate and loperamide are preferred as antidiarrheals.

5. **Cough** Though morphine is an effective antitussive, codeine is the preferred opioid for this purpose. But now many nonaddictive antitussives are available.

6. **Special anaesthesia**

- High doses of morphine can be used IV to produce general anaesthesia

- Neuroleptanalgesia - fentanyl with droperidol can be used to produce neuroleptanalgesia.

- Morphine can be used epidurally for the relief of postoperative and chronic pain.

7. **Sedative** Morphine relieves anxiety in threatened abortion without affecting uterine motility. It is an useful sedative in the presence of pain.

MIXED AGONISTS AND ANTAGONISTS

They include - pentazocine, cyclazocine nalbuphine, buprenorphine, butorphanol and nalorphine.

Pentazocine

In an attempt to develop an analgesic with less addiction liability and low adverse effects, pentazocine was developed. Pentazocine it is a κ receptor agonist.

- CNS effects of pentazocine are similar to morphine. 20 mg pentazocine = 10 mg morphine. Euphoria is seen only in low doses. With higher doses - above 60 mg dysphoria can occur due to κ receptor stimulation.

- Sedation and respiratory depression are less marked.

- It has weak antagonistic properties at μ receptors.

- Tolerance and dependance develop on repeated use.

- CVS - in contrast to morphine, pentazocine increases BP and heart rate and thereby increases cardiac work. It is therefore **not** suitable in MI.

- Biliary spasm and constipation are less severe.

Preparations Pentazocine can be given both orally and parenterally. It undergoes first pass metabolism.

Dose 50-100 mg oral; 30-60 mg IM (FORTWIN).

Adverse effects Sedation, sweating, dizziness, nausea, dysphoria with anxiety, nightmares and hallucinations which are unpleasant are seen above 60 mg. As it is an irritant, IM injection can be painful and cause sterile abscesses.

Uses

Pentazocine is a commonly used opioid analgesic especially in postoperative and chronic pain - abuse liability is less than morphine.

Cyclazocine is similar to pentazocine.

Nalbuphine

Nalbuphine is an agonist - antagonist - more potent than pentazocine. It is a good analgesic. Though it produces respiratory depression like morphine, it has a ceiling effect at 30 mg, i.e. an increase in dose beyond 30 mg does not increase respiratory depression further. Higher doses produce dysphoria.

Uses As analgesic - 10-20 mg IM.

Buprenorphine

Buprenorphine is a highly lipid soluble synthetic thebaine congener. It is a partial μ agonist, 25 times as potent as morphine. Though onset of action is slow, duration of analgesia is long. Other CNS effects are similar to morphine while respiratory depression is less marked. Patients exhibit lower degree of tolerance and dependence liability. Withdrawal syndrome appears late and is mild.

Dose 0.3-0.6 mg SC, IM or sublingual (oral not available).

Uses Chronic pain like in terminal cancer patients. Buprenorphine can also be used as a maintenance drug in opioid addicts as the withdrawal symptoms are mild.

Butorphanol is similar to pentazocine.

Nalorphine

Nalorphine is also an agonist - antagonist. At low doses, it is a good analgesic. But with increase in dose there is no increase in analgesia.

It causes dysphoria (κ agonist) and respiratory depression even in low doses. Hence it cannot be used as an analgesic. At high doses it acts as an antagonist and counters all the actions of opioids.

Uses Nalorphine may be used in acute opioid poisoning. It can also be used for the diagnosis of opioid addiction.

Newer agonist-antagonists

Meptazinol

Mepazinol is a short acting agonist - antagonist with additional anticholinergic effects. It produces short duration analgesia with less respiratory depression and is therefore suitable for obstetric analgesia.

Dezocine

Dezocine is a partial agonist at μ receptors. Its analgesic actions are similar to morphine but respiratory depression does not increase with an increase in dose-ceiling effect.

OPIOID ANTAGONISTS

Naloxone

Naloxone acts as a competitive antagonist to all types of opioid receptors. It is a pure antagonist. In normal individuals, it does not produce any significant actions. But in opium addicts, given IV, it promptly antagonises all the actions of morphine including respiratory depression and sedation and precipitates withdrawal syndrome. It also blocks the action of endogenous opioid peptides - endorphins, enkephalins and dynorphins. It blocks the analgesia produced by placebo and acupuncture. This suggests that endogenous opioid peptides are responsible for analgesia by these techniques.

Given orally it undergoes first pass metabolism and is metabolised by the liver. Hence it is given intravenously. Duration of action is 3-4 hours.

Dose 0.4 mg IV.

Uses

1. Naloxone is the drug of choice for morphine overdosage.
2. It is also used to reverse neonatal asphyxia due to opioids used in labour.
3. Naloxone can also be used for the diagnosis of opioid dependence - it precipitates withdrawal symptoms.
4. Hypotension seen during shock could be due to endogenous opioids released during such stress. Naloxone has been found to be beneficial in reversing hypotension.

Naltrexone

Naltrexone is another pure opioid antagonist. It is
- more potent than naloxone
- orally effective
- has a longer duration of action of 1-2 days.

Uses

1. Naltrexone is used for 'opioid blockade' therapy in post addicts (50-100 mg/ day orally) so that even if the addicts take an opioid, they do not experience the pleasurable effects and therefore lose the craving.
2. Alcohol craving is also reduced by naltrexone and is used to prevent relapse of heavy drinking (See page 192).

Nalmefene

Nalmefene is orally effective and longer acting. It has better bioavailability and is not hepatotoxic. It is used in opioid overdosage.

30 *Nonsteroidal anti-inflammatory Drugs (NSAIDs)*

- **Classification**
- **Mechanism of action**
- **Salicylates**
- **Para-aminophenol derivatives**
- **Pyrazolon derivatives**
- **Indole acetic acid derivatives**
- **Arylacetic acid derivatives**
- **Propionic acid derivatives**
- **Anthranilic acid derivatives**
- **Oxicams**
- **Selective COX-2 inhibitors**
- **Antagonists of leukotriene synthesis and leukotriene receptors**
- **Drug that block both cyclo-oxygenase and lipoxygenase**

Nonsteroidal anti - inflammatory drugs are aspirin-type or non - opioid analgesics. In addition, they have anti-inflammatory , antipyretic and uricosuric properties - without addiction liability.

The medicinal effects of the bark of the willow tree have been known since centuries. The active principle 'salicin' was isolated from the willow bark. This salicin is converted to glucose and salicylic acid in the body. In 1875, sodium salicylate was first used in the treatment of rheumatic fever. After its anti-inflammatory and uricosuric properties were established, efforts were made to synthesize derivatives which were less expensive. Now they have replaced the natural ones in the market.

CLASSIFICATION

A. NONSELECTIVE COX INHIBITORS

1. Salicylic acid derivatives
   Aspirin, sodium salicylate diflunisal

2. Para-aminophenol derivatives
   Paracetamol

3. Pyrazolone derivatives
   Phenylbutazone azapropazone

4. **Indole acetic acid derivatives**
   Indomethacin sulindac

5. **Arylacetic acid derivatives**
   Diclofenac, ketorolac, tolmetin

6. **Propionic acid derivatives**
   Ibuprofen, fenoprofen,
   carprofen, naproxen,
   ketoprofen, flurbiprofen
   oxaprozin

7. **Anthranilic acids (Fenamates)**
   Flufenamic acid
   mefenamic acid
   enfenamic acid
   meclofenamic acid

8. **Oxicams**   .
   Piroxicam, tenoxicam
   meloxicam

9. **Alkanones**
   Nabumetone

B. SELECTIVE COX-2 INHIBITORS
Nimesulide, celecoxib,
rofecoxib, etodolac

MECHANISM OF ACTION

During inflammation, arachidonic acid liberated from membrane phospholipids is converted to prostaglandins (PGs), catalysed by the enzyme cyclo-oxygenase (COX). These prostaglandins produce hyperalgesia - they sensitize the nerve endings to pain caused by other mediators of inflammation like bradykinin and histamine.

(Membrane) Phospholipids

| *Phospholipase A_2*

Arachidonic acid

Cyclooxygenase | *Lipoxygenase*

| Prostaglandins | | Leukotrienes |

NSAIDs inhibit the PG synthesis by inhibiting the enzyme cyclo-oxygenase.

Aspirin is an irriversible inhibitor of COX (by acetylation) while the others are reversible competitive COX inhibitors. There are two forms of cyclooxygenase viz., COX - 1 and COX - 2 (see page 274) COX - 1 is found in most of the normal cells (constitive) and is involved in maintaining tissue homeostasis. COX - 2 is induced in the inflammatory cells by cytokines and other mediators of inflammation. This COX -2 catalyses the synthesis of prostanoids which are the mediators of inflammation. Most NSAIDs inhibit both COX-1 and COX-2 while some newer agents like celecoxib and rofecoxib selectively inhibit only COX-2.

SALICYLATES

Salicylates are salts of salicylic acid, e.g. methyl salicylate, sodium salicylate, acetyl salicylic acid (aspirin). Aspirin is taken as the prototype.

Pharmacological Actions

1. Analgesia

Aspirin is a good analgesic and relieves pain of inflammatory origin. This is because PGs are formed during inflammation and they sensitize the tissues to pain and aspirin inhibits PG synthesis. Pain originating from the integumental structures like muscles, bones, joints, and pain in connective tissues is relieved. But in vague visceral pain, aspirin is relatively ineffective.

The pain is relieved without euphoria and hypnosis. Hence there is no development of tolerance and dependence. But aspirin is a weak analgesic when compared to morphine.

2.Antipyretic action

In presence of fever, salicylates bring down the temperature to normal level. But, in normal individuals, there is no change in temperature.

In fever, pyrogen - a protein, circulates in the body and this increases the synthesis of PGs in the hypothalamus, thereby raising its temperature set point. The thermostatic mechanism in the hypothalamus is thus disturbed. Aspirin inhibits PG synthesis in the hypothalamus and resets the thermostat at the normal level bringing down the temperature.

Enhanced sweating and cutaneous vasodilatation promote heat loss and assist in the antipyretic action.

3. Anti-inflammatory action

At higher doses of 4-6 g/day, aspirin acts as an anti-inflammatory agent. Signs of inflammation like tenderness, swelling, erythema and pain are all reduced or suppressed. But, the progression of the disease in rheumatoid arthritis, rheumatic fever or osteoarthritis is not affected.

Once again the mechanism involved is PG synthesis inhibition - PGs present in inflammatory tissues are responsible for oedema, erythema and pain. In addition, aspirin also interferes with the formation of chemical mediators of the kallikrein system. As a result, it decreases the adherence of granulocyte to the damaged vasculature, stabilizes lysosomes and decreases the migration of the polymorphonuclear leukocytes and macrophages into the site of inflammation.

4. Respiration

In therapeutic doses of 4-6 g/day - salicylates increase consumption of oxygen by skeletal muscles. As a result there is -CO_2 production. This -CO_2 stimulates respiratory centre. Salicylates also directly stimulate the medullary respiratory centre. Both these actions increase the rate and depth of respiration. These effects are dose dependent.

As a result of this stimulation of respiration, plasma CO_2 is washed out leading to respiratory alkalosis. With toxic doses, the respiratory centre is depressed leading to respiratory failure.

5. Acid-base and electrolyte balance

In anti-inflammatory doses, salicylates produce significant respiratory stimulation - CO_2 is washed out resulting in respiratory alkalosis; pH becomes alkaline. This is compensated by increased excretion of HCO_3^- in urine accompanied by Na^+, K^+ and water. pH then returns to normal. This stage is known as compensated respiratory alkalosis.

With toxic doses, salicylates depress the respiratory centre directly. As a result, CO_2 accumulates because more CO_2 is produced than is exhaled. Thus plasma CO_2 rises and pH decreases. Since the concentration of HCO_3^- is already low due to enhanced renal excretion, the change results in uncompensated respiratory acidosis. This is superimposed by metabolic acidosis caused by accumulation of acids.

Toxic doses also depress vasomotor centre. This vasomotor depression impairs renal function resulting in accumulation of strong acids of metabolic origin like lactic, pyruvic and acetoacetic acids.

The above effects are accompanied by dehydration due to:

- water lost in urine with HCO_3^-, Na^+ and K^+
- increased sweating
- water lost during hyperventilation.
  Thus there is severe dehydration with acidosis.

6. Metabolic effects

Salicylates enhance the cellular metabolism due to uncoupling of oxidative phosphorylation. More of O_2 is used and more CO_2 is produced, especially in skeletal muscles, leading to increased heat production.

In toxic doses, hyperpyrexia, increased protein catabolism with resultant aminoaciduria and negative nitrogen balance are seen. Enhanced utilization of glucose leads to mild hypoglycaemia.

But in toxic doses, hyperglycaemia occurs due to central sympathetic stimulation which increases adrenaline levels.

7. Gastrointestinal tract

Aspirin is a gastric irritant. Irritation of the gastric mucosa leads to epigastric distress, nausea and vomiting. Aspirin also stimulates the CTZ to produce vomiting.

Erosive gastritis, mucosal congestion, gastric ulceration and GI bleeding resulting in malaena and occasionally haematemesis can occur particularly in higher doses.

Mechanism

i. In the acidic pH of the stomach, salicylates remain unionised. These drug particles adhere to the mucosa producing irritation. These particles also promote local back diffusion of acid.

ii. Aspirin decreases prostaglandin synthesis. PGs inhibit gastric acid secretion, increase mucosal production and act as cytoprotectives in gastric mucosa. This defense mechanism is lost due to PG inhibition.

The above actions make aspirin ulcerogenic. In addition it decreases platelet aggregation which also increases the tendency to bleed.

With soluble aspirin, gastric irritation is less. The selective COX-2 inhibitors cause less gastric irritation.

8. CVS

In therapeutic doses no significant cardiovascular effects are seen. In toxic doses it depresses the VMC and thus depresses the circulation.

9. Immunological effects

In higher doses, salicylates suppress several antigen-antibody reactions including inhibition of antibody production, Ag-Ab aggregation and antigen induced release of histamine. These effects might also contribute to the beneficial effects in rheumatic fever.

10. Uric acid excretion

Uric acid is excreted by secretion from the distal tubules. In a dose of 1-2 g/day, aspirin increases plasma urate levels by urate retention because it interferes with urate secretion by the distal tubules.

Large doses of > 5 g/day increase urate excretion because it inhibits reabsorption of urate by proximal tubule causing uricosuria. But, its uricosuric effect cannot be used therapeutically because high doses are required and such doses result in prominent adverse effects.

11. Blood

Even in small doses aspirin irreversibly inhibits platelet cyclooxygenase and thereby TXA_2 synthesis by the platelets. It therefore interferes with platelet aggregation and prolongs the bleeding time. Even a single dose can irreversibly inhibit TXA_2 synthesis which is for the life of the platelets (8-11days). As platelets cannot synthesize proteins which means COX cannot be regenerated, fresh platelets have to be formed to restore TXA_2 activity. Moreover Aspirin inhibits platelet COX in the portal circulation itself and therefore even small doses (40mg daily) of aspirin is adequate for its antiplatelet aggregatory effect.

12. Local effects

Salicylic acid when applied locally is a keratolytic. It also has mild antiseptic and fungistatic properties. Salicylic acid is also an irritant for the broken skin.

Pharmacokinetics

Salicylates being acidic are absorbed from the stomach and the upper small intestine. But aspirin as such is poorly soluble, hence not well-absorbed. When administered as microfine particles, absorption increases. Thus particle size, pH of the GIT, solubility of the preparation and presence of food in the stomach influence the absorption.

Salicylic acid and methylsalicylate are absorbed from the intact skin. They are extensively bound to plasma proteins. Aspirin is deacetylated in the liver, plasma and other tissues to release salicylic acid which is the active form. Plasma t½ of aspirin is 3-5 hours. Elimination is dose dependent. It follows first order kinetics in small doses and zero order kinetics in higher doses. Therefore in anti-inflammatory doses, t½ increases to 12 hr. Salicylates are excreted in urine.

Adverse Effects

Analgesic doses are generally well tolerated but anti-inflammatory doses are usually associated with adverse effects especially when used over a long period.

- *GI tract* nausea, epigastric distress, vomiting, erosive gastritis, peptic ulcer, increased occult blood loss in stools are common.

- *Allergic reactions* are not common and may be manifested as rashes, urticaria, photo sensitivity, rhinorrhoea, angio-oedema, and asthma especially in those with a history of allergies.

As aspirin inhibits only cyclo-oxygenase pathway, arachidonic acid is available for conversion by lipoxygenase pathway into leukotrienes. Leukotrienes are powerful bronchoconstrictors. Hence aspirin can precipitate bronchial asthma in some individuals. Of the currently available NSAIDs, diclofenac and indomethacin inhibit the synthesis of both PGs and LTs.

- *Haemolysis:* Salicylates can cause haemolysis in patients with G_6PD deficiency.

- *Nephrotoxicity:* Almost all NSAIDs can cause nephrotoxicity after long-term use. Salt and water retention and impaired renal function can occur.

- *Hepatotoxicity* can also occur when high doses of NSAIDs are used over a long period. Plasma levels of liver enzymes are raised.

- *Reye's Syndrome* seen in children is a form of hepatic encephalopathy which may be fatal. It develops a few days after a viral infection especially influenza and varicella. An increased incidence of this syndrome has been noted when aspirin is used to treat fever. Hence aspirin is contraindicated in children

TABLE 30.1: Preparations and dosage of salicylates		
Drug	*Preparation*	*Dose*
Aspirin	300, 350 tab (ASABUF); DISPRIN (Aspirin 350 mg & Calcium carbonate 105 mg)	Analgesic - 300-600 mg every 6-8 hr Anti-inflammatory - 4-6 gm/day Antiplatelet effects - 75-300 mg/day
Sodium Salicylate	325, 650 mg tablets	325-650 mg every 4-8 hr
Salicylic acid	2% ointment; Whitfield's ointment- - Salicylic acid 3% - Benzoic acid 6%	For topical use
Methylsalicylate (Oil of wintergreen)	Ointment/liniment for topical use	As counter irritant
Diflunisal	250, 500 mg tab (DOLOBID)	250 mg every 8-12 hr

with viral fever.

- *Pregnancy and infancy* Aspirin when taken at term delays the onset of labour due to inhibition of PG synthesis (PGs play an important role in the initiation of labour). Premature closure of ductus arteriosus may occur in the foetus resulting in portal hypertension. It can also increase postpartum bleeding due to inhibition of platelet aggregation.

- *Salicylism* Higher doses given for a long time as in treatment of rheumatoid arthritis may cause chronic salicylate intoxication termed 'Salicylism'. The syndrome is characterised by headache, vertigo, dizziness, tinnitus, vomiting, mental confusion, diarrhoea, sweating, difficulty in hearing, thirst and dehydration. These symptoms are reversible on withdrawal of salicylates.

Acute salicylate intoxication Poisoning may be accidental or suicidal. It is more common in children, 15-30 g is the fatal dose of aspirin.

Symptoms and signs

Dehydration, hyperpyrexia, GI irritation, vomiting, sometimes haematemesis, acid-base imbalance, restlessness, delirium, hallucinations, metabolic acidosis, tremors, convulsions, coma and death due to respiratory failure and CV collapse.

Treatment is symptomatic and includes

1. Gastric lavage to eliminate unabsorbed drugs.

2. IV fluids to correct acid-base imbalance and dehydration.

3. Temperature is brought down by external cooling with alcohol or cold water sponges.

4. If haemorrhagic complications are seen, blood transfusion and vitamin K are needed.

5. The IV fluids should contain Na^+, K^+, HCO_3^- and glucose (to treat hypokalaemia and acidosis). Blood pH should be monitored.

6. In severe cases, forced alkaline diuresis with sodium bicarbonate and a diuretic like

NSAID	Preparation	Brand Name
TABLE 30.2: Topical preparations of NSAIDs		
Salicylic acid	6% W/W oint	KERALIN with hydrocortisone acetate and benzoic acid.
	3% oint	MYCODERM with benzoic acid and menthol
	2.2% ear drops	METHAZIL with 6% methanol
Diclofenac diethyl ammonium	1.16% gel	VOVERAN emulgel, RELAXYL gel, INAC gel.
Piroxicam	0.5 % gel	DOLONEX gel, PIROX gel.
Ibuprofen	50 mg gel	ACKS gel with mephenisin, methyl salicylate and menthol
Flurbiprofen	0.03% W/V eye drops	OCUFLUR
Indomethacin	1% W/V eye drops	INDOCAP ophthalmic drops.
Naproxen	10% gel	XENOLID gel.
Ketorolac tromethamine	0.5% W/V Eye drops	KETANOV eye drops KETLUR
Nimesulide	10 mg gel	NIZU gel with menthol 50 mg & Methyl salicylate 100 mg.
Rofecoxib	1% gel	ROFIZ gel, ROFECOXIB 1%.

frusemide is given along with IV fluids. Sodium bicarbonate ionizes salicylates making them water soluble and enhances their excretion through kidneys.

Precautions and Contraindications

Peptic ulcer, liver diseases, bleeding tendencies and viral fever in children contraindicate the use of aspirin/salicylates

Pregnancy - Aspirin should be avoided in pregnancy because it can cause premature closure of the ductus arteriosus in the foetus. Treatment with NSAIDs should be stopped one week before any surgery because of the risk of bleading due to antiplatelet effect.

Preparations

Preparations and dosage of salicylates (Table 30.1).

Uses

1. As analgesic

For headache, backache, myalgias, arthralgias, neuralgias, toothache and dysmenorrhoea. In headache PGs may be responsible for cerebral vasodilation. NSAIDs inhibit PG synthesis and relieve headache. - PG synthesis is responsible for dysmenorrhoea - aspirin effectively relieves pain. The NSAIDs are beneficial in a variety of painful conditions of integumental origin and all these are associated with PG synthesis.

2. Fever

NSAIDs are useful for the symptomatic relief of fever.

3. For inflammatory conditions

Aspirin is effective in a number of inflammatory conditions such as arthritis and fibromyositis.

4. Acute rheumatic fever

In a dose of 4-6 g/day (100 mg/kg/day) in 4-6 divided doses, aspirin brings about a dramatic relief of signs and symptoms in 24 to 48 hr. The dose is reduced after 4-7 days and maintenance doses of 50 mg/kg/day are given for 2-3 weeks.

5. Rheumatoid arthritis

Aspirin relieves pain, reduces swelling and redness of joints in rheumatoid arthritis. Joint mobility improves, fever subsides and there is a reduction in morning stiffness. But NSAIDs do not alter the progress of the disease. The relief is only symptomatic.

Dose: 4-6 g/day in 4-6 divided doses.

6. Osteoarthritis

NSAIDs provide symptomatic relief in osteo arthritis.

7. Postmyocardial infarction and post-stroke

Aspirin inhibits platelet aggregation and this may lower the incidence of reinfarction in a low dose of 50 to 300 mg/day. It also decreases the incidence of transient ischaemic attacks (TIA) and stroke in such patients.

Low dose aspirin is also given to patients with angina pectoris with the hope of preventing MI in such patients.

It is also given in deep vein thrombosis to prevent recurrence.

8. Miscellaneous uses

i. To delay labour - since PGs are involved in the initiation of labour, aspirin delays labour due to PG synthesis inhibition. But such use in associated with the risk of increased bleeding and premature closure of the ductus arteriosus.

ii. Some studies suggest that long-term use of aspirin at low doses is associated with a incidence of colon cancer.

nt Ductus Arteriosus. Aspirin may be en to bring about closure of PDA in the new born.

iv. Excess production of renal PGs is thought to be responsible for Bartter's syndrome characterised by raised plasma renin and aldosterone with hypokalemia. NSAIDs are useful in such patients.

v. Aspirin 60 - 100mg daily is recommended in pregnant women with 'high risk' of hyper tension. PGs are involved in the genesis of eclampsia and hypertension. Hence NSAIDs are useful in lowering BP in such patients.

9. Local

Salicylic acid is used as a keratolytic, fungistatic and mild antiseptic. Methylsalicylate is a counter-irritant used in myalgias. Mesalamine is used in inflammatory bowel disease (See page 336).

Drug Interactions

- Salicylates compete for protein binding sites and displace drug molecules resulting in toxicity with warfarin, heparin, naproxen, phenytoin and sulfonylureas. Inhibition of platelet aggregation may increase the risk of bleeding with oral anticoagulants.

- In low doses salicylates can counter the uricosuric actions of probenecid by decreasing uric acid excretion.

Diflunisal

Diflunisal is a difluorophenyl derivative of salicylic acid. Diflunisal is 3-4 times more potent than aspirin as an anti-inflammatory agent but is a poor antipyretic due to poor penetration into CNS. Gastrointestinal and antiplatelet effects are less intense than aspirin. Side effects are fewer.

Uses

Osteoarthritis, strain and sprains initial dose 500-1000 mg followed by 250 bd/tid.

PARA-AMINOPHENOL DERIVATIVES

Paracetamol (acetaminophen)

Phenacetin was the first drug used in this group. But, due to severe adverse effects it is now banned.

Paracetamol, a metabolite of phenacetin is found to be safer and effective.

Actions

Paracetamol has analgesic, good antipyretic and weak anti-inflammatory properties. Due to weak PG inhibitory activity in the periphery, it has poor anti-inflammatory actions.

Paracetamol is active on cyclo-oxygenase in the brain which accounts for its antipyretic action. In the presence of peroxides which are present at the site of inflammation, paracetamol has a poor ability to inhibit cyclo-oxygenase. It does not stimulate respiration, has no actions on acid-base balance, cellular metabolism, cardiovascular system and platelet function; it is not a uricosuric agent and gastric irritation is mild.

Pharmacokinetics

Paracetamol is well-absorbed orally and 30% protein bound; it is metabolised by the hepatic microsomal enzymes: by glucuronide conjugation (60%) and glutathione conjugation (20%).

Adverse effects

In antipyretic doses, paracetamol is safe and well-tolerated. Nausea and rashes may occur. But when large doses are taken, *acute paracetamol poisoning* results. Children are more susceptible because their ability to conjugate by glucuronidation is poor. 10-15 g in adults cause serious toxicity. Symptoms are - nausea, vomiting, anorexia and abdominal pain during first 24 hr. Paracetamol is hepatotoxic and causes severe hepatic damage. Manifestations are seen within 2-4 days and include increased serum transaminases, jaundice, liver tenderness and prolonged prothrombin time which may progress to liver failure in some patients. Hepatic lesions are reversible when promptly treated.

Nephrotoxicity may result in acute renal failure in some.

Mechanism

A small portion of paracetamol is metabolised to a highly reactive intermediate - N-acetyl-benzoquinone-imine which is detoxified generally by conjugation with glutathione. But when large doses of paracetamol are taken, hepatic glutathione is depleted and the toxic metabolite binds to sulphydryl groups in hepatic proteins resulting in hepatic necrosis.

Chronic alcoholics and infants are more prone to hepatotoxicity.

Treatment

Stomach wash is given. Activated charcoal prevents further absorption. Antidote is-N-acetylcysteine (150 mg/kg IV infusion over 15 min repeated as required; oral loading dose - 140 mg/kg followed by 70 mg/kg every 4 hr - 17 doses) - more effective when given early. N-acetylcysteine partly replenishes the glutathione stores of the liver and prevents binding of toxic metabolites to the cellular constituents.

Uses

- Paracetamol is used as an analgesic in painful conditions like toothache, headache and myalgia
- As an antipyretic.
- Chronic pulpitis, periodontal abscess, post-extraction - paracetamol is used with ibuprofen.

PYRAZOLONE DERIVATIVES

Phenylbutazone

Phenylbutazone has good anti-inflammatory activity, is more potent, but has poorer analgesic and antipyretic effects. It is a uricosuric agent.

Phenylbutazone causes retention of Na^+ and water. Thus after 1-2 weeks of use oedema results. It can also precipitate CHF.

Pharmacokinetics

Phenylbutazone is completely absorbed orally; IM injection is not recommended because its absorption is slow as it binds to local tissue proteins and also causes local tissue damage. It is 98% bound to plasma proteins; t½ is 60 hr.

Dose 100-200 mg, BD. Small doses may be given 3-4 times a day to avoid gastric irritation.

Adverse effects

- Phenylbutazone is more toxic than aspirin and is poorly tolerated - dyspepsia, epigastric distress, nausea and vomiting are common. Peptic ulceration and diarrhoea may occur. Oedema is a limiting factor and may precipitate CCF.
- Hypersensitivity reactions like rashes, serum sickness, stomatitis, hepatitis, nephritis, dermatitis and jaundice can occur. Phenylbutazone may cause serious haematological complications such as bone marrow depression, aplastic anaemia, agranulocytosis and thrombocytopenia.
- It may inhibit iodine uptake by thyroid, resulting in hypothyroidism and goitre on long-term use.
- CNS effects like insomnia, vertigo, optic neuritis, blurring of vision and convulsions may be encountered.

Because of its toxicity, phenylbutazone is withdrawn from the market in many western countries.

Uses

1. Rheumatoid arthritis
2. Ankylosing spondylitis
3. Osteoarthritis
4. Gout- phenylbutazone produces satisfactory relief from pain and inflammation in acute attacks
5. Other musculoskeletal disorders.

Azapropazone is structurally related to phenylbutazone but is less likely to cause agranulocytosis; t½ is 12-16 hr.

Metamizol is a potent analgesic and antipyretic, but poor anti-inflammatory agent and has no uricosuric properties (ANALGIN, NOVALGIN) 500 mg 3-4 times a day. It offers no advantages over aspirin. Not recommended in children upto 6 years.

Propiphenazone is similar to metamizol. *Dose* 300-600 mg 3-4 times a day (SARIDON).

INDOLE ACETIC ACID DERIVATIVES

Indomethacin is a potent anti-inflammatory agent, antipyretic and good analgesic. It is well-absorbed, 90% bound to plasma proteins; t½ - 4-6 hr.

Dose 25-50 mg BD-TDS.

Adverse effects are high Gastrointestinal irritation with nausea, GI bleeding, vomiting, diarrhoea and peptic ulcers can occur.

CNS effects include headache, dizziness, ataxia, confusion, hallucinations, depression and psychosis.

Hypersensitivity reactions like skin rashes, leukopenia, and asthma in aspirin sensitive individuals. It can also cause bleeding due to decreased platelet aggregation and oedema due to salt and water retention.

Drug interactions Indomethacin blunts the diuretic action of furosemide and the antihypertensive action of thiazides, furosemide, β-blockers and ACE inhibitors by causing salt and water retention.

Uses (Table 30.2)

- Rheumatoid arthritis
- Gout
- Ankylosing spondylitis
- Psoriatic arthritis
- For closure of patent ductus arteriosus (PDA).

Sulindac has weaker analgesic, antipyretic and anti-inflammatory actions but is less toxic. Does not antagonize the diuretic and antihypertensive actions of thiazides. It may be used as an alternative drug for inflammatory conditions.

ARYLACETIC ACID DERIVATIVES

Diclofenac is an analgesic, antipyretic and anti-inflammatory agent. Its tissue penetrability is good and attains good concentration in synovial fluid which is maintained for a long time. Adverse effects are mild.
Dose 50 mg BD-TDS. Gel is available for topical application (INAC GEL). Ophthalmic preparation is available for use in postoperative pain.

Uses

1. Treatment of chronic inflammatory conditions like rheumatoid arthritis and osteoarthritis.
2. Acute musculoskeletal pain, painful dental lesions.
3. Postoperatively for relief of pain and inflammation.

Ketorolac is another PG synthesis inhibitor having good analgesic and anti-inflammatory properties. It is used for its analgesic properties to relieve postoperative pain. It is mostly used parenterally though is can also be given orally.

TABLE 30.3: Properties of some commonly used NSAIDs

NSAID	Properties	Advantages	Uses
Aspirin	Good analgesic, antipyretic, anti-inflammatory and uricosuric agent	• Antiplatelet activity even in low doses; • Powerful anti-inflammatory activity	As analgesic-headache backache, neuralgias, dysmenorrhea; pyrexia, rheumatic fever, rheumatic, psoriatic and osteoarthritis, for antiplatelet activity in poststroke and post- MI; closure of PDA; to delay labour
Paracetamol	Good analgesic, antipyretic but poor anti-inflammatory *not a uricosuric agent*	• Less gastric irritation	As analgesic in fever
Diclofenac	Analgesic, antipyretic, anti-inflammatory	• Good concentration in synovial fluid; • Adverse effects mild	Chronic inflammatory conditions; rheumatoid arthritis, osteoarthritis, acute musculoskeletal pain and postoperative pain.
Piroxicam	Analgesic, antipyretic, anti-inflammatory	• Long-acting (given once a day) • Less ulcerogenic • Better tolerated	Arthritis, musculoskeletal pain, postoperative pain
Phenylbutazone	Good anti-inflammatory; poor analgesic, antipyretic; salt and water retention causes oedema; more toxic than aspirin	• Powerful anti-inflammatory agent	Rheumatoid and osteoarthritis; gout, ankylosing spondylitis
Indomethacin	Good analgesic, anti-inflammatory and antipyretic but toxicity is high	• Potent anti-inflammatory and analgesic	Rheumatoid, psoriatic and osteoarthritis, gout, ankylosing spondylitis, closure of PDA
Ibuprofen	Analgesic, anti-inflammatory, antipyretic all actions milder than aspirin	• Adverse effects milder therefore better tolerated	As analgesic in painful conditions, antipyretic, soft tissue injuries, fractures, postoperative pain, arthritis and gout

PROPIONIC ACID DERIVATIVES

Ibuprofen is better tolerated than aspirin. Analgesic, antipyretic and anti-inflammatory efficacy is slightly lower than aspirin. It is 99% bound to plasma proteins.

Adverse effects are milder when compared to other NSAIDs and the incidence is low. Nausea, vomiting, gastric discomfort, CNS effects, hypersensitivity reactions, fluid retention are all similar but **less severe** than phenylbutazone or indomethacin.

Dose Ibuprofen - 400-800 mg TDS (BRUFEN) ibuprofen + paracetamol (COMBIFLAM)

Uses

1. As an analgesic in painful conditions.

2. In fever.

3. Soft tissue injuries, fractures, following tooth extraction, to relieve postoperative pain, dysmenorrhoea and osteoarthritis.

4. Gout.

5. Surgical removal of impacted tooth - a combination of ibuprofen with a skeletal muscle relaxant like chlorzoxazone is recommended.

ANTHRANILIC ACID DERIVATIVES

Fenamates are analgesic, antipyretic, anti-inflammatory drugs with less efficacy, and are more toxic; contraindicated in children. They should not be used for more than one week. They are not preferred.

Adverse effects GI side effects are similar to aspirin but GI bleeding is less. Diarrhoea is common.

Uses Analgesic in myalgias, dysmenorrhoea, (250-500 mg TDS).

OXICAMS

Piroxicam is an oxicam derivative. It is long-acting, has good anti - inflammatory, analgesic and antipyretic activity. No clinically significant drug interactions are seen; better tolerated as it is less ulcerogenic. Dose 20 mg OD. It is **long-acting.** Piroxicam is used for rheumatoid arthritis, osteoarthritis, ankylosing spondylitis, acute musculoskeletal pain and postoperative pain and painful dental lesions.

Meloxicam is similar to piroxicam but in lower doses it causes less gastric irritation than piroxicam. It is therefore better tolerated. Dose 7.5-15mg once daily.

Many other oxicams are being developed with the idea of obtaining one which is nonulcerogenic. But most of them are prodrugs of piroxicam and in lower doses some of them are selective COX-2 inhibitors.

ALKANONES

Nabumetone is an anti - inflammatory agent with significant efficacy in rheumatoid arthritis and osteoarthritis. It shows a relatively low incidence of side effects, it is comparatively less ulcero genic. It is a prodrug and also selectively inhibits COX-2 - both account for the low ulcerogenic potential.

It is used in rheumatoid and osteoarthritis.

SELECTIVE COX-2 INHIBITORS

Celecoxib and rofecoxib - both diaryl substituted compounds are highly selective COX-2 inhibitors. They have good antiinflammatory, analgesic and antipyretic properties but do not affect platelet aggregation.

They are better tolerated because of milder gastric irritation (due to COX-2 selectivity) - but more long term studies are needed. Both celecoxib and rofecoxib can cause hypertension and edema which can be troublesome in patients with cardiovascular problems. They can be used in acute painful conditions like postoperative pain, dysmenorrhea and dental pain as well as in osteoarthritis and rheumatoid arthritis.

Dose:

Celecoxib - anti-inflammatory - 100-200mg once or twice daily.

Rofecoxib - analgesic - 50mg daily.
anti-inflammatory - 12.5-25 mg daily.

Nimesulide a sulfonamide compound is a sulfonanilide derivative. It is a weak inhibitor of PG synthesis with a higher affinity for COX-2 than COX-1. It inhibits leukocyte function, prevents the release of mediators and in addition has antihistaminic and antiallergic properties. Nimesulide has analgesic, antipyretic and anti-inflammatory actions like other NSAIDs.

Nimesulide is well-absorbed orally extensively bound to plasma proteins and has a t½ of 3 hours. It is excreted by the kidney.

Dose 50-100 mg BD

Adverse effects are mild; they are nausea, epigastric pain, rashes, drowsiness and dizziness. It is claimed to be better tolerated. Long-term use can cause hepatotoxicity.

Uses Nimesulide is used as an analgesic, antipyretic and anti-inflammatory agent for short periods as in headache, toothache, myalgia, dysmenorrhoea, sinusitis, postoperative pain and arthritis. It is beneficial in patients who develop bronchospasm with other NSAIDs. But because of the risk of hepatotoxicity, nimesulide is now banned.

ANTAGONISTS OF LEUKOTRIENE SYNTHESIS AND LEUKOTRIENE RECEPTORS

Zileuton, montelukast, pranlukast, docebenone, piriprost - Some of them inhibit 5-lipoxygenase preventing the synthesis of leukotrienes, while others act as competitive antagonists of LT receptor. They are useful in asthma and other inflammatory conditions.

Adverse effects Dyspepsia, diarrhea and headache.

Drugs that block both cyclo-oxygenase and lipoxygenase

Tenidap, diclofenac and indomethacin are drugs that block both cyclo-oxygenase and lipoxygenase. Tenidap also blocks IL-1 formation. These are less likely to precipitate acute attacks of bronchial asthma because they also inhibit leukotriene synthesis.

31 Drugs Used in Rheumatoid Arthritis and Gout

- • **Nonsteroidal anti-inflammatory drugs**
- • **Disease modifying drugs**
    - **- Gold salts**
    - **- d-Pencillamine**
    - **- Chloroquine and hydroxychloroquine**
    - **- Sulphasalazine**
    - **- TNF blocking agents**
    - **- Immunosuppressants**
    - **- Immunoadsorption apheresis**
- • **Diet and inflammation**
- • **Drugs used in gout**
    - **- NSAIDs**
    - **- Allopurinol**
    - **- Uricosuric drugs**
- • **Probenecid**
- • **Sulphinpyrazone**
- • **Benzbromarone**

Rheumatoid arthritis (RA) is a chronic, progressive, autoimmune, inflammatory disease, mainly affecting the joints and the periarticular tissues. Antigen-antibody complexes trigger the pathological process. Mediators of inflammation released in the joints initiate the inflammatory process. The earliest lesion is vasculitis, followed by synovial oedema and infiltration with inflammatory cells. There is local synthesis of prostaglandins and leukotrienes. Prostaglandins cause vasodilation and pain. The inflammatory cells release lysosomal enzymes which cause damage to bones and cartilage.

Drugs used in the treatment of rheumatoid arthritis

1. NSAIDs
2. DMDs

    Gold, d-penicillamine, chloroquine, hydroxychloroquine, sulphasalazine, TNF blocking drugs

3. Immunosuppressants

    Methotrexate, cyclophosphamide, azathioprine, leflunomide

4. Adjuvants

    Glucocorticoids

NONSTEROIDAL ANTI-INFLAMMATORY DRUGS

Nonsteroidal anti-inflammatory drugs (Chap. 30) are the first line drugs in RA. NSAIDs afford symptomatic relief but do not modify the course of the disease.

DISEASE MODIFYING DRUGS (DMDs)

Disease modifying drugs are also called disease modifying anti-rheumatic drugs (DMARDs). These are the second line drugs and are reserved for patients with progressive disease who do not obtain satisfactory relief from NSAIDs. They are capable of arresting the progress of the disease and inducing remission in these patients. Recent studies have shown that RA causes significant systemic effects that shorten life expectancy. This has renewed interest in the use of DMDs in RA. The effects of these drugs may take 6 weeks to 6 months to become evident and are therefore called slow-acting anti-rheumatic drugs (SAARDs).

Gold salts

Gold salts were introduced for the treatment of RA in 1920s, but only in 1960s their beneficial effects were clearly shown. They are considered to be the most effective agents for arresting the disease process.

On treatment, a gradual reduction of the signs and symptoms are seen. It brings about a decrease in the rheumatoid factor and immunoglobulins.

Mechanism of action is not exactly known - but gold depresses cell-mediated immunity (CMI). Gold salts concentrate in tissues rich in mononuclear phagocytes, selectively accumulate in the lysosomes of synovial cells and other macrophages in the inflamed synovium. They alter the structure and functions of the macrophages, depress their migration and phagocytic activity. They also inhibit lysosomal enzyme activity. Thus gold salts depress CMI.

Preparations

Aurothiomalate sodium (IM, IV) and aurothioglucose are given parenterally. Auranofin is given orally.

Adverse effects

Treatment with gold is associated with several adverse effects and only 60% of patients remain on treatment at the end of 2 years.

Adverse effects include -

1. *On skin and mucous membrane-* Dermatitis, pruritus, stomatitis, pharyngitis, glossitis, gastritis, colitis and vaginitis. A grey blue pigmentation on exposed parts of the skin may be seen.

2. *Kidney-* Haematuria, glomerulonephritis.

3. *Nervous system-* Encephalitis, peripheral neuritis.

4. *Liver -* Hepatitis, cholestatic jaundice.

5. *Blood-* Thrombocytopenia, leukopenia, agranulocytosis, aplastic anaemia.

6. *CVS -* Postural hypotension.

7. *Lungs -* Pulmonary fibrosis.

Contraindications

Kidney, liver and skin diseases; pregnancy and blood dyscrasias.

Uses

1. Rheumatoid arthritis - gold is used in active arthritis that progresses despite an adequate course of NSAIDs, rest and physiotherapy. In most patients gold salts arrest the progression of the disease, improve grip strength, reduce morning stiffness and prevent involvement of unaffected joints.

2. Gold is also beneficial in:
   - Juvenile rheumatoid arthritis
   - Psoriatic arthritis
   - Pemphigus
   - Lupus erythematosus.

d-Penicillamine

d-Penicillamine is an analog of the amino acid cysteine and a metabolite of penicillin. It is a chelating agent that chelates copper. Its actions and toxicities are similar to gold but is less effective than gold. Hence it is not preferred. It is used as an alternative to gold in early, mild and non-erosive disease.

Adverse effects

Adverse effects include drug fever, skin rashes, proteinuria, leucopenia, thrombocytopenia, aplastic anaemia, a variety of autoimmune diseases including lupus erythematosus, thyroiditis and haemolytic anaemia. Anorexia, nausea, vomiting, loss of taste perception and alopecia may also be seen.

Chloroquine and hydroxychloroquine

These antimalarial drugs are found to be useful in mild non-erosive rheumatoid arthritis. They induce remission in 50% of patients. They are less effective but are better tolerated than gold.

Mechanism of action is not exactly understood but they are known to depress cell-mediated immunity.

Toxicity

Chloroquine and hydroxychloroquine accumulate in tissues leading to toxicity. The most significant side effect is the retinal damage on long-term use. This toxicity is less common and reversible with hydroxychloroquine which is therefore preferred over chloroquine in rheumatoid arthritis. Every 3 months eyes should be tested. Other adverse effects include myopathy, neuropathy and irritable bowel syndrome.

Dose Hydroxychloroquine 400 mg/day for 4-6 weeks; maintenance dose is 200 mg/day.

Sulphasalazine

Sulphasalazine is a compound of sulphapyridine and 5-amino salicylic acid. In the colon, sulphasalazine is split by the bacterial action and sulphapyridine gets absorbed. This has anti-inflammatory actions though the mechanism is not known. *Adverse effects* include gastrointestinal upset and skin rashes.

TNF$_\alpha$ blocking agents

Cytokines, particularly tumor necrosis factor (TNF$_\alpha$) plays an important role in the process of inflammation. TNF$_\alpha$ produced by macrophages and activated T cells, acts through TNF$_\alpha$ receptors to stimulate the release of other cytokines. TNF$_\alpha$ blocking drugs are found to be useful in rheumatoid arthritis.

Infliximab

Infliximab a monoclonal antibody which specifically binds to human TNF$_\alpha$. When given in combination with methotrexate, it slows the progression of rheumatoid arthritis. It is given intravenously. Adverse effects of the combination include increased susceptibility to upper respiratory infections, nausea, headache, cough, sinusitis and skin rashes. Antinuclear and anti-DNA antibodies may develop.

Etanercept

Etanercept is a recombinant fusion protein that binds to TNF$_\alpha$ molecules. It is given subcutaneously and is found to slow the progression of the disease in rheumatoid arthritis patients. It is also found to be useful in psoriatic and juvenile arthritis. Etanercept is also given with methotrexate and the combination has a higher efficacy.

Pain, itching and allergic reactions at the site of injection, anti-etanercept antibodies and anti-DNA antibodies have been detected.

Immunosuppressants

Immunosuppressants are cytotoxic drugs and are reserved for patients with seriously crippling disease with reversible lesions after conventional therapy has failed. Among the immuno-suppressants, methotrexate is the best tolerated. Toxicity includes nausea, mucosal ulcers, bone marrow suppression and hepatotoxicity. Weekly regimens of low oral doses are better tolerated.

Leflunomide

Leflunomide is a prodrug. The active metabolite inhibits autoimmune T cell proliferation and production of autoantibodies by B cells. Leflunomide is orally effective, and has a long t½ of 5-40 days. *Adverse effects* include diarrhoea and raised hepatic enzymes.

Leflunomide is used with methotrexate in rheumatoid arthritis patients not responding to methotrexate alone.

Corticosteroids

Detailed pharmacology is discussed in chapter 64. Glucocorticoids have anti-inflammatory and immunosuppressant activity. They produce prompt and dramatic relief of symptoms but do not arrest the progress of the disease. However, long-term use of these drugs leads to several adverse effects. Moreover, on withdrawal of glucocorticoids, there may be an exacerbation of the disease. Therefore glucocorticoids are used as adjuvants. They may be used to treat exacerbations. Low dose long-term treatment with prednisolone is used in some patients (5-10 mg/day).

Intra-articular corticosteroids are helpful to relieve pain in severely inflamed joints.

Immunoadsorption Apheresis

Extracorporeal immunoadsorption of plasma for the removal of IgG - containing immuno complexes has been approved for the treatment of moderate to severe rheumatoid arthritis. The duration of benefit varies from a few months to several years. Adverse effects are mild and tolerable.

Diet and Inflammation

Clinical studies have shown that when patients of rheumatoid arthritis are given a diet rich in unsaturated fatty acids (such as marine fish), there is a decrease in morning stiffness, pain and swelling of the joints. Unsaturated fatty acids compete with arachidonic acid for uptake and metabolism. Moreover the metabolic products of unsaturated fatty acids are only weak inflammatory mediators when compared to the products of arachidonic acid metabolism. Adequate consumption of marine fish should be recommended. For people who do not eat fish, eicosapentaenoic acid 1-4 g/day may be given as tablets. It serves as an adjuvant.

PHARMACOTHERAPY OF GOUT

Gout is a familial metabolic disorder characterised by recurrent episodes of acute arthritis due to deposits of monosodium urate in the joints and cartilage. There is an inherent abnormality of purine metabolism resulting in over production of uric acid - a major end product of purine metabolism. As uric acid is poorly water soluble, it gets precipitated - especially at low pH and deposited in the cartilages of joints and ears, subcutaneous tissues, bursae and sometimes in kidneys. An acute attack of gout occurs as an inflammatory reaction to crystals of sodium urate deposited in the joint tissue. There is infiltration of granulocytes which phagocytize the urate crystals and release a glycoprotein that causes joint destruction. The joint becomes red, swollen, tender and extremely painful.

Secondary hyperuricaemia may be drug induced or may occur in lymphomas and leukaemias. Gout may also be due to decreased excretion of uric acid.

Strategy in the treatment of gout is either to decrease the biosynthesis of uric acid or enhance the excretion of uric acid.

Drugs used in gout are -

In acute gout

Colchicine, NSAIDs.

In chronic gout

- *Uric acid synthesis inhibitor*
  Allopurinol

- *Uricosuric drugs*
  Probenecid, sulphinpyrazone, benzbromarone.

Colchicine is an alkaloid of *Colchicum autumnale*. It is a unique anti-inflammatory agent effective only against gouty arthritis. It is not an analgesic.

Actions In gout, colchicine is highly effective in acute attacks and it dramatically relieves pain within a few hours.

Mechanism of action Colchicine inhibits the migration of granulocytes into the inflamed area and the release of glycoprotein by them.

Other actions Colchicine binds to microtubules and arrests cell division in metaphase. It increases gut motility by neurogenic stimulation.

Pharmacokinetics Colchicine is rapidly absorbed orally, metabolised in the liver and undergoes enterohepatic circulation.

Adverse effects are dose related. Nausea, vomiting, diarrhoea and abdominal pain are the earliest side effects and may be avoided by giving colchicine intravenously. Anaemia, leukopenia and alopecia may be seen. In high doses haemorrhagic gastroenteritis, nephrotoxicity, CNS depression, muscular paralysis and respiratory failure can occur.

Uses

1. Acute gout - colchicine 1 mg orally initially followed by 0.5 mg every 2-3 hours relieves pain and swelling within 12 hours. But diarrhoea limits its use.

2. Prophylaxis - Colchicine may also be used for the prophylaxis of recurrent episodes of gouty arthritis.

NSAIDs afford symptomatic relief in the treatment of gout. Indomethacin is the most commonly used agent in acute gout. Piroxicam, naproxen and other newer NSAIDs are also used. They relieve an acute attack in 12-24 hours and are better tolerated than colchicine. But NSAIDs are not recommended for long-term use due to their toxicity.

Allopurinol is an analog of hypoxanthine and inhibits the biosynthesis of uric acid.

Mechanism of action

Purine nucleotides are degraded to hypoxanthine. Uric acid is produced as shown in Figure 31.1. Allopurinol and its metabolite alloxanthine both inhibit the enzyme xanthine oxidase and thereby prevent the synthesis of uric acid. The plasma concentration of uric acid is reduced.

Pharmacokinetics

Allopurinol is 80% absorbed orally; t½ of allopurinol is 2-3 hr; t½ of alloxanthine 24 hr.

Adverse effects

Adverse effects are mild. Hypersensitivity reactions include fever and rashes. Gastrointestinal irritation, headache, nausea and dizziness may occur.

Attacks of acute gouty arthritis may be seen frequently during the initial months of treatment with allopurinol.

Drug interactions The anticancer drugs - 6-mercaptopurine and azathioprine are metabolised by xanthine oxidase. Hence when allopurinol is used concurrently the dose of these anticancer

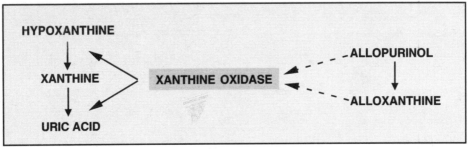

Fig. 31.1 Biosynthesis of uric acid. Both allopurinol and alloxanthine supress the enzyme xanthine oxidase.

drugs should be reduced.

Uses Allopurinol is used in chronic gout and secondary hyperuricaemia. Initial dose is 100 mg/day. and may be gradually increased to 300 mg/day depending on the response. Colchicine or an NSAID should be given during the first few weeks of allopurinol therapy to prevent the acute attacks of gouty arthritis. On treatment with allopurinol, tophi are gradually resorbed and the formation of renal stones are prevented. In patients with large tophaceous deposits, both allopurinol and uricosuric drugs can be given.

Uricosuric Drugs

Probenecid is an organic acid developed to inhibit the renal tubular secretion of penicillin in order to prolong its action.

Probenecid blocks tubular reabsorption of uric acid and thereby promotes its excretion. It is well-absorbed and well-tolerated. Adverse effects include gastrointestinal irritation and skin rashes.

Large amounts of water should be given to prevent the formation of renal stones.

Probenecid is indicated in chronic gout and secondary hyperuricaemia. It is started with 500 mg once a day and gradually increased to 1 g/day. Probenecid may also precipitate acute attacks of gout due to fluctuating urate levels.

Sulphinpyrazone

Sulphinpyrazone a pyrazolone derivative is another uricosuric drug which has actions and adverse effects similar to probenecid. It is used in chronic gout in an initial dose of 200 mg/day and gradually increased to 400-800 mg/day.

Benzbromarone

Benzbromarone is a uricosuric drug which acts by inhibiting renal tubular reabsorption of uric acid. It is a potent uricosuric given once daily 40-80mg., It is used as an alternative in patients allergic to other drugs. Benzbromarone can also be used in combination with allopurinol.

32 Drugs used in Psychiatric disorders - Antipsychotics and Antianxiety agents

- • **Organic mental disorders**
- • **Psychoses**
- • **Neuroses**
- • **Personality disorders**
- • **Antipsychotics (Neuroleptics)**
  - **- Classification**
  - **- Chlorpromazine (CPZ)**
  - **- Atypical antipsychotics**
- • **Anti-anxiety agents**
  - **- Benzodiazepines**
  - **- Buspirone**
  - **- β-blockers**
  - **- Others**

Since ages man has sought the help of drugs to modify behaviour, mood and emotion.

Psychoactive drugs were used both for recreational purposes and for the treatment of mental illnesses (Psyche = mind).

In 1931 Sen and Bose showed that *Rawolfia*

serpentina is useful in the treatment of insanity. ECT was introduced in 1937 for the treatment of depression. In 1950 chlorpromazine was synthesized in France and its usefulness in psychiatric patients was demonstrated in 1952. Since the second half of the twentieth century, extensive research has been carried out in psychopharmacology and we now have several useful drugs in this branch of pharmacology.

Psychiatric conditions are broadly divided into organic mental disorders, psychoses, neuroses and personality disorders.

Organic mental disorders

An organic cause is present in these disorders *ie.,* a definable toxic, metabolic or pathological change - as following head injury.

Psychoses

Of the psychiatric disorders, psychoses are the most severe forms and involve a marked impairment of behaviour, inability to think coherently, and to comprehend reality. Patients have no 'insight' into these abnormalities and have hallucinations and delusions. These include functional disorders where there is no organic cause like in schizophrenia, delusional disorders (paranoia) and affective (mood) disorders.

Schizophrenia

Schizophrenia affects about 1% of population, starts in an early age and is highly incapacitating. It has a strong hereditary tendency and is a disorder of thinking - earlier called split mind. Schizophrenia is characterised by delusions, hallucinations, irrational conclusions, interpretations and withdrawal from social contacts. Symptoms are grouped as positive and negative. *Positive symptoms* include delusions, hallucinations and disorders of thought while *negative symptoms* include poor concentration, social withdrawal, poverty of speech and lack of initiative and energy. Negative symptoms generally indicate poor prognosis and these symptoms do not respond to antipsychotics drugs. Patients with chronic schizophrenia have progressive shrinkage of the brain.

The pathology is not exactly understood but available evidence suggest overactivity of the neurotransmitters mainly dopamine and probably others including glutamate (NMDA receptors) and 5-HT in the brain.

Neuroses

Neuroses are the milder forms of psychiatric disorders and include anxiety, mood changes, panic disorders, obsessions, irrational fears and reactive depression as seen following tragedies.

Personality disorders

Personality disorders include paranoid, schizoid, histrionic, avoidant, antisocial and obsessive compulsive personality types.

Drugs used in psychiatric illnesses may be grouped as:

1. Antipsychotics or neuroleptics - used in psychoses.
2. Antidepressant drugs - used in affective disorders.
3. Mood stabilizers - used in bipolar mood disorders.
4. Antianxiety drugs - in anxiety related disorders.

Psychotropic drugs are drugs used in mental illnesses - they are drugs capable of affecting the mind, emotions and behaviour.

Neuroleptic is a drug that reduces initiative, brings about emotional quietening and induces drowsiness.

Tranquilliser is a drug that brings about tranquillity by calming, soothing and quietening effects. This is the older terminology. Neuroleptics or antipsychotics were called 'major traquillisers' and antianxiety drugs were called 'minor tranquillisers'. These terminologies are no longer used.

ANTIPSYCHOTICS (NEUROLEPTICS)

Classification

1. Classical/typical neuroleptics

A. *Phenothiazines* -

Chlorpromazine, triflupromazine, thioridazine, mesoridazine, trifluoperazine, fluphenazine.

B. *Butyrophenones* -
Haloperidol, droperidol, trifluperidol, penfluridol.

C. *Thioxanthenes* -
Thiothixene, chlorprothixene, flupenthixol

2. **Atypical neuroleptics -**
Clozapine, olanzapine, risperidone, quetiapine, ziprasidone, amisulpride, remoxipride.

3. **Miscellaneous -**
Reserpine, loxapine, pimozide.

CHLORPROMAZINE (CPZ)

Delay and Deniker demonstrated the antipsychotic effect of chlorpromazine. It has a wide variety of actions (hence the brand name Largactil) because it blocks the actions of several neurotransmitters including adrenaline, dopamine, histamine, acetylcholine and serotonine.

Mechanism of action

Typical neuroleptics act by blocking the dopamine D_2 receptors in the CNS. There are 5 subtypes of dopamine receptors - D_1 to D_5. They are all G-protien coupled receptors. Since dopaminergic overactivity mainly in the limbic area is thought to be responsible for pschizophrenia, DA receptor in the CNS helps in such patients. Some drugs like phenothiazines also block D_1, D_3, D_4 receptors. Dopamine receptor blockade also is responsible for the classical side effects of these

agents. There are 5 types of dopamine receptors. All are G protein coupled receptors.

Pharmacological actions

CNS: Behavioural effects - in normal subjects CPZ reduces motor activity, produces drowsiness and indifference to surroundings. In psychotic agitated patients, it reduces aggression, initiative and motor activity, relieves anxiety and brings about emotional quietening and drowsiness. It normalises the sleep disturbances characteristic of psychoses.

Other CNS actions

1. *Cortex* CPZ lowers seizure threshold and can precipitate convulsions in untreated epileptics.

2. *Hypothalamus* CPZ decreases gonado-trophin secretion and may result in amenorrhoea in women. It increases the secretion of prolactin resulting in galactorrhoea and gynaecomastia.

3. *Basal ganglia* CPZ acts as a dopamine antagonist and therefore results in extrapyramidal motor symptoms (drug induced parkinsonism).

4. *Brainstem* Vasomotor reflexes are

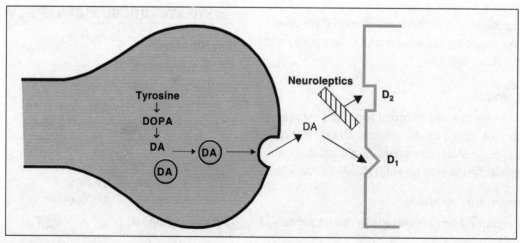

Fig. 32.1: Mechanism of action of neuroleptics. Neuroleptics block the Dopamine D_2 receptors and act as antipsychotics.

depressed leading to a fall in BP.

5. *CTZ* Neuroleptics block the dopamine (DA) receptors in the CTZ and thereby act as antiemetics.

Autonomic nervous system

The actions on the ANS are complex. CPZ is an alpha blocker. The alpha blocking potency varies with each neuroleptic. CPZ also has anticholinergic properties which leads to side effects like dryness of mouth, blurred vision, reduced sweating, decreased gastric motility, constipation and urinary retention. The degree of anticholinergic activity also varies with each drug.

CVS Neuroleptics produce orthostatic hypotension due to alpha blockade action and reflex tachycardia. CPZ also has a direct myocardial depressant effect like quinidine.

Local anaesthetic CPZ has local anaesthetic properties - but is not used for the purpose since it is an irritant.

Kidney CPZ depresses ADH secretion and has weak diuretic effects.

Tolerance develops to the sedative and hypotensive actions while no tolerance is seen to the antipsychotic actions.

Pharmacokinetics

CPZ is incompletely absorbed following oral administration and also undergoes significant first pass metabolism (bioavailability is 30%). It is highly protein bound; has a t½ of 20 to 24 hr and is therefore given once a day.

Adverse reactions

Antipsychotics have a high therapeutic index and are fairly safe drugs.

1. **Cardiovascular and autonomic effects** - postural hypotension, palpitation, blurred vision, dry mouth, constipation, nasal stuffiness and urinary retention result from blockade of a adrenergic and muscarinic receptors.

2. **CNS effects** - drowsiness and mental confusion are common, several neurological syndromes involving the extrapyramidal system are troublesome side effects.

Extrapyramidal symptoms

i. *Acute dystonias* - Facial grimacing, tics, muscle spasms, protruding tongue and similar involuntary movements can occur in the first few days of starting antipsychotics especially the high potency ones like haloperidol. They respond to anticholinergics.

ii. *Parkinsonism* - Bradykinesia, tremors and rigidity including the typical parkinsonian face' may be noticed in the first few weeks. It responds to anticholinergic antiparkinsonian drugs.

iii. *Perioral tremors* - also called 'rabbit syndrome' may occur after several months of antipsychotic therapy, Anticholinergics

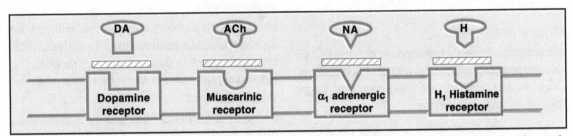

Fig. 32.2 : Chlorpromazine and other neuroleptics block dopamine receptor, muscarinic receptor, α_1 adrenergic receptor and H_1 histamine receptors which is responsible for their wide range of actions.

Seradase - don't put me to sleep

Rudresh a diabetic was an in-patient for drainage of an abscess. He was prescribed Seradase 10mg (serratiopeptidase) tablets. But the patient was found to be unusually drowsy the whole day and had extrapyramidal symptoms. On investigating the cause, it was found that the patient was given Seranase 10mg (haloperidol) in place of seradase. Such errors can put both the patient and the doctor including the nurse into trouble.

are useful.

iv. *Akathesia* - is a feeling of intense discomfort which compels the person to be continuously moving, like - constant walking. It necessitates a reduction in antipsychotic dosage and treatment with propranolol or other antianxiety drugs.

v. *Tardive dyskinesia* - appears after months or years of therapy and is characterised by involuntary movements of the face, tongue, eyelids, trunk and limbs. It can be disabling. Atypical antipsychotics like clozapine may be beneficial in such patients.

vi. *Malignant neuroleptic syndrome* is characterised by immobility, tremors and fever with autonomic effects like fluctuating blood pressure and heart rate. It can be fatal and requires immediate stopping of the neuroleptic. Dantrolene and bromocriptine may be useful.

3. Endocrine disturbances - gynaecoma stia, amenorrhoea and galactorrhoea due to DA receptor blockade.

4. Hypersensitivity reactions - jaundice, agranulocytosis and skin rashes.

Drug interactions

Neuroleptics enhance the sedative effects of CNS depressants, alpha blockers and of anticholinergic drugs. When combined with these groups of drugs, the effects may be additive.

Neuroleptics inhibit the actions of dopamine agonists and L-dopa.

Uses

Neuroleptics are given orally (chlorpromazine 100-800 mg). In acute psychosis they may be given intramuscularly and response is seen in 24 hr while in chronic psychosis it takes 2-3 weeks of treatment to demonstrate the beginning of obvious response.

1. *Psychiatric conditions* Psychoses including schizophrenia and organic brain syndromes like delirium and dementia all respond to antipsychotics.

2. *Nausea, vomiting* CPZ is a good antiemetic and is used in vomiting due to radiation sickness and drug induced vomiting.

3. *Hiccough* CPZ can control intractable hic- cough throughthe mechanism of action is not taken.

4. *Other neuropsychiatric syndromes* Neuroleptics are useful in the treatment of several syndromes with psychiatric features like psychoses associated with chronic alcoholism, Huntington's disease and Gilles de La Tourette's syndrome

Haloperidol

Haloperidol is a potent antipsychotic with actions similar to chlorpromazine. It differs from chlorpromazine in that it has lesser incidence of autonomic side effects and is therefore preferred in older patients.

Haloperidol is useful in acute schizophrenia, and is the drug of choice in Gilles de la Tourette's syndrome and Huntington's disease.

ATYPICAL ANTIPSYCHOTICS

The newer atypical antipsychotics like clozapine and others have the advantages of

1. causing fewer side effects

2. being effective in suppressing both positive and negative symptoms of schizopherinia and

3. being effective in resistant cases of pchoses.

Clozapine

Clozapine is an effective antipsychotic. It blocks the dopamine D_1 and D_4 receptors but has low affinity for D_2 receptors. Hence it has very low incidence of extrapyramidal side effects (EPS). Clozapine also blocks $5-HT_2$, alpha adrenergic and muscarinic receptors.

Clozapine has the following advantages over conventional antipsychotics:

1. Very low incidence of EPS.

2. Sedation is low.

3. No endocrine side effects - no galactorrhoea and gynaecomastia.

4. It is effective in patients not responding to conventional antipsychotics.

Adverse effects.

The most important disadvantages with clozapine is that it may cause agranulocytosis in some patients, which can be fatal. Hence its use should be restricted to patients not responding to other conventional drugs. Moreover, regular WBC counts are a must.

Clozapine can also cause sedation, weight gain and hypotension.

Olanzapine is similar to clozapine in actions and advantages. The incidence of EPS is negligible. It has the added advantage that it

Table 32.1: Therapeutic dosage of commonly used antipsychotics	
Drug	**Antipsychotic dose in mg/day**
Chlorpromazine	100-800
Triflupromazine	50-200
Thioridazine	100-400
Trifluroperazine	2-20
Fluphenazine	1-10
Haloperidol	2-20
Trifluperidol	1-8
Flupenthixol	3-15
Loxapine	20-100
Clozapine	50-300
Olanzapine	2.5-10
Risperidone	2-12
Pimozide	2-6
Sertindol	4-24

does not cause agranulocytosis.

Quetiapine is an effective antipsychotic, similar in actions to clozapine. Drowsiness and postural hypotension are seen.

Risperidone blocks serotonin ($5HT_{2A}$) and dopamine (D_2) receptors. It is effective against both positive and negative symptoms of schizophrenia.

Advantages

1. At low doses no EPS dysfunction

2. Low sedation

Ziprasidone is an effective antipsychotic with actions and mechanism of action similar to risperidone.

Amisulpride is a potent D_2 and D_3 antagonist. Its actions and advantages are similar to risperidone.

Reserpine acts by depleting monoamines i.e. NA and DA. It causes serious side effects including depression because of which it is not now used as an antipsychotic.

ANTIANXIETY DRUGS (ANXIOLYTICS)

Anxiety is tension or apprehension which is a normal response to certain situations in life. It is a universal human emotion. But when it becomes excessive and disproportionate to the situation, it becomes disabling and needs treatment.

Classification

Benzodiazepines

Diazepam, chlordiazepoxide, lorazepam, alprazolam.

5-HT agonist-antagonists

Buspirone, gepirone, ipsapirone.

Beta-blockers Propranolol.

Others Meprobamate, hydroxyzine.

Benzodiazepines

Benzodiazepines (Chap. 25) have good antianxiety actions and are the most commonly used drugs for anxiety. They are CNS depressants. Alprazolam in addition has antidepressant properties.

Buspirone

Buspirone is an azapirone with good anxiolytic properties. It is a selective 5-HT$_{1A}$ partial agonist 5-HT$_{1A}$ receptors are inhibitory autoreceptors and binding of buspirone inhibits the release of 5HT. Buspirone is also a weak D$_2$ antagonist. It is useful in mild to moderate anxiety. Antianxiety effect develops slowly over 2 weeks. Unlike diazepam, it is not a muscle relaxant, not an anticonvulsant, does not produce significant sedation, tolerance or dependence and is not useful in panic attacks.

Buspirone is rapidly absorbed and metabolised in the liver.

Dose: 5-15 mg OD or TDS.

Side effects are mild including headache, dizziness, nausea and, rarely, restlessness.

Uses Buspirone is used in mild to moderate anxiety and is particularly beneficial when sedation is to be avoided. Ipsapirone and gepirone are similar to buspirone.

OTHERS

Meprobamate

Meprobamate has anxiolytic property but is not used now as it is less effective and causes high sedation.

Hydroxyzine

Hydroxyzine is an antihistaminic with anxiolytic actions. But due to high sedation it is not used.

Beta-blockers

In patients with prominent autonomic symptoms of anxiety like tremors, palpitation and hypertension, propranolol (Chap. 13) may be useful. β-blockers are also useful in anxiety inducing states like public speaking and stage performance. They can be used as adjuvants to benzodiazepines.

33 *Antidepressants and Mood stabilizers*

- • **Antidepressants**
  - - **Classification**
  - - **Tricyclic antidepressants**
  - - **Selective serotonin reuptake inhibitors**
  - - **MAO inhibitors**
  - - **Atypical antidepressants**
- • **Mood stabilizers**

Mood disorders also called affective disorders are a group of psychoses associated with changes of mood, i.e depression and mania.

Depression is a common psychiatric disorder but the etiology of it is not clear.

Depression could be

1. Unipolar
   - • Reactive
   - • Endogenous
2. Bipolar mood disorder or manic depressive illness.

Unipolar depression

Reactive depression is due to stressful and distressing circumstances in life.

Endogenous depression is major depression and results from a biochemical abnormality in the brain. Deficiency of monoamine (NA, 5HT) activity in the CNS is thought to be responsible for endogenous depression.

Symptoms are:

- • Emotional symptoms - sadness, misery, hopelessness, low self esteem, loss of interest and suicidal thoughts.
- • Biological symptoms - fatigue, apathy, loss of libido, loss of appetite, lack of concentration and sleep disturbances.

Bipolar depression

Bipolar depression is characterised by alternate mania and depression. It was earlier called manic depressive psychosis (MDP) or manic depressive illness (MDI). The patient has cyclical mood swings. It is less common and is associated with a hereditary tendency. Mania can be considered opposite of depression with elation, over-enthusiasm, over-confidence, often associated with irritation and aggression.

Drugs used in affective disorders

Classification

1. *Tricyclic antidepressants (TCA) -*
   Imipramine, desipramine, clomipramine, amitriptyline, nortriptyline, doxepin

2. *Selective serotonin reuptake inhibitors (SSRI) -*
   Fluoxetine, fluoxamine, paroxetine, citalopram, sertraline, escitalopram

3. *Monoamine oxidase (MAO) inhibitors -*
   Phenelzine, tranylcypromine, isocarboxazid, moclobemide.

4. *Atypical antidepressants*
   Trazodone, nefazodone, venlafaxine, mianserine, bupropion, reboxetine, mirtazapine.

TRICYCLIC ANTIDEPRESSANTS

Pharmacological actions

1. CNS

In normal subjects, TCA cause dizziness, drowsiness, confusion and difficulty in thinking. In depressed patients, after 2-3 weeks of treatment, elevation of mood occurs; the patient shows more interest in the surroundings and the sleep pattern becomes normal.

Mechanism of action

TCAs block the reuptake of amines (noradrenaline or 5-HT) into the presynaptic terminal and thereby prolong their action on the receptors (Fig 33.1). Thus they potentiate amine neurotransmission in the CNS.

2. CVS

Postural hypotension and tachycardia (due to blockade of α_1 adrenergic and muscarinic receptors) can be severe in overdosage.

3. ANS

TCAs have anticholinergic properties and cause dry mouth, blurred vision, constipation and urinary retention.

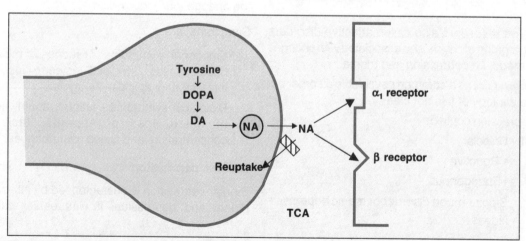

Fig. 33.1: Mechanism of action of of tricyclic antidepressents. 80% of noradrenaline released into the synaptic cleft enters into the synaptic neuron by reuptake. This reuptake is blocked by TCA.

Pharmacokinetics

TCAs are rapidly absorbed, extensively protein bound and metabolised in the liver. They have a long t½ and can be given once daily. On prolonged administration accumulation can occur resulting in cumulative toxicity.

Adverse effects

Sedation, postural hypotension, tachycardia, sweating and anticholinergic side effects like dry mouth, constipation, blurred vision and urinary retention are relatively common. TCA may precipitate convulsions in epileptics; may cause hallucinations and mania in some patients. Many TCAs may also cause weight gain due to increased appetite.

Acute toxicity is manifested by (mimic symptoms of atropine poisoning) delirium, excitement, hypotension, convulsions, fever, arrhythmias, respiratory depression and coma.

Treatment

Physostigmine is given to overcome atropine - like effects; sodium bicarbonate for acidosis, phenytoin for seizures and arrhythmias - with other supportive measures.

Tolerance and dependence

Tolerance develops gradually to the sedative and anticholinergic effects over 2-3 weeks. Starting with a low dose and gradually increasing the dose minimizes the side effects.

Following long-term treatment, TCAs should be gradually withdrawn, as withdrawal symptoms like headache, anxiety and chills can occur due to physical dependence.

Drug interactions

1. Tricyclics potentiate sympathomimetics - even small amounts of adrenaline used with local anaesthetics can cause serious hypertension.

2. Highly protein bound drugs like phenytoin, aspirin and phenylbutazone displace TCAs from binding sites resulting in toxicity.

3. TCAs potentiate the effects of alcohol and other CNS depressants.

SELECTIVE SEROTONIN REUPTAKE INHIBITORS (SSRIs)

SSRIs include fluoxetine, fluoxamine, paroxetine, citalopram, sertraline, escitalopram. Antidepressant actions and efficacy of SSRIs are similar to TCAs.

Mechanism of action

SSRIs block the reuptake of serotonin into the serotonergic nerve endings. Hence they enhance serotonin levels in these synapses (Fig 33.2).

SSRIs have the following advantages over TCAs.

- Low cardiovascular side effects
- Anticholinergic side effects are negligible
- Less sedation
- Preferred in elderly because of low anticholinergic effects (anticholinergic effects like constipation and urinary retention may be troublesome in the elderly)
- Safer in overdose (this is particularly advantageous in patients with depression who may have suicidal tendencies.)
- Due to low side effect profile, SSRIs are generally well accepted by patients.
- Escitalopram is 1000 times more potent than citalopram. Moreover, unlike with other SSRIs, drug interactions are uncommon with escitalopram.

Adverse effects to SSRIs include nausea, vomiting, insomnia, anxiety and sexual dysfunction.

Among the SSRIs, fluoxetine is the most commonly used.

MAO INHIBITORS

Monoamine oxidase (MAO) is an enzyme which metabolizes NA, 5-HT and DA. Drugs which inhibit this enzyme enhance the neuronal levels of NA, DA and 5HT. MAO exists as two isozymes - MAO_A and MAO_B. MAO_A is selective for 5-HT. Reversible and MAO_A selective inibitors like moclobemide are now developed. Nonselective and irreverible MAO inhibitors- phenelzine and tranylcypromine are associated with several side effects and many food-drug interactions.

Tranylcypromine and phenelzine

- Irreversibly inhibit the enzyme MAO and enhance neuronal levels of noradrenaline, dopamine and 5-HT.

- Antidepressant actions develop slowly over weeks of treatment.

- Most of them are long acting and require 1-2 weeks for recovery of MAO activity after stopping the drug.

- Side effects are hypotension, weight gain, restlessness, insomnia (due to CNS stimulation), anticholinergic effects and, rarely, liver dysfunction.

- They interact with many drugs and food.

- Patients on MAO inhibitors taking tyramine containing foods like cheese, beer, wines, yeast, buttermilk and fish - develop severe hypertension and is known as *'cheese reaction.'* Tyramine is normally metabolised by MAO in the gut wall. On inhibition of MAO by drugs, tyramine escapes metabolism and displaces NA from nerve endings leading to hypertension.

- Similar interaction with SSRI can result in severe hypertension (serotonin syndrome).

- Because of the side effects and drug interactions, MAO inhibitors are not the preferred antidepressants.

Moclobemide

Moclobemide is a reversible, competitive, selective MAO_A inhibitor. It is short acting and MAO activity recovers within 1-2 days after stopping the drug. It is found to be an effective antidepressant and has the advantages that it is not a sedative, does not produce cardiovascular and anticholinergic side effects. Hence it is well tolerated. No significant drug interactions are seen.

Adverse effects include nausea, insomnia, headache and dizziness.

Moclobemide is used in mild to moderate depression as an alternative to TCA. It is also useful in anxiety related mood disorders.

ATYPICAL ANTIDEPRESSANTS

Atypical antidepressants include trazodone, nefazodone, venlafaxine, bupropion, mianserin, and mirtazapine.

Advantages

- Fewer side effects - particularly sedation and anticholinergic effects

- Safer in overdose

- Effective in patients not responding to TCA.

Trazodone is a weak serotonin reuptake inibitor. It is short acting (t½ - 6 hr) and lacks anticholinergic activity. It is well tolerated and safe in overdosage. It can cause postural hypotension and priapism due to its α_1 blocking effects.

Nefazodone blocks serotonin reuptake and is an effective antidepressant. It is well tolerated - causes sedation and mild postural hypotension. Nefazodone is used in the prophylaxis of recurrent depression.

Venlafaxine inhibits the reuptake of noradrenline in addition to 5 HT (serotonin and noradrenaline reuptake inhibitor - SNRI) at the presynaptic neurons. It is thought to be faster acting and may be useful in patients not responding to other antidepressants. Venlafaxine has a short t ½ (~5 hrs) and needs to be given twice daily, it is safe in overdosage. If abruptly stopped or if doses are missed withdrawal symptoms are common. Venlafaxine is better tolerated than the TCAs because it does not block alpha adrenergic, muscarinic and histamine H_1 receptors and therefore devoid of the related adverse effects.

Mirtazapine blocks $5HT_2$, $5HT_3$ and α_2 receptors and enhances the release of NA and 5HT. It is faster acting - action starts by one week of treatment. It causes sedation but other side effects are negligible.

Bupropion is a weak DA reuptake inhibitor and has CNS stimulant effects. It is used in depression with anxiety. Bupropion is also used to help stop smoking (along with nicotine patch).

Mianserin acts by blocking presynaptic α_2 receptors but toxicity including blood dyscrasias, seizures and liver damage has limited its use

Uses of Antidepressants

1. *Endogenous depression* Antidepressants are used over a long period. The response appears after 2-3 weeks of treatment. The choice of drug depends on the side effects and patient factors like age. In severe depression with suicidal tendencies, electroconvulsive therapy (ECT) is given.

2. *Panic attacks* Post-traumatic stress disorders and other anxiety disorders - all respond to antidepressants (acute episodes of anxiety are known as panic attacks).

3. *Obsessive compulsive disorders* SSRIs and clomipramine are effective.

4. *Nocturnal enuresis* in children may be treated with antidepressants only when other measures fail and drugs are indicated.

5. *Psychosomatic disorders* Newer antidepressants are tried in fibromyalgia, irritable bowel syndrome, chronic fatigue, tics, migraine and sleep apnoea.

6. *Other indications* Attention deficit hyperactivity disorder, chronic pain and chronic alcoholism - may result in depression - antidepressants are tried.

MOOD STABILIZERS

Mood stabilzers control the mood swings that are seen in bipolar mood disorders. They are also called *antimanic drugs*. Lithium salts (Lithium carbonate and lithium citrate) have been used for several decades but several antiepileptics like carbamazepine, valproic acid and gabapentin are now being tried. Antipsychotics like chlorpromazine and haloperidol are used in acute episodes of mania.

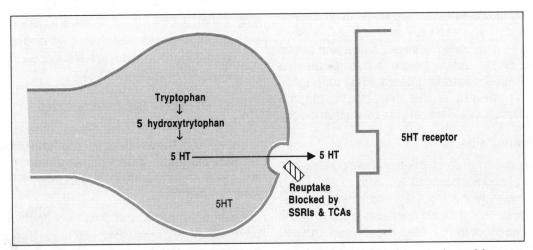

Fig. 33.2: Mechanism of action of SSRIs. They block the reuptake of serotonin and improve serotonergic transmission.

LITHIUM

Lithium is a monovalent cation. On prophylactic use in bipolar mood disorder (manic-depressive illness), lithium acts as a mood stabilizer. It prevents swings of mood and thus reduces both the depressive and manic phases of the illness. Given in acute mania, it gradually suppresses the episode over weeks.

Mechanism of action of lithium is complex and not fully understood. It is thought that lithium acts by the following mechanisms -

- It inhibits the synthesis of second messengers IP_3 and DAG by blocking the phospho tidyl inositol (PI) pathway.

- Lithuim blocks the formation of inositol from IP_3 and thereby inhibits the regeneration of PI. Depletion of membrane phosphotidyl inositol results in inhibition of receptor mediated effects through IP_3 and DAG. This is the accepted mechanism of action.

- Lithium also decreases hormone - induced cAMP production but the actual significance of this effect in the brain is not well understood.

Pharmacokinetics Lithium is a small ion and mimics the role of sodium in excitable tissues. Given orally it is well-absorbed. It is filtered at the glomerulus but reabsorbed like sodium. Steady state concen tration is reached in 5 - 6 days. Lithium is secreted in sweat, saliva and breast milk. Since safety margin is narrow, **plasma lithium concentration needs to be monitored** (0.5-1 mEq/lit is the therapeutic plasma concentration) 3-5 mEql/lit can cause fatal toxicity.

Adverse effects

Lithium is a drug of low therapeutic index and side effects are common. Nausea, vomiting, mild diarrhoea, thirst and polyuria occur initially in most patients. Weight gain can also occur. As the plasma concentration rises, hypothyroidism, CNS effects like coarse tremors, drowsiness, giddiness, confusion, ataxia, blurred vision and nystagmus are seen. In severe overdosage, delirium, muscle twitchings, convulsions, arrhythmias and renal failure develop.

Precautions

1. Minimum effective dose should be used.
2. Patients should always use the same formulation.
3. Patients should be made aware of the first symptom of toxicity.
4. Lithium is contraindicated in pregnancy.

Drug Interactions

1. Diuretics enhance Na^+ loss and lithium absorption from the kidney. This increases plasma lithium levels resulting in toxicity.
2. NSAIDs decrease lithium elimination and enhance toxicity.

Uses

1. Prophylaxis of bipolar mood disorder - episodes of mania and depression and their severity are reduced.
2. Acute mania - since the response to lithium is slow, neuroleptics are preferred.
3. Depression - Lithium is tried along with other antidepressants as an add-on drug in the treatment of severe recurrent depression.
4. Other uses - lithium is tried in recurrent neuropsychiatric disorders, childhood mood disorders, hyperthyroidism and inappropriate ADH secretion syndrome.

OTHER MOOD STABILIZERS

Because of difficulty in using lithium, other drugs are being tried. The antiepileptics *carbamazepine, sodium valproate, gabapentin and lamotrigine* are found to be useful, less toxic alternatives. (See Chap 27).

Carbamazepine is found to be effective in preventing the relapses of bipolor mood disorder and in the treatment of acute mania. It can be combined with lithium for better therapeutic effects but lithium can enhance the toxicity of carbamazepine.

Mechanism of action is not understood. Carbamazepine may be used alone in mild cases as a mood stabilizer. **Dose:** started with 200mg twice daily and may be increased if required.

Sodium valproate can be tried alone in mild to moderate cases or along with lithium in refractory cases. It is now known that sodium valproate has antimanic effects. It has several advantages.

- It is almost as effective as lithium.
- It may be effective in patients not responding to lithium.

- It is well tolerated and adverse effects are milder as compared to lithium. Nausea may be experienced in some patients.

- It can be combined with other antipsychotics and the combination is well tolerated.

- Valproic acid is now considered as the first line drug in the initial treatment of mania.

Dose : started with 750mg/ day and may be increased to 1500 - 2000mg/day if required.

Lamotrigine, gabapentin and other newer anteipileptics are being tried in the prophylaxis of bipolar mood disorder as alternatives to lithium.

34 CNS Stimulants & Drugs of Abuse

- • **Respiratory stimulants**
  - **- Doxapram**
  - **- Nikethamide**
- • **Psychomotor stimulants**
  - **- Amphetamine**
  - **- Cocaine**
  - **- Methylxanthines**
- • **Nootropics**
- • **Drugs of Abuse**

Drugs that have a predominantly stimulant effect on the CNS may be broadly divided into:

1. **Respiratory stimulants**
   Doxapram, nikethamide

2. **Psychomotor stimulants**
   Amphetamine, cocaine, methylxanthines

3. **Convulsants**
   Leptazol, strychnine.

Respiratory stimulants are also called *analeptics*. These drugs stimulate respiration and are sometimes used to treat respiratory failure. Though they may bring about temporary improvement in respiration, the mortality is not reduced. They have a low safety margin and may produce convulsions.

Doxapram appears to act mainly on the brainstem and spinal cord and increase the activity of respiratory and vasomotor centres.

Adverse effects are nausea, cough, restlessness, hypertension, tachycardia, arrhythmias and convulsions.

Uses

1. Doxapram is occasionally used IV as an analeptic in acute respiratory failure

2. Apnoea in premature infants not responding to theophylline.

Nikethamide is not used because of the risk of convulsions.

Psychomotor stimulants

Amphetamine and dextroamphetamine are sympathomimetic drugs (Chap. 12).

Cocaine is a CNS stimulant, produces euphoria and is a drug of abuse (Page 178).

Methylxanthines

Caffeine, theophylline and theobromine are the naturally occurring xanthine alkaloids. The beverages - coffee contains caffeine; tea contains theophylline and caffeine; cocoa has caffeine and theobromine.

Actions

CNS Caffeine and theophylline are CNS stimulants. They bring about an increase in mental alertness, a reduction of fatigue, produce a sense of well being and improve motor activity and performance with a clearer flow of thought. Caffeine stimulates the respiratory centre. Higher doses produce irritability, nervousness, restlessness, insomnia, excitement and headache. High doses can result in convulsions.

CVS Methylxanthines increase the force of contraction of the myocardium and increase the heart rate and therefore increase the cardiac output. But, they also produce peripheral vasodilatation which tends to decrease the BP. The changes in BP are therefore not consistent. Caffeine causes vasoconstriction of cerebral blood vessels.

Kidneys The xanthines have a diuretic effect and thereby increase the urine output.

Smooth muscle Xanthines cause relaxation of smooth muscles especially the bronchial smooth muscle (Page 283).

Skeletal muscle Xanthines enhance the power of muscle contraction and thereby increase the capacity to do muscular work by both a central stimulant effect and the peripheral actions.

GI tract Xanthines increase the secretion of acid and pepsin in the stomach and are gastric irritants.

Adverse effects

Include nervousness, insomnia, tremors, tachycardia, hypotension, arrhythmias, headache, gastritis, nausea, vomiting, epigastric pain and diuresis. High doses produce convulsions. Tolerance develops after sometime. Habituation to caffeine is common.

Uses

i. *Headache* Because of the effect of caffeine on cerebral blood vessels, it is combined with ergotamine for the relief of migraine headache. Caffeine is also combined with aspirin/paracetamol for the treatment of headache.

ii. *Bronchial asthma* Theophylline is used in the treatment of bronchial asthma.

NOOTROPICS

Nootropics are drugs that improve memory and cognition. They are also called cognition enhancers.

S – described as a 'nootropic agent' is thought to protect cerebral cortex from hypoxia and improve learning and memory. In higher doses it also inhibits platelet aggregation. Adverse effects include insomnia, weight-gain, nervousness, depression and gastrointestinal disturbances.

Piracetam and aniracetam have been tried in dementia, myoclonus, stroke and other cerebrovascular accidents; alcoholism, Alzhemer's disease (See page 208) behavioural disorders and learning problems in children and in vertigo. The beneficial effects in all these are not proved.

DRUGS OF ABUSE

Several drugs have been used for recreational purposes - for their pleasurable effects. Drug abuse is often closely associated with drug dependence. Dependence may by physical or psychological. (See page 50). Sudden withdrawal of such drugs of dependence can results in withdrawal symptoms which are difficult to tolerate. The word drug addiction is used to mean a drug dependence.

Drugs of dependence include (some examples)

• Opioids	Morphine, Heroin, Pethidine
• CNS stimulants	Amphetamines, cocaine, caffeine, nicotine
• CNS depressants	Ethylalcohol, Barbiturates, Benzodiazepines, Methaqualone.
• Hallucinogens	LSD, Mescaline, Phencyclidine (PCP), Psilocybine, psilocin, dimethyl tryptamine (DMT) diethyltryptamine (DET) Cannabinoids.

Drugs which are not discussed in the respective chapters have been dealt here.

CNS Stimulants

Cocaine, amphetamines and their analogs including methamphetamine methylphenidate and methylene dioxymethamphetamine (MDMA, 'ecstasy') are CNS stimulants. Long term abuse of these stimulants can result in changes in the personality, paranoid behaviour and even psychosis.

Caffeine - Long term intake of caffeine can cause dependence. Withdrawal symptoms like headache and lethargy can occur.

Nicotine is an alkaloid present in tobacco and is a commonly used drug of dependence. Tobacco is used for smoking (as cigarettes) as well as by other routes (like nasal insufflation of snuff) and by chewing.

CNS depressants

Sedative hypnotics like barbiturates, benzodiazepenes and meprobamate are abused for their pleasurable effects and anxiolytic properties. Barbiturate over dosage can often be fatal.

Ethanol is the most common and oldest agent of abuse. Chronic drinkers develop withdrawal symptoms on suddenly stopping alcohol and develop a craving for the drug (See page192).

HALLUCINOGENS

Hallucinogens or psychotogenic drugs are drugs that can produce psychosis. They are also called psychotomimetics, psychedelics or psychodysleptics.

Hallucinogens include -

Lysergic acid diethylamide (LSD) is a semisynthetic derivative related to the ergot alkaloid ergometrine. Like ergometrine it also is an uterine stimulant. It was synthesized by Hoffmann in 1938.

Pharmacological Effects: LSD is very potent and a dose of 20 - 30 mcg can bring about its effects. It produces euphoria, emotional out bursts, visual illusions, altered perception, terror, impairment of judgement, mood and thinking ability. Mood swings and a feeling of disintegration of the person can be highly frightening. LSD also produces sympathetic stimulation, anxiety tremors and nausea. The symptoms last from 8 to 12 hours. LSD is effective both orally and parenterally - but is usually taken orally is obtained from a mushroom while mescaline is obtained from a cactus.

Phencyclidine (PCP) causes CNS stimulation, hallucinations (mainly auditory), psychotic behaviour and dissociative anaesthesia (ketamine, a PCP derative is used for dissociative anaesthesia), sweating, tachycardia, hypertension and nystagmus. Overdosage with PCP and ketamine can be fatal.

Tolerance and dependence - The development of tolerance to the effects of hallucinogens is rapid - even after 3 - 4 doses tolerance can be evident. Fortunately there are no physical withdrawal symptoms and no craving for these hallucinogens - therefore there is no dependence.

Cannabinoids:

Cannabis obtained from the hemp plant (*Cannabis sativa*) has been used for its pleasurable effects since several centuries. **Marijuana** is the name given for dried leaves and flowering heads of the plant, while **Hashish** or **charas** is the dried solid, black resinous substance obtained from the leaves of the plant. **Ganja** is the dried female inflorescence. All these forms are used for smoking while **Bhang** is taken orally and consists of dried leaves of cannabis. A^9 tetrahydrocannabinol (THC) is the principal constituent of cannabis that is responsible for psychopharmacological effects. On smoking, THC is rapidly absorbed. It produces euphoria, uncontrolled laughing, a feeling of relaxation, altered time sense, a dream-like state followed by drowsiness and poor motor co-ordination. These effects may vary from person to person based on the personality of the individual.

Mechanism of action

Cannabinoids act on the cannabinoid receptors (CB_1) present in the CNS. **Anandamide** is an endogenous substance that binds the cannabinoid receptors. Its physiological role is not clear.

Other actions

Cannabinoids also produce tachycardia, vasodilation. The conjunctiva are red because of vasodilation. hypotension, bronchodilation and reduce intraocular pressure. They also have analgesic and antiemetic properties (dronabinol see page 329). Chronic heavy marijuana smokers may experience bronchitis, airway obstruction, precancerous changes in the lung and worsening of angina.

35 *Histamine and Antihistamines*

- **Histamine**
- **Histamine substitutes**
- **Antihistamines**
- **Newer non - sedative antihistamines**
- **Other Drugs**
- **Uses of antihistamines**

Autocoids are -

- Amines
  Histamine, 5-hydroxytryptamine

- Peptides
  Angiotensin, kinins

- Phospholipid derived autacoids
  Prostaglandins, leukotrienes,
  platelet activating factor (PAF).

Autacoids Autacoids are substances formed in various tissues, have complex physiologic and pathologic actions and act locally at the site of synthesis. They have a brief action and are destroyed locally. Hence they are called '*local hormones*'. They differ from true hormones which are produced by specific cells and reach their target tissues through circulation. The word autacoid is derived from Greek: *autos* = self *akos* = remedy.

HISTAMINE

Histamine (tissue amine) (*Histos* = tissue) is a biogenic amine formed in many tissues. It is also found in the venoms of bees, wasps and other stinging secretions.

Synthesis, storage, distribution and degradation

In humans, histamine is formed by the decarboxylation of the amino acid histidine.

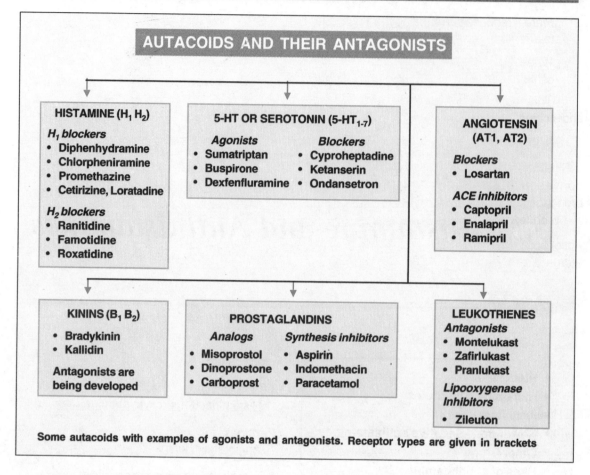

AUTACOIDS AND THEIR ANTAGONISTS

HISTAMINE (H_1 H_2)

H_1 blockers
- Diphenhydramine
- Chlorpheniramine
- Promethazine
- Cetirizine, Loratadine

H_2 blockers
- Ranitidine
- Famotidine
- Roxatidine

5-HT OR SEROTONIN (5-HT_{1-7})

Agonists
- Sumatriptan
- Buspirone
- Dexfenfluramine

Blockers
- Cyproheptadine
- Ketanserin
- Ondansetron

ANGIOTENSIN (AT1, AT2)

Blockers
- Losartan

ACE inhibitors
- Captopril
- Enalapril
- Ramipril

KININS (B_1 B_2)

- Bradykinin
- Kallidin

Antagonists are being developed

PROSTAGLANDINS

Analogs
- Misoprostol
- Dinoprostone
- Carboprost

Synthesis inhibitors
- Aspirin
- Indomethacin
- Paracetamol

LEUKOTRIENES
Antagonists
- Montelukast
- Zafirlukast
- Pranlukast

Lipooxygenase Inhibitors
- Zileuton

Some autacoids with examples of agonists and antagonists. Receptor types are given in brackets

Large amounts of histamine are found in the lungs, skin and intestines. It is stored in the granules of the mast cells and basophils in an inactive form. Non-mast cell histamine found in brain, serves as a neurotransmitter. Degranulation of the mast cells releases histamine which is quickly degraded by deamination and methylation.

Mechanism of Action

Histamine produces its effects by acting on the histamine receptors. Three subtypes are known.

- H_1 - present in lungs, gut, blood vessels, nerve endings and brain.

- H_2 - stomach (gastric glands), heart, blood vessels and brain.

- H_3 - CNS.

Actions

1.CVS

Histamine dilates small blood vessels resulting in hypotension accompanied by reflex tachycardia. Cerebral blood vessels dilate producing severe throbbing headache.

Triple response

Intradermal injection of histamine elicits triple response comprising of:

- *Red spot at the site* (flush) - due to local capillary dilation.

- *Flare* - redness surrounding the 'flush' due to arteriolar dilatation.

- *Wheal* - local oedema due to the escape of fluid from the capillaries.

This response is accompanied by pain and itching.

2. Smooth muscle

Histamine causes contraction of the nonvascular smooth muscles. Thus bronchospasm and increased intestinal motility are produced.

Actions on other visceral smooth muscles like uterus are insignificant in humans.

3. Glands

Histamine is a powerful stimulant of the gas tric acid secretion-acts through H_2 recep tors (See page 317). It also stimulates pepsin and intrinsic factor secretion.

4. CNS

Histamine functions as a neuro-transmitter in the CNS.

5. Nerve endings

Histamine stimulates sensory nerve end ings causing pain and itching.

Adverse reactions include hypotension, flushing, tachycardia, headache, wheal, bronchospasm and diarrhoea.

Uses

Histamine is of no therapeutic value. It is occasionally used in some diagnostic tests like

1. Testing gastric acid secretion: To test the acid secreting ability of the stomach. But now pentagastrin is preferred for this purpose.

2. Diagnosis of pheochromocytoma: His tamine releases catecholamines and raises

BP - now not used.

3. Pulmonary function: To test for bronchial hyperreactivity.

Histamine Substitutes

Betazole is a H_2 agonist and can be used in gastric function tests. *Betahistine* is a H_1 agonist used to control vertigo in Meniere's disease.

ANTIHISTAMINES

Histamine antagonists can be H_1 receptor blockers and H_2 receptor blockers.

Drugs that competitively block H_1 histamine receptors are conventionally called the '*antihistamines*'. H_2 blockers (cimetidine, ranitidine, famotidine) are used in the treatment of peptic ulcer (see Chapter 43).

Classification

Sedative (I generation agents)

- Diphenhydramine, dimenhydrinate, promethazine

Less sedative (I generation agents)

- Pheniramine, chlorpheniramine, cyclizine, meclizine, buclizine, mepyramine, tripelennamine.

Newer non - sedative (II generation agents)

- Terfenadine, astemizole, loratadine, cetirizine, fexofenadine, acrivastine, azelastine, mizolastine, levocabastine, mequitazine

Actions

1. Blockade of actions of histamine

H_1 receptor antagonists block the actions of histamine on H_1 receptors. They block the histamine induced effects on smooth muscles of the gut, bronchi, blood vessels and triple response.

2. Sedation

Antihistamines cause CNS depression; sedation, dizziness, inability to concentrate and disturbances of coordination are common. Alcohol and other CNS depressants potentiate this action. Some patients may experience CNS stimulation resulting in tremors, restlessness and insomnia.

3. Antimotion sickness effects

Several antihistamines prevent motion sickness and vomiting due to other labyrinthine disturbances. Some of them also control vomiting of pregnancy.

4. Antiparkinsonian effects

Some of them suppress tremors, rigidity and sialorrhoea probably due to their anticholinergic properties.

5. Anticholinergic actions

Many of the H_1 blockers have anticholinergic property. This accounts for both useful and adverse effects. Such antihistamines have antisecretory, antiemetic and antiparkinsonian effects.

6. Other actions

Antihistamines also have local anaesthetic effects in high doses. Some of them also block α_1 adrenergic and 5-HT receptors.

Pharmacokinetics

Antihistamines are well - absorbed, widely distributed in the body, metabolised in the liver and are excreted in the urine. Dose and route of administration are given in Table 6.1.

Adverse reactions are mild and on continued use tolerance develops.

Sedation, dizziness, motor incoordination and inability to concentrate make driving dangerous while on antihistamines. Anticholinergic effects like dryness of mouth, blurred vision, constipation and urinary retention may be troublesome. Epigastric distress, allergic

TABLE 35.1: Dose and preparations of some antihistamines

Antihistamine	Dose and route	Trade name
First generation antihistamines		
Diphenhydramine HCl	25-50 mg oral, 10 mg IM	BENADRYL Cap, Syr
Dimenhydrinate	25-50 mg oral, IM	DRAMAMINE Tab, Syr, Inj
Promethazine	25-50 mg oral, IM	PHENERGAN Tab, Syr, Inj
Promethazine chlortheophyllinate	25-75 mg oral	AVOMINE Tab
Pheniramine maleate	25-50 mg oral, IM	AVIL Tab, Syr, Inj
Chlorpheniramine	4-20 mg oral, IM	ZEET Tab, Syr, Inj
Cyclizine HCl	50 mg oral	MAREZINE Tab
Meclizine HCl	25-50 mg oral	ANCOLAN Tab
Buclizine	25-50 mg oral	LONGIFENE Tab, Syr
Cinnarizine	25-50 mg oral	STUGERON Tab
Second generation (Nonsedative) antihistamines		
Loratadine	10 mg oral	LORFAST, Tab, Syr
Desloratadine	5 mg oral	DESLOR, Tab
Cetirizine	10 mg oral	ALERID, Tab, Syr
Fexofenadine	120 mg oral	ALLEGRA, Tab
Acrivastine	8 mg oral	SEMPRAX, Tab

reactions and headache can also occur. Many of them are teratogenic.

Drug interactions

1. Drugs that can produce sedation and CNS depression like alcohol, barbiturates, clonidine, benzodiazepines and antidepressants should not be combined with sedative antihistamines because sedation gets added up.

2. When terfenadine or astemizole are combined with microsomal enzyme inhibitors like erythromycin, ketoconazole or grape fruit juice , plasma levels of antihistamines raise - resulting in ventricular arrhythmias. Some of them have been fatal.

3. Antimuscarinic effects of older antihistamines get added up when combined with other drugs having antimuscarinic effects.

Newer non-sedative antihistamines

Newer non-sedative antihistamines also called second generation antihistamines have the following advantages over classical antihistamines:

- No sedation because they poorly cross the blood - brain barrier.

- No anticholinergic side effects as these agents are pure H_1 blockers and do not block cholinergic receptors.

- Some of them like astemizole are long-acting.

However, the therapeutic indications of these agents are limited to allergic disorders like allergic rhinitis and chronic urticaria. They are more expensive than conventional antihistamines. Terfenadine and astemizole can sometime' cause *torsades de pointes* and fatal ventricular arrhythmias; erythromycin, ketoconazole and itraconazole potentiate this cardiotoxicity. Terfenadine and astemizole are therefore withdrawn now. Loratadine and fexofenadine appear to be free from this toxic effect. Though considered nonsedative, cetirizine can cause some sedation when compared to other second generation agents.

Other drugs

Doxepine

Doxepine a tricyclic antidepressant also blocks H_1 receptors. Hydroxyzine is a good antipruritic and has a long duration of action- it is used in skin allergies- but it causes significant sedation. Cyproheptadine blocks both H_1 histamine and $5HT_2$ serotonin receptors.

Uses of antihistamines

1. **Allergic reactions:** Antihistamines are useful for the prevention and treatment of symptoms of allergic reactions. They are effective in allergic rhinitis, conjunctivitis, hayfever, urticaria, pruritus, some allergic skin rashes and pollinosis.

   Though they prevent bronchospasm induced by histamine, antihistamines are *not* useful in bronchial asthma because many other mediators are also involved in the pathogenesis of bronchial asthma. Moreover antihistamines render the respiratory secretions more thick making it difficult to cough it out.

2. **Common cold:** Antihistamines reduce rhinorrhoea and afford symptomatic relief in common cold.

3. **Motion sickness:** Given 30-60 minutes before journey, antihistamines prevent motion sickness - promethazine, dimenhydrinate, flunarizine, meclizine and cyclizine are useful. They are also useful in treating vertigo of Meniere's disease and other vestibular dis t u r b a n c e s - dimenhydrinate, meclizine and cinnarizine are preferred.

4. **Antiemetic:** Promethazine is used to prevent drug induced and postoperative vomiting. It has also been used in 'morning sickness'.

5. **Preanaesthetic medication:** For the sedative, anticholinergic and antiemetic properties, promethazine has been used as pre-anaesthetic medication.

6. **Hypnotic:** The sedative antihistamines are sometimes used to induce sleep. Hydroxyzine has been used as an anxiolytic.

7. **Parkinsonism:** Diphenhydramine, orphenadrine, promethazine are useful in drug induced parkinsonism due to their anticholinergic action.

8. **Cough:** due to postnasal drip can be controlled by antihistamines like diphenhydramine.

36 5-Hydroxytryptamine, Ergot Alkaloids, Angiotensin and Kinins

- 5 - Hydroxytryptamine
- Serotonin Agonists
- Serotonin Antagonists
- Drugs used in the treatment of migraine
- Angiotensin
- Kinins
- Cytokines

5-HYDROXYTRYPTAMINE

5-Hydroxytryptamine (serotonin) was isolated in 1948. A large volume of information on 5-HT is now available and has been of great pharmacological interest. It is found in various plant and animal tissues.

Distribution, synthesis and degradation

In human body, 5-HT is present in the intestines, platelets and brain. It is synthesized from the amino acid tryptophan and stored in granules. It is degraded mainly by MAO.

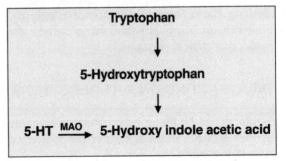

5-HT Receptors

The actions of serotonin are mediated through its receptors. Seven types of 5-HT receptors ($5\text{-HT}_{1\text{-}7}$) with further subtypes of 5-HT_1 and 5-HT_2 receptors are presently known. Many receptor - selective agonists and antagonists are being developed.

Actions

1. **CVS:** The action on blood vessels is

complex. Large vessels are constricted while arterioles dilate. A characteristic triphasic response is seen on blood pressure following IV injection.

- Initial fall in BP is due to increased vagal activity
- Rise in BP - due to vasoconstriction of large vessels, followed by
- Fall in BP - due to arteriolar dilation.

2. **GI tract:** Increases GI motility and contraction resulting in diarrhoea.

3. **Other actions:** Weak bronchoconstriction, platelet aggregation; stimulation of sensory nerve endings - causes pain if injected into the skin. 5-HT is a neurotransmitter in the CNS. Selective serotonin reuptake inhibitors (SSRIs) are used in the treatment of depression (See page 251).

Physiological and pathophysiological role

5-HT is postulated to be having a role in peristalsis, vomiting, platelet aggregation, homoeostasis and inflammation. It is also thought to initiate the vasoconstriction in migraine.

DRUGS ACTING ON 5-HT RECEPTORS

Serotonin has no therapeutic uses. However, its receptor agonists and antagonists have been used in various conditions.

Serotonin Agonists

Sumatriptan - a 5-HT$_{1D}$ agonist is effective in the treatment of acute migraine and cluster headache. Given orally/SC at the onset of an attack, sumatriptan relieves headache and also suppresses nausea and vomiting of migrane. It is short-acting.

Adverse effects include dizziness, altered sensations, weakness, chest discomfort and neck pain. It is contraindicated in coronary artery disease.

Other Agonists

Buspirone (See page 247) is a 5-HT$_{1A}$ agonist-antagonist used as an antianxiety agent.

Dexfenfluramine (See page 99) is used as an appetite suppressant.

Serotonin Antagonists

Cyproheptadine blocks 5-HT$_2$, H$_1$ histamine and cholinergic receptors. It increases appetite and is used to promote weight gain especially in children. It is also used in carcinoid tumours.

Ketanserin blocks 5-HT$_2$ receptors and antagonises vasoconstriction and platelet aggregation promoted by 5-HT. It is used in hypertension.

Ondansetron is a 5-HT$_3$ antagonist (See page 327) used in the prevention and treatment of vomiting due to radiation and cancer chemotherapy.

Many other drugs including some antihistamines also block serotonin receptors.

Ergot alkaloids

Ergot alkaloids are produced by *Claviceps purpurea,* a fungus that infects rye, millet and other grains. Consumption of such grains results in 'ergotism' manifested as gangrene of hands and feet, hallucinations and other CNS effects. Barger and Dale isolated ergot alkaloids in 1906.

Natural ergot alkaloids include ergometrine, ergotamine and ergotoxine. The semisynthetic dehydrogenated derivatives are also available.

Actions

Ergot alkaloids have agonist, partial agonist and antagonistic actions at 5-HT and alpha adrenergic receptors and agonistic actions at CNS dopamine receptors. Thus their actions are complex. Some of them are powerful hallucinogens, *e.g.* lysergic acid diethylamide (LSD). They cause stimulation of smooth muscles - some stimulate mainly vascular smooth muscles and others mainly uterine smooth muscles. The vasoconstrictor effect is responsible for gangrene.

Adverse effects like nausea, vomiting and diarrhoea are common. Prolonged use results in gangrene due to persistent vasospasm. Methysergide causes retroperitoneal and mediastinal fibrosis.

Uses (Table 36.1)

1. Migraine (See below)

2. Postpartum haemorrhage - ergometrine is used (See page 498) for the prevention and treatment of post partum haemorrhage.

DRUGS USED IN THE TREATMENT OF MIGRAINE

Migraine is a common disorder characterised by severe, throbbing and unilateral headache often associated with nausea, vomiting and fatigue lasting for several hours. In the classical migraine, a brief 'aura' of visual disturbances occurs prior to the headache. An attack is triggered by factors like stress, anxiety, excitement, food (like chocolate and cheese) and hormonal changes. These triggering factors stimulate the release of vasoactive substances from nerve endings which are responsible for the events that follow. However, the exact pathophysiology is not understood and several hypotheses have been put forward.

Drugs used in acute attacks

Aspirin, paracetamol or other NSAIDs are effective. Drug should be taken at the initiation of

TABLE 36.1: Serotonin agonists, antagonists and their therapeutic uses			
	Receptor	*Uses*	*Comments*
AGONISTS			
Sumatriptan	$5\text{-}HT_{1D}$	• Acute migraine • Cluster headache	Short-acting; may need repetition of dose
Buspirone	$5\text{-}HT_{1A}$ (Agonist-antagonist)	Anxiolytic	—
Dexfenfluramine	5-HT	Appetite suppressant	Patients should be carefully monitored for risk of pulmonary hypertension
ANTAGONISTS			
Cyproheptadine	$5\text{-}HT_2$; H_1-histamine and muscarinic receptors	• Appetite stimulant • Carcinoid tumours	—
Ketanserin	$5\text{-}HT_1$ and $5\text{-}HT_2$	Hypertension	Also antagonises platelet aggregation promoted by 5 - HT
Ondansetron	$5\text{-}HT_3$	Antiemetic	—
ERGOT ALKALOIDS			
Ergotamine	$5\text{-}HT_1$ partial agonist/ antagonist	Acute attack of migraine	—
Ergometrine	$5\text{-}HT_1$ partial agonist/ antagonist	Postpartum haemorrhage	—
Methysergide	$5\text{-}HT_2$ partial agonist/ antagonist	Prophylaxis of migraine	Not preferred due to risk of retroperitoneal and mediastinal fibrosis

attack. Metoclopramide can be combined with aspirin as it is an antiemetic and also speeds up absorption of aspirin.

Ergotamine given orally (or sublingual/rectal when vomiting is present) is an effective alternative.

Sumatriptan is very effective but short-acting.

Prophylaxis

When the attacks are frequent and severe, prophylaxis is needed. Drugs used for the prophylaxis are:

β- adrenergic blockers

Propranolol reduces frequency and severity of attacks. The initial dose is 40 mg twice daily and is gradually increased to a maximum of 160 mg twice daily. The mechanism of action is not exactly known.

Ca^{++} channel blockers

Flunarizine may be useful. It has weak Ca^{++} channel blocking properties and is thought to be selective for the CNS. Adverse effects include hypotension, flushing, drymouth, constipation and sedation.

Pizotifen and cyproheptadine

Pizotifen and cyproheptadine Block 5-HT and H_1 histamine receptors; may be used as alternatives.

Tricyclic antidepressants

Amytriptyline may be tried but it is associated with many adverse effects (See page 250).

Methysergide

Methysergide blocks 5-HT receptors but due to adverse effects like retroperitoneal fibrosis, it is not preferred.

ANGIOTENSIN

Angiotensins are peptides synthesized from the precursor angiotensinogen. Angiotensinogen, a circulating protein synthesized in the liver is converted sequentially to angiotensin I, angiotensin II and angiotensin III (Fig. 36.1). Angiotensin converting enzyme is widely distributed in the body. It is present in blood vessels, kidneys, heart, brain, lungs, adrenals and other tissues. Angiotensin II, the most potent angiotensin acts through angiotensin receptors (AT_1 and AT_2) present on the tissues.

Angiotensinogen
$\downarrow$ *Renin*
Angiotensin I
$\downarrow$ *Converting enzyme*
Angiotensin II
$\downarrow$ *Aminopeptidase*
Angiotensin III
$\downarrow$ *Angiotensinases*
Peptide fragments

Fig. 36.1 Synthesis and metabolism of angiotensins

Actions

Angiotensin II causes vasoconstriction resulting in increased blood pressure. It stimulates the synthesis of aldosterone by the adrenal cortex, increases sodium reabsorption by the kidneys and increases secretion of vasopressin. Angiotensin II also promotes the growth of vascular and cardiac muscle cells and may play a role in the development of cardiac hypertrophy as in hypertension. By these actions, renin- angiotensin system regulates the fluid and electrolyte balance as well as blood pressure.

Inhibitors of ACE and blockers of angiotensin II receptors are now used in the

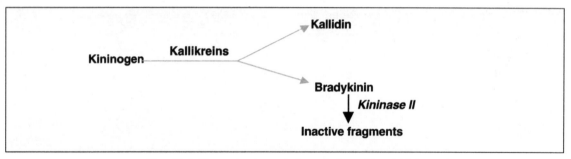

Fig. 36.2 Biosynthesis and degradation of bradykinin

treatment of hypertension, congestive heart failure and other conditions that are due to excess of angiotensin II activity (see Section 4).

KININS

Kinins are vasodilator peptides formed from the precursor kininogen by the action of the enzymes called kallikreins. Kallikreins are present in the plasma, kidneys, pancreas, intestines, salivary glands and other tissues.

Kinins are rapidly degraded by kininase II (Fig. 36.2) which is same as ACE and has a very short t½ (< 15 seconds).

Actions

Kinins are potent vasodilators and cause a brief fall in BP. They stimulate contraction of other smooth muscles - thus they induce bronchospasm in asthmatics, slow contraction of intestines (*Brady* = slow) and uterus. Kinins mediate inflammation, and stimulate the pain nerve endings. Kinins produce their actions by acting through β_1 and β_2 receptors.

Drugs affecting the kallikrein-kinin system - β_1 and β_2 antagonists are now being developed.

CYTOKINES

Cytokines are also considered as autacoids. They are peptides released from the inflammatory cells. They are classified into 5 families.

- Interleukins
- Colony stimulating factors
- Chemokines
- Growth factor and tumor necrosis factors
- Interferons

Cytokines stimulate specific receptors to bring about their effects. IL-1 and TNF - α are involved in inflammation - they are pro-inflammatory cytokines while IL-4, IL-10 and IL-13 inhibit inflammatory activity - they are anti-inflammatory cytokines. The interferons α and β have antiviral activity (See page 406, 444). while interferon γ has immunoregulatory activity (See page 448) and is used in multiple sclerosis.

37 Eicosanoids

- **Biosynthesis**
- **Prostaglandins and Thromboxanes**
- **Prostanoid receptors**
- **Actions**
- **Adverse effects**
- **Uses**
- **Leukotrienes**

Eicosanoids are 20-carbon (eicosa referring to the 20-C atoms) unsaturated fatty acids derived mainly from arachidonic acid in the cell walls. The principal eicosanoids are the prostaglandins (PG), the thromboxanes (TX), and the leukotrienes (LT).

Biosynthesis

Eicosanoids are synthesized locally in most tissues from arachidonic acid. The pathway for synthesis is shown in Figure 37.1.

The cyclo-oxygenase (COX) pathway generates PGs and TXs while lipoxygenase (LOX) pathway generates LTs. There are 2 cyclo-oxygenase isozymes *viz.* COX-1 and COX-2. COX-1 is present in almost all cells and prostanoids (PGs and TXs) obtained from COX-1 mainly take part in physiological functions. COX-2 is induced by inflammation in the inflammatory cells and the prostanoids produced by COX-2 are involved in inflammatory and pathological changes. All products of COX pathway are metabolised by oxidation and excreted in urine.

PROSTAGLANDINS AND THROMBOXANES

In 1930s it was found that human semen contains a substance that contracts uterine smooth muscle. As this substance was thought to originate in the prostate, they called it 'Prostaglandin' but it was later found to be produced in many tissues.

Prostanoid receptors

The prostanoids bring about their effects by acting on prostanoid receptors, which are G-protein coupled receptors. There are five classes of prostanoid receptors. They are -

- DP (for PGD_2)
- EP (for PGE_2)
- FP (for $PGF_{2\alpha}$)
- IP (for PGI_2)
- TP (for TXA_2)

Actions

The prostanoids act on many tissues to bring about the following effects.

1. **CVS:** Prostacyclin causes vasodilation while TXA_2 causes vasoconstriction. PGE_2 and $PGF_{2\alpha}$ are weak cardiac stimulants.

2. **GIT:** Most PGs and TXs stimulate gastrointestinal smooth muscle resulting in colic and watery diarrhoea. PGE_2 inhibits gastric acid secretion and enhances

---

Keybox 37.1

Prostaglandins

- 20-carbon unsaturated fatty acids synthesized from arachidonic acid through cyclo-oxygenase pathway

- PGI_2 causes vasodilation while TXA_2 causes vasoconstriction

- PGs contract g.i. and bronchial (TXA_2, $PGE_{2\alpha}$) smooth muscles. TXA_2 induces platelet aggregation (PGI_2 inhibits); PGE_2 and $PGF_{2\alpha}$ contract uterus. PGs stimulate bone turnover and sensitize the nerve endings to pain

- *Uses* Abortion, facilitation of labour, cervical priming, PPH, to maintain the patency of ductus arteriosus, for prevention of platelet aggregation, open angle glaucoma and peptic ulcer.

---

mucous production. Thus they have a protective effect on gastric mucosa.

3. **Airways:** PGE_2 and PGI_2 relax bronchial smooth muscles while TXA_2 and $PGF_{2\alpha}$ contract them. They may have a role in the pathophysiology of bronchial asthma.

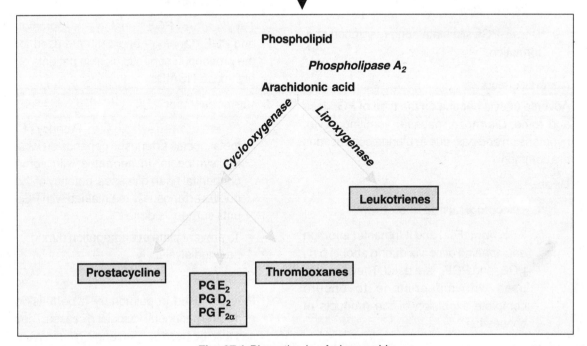

Fig. 37.1 Biosynthesis of eicosanoids

4. **Platelets:** TXA_2 induces platelet aggregation while PGI_2 inhibits platelet aggregation.

5. **Uterus** PGE_2 and $PGF_{2\alpha}$ contract human uterus (See page 499) which is more sensitive to PGs during pregnancy. They also soften the cervix. Thus PGs may be involved in the initiation and progression of labour. PGs are produced by foetal tissues during labour. PGs present in the semen may facilitate movement of sperms and fertilization by coordinating the movement of the uterus. They also play a role in dysmenorrhoea and menorrhagia.

6. **Kidneys:** PGE_2 and PGI_2 cause renal vasodilation and have a diuretic effect.

7. **CNS:** PGs increase body temperature when administered into cerebral ventricles. They also induce sleep.

8. **Nerves:** PGs sensitize sensory nerve endings to pain and on intradermal injection cause pain. They have a role in the genesis of inflammation.

9. **Bone:** PGs stimulate bone resorption and formation.

Adverse effects

Adverse effects depend on the type of PG, dose and route. Diarrhoea, nausea, vomiting, fever, hypotension and pain due to uterine contractions are common.

Uses

1. **Gynaecological and obstetrical**

   • **Abortion:** For I and II trimester abortion and ripening of cervix during abor t i o n , PGE_2 and $PGF_{2\alpha}$ are used. They are also used with mifepristone to ensure complete expulsion of the products of conception.

   • **Facilitation of labour:** As alternative to

Keybox 37.2	
PG analogs used therapeutically	
Misoprostol	PGE_1
Gemeprost	PGE_1
Rioprostil	PGE_1
Alprostadil	PGE_1
Enprostil	PGE_2
Dinoprostone	PGE_2
Carboprost	15-Methyl $PGF_{2\alpha}$
Latanoprost	$PGF_{2\alpha}$
Dinoprost	$PGF_{2\alpha}$
Epoprostenol	PGI_2

   oxytocics in patients with renal failure.

   • **Cervical priming:** Intravaginal PGE_2 is used.

   • **Postpartum haemorrhage:** Intramuscular $PGF_{2\alpha}$ is used as an alternative to ergometrine.

2. **Gastrointestinal**

   Peptic ulcer PGE_1 (analog - misoprostol) and PGE_2 (analog - enprostil) are used for the prevention of peptic ulcer in patients on high dose NSAIDs.

3. **Cardiovascular**

   • **Patent ductus arteriosus:** Patency of foetal ductus arteriosus depends on local PG synthesis. In neonates with some congenital heart diseases, patency of the ductus arteriosus is maintained with PGs until surgery is done.

   • To prevent platelet aggregation during haemodialysis.

4. **Other uses**

   PGs are used in pulmonary hypertension and some peripheral vascular diseases. They can also be used in open angle glaucoma to lower intraocular pressure.

LEUKOTRIENES

Leukotrienes (LT) are products of arachidonic acid metabolism synthesized by the lipoxygenase pathway and are found in the lungs, platelets, mast cells and white blood cells. ('Leuko' - because they are found in white cells; 'trienes' - they contain three double bonds). LTA_4 is the precursor from which LTB_4, LTC_4, LTD_4, LTE_4 and LTF_4 are derived. LTC_4, LTD_4 and LTE_4 are together known as slow reacting substances (SRS-A) of anaphylaxis. The LTs produce their effects through specific receptors.

Actions

Leukotrienes cause vasoconstriction, alter vascular permeability leading to edema, increase airway mucous secretion and are potent bronchiolar spasmogens. Given subcutaneously they cause wheal and flare. Leukotrienes have a role in inflammation including rheumatoid arthritis, psoriasis and ulcerative colitis. They also contribute to bronchial hyper-responsiveness in bronchial asthma.

Drugs that inhibit lipoxygenase like zileuton and thus block the synthesis of leukotrienes are useful in the treatment of bronchial asthma and allergic rhinitis.

Leukotriene receptor antagonists

Montelukast, zafirlukast and pranlukast block the actions of LTC_4 and LTD_4 on the bronchial and vascular smooth muscles. They are useful as adjuvants in bronchial asthma. They are all effective orally.

PLATELET ACTIVATING FACTOR (PAF)

PAF is an important mediator in acute and chronic, allergic and inflammatory phenomena. PAF is a lipid released from inflammatory cells on stimulation and acts on specific receptors. It causes local vasodilatation resulting in edema, hyperalgesia and wheal formation. It is a potent chemotaxin for leukocytes and a spasmogen on bronchial and intestinal smooth muscles. It is a mediator of inflammation.

RESPIRATORY SYSTEM

- Drugs used in the treatment of bronchial asthma
- Drugs used in the treatment of cough

Drugs used in the treatment of Bronchial Asthma

- **Sympathomimetic Drugs**
    - **Short acting β_2 agonists**
    - **Longer acting β_2 agonists**
    - **Adrenaline, ephedrine and isoprenaline**
- **Methylxanthines**
- **Anticholinergics**
- **Anti-inflammatory Drugs**
- **Mast cell stabilizers**
- **Cromolyn sodium**
- **Leukotriene receptor antagonists**
- **Treatment of Asthma**
    - **Mild asthma**
    - **Moderate asthma**
    - **Acute severe asthma**

Bronchial asthma is characterised by dyspnoea and wheeze due to increased resistance to the flow of air through the bronchi. Bronchospasm, mucosal congestion and oedema result in increased resistance. The tracheobronchial smooth muscle is hyper-responsive to various stimuli like dust, allergens, cold air, infection and drugs. These trigger factors trigger an acute attack.

Antigen-antibody interaction on the surface of mast cells cause (Fig. 38.1):

i. Degranulation of mast cells releasing stored mediators of inflammation

ii. Synthesis of other inflammatory mediators which are responsible for bronchospasm, mucosal congestion and oedema.

Inflammation is the primary pathology.

Clinically 2 types of asthma are identified.

- Extrinsic asthma: Starts at an early age, occurs in episodes; the patient has a family history of allergies.

- Intrinsic asthma: Starts in the middle age and assumes chronic form. There is no family history of allergies.

Drugs used in the bronchial asthma may be grouped as follows -

CLASSIFICATION

1. **Bronchodilators**
   a. *Sympathomimetics*
      i. Selective β_2 agonists

Short acting	- Salbutamol,terbutaline.
Longer acting	- Salmeterol, fenoterol, formoterol, pirbuterol.

      ii. Nonselective agents

	- Adrenaline, isoprenaline, ephedrine.
b. *Methylxanthines*	- Theophylline, aminophylline.
c. *Anticholinergics*	- Ipratropium bromide, atropine.

2. **Anti-inflammatory agents**

a. *Systemic*	- Glucocorticoids, (Hydrocortisone, Prednisolone).
b. *Inhalational*	- Beclomethasone, Budesonide, Fluticasone, Triamcinolone

3. **Mast cell stabilizers** - Disodium cromoglycate, Nedocromil, Ketotifen.

4. **LT receptor antagonists** - Montelukast, zafirlukast.

SYMPATHOMIMETIC DRUGS

Sympathomimetics (See Chap.11) are potent bronchodilators and are the most useful drugs to relieve bronchospasm.

Mechanism of action

Adrenergic agonists stimulate β_2 receptors in the bronchial smooth muscles which in turn cause activation of adenyl cyclase resulting in increased cAMP levels (Fig 38.2). This increased cAMP leads to bronchodilatation. The increased cAMP in mast cells inhibit the release of inflammatory mediators. They also reduce bronchial secretions and congestion (by acting on α receptors).

Short acting β_2 agonists

Salbutamol (albuterol) and terbutaline are short acting and selective β_2 agonists. Given by inhalation, they are fastest-acting bronchodilators with peak effect in 10 minutes. The action lasts for 6 hours. Adverse effects to β_2 agonists include muscle tremors, palpitation and nervousness.

Selective β_2 agonists are the most commonly used bronchodilators as they are the

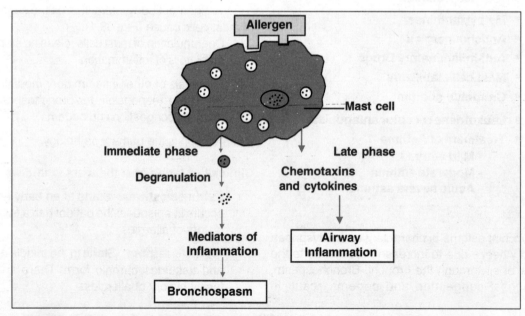

Fig. 38.1 Immediate and late responses of mast cell activation by antigen or allergen

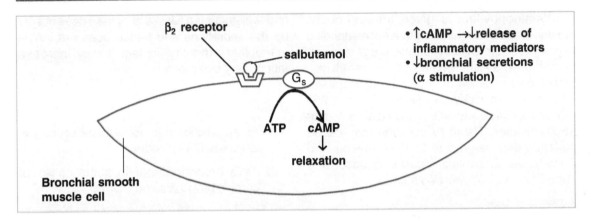

Fig 38.2 Mechanism of action of β_2 agonists in bronchial asthma

most effective, fast-acting, convenient and relatively safe bronchodilators. They are available as metered dose inhalers (Table 38.1), nebulizers, injections and also tablets for oral use. The proper technique in using the inhaler should be taught. 'Spacers' (Fig. 38.3) can be used in children and adults who cannot follow the right technique of inhalation.

Oral β_2 agonists have higher adverse effects than inhaled ones and are used only in small children who cannot use inhalers and have occasional wheezing (1-4 mg 6 hrly).

Longer acting β_2 agonists

Salmeterol is a long-acting selective β_2 agonist. The onset of action is slow (hence not useful in acute attacks) but the effect remains for 12 hours. It is therefore used for long-term maintenance and for prevention of nocturnal asthmatic attacks.

Other longer acting agents are also available for use - they are **formoterol, fenoterol, bambuterol and pirbuterol**. Bambuterol is a prodrug of terbutaline which is effective for 24 hours. Formoterol is fast acting and long acting. But the long term use of β_2 agonists may result in reduced response due to development of tolerance. Management of acute bronchospasm becomes a problem in such patients.

Others

Adrenaline, ephedrine **and** isoprenaline Though adrenaline and isoprenaline produce prompt bronchodilation, they are not preferred due to the risk of adverse effects like palpitation, anxiety, restlessness and tremors (See page 93)

Ephedrine produces bronchodilation but is slow in onset. Because of low efficacy, side effects and availability of better drugs, ephedrine is not preferred.

METHYLXANTHINES

Theophylline (See page 257) and its derivatives like **aminophylline** are good bronchodilators.

Mechanism of action

Phosphodiesterase (PDE) is the enzyme that degrades cyclic AMP. Methylxanthines inhibit PDE and thereby enhance cAMP levels which brings about bronchodilation. cAMP also inhibits the release of mediators of inflammation.

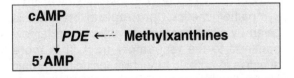

Aminophylline is given intravenously, **slowly**, in acute attacks of asthma not responding to β_2 agonists. In an acute attack, drugs given by inhalation may sometimes fail to reach the bronchioles because of severe bronchospasm. Intravenous aminophylline may then be tried. 250 mg aminophylline should be injected slow IV over 15-20 minutes. Rapid IV injection may cause collapse and death due to hypotension and arrhythmias. Convulsions can also occur and should be carefully watched for.

Adverse effects

Theophylline is a drug of low therapeutic index. Gastric irritation, vomiting, insomnia, tremors, diuresis, palpitation, and hypotension are quite common. Higher doses cause restlessness, delirium, convulsions and arrhythmias. Children may develop behavioural abnormalities on prolonged use - should be avoided.

Status in bronchial asthma

Theophylline is a second line drug in bronchial asthma.

1. *Chronic asthma:* Oral theophylline can be used to control mild to moderate asthma. Etophylline + 80% theophylline (Deriphylline) injections (IM) are used to relieve acute attacks. When used over a long-term, plasma levels should be monitored.

2. *Acute severe asthma (status asthmaticus):* Intravenous aminophylline is tried when sympathomimetics fail to relieve bronchospasm - but is found to be less effective.

ANTICHOLINERGICS

Anticholinergics (See chap. 9) relax bronchial smooth muscles but response is slower than sympathomimetics. **Ipratropium bromide** is given by inhalation and its actions are largely confined to the respiratory tract. It is more effective in chronic bronchitis including chronic obstructive pulmonary disease (COPD). It is safe

and well-tolerated. Unlike atropine it does not dry up the secretions and hence does not inhibit mucociliary motility. In fact it may increase mucociliary clearance.

Uses

1. As an adjunct to β_2 agonists particularly in severe acute episodes.

2. As a bronchodilator in some cases of chronic bronchitis and COPD.

ANTI-INFLAMMATORY DRUGS

Glucocorticoids

Since inflammation is the primary pathology in bronchial asthma, antiinflammatory agents afford significant benefit (See chap. 64).

Mechanism of action

Steroids are not bronchodilators. They suppress the inflammatory response to antigen-antibody reaction and thereby reduce mucosal oedema and hyperirritability. They bind to steroid receptors in the cytoplasm, drug receptor complex moves to the nucleus, bind to DNA and induce the synthesis of specific mRNA, to bring about the following effects -

1. They decrease the formation of cytokines. These cytokines activate eosinophils and also promote the IgE antibody production.

2. ↓ PG synthesis by inhibiting induction of COX-2

3. induce lipocortin and thereby inhibit the production of leukotrienes and PAF.

4. reduce the influx of eosinophils into the lungs and thus release of mediators from them.

5. ↓ IL-3 synthesis.

6. restore response to β_2 agonist if tolerance

has developed - by upregulating the β_2 receptors.

Glucocorticoids may be given systemically in acute episodes. Oral prednisolone is commonly used (dose 30-60 mg/day). The onset of response requires about 12 hours. Chronic asthma requires prophylaxis with inhaled steroids.

Steroids for inhalation

The use of inhalational steroids largely minimizes the adverse effects of steroids because of the small dose required, but they are not effective in acute attacks and are only of prophylactic value. They prevent episodes of acute asthma, reduce bronchial hyperreactivity and effectively control symptoms. The effect develops after one week of treatment.

Side effects of inhaled steroids include hoarseness of voice - (by a direct effect on vocal cords), sore throat and oropharyngeal candidiasis. Rinsing the mouth and throat with water after each use can reduce the incidence of candidiasis and sore throat. HPA axis suppression is generally not seen in the recommended doses. But, the drug that is swallowed may be systemically absorbed. Large doses given for a long time may occasionally result in systemic effects of steroids particularly in children. The use of a **'spacer'** reduces this risk and the adverse effects are also less common when a spacer is used (Fig. 38.3).

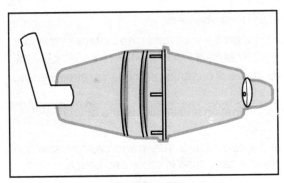

Fig 38.3 Spacer

Beclomethasone dipropionate, budesonide, triamcinolone and fluticasone are used as inhalers.

Beclomethasone dipropionate is available as metered dose inhaler and as rotacaps. It is also available in combination with salbutamol.

Budesonide has the advantage of having high topical activity and the absorbed portion is rapidly metabolised. Budesonide is used in the prophylaxis of bronchial asthma and as nasal spray in allergic rhinitis. (Flunisolide is available as nasal spray for allergic rhinitis).

Fluticasone is available as metered dose inhaler. It has the advantages that it is poorly absorbed from the gut and also undergoes high first pass metabolism. Hence even when swallowed, systemic adverse effects are unlikely with fluticasone.

Dose: Fluticasone (FLOHALE) is available as 25, 50, 125mcg/metered dose - 2 - 3 puffs twice daily. It is not recommended in children below 4 years of age.

Status of glucocorticoids in asthma

1. Acute exacerbation A short course (5-7 days) of oral prednisolone 30-60 mg/day for 7 days is given in addition to β_2 agonists.

2. Chronic asthma Steroid inhalation (2-4 times a day) for a long period as prophylaxis.

3. Status asthmaticus Intravenous hydrocortisone hemisuccinate (100-200 mg) followed by oral prednisolone.

MAST CELL STABILIZERS

Cromolyn sodium (disodium cromoglycate) was synthesized in 1965.

Mechanism of action

- Cromolyn inhibits the degranulation of mast cells and thereby inhibits the release of mediators of inflammation. particularly histamine.

- It also inhibits the release of cytokines.

- It may depress the neuronal reflexes which are exaggerated. But the exact mechanism of action is not known.

We know that cromolyn prevents bronchospasm and inflammation following exposure to allergens and decreases bronchial hyper-reactivity. It is therefore used for **prophylaxis**. It is **not** a bronchodilator - hence **not** useful in acute episodes.

Cromolyn sodium is used as an inhaler; it takes 2-4 weeks of treatment for the beneficial effects to develop. All patients do not respond but it should be tried in all suitable patients. Children are more likely to respond.

Adverse effects are rare. Throat irritation, cough and sometimes bronchospasm can occur on inhalation due to deposition of the fine powder. Allergic reactions are rare.

Uses

1. Prophylaxis of bronchial asthma -

cromolyn sodium used over a long period - 2 puffs - 3-4 times daily reduces episodes of acute asthma. Young patients with extrinsic asthma are more likely to be benefitted. Chromolyn can also be used for prophylaxis before exposure to a known allergen.

2. Allergic rhinitis - Prophylactic nasal spray is used.

3. Allergic conjunctivitis - Eye drops are used prophylactically- 1-2 drops, 3-4 times a day.

Preparations

FINTAL inhaler (1mg), eye drops 2%, nasal spray 2%, CROMAL inhaler 1 mg, 2mg and 5 mg / metered dose, eye drops 2%, nasal spray 2%.

Nedocromil is similar to cromolyn sodium in its actions and uses. It is given twice daily.

Ketotifen is an antihistaminic with actions like cromolyn sodium. It inhibits airway inflammation but it is not a bronchodilator. It is given orally.

Keybox 38.1
Aerosols in asthma

- β_2 agonists, ipratropium bromide, cromolyn sodium and some glucocorticoids are available for inhalation.
- Use of aerosols largely reduces systemic effects.
- Inhalation can be given by - metered dose inhalers and nebulizers.
- Metered dose inhalers deliver a particular dose of the drug on activation. Advantages - cheaper and portable. But breathing coordination and correct technique of using inhaler should be taught.
- Factors like particle size, breath holding period and rate of breathing all influence effectiveness of inhalers.
- Use of spacers reduces the need for breathing coordination and increases the amount of drug reaching the lungs.
- Dry powder inhalers - rotacaps - have the disadvantages of requiring deep and forceful inspiration which is not possible in children. Morover the powder can cause irritation and cough.
- Nebulizers do not require breathing coordination. But the device is expensive.

TABLE 38.1 : Aerosols in bronchial asthma

Drug	Preparation	Dose
1. Salbutamol	MDI -100mcg/m.d. RC - 200mcg Neb soln - 5mg/ml	1-2 puffs 3-4 times a day 3-4 times a day 2.5mg 3-4 times a day
2. Salmeterol	MDI - 25mcg/m.d. RC - 50mcg	50mcg twice daily
3. Terbutaline	MDI - 250mcg/m.d. Neb soln -10mg/ml	1-2 puffs 3-4 times a day 5mg 2-4 times a day
4. Ipratropium bromide	MDI - 20, 40mcg/m.d. RC - 40mcg	1-2 puffs 3-4 times a day
5. Cromolyn sodium	MDI - 1, 2, 5mg/m.d.	1-2 puffs 3-4 times a day
6. Beclomethasone	MDI - 50, 100, 200mcg/m.d. RC - 100, 200, 400mcg	400-800mcg/day in 2-3 divided doses
7. Budesonide	MDI - 100, 200mcg/m.d.	100-200mcg twice a day
8. Fluticasone	MDI - 25, 50, 125mcg/m.d. RC - 50, 100, 250mcg	100-250mcg twice a day

MDI - metered dose inhaler   m.d. - metered dose   Neb soln - Nebulizer solution   RC - Rotacaps

Beneficial effects are seen after 6-12 weeks of use. It is used for the prophylaxis of bronchial asthma and other allergic disorders like allergic rhinitis, atopic dermatitis, urticaria and conjunctivitis. Drowsiness and dry mouth are common side effects. It can also cause dizziness and weight gain.

LEUKOTRIENE RECEPTOR ANTAGONISTS

Leukotrienes are important mediators of inflammation. They bring about bronchospasm, mucosal edema, increase the influx of inflammatory cells and respiratory mucus production by their actions on leukotriene receptors particularly LTB_4. Zafirlukast, montelukast and pranlukast are highly selective

and competitive antagonists of leukotriene receptors. They block the effects of leukotrienes and thereby reduce mucosal edema and relieve bronchospasm. They decrease the response to allergens. They inhibit exercise-induced and aspirin - induced bronchospasm. Adverse effects are rare - headache, rashes and gastrointestinal disturbances can occur.

Montelukast and zafirlukast can be used in the prophylaxis of mild to moderate asthma as alternatives or as add - on drugs. They also reduce the dose of steroid required. Bronchodilator effect is additive with β_2 agonists. Their place in asthma is yet to be clearly known.

Zileuton inhibits leukotriene synthesis by inhibiting the enzyme lipoxygenase. But it causes a rise in liver enzymes. Hence not preferred.

TREATMENT OF ASTHMA

Mild asthma

Rapidly acting, inhaled β_2 stimulants like salbutamol.

Moderate asthma

Regular prophylaxis with cromoglycate. If symptoms persist *i.e.* if the patient does not respond to cromolyn - inhaled steroids are given for prophylaxis. Acute episodes are managed with inhaled β_2 agonists.

Severe asthma

a. Regular inhaled steroids

b. Inhaled β_2 agonists 3-4 times a day

c. Oral steroids may be considered

d. Additional inhaled ipratropium bromide or oral theophylline may be given.

Acute severe asthma **or** status asthmaticus is an acute exacerbation. It is a medical emergency; may be triggered by an acute respiratory infection, abrupt withdrawal of steroids after prolonged use, by drugs, allergens or emotional stress.

Treatment

1. Nebulization of β_2 agonist and ipratropium alternately - every 30 minutes. Additional salbutamol 0.4 mg IM/SC may be given. Severe tachycardia should be watched for.

2. Hydrocortisone hemisuccinate IV 100 mg stat followed by 100 mg every 8 hours infusion followed by a course of oral prednisolone.

3. Oxygen inhalation.

4. Antibiotics - if infection is present

5. IV fluids to correct dehydration and acidosis.

6. Aminophylline 250 mg slow IV over 15 - 20 minutes may be given carefully - watching for adverse effects but is now not preferred.

7. Artificial ventilation may be required in extreme cases.

39 *Drugs used in the treatment of Cough*

- • **Central Cough suppresants**
- • **Pharyngeal Demulcents**
- • **Expectorants**
  - **- Direct stimulants**
  - **- Reflex expectorants**
- • **Bronchodilators**
- • **Mucolytics**

Cough is a protective reflex that removes the irritant matter and secretions from the respiratory tract. It could be due to infection, allergy, pleural diseases and malignancy. Since it is a protective mechanism, undue suppression of cough can cause more harm than benefit. In some conditions, as in dry annoying cough, it may serve no useful purpose. In such situations, antitussives or cough suppressants may be used. Antitussives only provide symptomatic relief and do not alter the cause.

Antitussives

1. Central cough suppressants
   Codeine, pholcodeine, noscapine, dextromethorphan, antihistamines, benzonatate.

2. Pharyngeal demulcents
   Lozenges, cough drops, linctuses

3. Expectorants
   Potassium iodide, Guaiphenesin, ammonium chloride, ipecacuanha

Central cough suppressants

Central cough suppressants act by inhibiting cough centre in the medulla.

Codeine is a good antitussive with less addiction liability. However, nausea, constipation and drowsiness are common. **Dose** 10-15 mg every 6 hours (See page 215).

Noscapine is a natural opinum alkaloid which is a potent antitussive. No other CNS effects are prominent in therapeutic doses (See page 215). Nausea is the only occasional side effect. **Dose** 15-30 mg every 6 hours.

Dextromethorphan and pholcodeine are synthetic opioid derivatives with antitussive actions like codeine but with lesser side effects. Pholcodeine is longer-acting - given twice daily.

Benzonatate is chemically related to the local anaesthetic procaine. It acts on the cough receptors in the lungs and also has a central effect. It is given orally - 100 mg thrice daily.

Antihistamines are useful in cough due to allergy except that due to bronchial asthma. They thicken the secretions which may be difficult to cough out. An antihistamine is generally one of the components of cough syrups. Their sedative property may be of additional value in suppressing cough.

Other centrally acting antitussives include carbetapentane, chlophedianol and caramiphen. More extensive studies are required to prove their efficacy.

Pharyngeal Demulcents

Pharyngeal demulcents (**demulcere** = to caress soothingly - in LATIN) increase the flow of saliva which produces a soothing effect on the pharyngeal mucosa and reduce afferent impulses arising from the irritated mucosa. Dry cough due to irritation of the pharyngeal mucosa is relieved. Candy sugar or a few drops of lemon also serve this purpose.

Expectorants

Expectorants (Latin - *expectorare* = to drive from the chest) increase the production of respiratory tract secretions which cover the irritated mucosa. As the secretions become thin and less viscid, they can be easily coughed out. Expectorants may increase the secretions directly or reflexly.

• **Direct stimulants** Volatile oils like eucalyptus oil; creosotes, alcohol, cidar wood oil - when administered by inhalation with steam can increase respiratory secretions.

• **Reflex expectorants** are given orally, they are gastric irritants and reflexly increase respiratory secretions.

Potassium iodide acts both directly and reflexly.

Ipecacuanha is an emetic. In sub-emetic doses it is used as an expectorant.

Bronchodilators

Bronchodilators like salbutamol and terbutaline relieve cough that results from bronchospasm.

The antitussive preparations generally have a combination of a central cough suppressant, an expectorant, an antihistaminic and sometimes a bronchodilator and a mucolytic agent.

Mucolytics

Normally the respiratory mucous is watery. The glycoproteins in the mucous are linked by disulphide bonds to form polymers making it slimy. In respiratory diseases, the glycoproteins form larger polymers with plasma proteins present in the exudate and the secretions become thick and viscid. Mucolytics liquefy the sputum making it less viscid so that it can be easily expectorated.

The following are mucolytics -

Bromhexine

Bromhexine, a semisynthetic compound related to vasicine (an alkaloid from the plant *Adhatoda vasica*) is a good mucolytic. It depolymerises the mucopolysaccharides in the mucus. It is given orally (8-16 mg thrice daily). Side effects are minor - may cause rhinorrhoea.

Ambroxol

Ambroxol is a metabolite of bromhexine with actions similar to it. Ambroxol may be given orally or by inhalation. It can be used as an alternative to bromhexine.

Acetylcysteine

Acetylcysteine opens disulfide bonds in mucoproteins of the sputum reducing its viscosity. It is given by aerosol. Side effects are common and hence not preferred.

Carbocysteine

Carbocysteine is similar to acetylcysteine and is used orally.

Pancreatic dornase

Deoxyribonucleoprotein is a major component of the purulent respiratory tract secretions. Pancreatic dornase is a deoxyribonuclease obtained from the beef pancreas. It breaks the deoxyribonucleic acid (DNA) into smaller parts thus making the secretions thin and less viscid. It is administered by inhalation.

Pancreatic dornase can cause allergic reactions.

Steam inhalation

Steam inhalation offers an effective and inexpensive alternative to drugs. It humidifies the sputum as well as respiratory mucosa. This helps in reducing the irritation and for easier expectoration of the sputum. In presence of dehydration, just rehydrating the patient is found to be beneficial.

BLOOD

- ◆ Haematopoietic System
- ◆ Drugs used in the Disorders of Coagulation
- ◆ Hypolipidaemic Drugs

40   *Heamatopoietic System*

- **Haematinics**
  - **Iron**
  - **Vitamin B$_{12}$ and Folic Acid**
- **Haematopoietic growth factors**
  - **Erythropoietin**
  - **Myeloid growth factors**
  - **Megakaryocyte growth factors**

HAEMATINICS

Haematinics are compounds required in the formation of blood and are employed in the treatment of anaemias. Haematinics include iron, vitamin B$_{12}$ and folic acid. Haematopoietic growth factors are also discussed here.

IRON

Iron, vitamin B$_{12}$ and folic acid are essential for normal erythropoiesis.

Iron is essential for haemoglobin production. Total body iron is about 2.5 to 5 grams, two-thirds of which is present in haemoglobin. Each molecule of haemoglobin has 4 iron containing residues. It is also present in myoglobin, the cytochromes and other enzymes.

Distribution of iron in the body

Haemoglobin	66%
Ferritin, haemosiderin	25%
Myoglobin (in muscles)	03%
Enzymes (cytochromes, etc.)	06%

Daily requirement of iron

Adult male	0.5-1 mg
Adult female	1-2 mg
Pregnancy and lactation	3-5 mg

Dietary sources of iron

Food items that are rich in iron are liver, egg yolk, meat, fish, chicken, spinach, dry fruits, wheat and apple.

Absorption

The average Indian diet provides about 10-20 mg of iron. Ten per cent of this iron is absorbed. Dietary iron may be present as haeme or as inorganic iron. It is mostly absorbed from the upper gut in the ferrous form. During deficiency, absorption is better. Haeme iron is better absorbed than inorganic iron.

Factors that influence iron absorption

Ascorbic acid, amino acids, meat, ↑gastric acidity } **Increase absorption**

Antacids, phosphates, phytates, tetracyclines presence of food in the stomach } **Decrease absorption**

Transport and distribution

Iron is transported with the help of a glycoprotein **transferrin** and stored as **ferritin** and **haemosiderin**, in liver, spleen and bone marrow.

Excretion

Daily 0.5-1 mg of iron is excreted. A large part is lost in shedding of intestinal mucosal cells and small amounts in the bile, desquamated skin and urine. In females, iron is also lost in menstruation.

Preparations of Iron

Iron is generally given orally - but can be given parenterally.

Oral iron preparations

1. Ferrous sulphate - 200 mg tab
2. Ferrous fumarate - 200 mg tab
3. Ferrous gluconate - 300 mg tab
4. Ferrous succinate - 100 mg
5. Iron calcium complex - 5% iron
6. Ferric ammonium citrate - 45 mg.

- Ferrous salts are better absorbed than ferric salts and are cheaper.

- The last three preparations are claimed to be better tolerated but are more expensive.

- Expensive preparations of iron with vitamins, liver extract, amino acids, etc. are available but offer no obvious benefits.

- **Dose** Ferrous sulphate 200 mg - 3-4 tablets daily. The elemental iron content of different salts varies.

Adverse effects of oral iron

Epigastric pain, nausea, vomiting, gastritis, metallic taste, constipation (due to astringent effect) or diarrhoea (irritant effect) are the usual adverse effects. Liquid preparations of iron cause staining of the teeth.

Parenteral iron

Intramuscular injection of iron is given deep IM in the gluteal region using 'Z' technique to avoid staining of the skin. Intravenous iron is given slowly over 5-10 minutes or as infusion after a test dose.

Indications

1. When oral iron is not tolerated

2. Failure of absorption - as in malabsorption, chronic bowel disease

3. Noncompliance

4. Severe deficiency with bleeding.

Preparations

1. Iron dextran - has 50 mg elemental iron/ml (2 ml ampoule) - it is the only preparation that can be given intravenously. It can also be given IM.

2. Iron-sorbitol-citric acid complex - contains 50 mg elemental iron/ml; given only IM. This preparation should not be given IV

because it quickly saturates the transferrin stores. As a result free iron levels in the plasma rises and can cause toxicity.

Dose is to be calculated using a formula.

Formula

$$\text{Iron requirement} = 4.4 \times \text{body weight} \times \text{Hb deficit}$$
$$\quad\text{(mg)} \qquad\qquad \text{(kg)} \qquad\qquad \text{(g/dl)}$$

This also includes iron needed for replenishment of stores.

Adverse Effects

- **Local**

  Pain at the site of injection, pigmentation of the skin and sterile abscess.

- **Systemic**

  Fever, headache, joints pain, palpitation, difficulty in breathing, lymph node enlargement and rarely, anaphylaxis.

Acute iron poisoning

Acute iron poisoning (See Chap. 76) is common in infants and children in whom about 10 tablets (1-2 g) can be lethal. Manifestations include vomiting, abdominal pain, haematemesis, bloody diarrhoea, shock, drowsiness, cyanosis, acidosis, dehydration, cardiovascular collapse and coma. Immediate diagnosis and treatment are important as death may occur in 6-12 hr.

Treatment

- Gastric lavage with sodium bicarbonate solution.
- Desferrioxamine is the antidote. It is instilled into the stomach after lavage, to prevent iron absorption; injected IV/IM.
- Correction of acidosis and shock.

Indications for Iron

Iron deficiency anaemia - both for the prophylaxis and treatment. The cause for iron deficiency should be identified. Treatment should be continued depending on the response for 3-6 months to replenish iron stores. Prophylactically iron is given in conditions with increased iron requirement as in pregnancy, infancy and professional blood donors.

VITAMIN B$_{12}$ AND FOLIC ACID

Vitamin B$_{12}$ and folic acid are water soluble vitamins, belonging to the B-complex group. They are essential for normal DNA synthesis. Their deficiency leads to impaired DNA synthesis and abnormal maturation of RBCs and other rapidly dividing cells. This results in megaloblastic anaemia, characterised by the presence of red cell precursors in the blood and bone marrow. Vitamin B$_{12}$ and folic acid are therefore called maturation factors. Other manifestations of deficiency include glossitis, stomatitis and malabsorption. Neurological manifestations can also result.

Vitamin B$_{12}$

Vitamin B$_{12}$ (Cyanocobalamin) is synthesized by microorganisms. Liver, fish, egg yolk, meat, cheese and pulses are the dietary sources of B$_{12}$.

Vitamin B$_{12}$ or extrinsic factor is absorbed with the help of intrinsic factor, a protein secreted by the stomach. It is carried in the plasma by B$_{12}$ - binding proteins called **transcobalamin** and is stored in the liver.

Functions

Vitamin B$_{12}$ is converted in the tissues to the active coenzyme form. It is involved in several vital metabolic reactions and is essential for the synthesis of purine which is needed for the DNA synthesis.

Vitamin B$_{12}$ acts as a cofactor in the following important enzymatic reactions -

TABLE 40.1 Daily requirement of vitamin B_{12} and folic acid		
	Adults	Pregnancy and lactation
Vitamin B_{12}	1-3 µg	3-5 µg
Folic acid	50-100 µg	200-400 µg

As 50% of ingested drug is lost, double the amount is recommended for daily dietary intake

1. Homocysteine + methyl FH_4*

$$\text{Vitamin } B_{12} \downarrow \text{Methionine synthetase}$$

Methionine + FH_4

2. Methylmalonyl CoA

$$5 \text{ deoxyadenosyl } B_{12} \downarrow \text{Methyl malonyl CoA}$$

Succinyl CoA

(FH_4 - tetrahydrofolate)

The above reactions show that vitamin B_{12} and folic acid metabolism are linked. Tetrahydrofolate is essential for the biosynthesis of purines.

Deficiency

Vitamin B_{12} deficiency may be due to:

1.Addisonian pernicious anaemia

Thomas Addison first described cases of anaemia not responding to iron. There is deficiency of intrinsic factor due to destruction of partietal cells resulting in failure of B_{12} absorption.

2.Other causes

Gastrectomy, chronic gastritis, malabsorption and fish tapeworm infestation (fish tapeworm consumes B_{12}).

Preparations

- Cyanocobalamin - 100 mcg/ml injection may be given IM or deep SC - hypersensitivity reactions can occur.

- Hydroxocobalamin - 100, 500, 1000 mcg/ml injection - has longer lasting effect because

of its protein binding but hydroxocobalamin administration can result in the formation of antibodies.

- Multivitamin preparations contain variable amounts of vitamin B_{12} with or without intrinsic factor for oral use.

Uses

1. **Vitamin B_{12} deficiency**

- *Treatment of megaloblastic anaemia due to B_{12} deficiency* - If B_{12} deficiency is due to lack of intrinsic factor, vitamin B_{12} is given IM or SC. Pernicious anaemia needs life long treatment with parenteral B_{12} because in pernicious anaemia, orally given vitamin B_{12} cannot be absorbed due to intrinsic factor deficiency. Patients with severe deficiency and with neurological manifestations require immediate treatment with cyanocobalamin 100 mcg IM and 5mg folic acid. Cyanocobalamin 100mcg should be given daily with 5 mg oral folic acid for the next two weeks and then continued over three to four weeks but neurological improvement depends on the severity. Though there is a feeling of overall subjective improvement with better appetite, complete neurological recovery particularly of the mental functions may not be seen at all. Oral folic acid should be added because B_{12} induced brisk haemopoiesis may also increase the demand for folic acid. It is also essential to supplement iron because such active haemopoiesis generally precipitates iron deficiency as available iron is used up.

- *Prophylaxis of B_{12} deficiency* - prophylactic dose of vitamin B_{12} is 3-10 mcg daily.

2. Neuropathies

Neuropathies thought to be due to B_{12} deficiency like tropical neuropathy respond to vitamin B_{12} but the mechanism is not clear. Vitamin B_{12} is also given in many other conditions like trigeminal neuralgia, multiple sclerosis, some psychiatric disorders and even for general weakness. There is no evidence to recommend such use for vitamin B_{12}.

FOLIC ACID

Folic acid is pteroylglutamic acid. It was first isolated from spinach and therefore named as folic acid (from leaf).

Dietary source Green vegetables, liver, yeast, egg, milk and some fruits. Prolonged cooking with spices destroys folic acid.

Absorption takes place in the duodenum and jejunum and is transported in the blood by active and passive transport, widely distributed in the body and is stored in the liver.

Functions Folic acid is converted to dihydrofolic acid and then to tetrahydrofolic acid which serves as a coenzyme for many vital (one-carbon transfer) reactions necessary for DNA synthesis.

Deficiency Folate deficiency may be due to dietary folate deficiency, malabsorption and other diseases of the small intestine or drug induced. Phenytoin, phenobarbitone, oral contraceptives, methotrexate and trimethoprim can induce folate deficiency. Increased requirement, as in growing children, pregnancy and lactation, can also cause deficiency. Manifestations include megaloblastic anaemia, glossitis, diarrhoea and weakness.

Uses

1. Megaloblastic anaemia due to folate as well

as B_{12} deficiency - folic acid 2-5 mcg/day is given orally along with vitamin B_{12}. In folic acid deficiency due to malabsorption syndromes, folic acid is given IM.

2. Prophylactically in pregnancy, lactation, infancy and other situations with increased requirement of folic acid - 500 mcg daily orally.

Folinic acid (citrovorum factor, leucovorin) is N-formyl tetrahydrofolic acid and is the active coenzyme form which overcomes methotrexate toxicity (See page 439).

HAEMATOPOIETIC GROWTH FACTORS

Haematopoietic growth factors are hormones that regulate erythropoiesis. Many of these glycoproteins have now been produced for clinical use by recombinant DNA technology. Frequent blood counts are needed to monitor therapy with these growth factors.

Haemotopoietic growth factors

- Erythopoietin
- Myeloid growth factors

 GM-CSF

 G-CSF

 M-CSF

- Megakaryocyte growth factors

 Thrombopoietin

 Interleukin-II

Erythropoietin

Erythropoietin is produced by the kidney in response to hypoxia and anaemia. It binds to erythropoietin receptors on red cell progenitors and stimulates red cell production.

Adverse effects

If the rise in haemotocrit and haemoglobin is too rapid, hypertension and thrombosis can complicate erythropoietin therapy. Allergic reactions are mild. Parenteral iron may be needed to prevent iron deficiency that is precipitated by rapid erythropoiesis.

Uses

Erythropoietin is useful in the treatment of anaemia seen in chronic renal failure, bone marrow disorders, malignancies, chronic inflammation and anaemia associated with AIDS.

Myeloid Growth Factors

Myeloid growth factors include Granulocyte - Macrophage colony stimulating factor (GM-CSF), Granulocyte colony stimulating factor (G-CSF) and Monocyte colony stimulating factor (M-CSF).

Sargramostim Recombinant human GM-CSF is sargramostim. This glycoprotein binds to specific receptors on the myeloid progenitor cells and stimulates the proliferation and differentiation of neutrophils and monocytes.

Sargramostim is given as SC or IV infusion. There is an increase in leucocyte count over 7 to 10 days. On stopping the drug, the count returns to baseline in 2-7 days. **Molgramostim** is another recombinent GM-CSF preparation.

Adverse effects include bone pain, fever, arthralgia, myalgia and dyspnoea. Higher doses sometimes can cause a capillary leak syndrome with edema, pericardial and pleural effusion and heart failure.

Filgrastim is human recombinant G-CSF. It stimulates the production of neutrophils. Filgrastim is given as SC injection or IV infusion.

Adverse effects Filgrastim is better tolerated than sargramostim. It can cause bone pain and rarely allergic reactions.

Uses

Sargramostim and filgrastim are used to shorten neutropenia in bone marrow transplantation, following cancer chemotherapy, aplastic anaemia, congenital neutropenia, myelodysplasia and in AIDS patients with neutropenia.

M-CSF Stimulates the production of monocytes and macrophages. It can cause splenomegaly and thrombocytopenia.

Megakaryocyte growth factors

Thrombopoietin

Thrombopoietin increases the production of platelets by binding to the receptors on the platelet progenitor cells. Recombinant thrombopoietin is available for therapeutic use. It is being tried in severe thrombocytopenia that occurs following cancer chemotherapy.

Interleukins

Oprelvekin is the recombinant form of interleukin - II. It stimulates the production of megakaryocytes and platelets by activating the interleukin - II receptors on the platelet progenitor cells. Oprelvekin is used for the secondary prevention of thrombocytopenia in patients receiving cancer chemotherapy. Oprelvekin can cause sodium retention resulting in edema.

41

Drugs used in the Disorders of Coagulation

- • **Classification**
- • **Heparin**
- • **Oral anticoagulants**
- • **Thrombolytics (Fibrinolytics)**
- • **Antifibrinolytics**
- • **Antiplatelet drugs**
- • **Coagulants**
- • **Sclerosing agents**

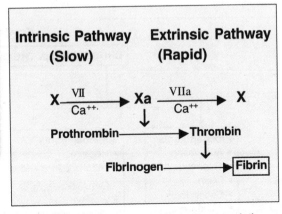

Fig. 41.1 Major reactions of blood coagulation

Haemostasis is the spontaneous arrest of bleeding from the damaged blood vessels. In the process, complex interactions take place between the injured vessel wall, platelets and clotting factors.

Following injury, there is local vasoconstriction and platelet adhesion - forming a plug which temporarily stops bleeding. This is reinforced by fibrin for long-term haemostasis.

Clotting factors are proteins synthesized by the liver. Two systems - the extrinsic and the intrinsic system are involved in the process of coagulation. Several proteins interact in a cascading series to form the clot (Fig. 41.1).

Anticoagulants are drugs that reduce the coagulability of the blood.

301

CLASSIFICATION

Anticoagulants used *in vivo*

1. Fast acting
   - Heparin
   - Low mol. wt. heparins
     Enoxaparin, Dalteparin
   - Heparinoids
     *Heparan sulphate, Dextran sulphate
     Danaparoid, Lepirudin*

2. Slow acting (oral anticoagulants)

   - Coumarin derivatives
     *Bishydroxycoumarin
     Warfarin sodium, Nicoumalone*

   - Indandione derivatives:
     Phenindione, Diphenadione

Anticoagulants used *in vitro*

- Heparin
- Oxalates
- Citrates
- Sodium edetate.

HEPARIN

Heparin was discovered by McLean, a medical student in 1916. It was named 'heparin' as it was first extracted from the liver. It is a mucopolysaccharide found in the mast cells of the liver, lungs and intestinal mucosa. Heparin is the strongest acid in the body. It is a glycosaminoglycan.

Actions

Heparin is a powerful anticoagulant that acts instantaneously both *in vivo* and *in vitro*.

Mechanism of Action

Antithrombin III is a peptide that is synthesized in the liver and circulates in the plasma. Heparin activates plasma antithrombin III (Fig 41.2). Antithrombin III binds to and inhibits the activated

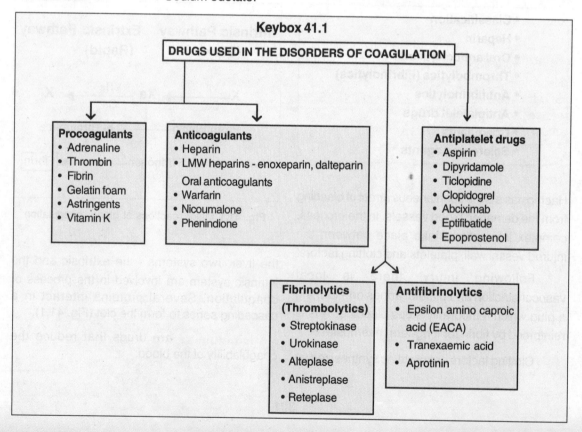

Keybox 41.1

DRUGS USED IN THE DISORDERS OF COAGULATION

Procoagulants
- Adrenaline
- Thrombin
- Fibrin
- Gelatin foam
- Astringents
- Vitamin K

Anticoagulants
- Heparin
- LMW heparins - enoxeparin, dalteparin

  Oral anticoagulants
- Warfarin
- Nicoumalone
- Phenindione

Antiplatelet drugs
- Aspirin
- Dipyridamole
- Ticlopidine
- Clopidogrel
- Abciximab
- Eptifibatide
- Epoprostenol

Fibrinolytics (Thrombolytics)
- Streptokinase
- Urokinase
- Alteplase
- Anistreplase
- Reteplase

Antifibrinolytics
- Epsilon amino caproic acid (EACA)
- Tranexaemic acid
- Aprotinin

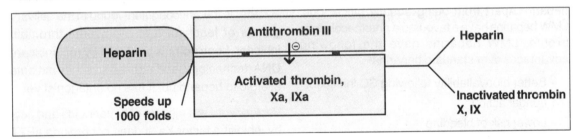

Fig 41.2 Mechanism of action of heparin

thrombin and coagulation factors (Xa and IXa). This is a physiological reaction, but heparin accelerates it by 1000 times. Clotting time is prolonged. The heparin-antithrombin III complex inhibits activated factor X and thrombin, while low molecular weight (LMW) heparin only inhibits factor X and not thrombin.

Other actions

Heparin activates lipoprotein lipase which hydrolyses triglycerides present in the plasma and thus clears the plasma of lipids.

Pharmacokinetics

Heparin is not effective orally. It is given IV or SC. It should not be given IM because it may cause haematomas. Given intravenously the onset of action is immediate, reaches peak in 5-10 minutes and clotting time returns to normal in 2-4 hours. Treatment is monitored by the aPTT (preferable) or clotting time. Heparin is metabolised by heparinase in the liver.

Because of its large molecular size, heparin does not cross the placental barrier. Therefore heparine can be used in pregnancy if an anticoagulant is needed.

Heparin is given as a bolus dose of 5000 units followed by a maintenance dose of 1000 units/hour as infusion.

Adverse reactions

1. Bleeding is the most common, major adverse effect of heparin. Careful monitoring and dose control will prevent this to a great extent.

2. Hypersensitivity reactions: For commercial use heparin is obtained from bovine lung or porcine intestine. Because of its animal origin allergic reactions are quite common.

3. Thrombocytopenia: Heparin induced platelet aggregation and formation of antiplatelet antibodies both result in thrombocytopenia. The antigen antibody complexes may damage the vessel wall triggering thrombosis and disseminated intravascular coagulation. This paradoxical complication of heparin therapy is rare but can be serious. Heparin should be stopped immediately at the first sign of thrombocytopenia.

4. Alopecia is reversible.

5. Osteoporosis - can occur on long-term use of heparin - the cause is unknown.

6. Hypoaldosteronism - Heparin can inhibit the synthesis of aldosterone and may result in hyperkalemia.

Contraindications to heparin therapy

Bleeding disorders, thrombocytopenia, haemophilia, severe hypertension, intracranial haemorrhage, cirrhosis, ulcers in the gut, renal failure and neurosurgery.

Low molecular weight (LMW) heparins *e.g.* enoxaparin, dalteparin. LMW heparins are obtained by chemical/enzymatic treatment of standard heparin. Apart from being equally efficacious, LMW heparins have a favourable pharmacokinetic profile. LMW heparins have the following advantages over standard heparins-

- Better bioavailability following SC injection.
- Longer action
- Lower risk of bleeding
- Lower risk of osteoporosis
- Lower incidence of thrombocytopenia and thrombosis

Uses

LMW heparins are used in the prevention and treatment of venous thrombosis and pulmonary embolism; they are also useful in unstable angina and to maintain the patency of tubes in dialysis patients.

Dose: Enoxaparin - 1 mg / kg SC twice daily.
Prophylaxis - 40 mg once daily.
Dalteparin - 200 U / kg SC once daily.
Prophylaxis - 5000 U / SC once daily.

Heparin antagonist

Mild heparin overdosage can be treated by just stopping heparin because heparin is short acting. In severe heparin overdose, an antagonist may be needed to arrest its anticoagulant effects. **Protamine sulphate** is a protein obtained from the sperm of certain fish. Given intravenously, it neutralises heparin (1 mg for every 100 units of heparin). In the absence of heparin, protamine sulphate can itself act as a weak anticoagulant. Hence overdose should be avoided. Protamine sulphate is a strongly basic protein which binds with the strongly acidic groups of heparin forming a stable complex which is devoid of anticoagulant activity.

Whole blood transfusion may be needed.

Heparinoids

Heparan sulfate present in some tissues is similar to heparin. It is believed to be responsible for antithrombotic activity on the vascular endothelium.

Hirudin is the anticoagulant found in the salivary glands of leeches. It is a powerful thrombin inhibitor. **Lepirudin** is produced by recombinant DNA technology and can be used in patients allergic to heparin but it has no antagonist yet.

Danaparoid is a mixture of heparinoids and acts by inhibiting factor Xa. It does not prolong aPTT and is longer acting. It is used subcutaneously in the treatment of deep vein thrombosis and in other conditions as an alternative to heparin.

ORAL ANTICOAGULANTS

Cattle that were fed on spoiled sweet clover hay, developed a haemorrhagic disease in North America in 1924. This turned out to be due to bishydroxycoumarin, an anticoagulant in the spoiled sweet clover. Many related compounds were then developed and are also being used as rat poison.

Mechanism of action

Warfarin and its congeners act as anticoagulants only *in vivo* because they act by interfering with the synthesis of vitamin K dependent clotting factors in the liver. They block the gama carboxylation of glutamate residues in prothrombin, factors VII, IX and X. Gama carboxylation is necessary for these factors to participate in coagulation.

The onset of action is slow; it develops over 1-3 days because oral anticoagulants do not destroy the already circulating clotting factors. Prothrombin time (PT) is measured to monitor the treatment. It takes 5-7 days for PT to return to normal after stopping oral anticoagulants.

Pharmacokinetics

Warfarin is completely absorbed orally and is 99% bound to plasma proteins.

Factors influencing oral anticoagulant activity	
Factors enhancing activity	*Factors reducing activity*
Poor diet, bowel disease, liver disease and chronic alcoholism—result in vitamin K deficiency	**Pregnancy—there is increased synthesis of clotting factors** **Hypothyroidism—there is reduced degradation of clotting factors.**

Adverse effects

1. *Haemorrhage* is the main hazard. Bleeding in the intestines or brain can be troublesome. Minor episodes of epistaxis and bleeding gums are common.

Treatment depends on the severity

- Stop the anticoagulant.
- Fresh blood transfusion is given to supply clotting factors.
- **Antidote** The specific antidote is **vitamin K$_1$ oxide.** It allows synthesis of clotting factors. But even on IV administration, the response to vitamin K$_1$ oxide needs several hours. Hence in emergency, **fresh whole blood** is necessary to counter the effects of oral anticoagulants.

2. *Other adverse effects* include allergic reactions, gastrointestinal disturbances and teratogenicity.

Drug interactions

Many drugs **potentiate** warfarin action

1. Drugs that inhibit platelet function - NSAIDs like aspirin increase the risk of bleeding.

2. Drugs that inhibit hepatic drug metabolism like cimetidine, chloramphenicol and metronidazole enhance plasma levels of warfarin.

Some drugs **reduce** the effect of oral anticoagulants.

1. Drugs that enhance the metabolism of oral anticoagulants - microsomal enzyme inducers like barbiturates, rifampicin, griseofulvin enhance the metabolism of oral anticoagulants. When these drugs are suddenly withdrawn, excess anticoagulant activity may result in haemorrhages.

2. Drugs that increase the synthesis of clotting factors - oral contraceptives.

Uses of anticoagulants

Anticoagulants can prevent the extension of thrombus but cannot destroy the existing clots. Heparin has rapid and short-action which makes it suitable for initiating treatment while warfarin is suitable for long-term maintenance due to its slow and prolonged action and convenience of oral use.

1. Venous thrombosis and pulmonary embolism - anticoagulants prevent extension of thrombus and recurrence of embolism.

2. Postoperative, post-stroke patients; bedridden patients due to leg fractures and other causes - who cannot be ambulant for several months - anticoagulants prevent venous thrombosis and pulmonary embolism in such patients.

3. Rheumatic valvular disease - anticoagulants prevent embolism.

4. Unstable angina - heparin reduces the risk of myocardial infarction in patients with unstable angina.

5. Vascular surgery, artificial heart valves and haemodialysis - anticoagulants prevent thromboembolism.

Contraindications to anticoagulant therapy

- Bleeding disorders including thrombocytopenia
- Severe hypertension
- Malignancies
- Bacterial endocarditis
- Liver and kidney diseases.

THROMBOLYTICS (Fibrinolytics)

Thrombolytics lyse the clot or thrombi by activating the natural fibrinolytic system.

Plasminogen circulates in the plasma and also some of it is bound to fibrin. Tissue plasminogen activator (tPA) activates plasminogen which is converted to plasmin. Plasmin degrades fibrin thereby dissolving the clot. Thrombolytic agents are

First generation agents
Streptokinase, urokinase,

Second generation agents
Alteplase, duteplase, tenecteplase, reteplase, anistreplase.

Streptokinase obtained from β-haemolytic streptococci activates plasminogen. Antistreptococcal antibodies present in the blood due to previous streptococcal infections inactivate a large amount of streptokinase.

Streptokinase is antigenic and can cause allergy. The antibodies formed may persist for five years. Hence if thrombolytics are required during that period, others like tPa or urokinase should be used. Streptokinase also causes hypotension.

Anistreplase (Anisoylated plasminogen streptokinase complex) is a form of streptokinase which is long acting and can be injected in a single IV bolus. Hence it is more convenient to use. Coronary reperfusion is better than with streptokinase but it also causes fibrinogenolysis and allergic reactions.

Urokinase is an enzyme prepared from cultures of human kidney cells (it was first isolated from human urine - hence the name). It activates plasminogen. It is more expensive than streptokinase.

Tissue plasminogen activator (tPA) preferentially activates plasminogen that is bound to fibrin which means circulating plasminogen is largely spared. Chances of reocclusion may be reduced by use of heparin and antiplatelet drugs.

Alteplase, duteplase are tPA produced by recombinant DNA technology. They are very expensive.

Reteplase is modified human tPA obtained by genetic engineering. It is claimed to have the following advantages over tPA -

- Faster reperfusion
- Bleeding tendency is negligible.

Tenecteplase is longer acting and can be given as an IV bolus injection. Its ability to bind fibrin is better than that of alteplase.

Adverse effects of thrombolytics

Bleeding is the major toxicity of all thrombolytics. Hypotension and fever can occur. Allergic reactions are common with streptokinase.

Uses

Fibrinolytics are all expensive drugs.

1. Acute myocardial infarction - Intravenous thrombolytics given immediately reduce the mortality rate in acute MI. They should be

given within 12 hours but preferrably immediately because early treatment largely reduces mortality (See page 141).

2. Deep vein thrombosis and large pulmonary emboli are also treated with fibrinolytics.

Contraindications to thrombolytic therapy

- Recent surgery, injury, gastrointestinal bleeding, stroke.
- Severe hypertension.
- Bleeding disorders.

ANTIFIBRINOLYTICS

Antifibrinolytics inhibit plasminogen activation and thus prevent fibrinolysis.

Epsilon aminocaproic acid (EACA) and its analog **tranexaemic acid** are antifibrinolytics. **Aprotinin** is another antifibrinolytic drug which acts by inhibiting proteolytic enzymes.

Antifibrinolytics are used in overdose of fibrinolytics and to reduce bleeding after prostatic surgery and some patients undergoing cardiac surgeries or after tooth extraction in haemophiliacs - but the beneficial effect is uncertain.

ANTIPLATELET DRUGS

Platelets form the initial haemostatic plug at the site of vascular injury and are also involved in the formation of atherosclerosis. By inhibiting the platelet function, thrombosis and atherosclerotic vascular disease can be largely prevented.

Antiplatelet drugs or drugs interfering with platelet function include -

1. PG synthesis inhibitors
   - Aspirin
2. Phosphodiesterase inhibitor
   - Dipyridamole
3. ADP antagonists
   - Ticlopidine

- Clopidogrel

4. Glycoprotein IIb/IIIa receptor antagonists
   - Abciximab
   - Eptifibatide
   - Tirofiban

5. Others
   - $PG1_2$

Aspirin

Thromboxane A_2 promotes platelet aggregation. Aspirin inactivates cyclo-oxygenase (COX) (See Chapter 30) and thereby inhibits the synthesis of thromboxane A_2 even in low doses (75 mg/day). The COX inhibition is irreversible and the effect lasts for 7 to 10 days - till fresh platelets are formed.

Dipyridamole

It is a phosphodiesterase inhibitor which interferes with platelet function by increasing platelet cyclic AMP levels. It is used along with aspirin for the prophylaxis of thromboemboli in patients with prosthetic heart valves.

ADP antagonists

Ticlopidine ADP binds to receptors on platelets to bring about platelet aggregation. Ticlopidine is a prodrug. Its active metabolite blocks ADP receptors and prevents platelet aggregation. Onset of action is slow (7-11days) and the antiplatelet effect remains for some days even after stopping the drug. Dose: 250mg twice daily. Adverse effects include dyspepsia, diarrhoea, bleeding and leukopenia. It is used in patients who cannot tolerate aspirin.

Clopidogrel has structural similarity to ticlopidine with similar mechanism of action. Like ticlopidine it is a prodrug and the active metabolite blocks ADP receptors. Its actions are additive with aspirin as the mechanisms are different. Toxicity is milder with lesser incidence of leukopenia and thrombocytopenia.

Clopidogrel is used as an alternative when

aspirin cannot be used. It can also be used with aspirin for additive effects.

Glycoprotein IIb/IIIA receptor antagonists

Fibrinogen and von Willebrand factor bind to glycoprotein IIb/IIIA receptors on the platelets and mediate platelet aggregation by platelet agonists like thrombin, collagen and TXA_2. Drugs that block these receptors inhibit platelet aggregation induced by all platelet agonists.

Abciximab is a monoclonal antibody which binds GP IIb/IIIA receptors and inhibits platelet aggregation. It can cause bleeding and allergic reactions. It is used in patients undergoing coronary angioplasty.

Eptifibatide and tirofiban are peptides given as IV infusion. They are short acting and are tried in unstable angina and myocardial infarction.

Others

Epoprostenol (PGI_2) can be used during hemodialysis to prevent platelet aggregation as an alternative to heparin.

Uses of antiplatelet drugs

1. Myocardial infarction Aspirin with thrombolytics improves survival in acute MI. Long-term treatment with aspirin reduces reinfarction in post MI patients.

2. Unstable angina and stable angina pectoris - Aspirin reduces the risk of acute MI. Clopidogrel may be added to aspirin in unstable angina.

3. In patients with prosthetic heart valves, valvular heart disease, coronary artery by-pass surgery - long-term use of low dose aspirin is recommended.

4. Cerebral thrombosis and TIA In patients with transient ischaemic attacks aspirin reduces the incidence of stroke and mortality. In cerebral thrombosis aspirin prevents recurrence.

5. Atrial fibrillation If oral anticoagulants cannot be given, aspirin is useful.

COAGULANTS

Coagulants are drugs that promote coagulation (procoagulants) and control bleeding. They are also called **haemostatics.** They may be used locally or systemically. Local haemostatics are called **styptics.** Physical methods like application of pressure, tourniquet or ice can control bleeding.

Styptics are local haemostatics that are used on bleeding sites like tooth socket and wounds.

They are

1. Adrenaline Sterile cotton soaked in 1:10,000 solution of adrenaline is commonly used in tooth sockets and as nasal packs for epistaxis. Adrenaline arrests bleeding by vasoconstriction.

2. Thrombin powder is dusted over the bleeding surface following skin grafting. It is obtained from bovine plasma.

3. Fibrin obtained from human plasma is available as sheets. It is used for covering or packing bleeding surfaces.

4. Gelatin foam is porous spongy gelatin used with thrombin to control bleeding from wounds. It gets completely absorbed in 4 to 6 weeks and can be left in place after suturing of the wound.

5. Thromboplastin powder is used in surgery as a styptic.

6. Astringents like tannic acid are used on bleeding gums.

Coagulants used systemically

Vitamin K

Vitamin K is a fat-soluble vitamin essential for the biosynthesis of clotting factors. There are three compounds: vitamin K_1 - present in food from plant source, vitamin K_2 - produced in the gut by

Sclerosing agent IV!

Rajan a 45 year old man suffering from esophageal varices was prescribed a sclerosing agent for local injection. The drug was injected intravenously in the arm instead of local injection. Sclerosing agents are irritants. Therefore IV injection resulted in severe thrombophlebitis and the patient was in great pain. Though it is the nurse who gave the injection in this case, it is the responsibility of the doctor to ensure proper administration of the medicine.

bacteria and vitamin K_3 - a synthetic compound used therapeutically.

Actions

Vitamin K is essential for the biosynthesis of clotting factors - prothrombin and factors VII, IX and X by the liver.

Vitamin K deficiency results from liver diseases, malabsorption, long-term antibiotic therapy and rarely by dietary deficiency. It is manifested as bleeding tendencies.

Adverse reactions are seen on parenteral administration - allergic reactions and jaundice can occur.

Uses

1. Vitamin K deficiency

2. Newborn babies lack intestinal flora and have low levels of prothrombin and other clotting factors. Routine administration of vitamin K - 1 mg IM prevents haemorrhagic disease of the newborn.

3. Oral anticoagulant toxicity.

Other Coagulants

Fresh plasma or whole blood is useful in most coagulation disorders as it contains all the clotting factors. Other concentrated plasma fractions like fibrinogen, factors VIII, II, VII, IX and X are available for the treatment of specific deficiencies.

Snake venom

Some snake venoms like Russels viper venom stimulate thrombokinase and promote coagulation (See page 537).

SCLEROSING AGENTS

Sclerosing agents are irritant substances. They are injected locally to the varicose veins, esophageal varices and into piles. They cause local inflammation and obliterate these veins. The compounds used are -

- Sodium tetradecyl sulfate - a detergent used as 3% solution (SETROL Inj.) for sclero therapy.

- Phenol 5% in vegetable oil - 2-5ml is injected into the vein.

- Ethanolamineoleate 5% - 1-5ml.

- Polydocanol 3% - is a detergent - 2ml injection (AETHOXYSKLEROL, ASKLEROL Inj.)

- Sodium Linoleate - 2-5 ml injection.

42 *Hypolipidaemic drugs*

- **HMG CoA reductase inhibitors**
- **Fibric acids**
- **Bile acid binding resins**
- **Antioxidant**
- **Miscellaneous**

Hyperlipoproteinaemias (HPL) are conditions in which the concentration of cholesterol or triglyceride (TG) carrying lipoproteins in the plasma is elevated above normal (Table 42.1) Increase in lipoproteins can hasten the development of atherosclerosis and is a risk factor for myocardial infarction.

Lipids and proteins form complexes called lipoproteins and circulate in the blood vessels. There are four types of lipoproteins-

- Low density lipoproteins (LDL)
- High density lipoproteins (HDL)
- Very low density lipoproteins (VLDL)
- Chylomicrons.

LDL is the primary carrier of cholesterol while VLDL is of triglycerides. There are different pathways for the transport of endogenous and exogenous lipids. In the exogenous pathway, cholesterol and triglycerides absorbed from the gut are transported as chylomicrons. They are hydrolysed to chylomicron remnants by the action

TABLE 42.1: Plasma lipid levels (mg/dl)		
Grade	Total cholesterol	Triglycerides
Normal	< 200	< 200
Borderline	200-240	200-400
High	> 240	> 400

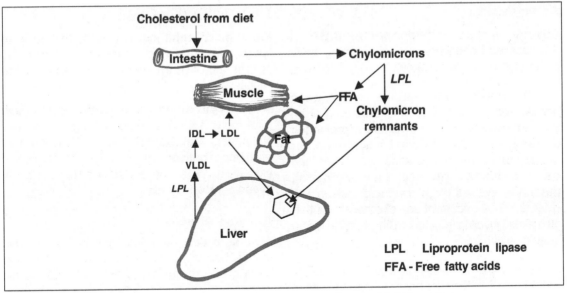

Fig. 42.1 Endogenous and exogenous pathway of lipid transport

of lipoprotein lipase (LPL) and free fatty acids are released which are taken up by muscle and adipose tissue. The chylomicron remnants are transported to the liver.

In the endogenous pathway cholesterol and triglycerides from the liver are carried as VLDL to the muscle and adipose tissue. Here the triglycerides in VLDL are hydrolysed and free fatty acids released. Thus IDL and then LDL are formed by the action of lipoprotein lipase. Cells have LDL receptors and LDL is taken up into the cell.

HYPOLIPIDAEMICS

1. **HMG CoA reductase inhibitors -**
   - Lovastatin
   - Simvastatin
   - Pravastatin
   - Atorvastatin

2. **Fibric acids**
   - Gemfibrozil
   - Clofibrate
   - Fenofibrate
   - Bezafibrate
   - Ciprofibrate

3. **Bile acid binding resins**
   - Cholestyramine
   - Colestipol

4. **Antioxidant**
   - Probucol

5. **Miscellaneous**
   - Nicotinic acid
   - Neomycin
   - Gugulipid

HMG CoA Reductase Inhibitors (Statins)

Hydroxymethylglutaryl-CoA (HMG-CoA) is the rate-controlling enzyme in the biosynthesis of cholesterol. Lovastatin and its congeners are competitive inhibitors of the enzyme HMG-CoA reductase. They lower plasma LDL cholesterol and triglycerides. The concentration of HDL-cholesterol (the protective lipoprotein) increases by 10%.

Pharmacokinetics

Statins are well absorbed when given orally but may undergo extensive first pass metabolism in the liver. Simvastatin is a prodrug converted to its active metabolite in the liver.

Adverse effects

Adverse effects include gastrointestinal disturbances, headache, insomnia, rashes, rarely myopathy and angio-oedema.

Treatment with statins can cause hepatotoxicity though not very common. Serum transaminases may be elevated on prolonged therapy. Patients should be watched for hepatotoxicity while on statins. All statins can cause **myopathy** (with myalgia and weakness), rhabdomyolysis though the incidence is low (<0.1-0.1%). Concurrent use of other drugs that also cause myopathy including fibrates and niacin should be avoided.

Statins are contraindicated in pregnancy and lactation as they are not proved to be safe in them.

Uses

1. Several large scale studies have shown statins to be useful in lowering morbidity and mortality in patients with coronary heart disease. Hence they are used in patients with MI, angina, stroke and transient ischemic attacks to lower cholesterol levels.

2. HMG CoA reductase inhibitors are the first line drugs for hyperlipidaemias (Table 42.2)- both for familial and secondary hyperlipidaemias as in diabetes mellitus.

Fibric acids (fibrates)

Fibric acids enhance activity of the enzyme lipoprotein lipase which degrades VLDL resulting in lowering of triglycerides. They also increase HDL levels.

Fibrates also inhibit coagulation and promote thrombolysis which also account for their beneficial effects. **Gemfibrozil** 600 mg BD is the drug of choice in patients with increased TG levels and in type III, type IV and type V hyperlipoproteinaemias.

Adverse effects

Adverse effects like gastrointestinal upset, skin rashes, headache, myositis, muscle cramps and blurred vision can occur. Fibrates can cause rhabdomyolysis particularly in patients with renal failure.

Bezafibrate is similar to gemfibrozil and has greater LDL lowering effects.

Bile Acid Binding Resins

Bile acid binding resins - are not absorbed but they bind bile acids in the intestine and increase their excretion. Bile acids are required for intestinal absorption of cholesterol. Plasma cholesterol and LDL levels fall. Bile acid binding resins are unpleasant to take; they may cause gastrointestinal upset, constipation and piles.

TABLE 42.2 : Types of primary hyperlipoproteinemias		
Type	*Disorder*	*Plasma lipids raised*
I	Familial LPL deficiency	C, TG
IIa	Familial hypercholesterolemia	C
IIb	Polygenic hypercholesterolemia	C
III	Familial dysbetalipoproteinemia	C, TG
IV	Hypertriglyceridemia	TG
V	Familial combined hyperlpidemia	C, TG
C - Cholesterol	*TG - Triglycerides*	*LPL - Lipoprotein lipase*

They also bind fat soluble vitamins and many drugs like warfarin, chlorothiazide and digoxin in the intestines thereby reducing their absorption.

Bile acid binding resins can be used in patients with raised LDL levels; they can be used along with lovastatin or nicotinic acid.

Antioxidant

Probucol lowers LDL and HDL cholesterol and has antioxidant properties. It is generally not preferred.

Miscellaneous

Nicotinic acid a B group vitamin (See page 526), in large doses inhibits triglyceride synthesis in the liver and VLDL production resulting in a decrease in LDL and increase in HDL cholesterol. Adverse effects include flushing, dyspepsia, dryness and pigmentation of the skin.

Niacin is used in hypertriglyceridemia with low HDL levels.

Gugulipid obtained from 'gum guggul' lowers plasma cholesterol and triglycerides. It is well tolerated but can cause diarrhoea.

GASTROINTESTINAL TRACT

◆ Drugs used in peptic ulcer

◆ Prokinetic agents

◆ Emetics and antiemetics

◆ Drugs for constipation and diarrhoea

43 *Drugs Used in Peptic Ulcer*

- • **Classificaton**
- • **Antacids**
- • **H₂ receptor blockers**
- • **Proton Pump Inhibitors**
- • **Anticholinergics**
- • **Ulcer Protectives**
- • **Treatment of *H.Pylori* infection**

Acid-peptic disease is common in the present days that are full of tension and anxiety. Peptic ulcer is thought to result from an imbalance between acid-pepsin secretion and mucosal defense factors. The stomach secretes about 2.5 litres of gastric juice daily. The chief cells secrete pepsinogens while the parietal cells secrete HCl and intrinsic factor. The factors that protect the mucosa are its ability to secrete mucus, bicarbonate and prostaglandins. The mucous and bicarbonate form a layer which protects the gastric mucosa from gastric acid. Prostaglandins (PGE$_2$ & PGI$_2$) stimulate the secretion of mucus and bicarbonate, bring about vasodilation and also inhibit acid secretion. They act on the PG receptors present on the parietal cell. Gastric acid secretion is regulated by three pathways - vagus (ACh), gastrin and local release of histamine - each acting through its own receptors (Fig. 43.1). These activate H$^+$ K$^+$ ATPase (proton pump) on the parietal cells resulting in the secretion of H$^+$ into the gastric lumen where it combines with Cl$^-$ (drawn from plasma) and HCl is secreted. Acetylcholine and gastrin act both directly on the parietal cells and indirectly by releasing histamine from the enterochromaffin cells. Histamine acts through H$_2$ receptors on parietal cells while acetylcholine through M$_1$ muscarinic and gastrin through G receptors.

The exact etiopathogenesis of peptic ulcer is not known. Infection of the stomach mucosa with *Helicobacter pylori* is now known to be associated with chronic gastritis, peptic ulcers and their recurrence.

317

Drugs used in peptic ulcer are -

CLASSIFICATION

1. **Drugs that neutralise gastric acid** - ***Antacids*** - Magnesium hydroxide, aluminium hydroxide, calcium carbonate, sodium bicarbonate

2. **Drugs that reduce gastric acid secretion**

   a. *H_2 receptor blockers* - Cimetidine, ranitidine, famotidine, roxatidine, nizatidine

   b. *Proton pump inhibitors* - Omeprazole, lansoprazole, pantoprazole, rabeprazole

   c. *Muscarinic antagonists* - Pirenzepine, telenzepine
3. **Ulcer protectives** - Sucralfate, bismuth compounds
4. **Other drugs** - Carbenoxolone, cisapride, prostaglandins.

ANTACIDS

Antacids are basic substances. Given orally they neutralize the gastric acid and raise the pH of gastric contents. Peptic activity is also reduced, as pepsin is active only below pH 4. Thus antacids provide rapid relief of symptoms in hyperacidity as they chemically neutralise the acid already present in the stomach.

Antacids are of 2 types

1. Systemic
   - Sodium bicarbonate

2. Nonsystemic
   - Aluminium hydroxide
   - Magnesium trisilicate,
   - Magnesium hydroxide
   - Calcium carbonate.

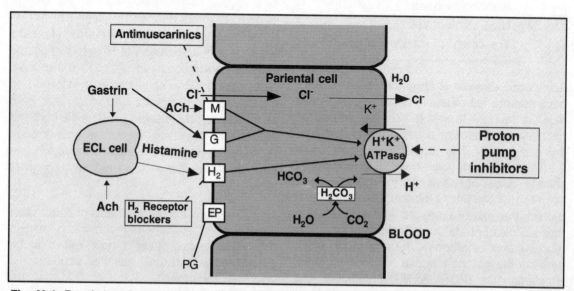

Fig. 43.1 Regulation of gastric secretion: ECL - Enterochromaffin cell; M - Muscarinic receptor (chiefly M_1); G - Gastrin receptors; H_2 - Histamine H_2 receptor, EP - Prostanoid receptor.

Systemic Antacids

Sodium bicarbonate is rapid but short-acting. CO_2 that is released in the stomach escapes as eructation. Sodium bicarbonate gets absorbed from the intestines leading to systemic alkalosis. There is 'rebound' hyperacidity as gastrin levels increase due to raised gastric pH. Sodium load may increase. It is not preferred for long term use because of the above disadvantages.

Sodium bicarbonate is used with other antacids in peptic ulcer. Other uses are to alkalinise the urine in poisoning and to treat metabolic acidosis.

Non-systemic Antacids

Non-systemic antacids are insoluble compounds that react in the stomach with HCl to form a chloride salt and water. They are not absorbed.

Aluminium hydroxide is slow acting. Food further slows its neutralizing capacity. It is also an astringent and demulcent - forms a protective coating over the ulcers. The aluminium ions relax the smooth muscles resulting in delayed gastric emptying and constipation. Aluminium hydroxide binds phosphate and prevents its absorption resulting in hypophosphataemia on prolonged use.

Magnesium salts The action is quick and prolonged. Rebound acidity is mild. Magnesium salts are osmotic purgatives and the dose used as antacids may cause mild diarrhoea.

Calcium carbonate acts quickly and has prolonged action but liberates CO_2 which may cause discomfort. Calcium salts also have a chalky taste. They may cause constipation and hypercalcaemia. Increased plasma Ca^{++} levels may result in rebound hyperacidity. Long term use may also result in renal Ca^{++} stones.

Antacid combinations are given to obtain maximum effects with least adverse effects as follows -

1. Quick and prolonged effect

   Fast-acting $[Mg(OH)_2]$ and slow as well as long acting $[Al(OH)_3]$ compounds are combined (Table 43.1).

2. Neutralising side effects

   Magnesium salts have a laxative effect while aluminium salts are constipating - combination neutralizes each other's side effects.

3. Gastric emptying

   Magnesium salts hasten while aluminium salts delay gastric emptying.

4. Additive effect

   Given together, aluminium & magnesium salts have additive effect and the dose of each compound required is lower.

All antacid tablets should be chewed and swal-

TABLE 43.1: Some antacid combination preparations	
Brand name	*Combination*
1. GELUSIL liquid	Aluminium hydroxide gel 312 mg + Magnesium trisilicate 625 mg in every 5 ml
2. GELUSIL tablet	Aluminium hydroxide gel 250 mg + Magnesium trisilicate 500 mg
3. DIGENE gel	Magnesium hydroxide 185 mg + Aluminium hydroxide gel 830 mg + Carboxymethyl cellulose sodium 100 mg + Methylpolysiloxane 25 mg - in every 10 ml
4. DIGENE tablet	Dried aluminium hydroxide gel 30 mg + Magnesium silicate 50 mg + Magnesium hydroxide 25 mg+Methylpolysiloxane 10 mg

lowed as they do not disintegrate well in the stomach. Gels are more effective than tablets. One dose given 1 hr after food neutralizes the acid for 2 hours.

Uses

Antacids are used as adjuvants in hyperacidity, peptic ulcer and reflux oesophagitis.

Drug interactions

Antacids form complexes with iron, tetracyclines, digoxin, ranitidine, fluoroquinolones, sulfonamides and antimuscarinic drugs. To avoid these, antacids should be taken 2 hours before or 2 hours after other drugs.

H_2 RECEPTOR BLOCKERS

Cimetidine, ranitidine, famotidine, roxatidine. nizatidine are the H_2 receptor blockers available.

These drugs competitively inhibit the action of histamine on H_2 receptors and thereby reduce gastric secretion. Both volume and acidity of basal, nocturnal and food induced secretion are reduced. They can cause 90% reduction in gastric secretion by a single dose. Gastrin induced HCl secretion and pepsin is also reduced. These actions, particularly their ability to suppress nocturnal acid secretion, hasten the healing of peptic ulcers.

Pharmacokinetics

H_2 blockers are rapidly and well-absorbed. Cimetidine acts for 5-8 hours, ranitidine and famotidine for 12 hours. They are partly metabolised in the liver and excreted by the kidneys. Dose - Table 43.2.

Adverse effects

The H_2 blockers are well-tolerated with minor side effects like diarrhoea, dizziness, muscle pain and headache. Because the H_2 receptors do not have any significant functions in other tissues (except stomach), H_2 receptor blockers are fairly safe drugs.

Cimetidine has antiandrogenic actions (it displaces testosterone from its binding sites); it increases plasma prolactin levels and inhibits estrogen metabolism in the liver. On prolonged use it may result in gynaecomastia, decreased sperm count, impotence and loss of libido in men. CNS effects include confusion, delirium and hallucinations in the elderly. Headache, dizziness, rashes and diarrhoea can result.

TABLE 43.2: Dosage and frequency of administration of drugs used in peptic ulcer	
Drug	*Dose and Frequency*
Ranitidine (RANTAC)	150 mg BD/300 mg HS
Famotidine (FAMOTIN)	20 mg BD/40 mg HS
Roxatidine (ROTANE).	75 mg BD/150 mg HS
Cimetidine (CIMET)	400 mg BD/800 mg HS
Omeprazole (OMEZ, LOMAC)	20-40 mg OD
Lansoprazole (LANZOL)	15-30 mg OD
Rabeprazole (VELOZ)	20 mg OD
Sucralfate (SUCRACE)	1 g 1 hr before each meal
Colloidal bismuth subcitrate (PYLOCID)	120 mg 1 hr before meals and at bed time
Carbenoxolone (GASTRIULCER)	50-100 mg TDS
Misoprostol	200 mcg BD-QID

Cimetidine inhibits microsomal enzymes (cytochrome P_{450}) and interferes with the metabolism of many drugs. This can result in several drug interactions.

Ranitidine is the preferred H_2 blocker as it has several advantages over cimetidine. Ranitidine is more potent, longer acting, has no antiandrogenic effects, no CNS effects as it does not cross BBB and does not inhibit microsomal enzymes significantly. Only adverse effects are headache and dizziness.

Famotidine is similar to but more potent than ranitidine. Headache and rashes can occur.

Roxatidine is similar to ranitidine but is more potent and longer-acting.

Nizatidine is similar to ranitidine. About 90% of the dose is excreted through the kidneys.

Uses of H_2 blockers

H_2 blockers are used in the treatment of peptic ulcer, gastritis, reflux oesophagitis (GERD) and as preanaesthetic medication - to prevent damage to the respiratory mucosa if aspiration occurs during surgery (See page 173). Ranitidine is the most preferred. It is given for 4-8 weeks in peptic ulcers - 150mg BD or 300mg HS. It may be continued for 6 months to prevent recurrence.

PROTON PUMP INHIBITORS

Dr.George Sachs putforth the idea that proton pump was the final common pathway in acid secretion and drugs that inhibit the proton pump could control acid secretion. **Omeprazole** was discovered in 1978 and was approved for use in 1989 after clinical trials. Proton pump (PP) inhibitors are the most efficacious inhibitors of the gastric acid secretion. Of the PP inhibitors, omeprazole was the first to be developed but we now have lansoprazole, pantoprazole and rabeprazole with minor pharmacokinetic variations.

Omeprazole is the most commonly used PP inhibitor.

Mechanism of Action

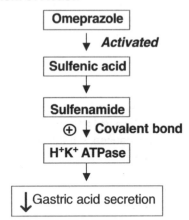

The parietal cells of the stomach secrete H^+ with the help of an enzyme H^+K^+ ATPase (proton pump) present in its plasma membrane. This is the final step in gastric acid secretion due to any stimuli. Proton pump inhibitors accumulate in the parietal cells where they specifically and irreversibly inhibit H^+K^+ATPase and thereby inhibit gastric secretion. Omeprazole and other proton pump inhibitors are prodrugs, get activated in the acidic environment of the stomach to sulfenamide which binds covalently with (SH groups on) H^+K^+ ATPase. The binding is irreversible. A single dose can almost totally (95%) inhibit gastric secretion. Acid secretion starts only after new H^+K^+ATPase enzyme is synthesized. Ulcer heals rapidly even in resistant cases.

Pharmacokinetics

PP inhibitors are given as enteric coated granules to avoid degradation by the acid in the stomach. Omeprazole is rapidly absorbed and reaches the parietal cells; it is highly protein bound and is metabolised in the liver by the microsomal enzymes (cytochrome P450). Though the $t\frac{1}{2}$ of omeprazole is 1-2 hours, the effect of a single dose remains for 2-3 days because of its accumulation in the pareital cell canaliculi. PP inhibitors are microsomal enzyme inhibitors and can result in many drug interactions - they may enhance the plasma levels of drugs like benzodiazepines, warfarin and phenytoin – precipitating toxicity.

Adverse effects

Omeprazole is well-tolerated. Prolonged acid suppression may allow bacterial over growth in the stomach. Dizziness, headache, diarrhoea, abdominal pain, nausea, arthralgia and rashes are rare.

Long term administration may result in-

- Vitamin B_{12} deficiency due to its reduced absorption.
- ↑Gastrin levels.
- Atrophic changes in the stomach have been noticed after 3-4 years of use.

Lansoprazole is similar to omeprazole but is longer-acting.

Pantoprazole is more acid stable and an intravenous formulation is also available for use. It does not inhibit microsomal enzymes. All other features are similar to omeprazole.

Rabeprazole is shorter acting.

Uses of PP inhibitors

- Proton pump inhibitors are used in peptic ulcers and in severe gastroesophageal reflux disease that is not responding to H_2 blockers. Ulcers heal fast and pain is relieved. They are given for 4-8 weeks.
- They also form a component in *H. pylori* treatment regimen.
- PP inhibitors are useful in Zollinger Ellison syndrome associated with gastrin secreting tumors.

Anticholinergics

Though atropine reduces gastric secretion, the

Keybox 43.1

PP Inhibitors

- PP inhibitors require acid for their activation and therefore should be given with or before food as food stimulates the secretion of acid.
- Antacids, H_2 receptor blockers and other drugs which reduce gastric acidity reduce the efficacy of proton pump inhibitors.
- Omeprazole inhibits the microsomal enzyme activity which can result in many drug interactions.

---

dose needed results in several adverse effects. A derivative of atropine - pirenzepine selectively blocks gastric M_1 receptors and inhibits gastric secretion by 40-50% without significant side effects. It also inhibits the secretion of gastrin, mucous and bicarbonate. As it does not cross BBB, it does not cause CNS side effects unlike atropine. Dryness of mouth and blurring of vision can occur. Pirenzepine is used as an adjuvant. Telenzepine is more potent than pirenzepine.

Ulcer Protectives

Sucralfate

In acidic medium (pH < 4), sucralfate polymerizes to form a sticky, viscid gel which firmly adheres to the base of the ulcers. It remains there for over 6 hours acting as a physical barrier and prevents contact with acid and pepsin. It also stimulates the PG synthesis in gastric mucosa. It thus promotes healing by protecting the ulcer. Sucralfate is not absorbed and is well-tolerated.

One tablet is given 1 hr before each meal and one at bed time for 4-8 weeks and then 1 gram BD is continued for 6 months to prevent recurrence.

Side effects are rare and include constipation and dryness of mouth.

Drug interactions

- Sucralfate needs acidic pH for activation. Hence antacids should not be given with it.

- Sucralfate adsorbs and interferes with the absorption of tetracyclines, digoxin, phenytoin and cimetidine.

Bismuth salts

Colloidal bismuth subcitrate on oral administration chelates proteins in the ulcer base and forms a protective coating over the gastric mucosa. It also inhibits the growth of *H. pylori* on gastric mucosa and stimulates the mucous production and PG synthesis. By these actions it promotes ulcer healing in 4-8 weeks. It may cause constipation and black stools.

Other Drugs

Carbenoxolone is a steroid like compound obtained from glycyrrhizic acid found in the root of liquorice. On ingestion, it alters the composition of mucous so that it is more viscid and adheres to gastric mucosa to protect the ulcer base. It also inhibits pepsin activity and prolongs the life of PGs. Because of its steroid like effects, it causes salt and water retention. It is therefore not preferred.

Prostaglandins PGE_2 and PGI_2 synthesized by the gastric mucosa inhibit gastric secretion, enhance mucous production, mucosal blood flow and exert a cytoprotective effect. They act by binding to the PG receptor (EP_3) present on the parietal cells and inhibit cAMP production.

Misoprotol is a synthetic PGE_1 analog given orally. It is of special value in preventing NSAID induced gastric ulceration because NSAIDs are PG synthesis inhibitors. Diarrhoea and muscle cramps are common.

Treatment of *H. pylori* Infection

The gram negative bacterium *H. pylori* is adapted to living in the stomach. Infection with *H. pylori* is associated with gastroduodenal disease including gastritis and peptic ulcer. It is also thought to be responsible for recurrence of peptic ulcer disease and is considered as a major risk factor for stomach cancer. Eradication of *H. pylori* with drugs that reduce acid secretion has shown to reduce the relapse rate.

Various combination regimens are tried with clarithromycin, amoxicillin or tetracycline; metronidazole and omeprazole or a H_2 receptor blocker for 1-2 weeks. Use of a PP inhibitor in the regimen improves the efficacy of the antibiotics in eradicating *H. Pylori* by raising gastric pH and enhancing antibiotic stability - activity of amoxillin and clarithromycin are pH dependent. Some regimens are:

1. Clarithromycin 250 mg BD + metronidazole 400 mg BD + Omeprazole 20 mg BD - for one week.

2. Clarithromycin 500 mg TDS/amoxycillin 750 mg TDS + Omeprazole 20 mg BD - for two weeks.

44 *Prokinetic Agents*

- • **Metoclopramide**
- • **Domperidone**
- • **Cisapride**
- • **Gastroesophageal reflux disease**

Drugs that enhance gastroduodenal motility and hasten gastric emptying are called **prokinetic agents.** Metoclopramide, domperidone and cisapride are some prokinetic agents.

METOCLOPRAMIDE

Actions

GIT Metoclopramide promotes forward movement of contents of the upper GI tract. It raises lower oesophageal sphincter pressure, speeds up gastric emptying, prevents reflux oesophagitis and also slightly enhances intestinal peristalsis.

CNS Metoclopramide acts as an antiemetic by its actions on CTZ and by speeding up gastric emptying.

Mechanism of action

Prokinetics act -

- • by blocking D_2 dopamine receptors (Fig 44.1). Antiemetic action is due to blockade of D_2 receptors in the CTZ.

- • by enhancing acetylcholine release from the cholinergic neurons in the gut.

Adverse effects

Adverse effects are sedation, dystonia and diarrhoea; gynaecomastia, galactorrhoea and parkinsonism (extrapyramidal symptoms) can occur on long-term use.

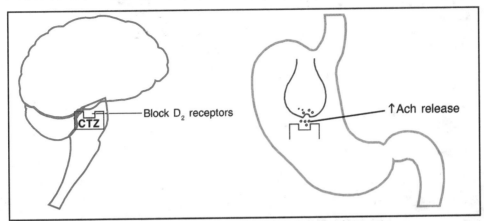

Figure 44.1 Mechanism of action of prokinetic agents.

Uses

1. Reflux oesophagitis - 'heart burn' due to reflux of acid into the oesophagus is benefited by prokinetic agents.

2. As antiemetics - in postoperative period and vomiting due to anticancer drugs.

3. As preanaesthetic medication to promote gastric emptying before induction of general anaesthesia in emergency.

4. In endoscopy - to assist passage of tubes into the duodenum.

Domperidone is a D_2 dopamine receptor blocker like metoclopramide. It blocks the dopamine receptors in the CTZ and thereby acts as an antiemetic. Domperidone differs from metoclopramide in that it does not cross the blood-brain barrier and hence extrapyramidal side effects are rare. Because CTZ is outside the BBB, domperidone can still produce its effects. Side effects are rare and include headache, dryness of mouth, diarrhoea and rashes.

Domperidone can be used in place of metoclopramide.

Cisapride enhances gastric motility by promoting the release of acetylcholine in the gut wall. It does not block dopamine receptors - hence is not an antiemetic and there are no antidopaminergic side effects. It also promotes colonic motility which may result in diarrhoea. It was used in reflux oesophagitis. Cisapride is now **banned** because it can cause serious cardiac adverse effects. Cardiac arrhythmias including ventricular tachycardia, atrial fibrillation and QT prolongation can occur- particularly when used with microsomal enzyme inhibitors like erythromycin, fluconazole, ketoconazole, indinavir and ritonavir.

Tegaserod is a $5HT_4$ partial agonist which promotes gastric emptying. It is free of the drug interactions and cardiotoxicity that is seen with cisapride (See page 335).

Gastroesophageal reflux disease (GERD)

Reflux of acidic gastric contents into the esophagus results in 'heart burn' due to esophagitis. Chronic esophagitis can result in changes in the esophageal mucosa which could be a premalignant condition. Based on severity, GERD may be treated with antacids, metoclopramide or drugs that reduce acid secretion. Uncomplicated, mild GERD may be relieved with antacids, H_2 receptor blockers or prokinetic agents. In moderate to severe cases, proton pump inhibitors like omeprazole are the drugs of choice. They effectively relieve symptoms and promote the healing of esophagitis in 4-8 weeks. Avoiding - heavy meals, late night dinner, smoking and alcohol - all help.

45 Emetics and Antiemetics

- Emetics
- Antiemetics
    - Classification
    - Dopamine D_2 antagonists
    - 5-HT_3 antagonists
    - Antimuscarinics
    - Neuroleptics
    - Other antiemetics
    - Antiemetic combinations

EMETICS

Emetics are drugs that produce vomiting. When a noxious substance is ingested, vomiting has to be induced. Mustard powder (1 teaspoon) with water or hypertonic salt solution can evoke vomiting.

Apomorphine is a derivative of morphine. Given SC/IM, it produces vomiting in 5-10 minutes. It acts by stimulating the CTZ.

Ipecacuanha contains an alkaloid emetine. Given as a syrup (15- 20 ml), it produces vomiting in 15 minutes. It is safe even in children.

ANTIEMETICS

Vomiting is a protective mechanism aimed at eliminating the unwanted harmful material from the stomach. But in some situations, vomiting may not serve any useful purpose and may only be troublesome. It can cause dehydration, weakness and electrolyte imbalance. In such circumstances, vomiting needs to be suppressed with drugs.

Stimulation of the vomiting centre in the medulla oblongata results in vomiting. The vomiting centre receives afferents from the chemoreceptor trigger zone (CTZ), vestibular apparatus, GI tract and centres in the brain (Fig.45.1). CTZ is not protected by the blood-brain barrier and is stimulated by various drugs, chemicals and radiation.

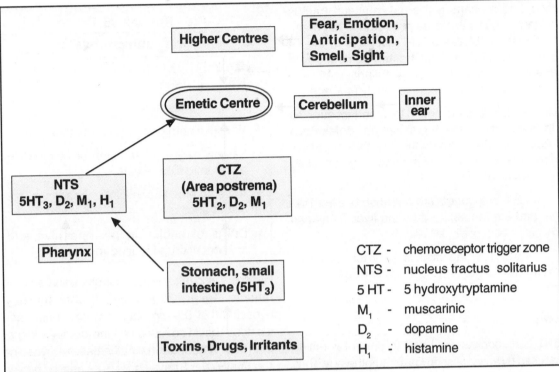

Fig 45.1: The stimuli, pathways and centres mediating emetic reflex and the receptors involved.

CLASSIFICATION

1. Dopamine D_2 antagonists - prokinetics-
   - Metoclopramide, domperidone

2. $5HT_3$ antagonists
   - Ondansetron, granisetron dolasetron, tropisetron

3. Antimuscarinics
   - Hyoscine
   - Cyclizine
   - Promethazine
   - Diphenhydramine.

4. Neuroleptics
   - Chlorpromazine, prochlorperazine, haloperidol

5. Other agents
   - Cisapride, corticosteroids.

Dopamine D_2 antagonists

Metoclopramide (See page 324) acts centrally by blocking dopamine D_2 receptors in the CTZ. It enhances the tone of the lower oesophageal sphincter and enhances gastric peristalsis. It is used in nausea and vomiting due to gastrointestinal disorders, migraine, in postoperative period and vomiting due to cytotoxic drugs and radiotherapy.

Domperidone acts like metoclopramide with fewer side effects (See page 325).

5-HT₃ Antagonists

Ondansetron

5-Hydroxytryptamine released in the gut is an important inducer of emesis. It is believed that anticancer drugs induce the release of 5HT in the gut which initiates emetic reflex through $5HT_3$

receptors present in the gut, nucleus tractus solitarius (NTS) and area postrema in the brain. Ondansetron blocks 5 HT_3 receptors in the GI tract, CTZ and nucleus tractus solitarius and prevents vomiting. It is a powerful antiemetic and can be given orally or intravenously (4-8 mg).

Granisetron is more potent than ondansetron as an antiemetic. Though granisetron, **dolasetron** and **tropisetron** have longer t ½, their biological effect t ½ remains the same and they can all be given once daily.

5HT_3 antagonists are well absorbed from the gut and are metabolised by the liver .They can be given both orally, IM and IV.

All 5HT_3 antagonists are well tolerated with minor adverse effects like headache and constipation.

Uses

5HT_3 antagonists are used to control vomiting induced by anticancer drugs or radiotherapy. They are also useful in postoperative vomiting and other drug induced vomiting.

Antimuscarinics

Hyosine (See chap. 9) is a labyrinthine sedative very effective in motion sickness. Motion sickness or travelling sickness is due to over stimulation of the vestibular apparatus along with psychological and environmental factors.

Hyoscine also relaxes the gastrointestinal smooth muscle. Taken 30 minutes before journey, hyoscine (0.4-0.6 mg oral) acts for 6 hours and the dose should be repeated if the journey is longer than that. A transdermal patch delivers hyoscine constantly over 3 days and is to be applied behind the ear. Sedation and dry mouth are common side effects.

Dicyclomine is used to control vomiting in morning sickness and motion sickness (Table 45.1).

H_1 antihistamines (See Chap. 35) like promethazine, diphenhydramine, cyclizine and cinnarizine have anticholinergic properties. Antihistamines block H_1 receptors in the area

TABLE 45.1 Preferred drugs for vomiting due to various causes	
Conditions	*Drugs*
Motion sickness	Hyoscine, Cyclizine, Promethazine, Cinnarizine
Vomiting due to cytotoxic drugs	1. Ondansetron + Dexamethasone 2. Metoclopramide + dexamethasone + diphenhydramine+ lorazepam.
Vomiting due to other drugs	Chlorpromazine, Metoclopramide
Postoperative vomiting	Ondansetron, Metoclopramide
Vomiting in pregnancy	Dicyclomine, Pyridoxine, Cyclizine, Meclizine, Metoclopramide

postrema as well as muscarinic receptors in the CNS. They probably also act on the GI tract. Some of them are useful in motion sickness and postoperative vomiting.

Neuroleptics (See chap. 32) also block D_2-receptors in the CTZ and are useful in vomiting due to most causes except motion sickness. Sedation and extrapyramidal symptoms are the common side effects. Prochlorperazine is mainly used as an antiemetic in vomiting and is also effective in vertigo associated with vomiting.

Other antiemetics

Corticosteroids are used in combination with other antiemetics like ondansetron or metoclopramide. Corticosteroids control delayed vomiting following anticancer drug therapy.

Pyridoxine is used in the prevention of vomiting in pregnancy without any known pharmacological basis

Sedative hypnotics – Barbiturates and benzodiazeapines may raise the threshold for vomiting by depressing the CNS. Their anxiolytic and sedative properties also help. Sedative hypnotics are used as adjuvants to other antiemetics in treating anticancer drug - induced vomiting.

Cannabinoids Dronabinol, a cannabinoid has antiemetic properties. It may act by the stimulation of the cannabinoid receptors (CB_1) in the vomiting centre. It also increases appetite. Dronabinol can cause behavioural abnormalities and dependence. It can be used as an alternative in the prevention of vomiting when other drugs are ineffective.

Antiemetic combinations

Severe retching and vomiting like that induced by anticancer drugs are treated with a combination of antiemetics including ondansetron, metoclopramide, glucocorticoids and sedative-hypnotics.

Later cycles of anticancer drug regimens can cause 'anticipatory' vomiting *i.e.*vomiting at the sight or even the thought of receiving anticancer drugs. This can be avoided by using appropriate antiemetics in the earlier cycles of anticancer therapy.

46 Drugs for Constipation and Diarrhoea

- **Purgatives**
  - Classification
  - Bulk laxatives
  - Faecal softeners
  - Osmotic purgatives
  - Stimulant purgatives
  - Enema
  - Use of laxatives in constipation
  - Drug induced constipation
  - Laxative abuse
- **Drugs used in the treatment of diarrhoea**
- **Irritable bowel syndrome**
- **Inflammatory bowel diseases**

Purgatives are drugs that promote defecation. They are also called **laxatives** or **cathartics**. **Laxatives** have milder action while cathartics or purgatives are more powerful evacuants. Purgatives may be classified as

CLASSIFICATION

1. **Bulk laxatives**
   - Bran, plantago seeds, agar, methylcellulose, ispaghula husk.

2. **Faecal softeners**
   - Docusate sodium, liquid paraffin (emollients)

3. **Osmotic purgatives**
   - Magnesium sulphate, Magnesium hydroxide, Sodium phosphate, Sodium sulphate, Magnesium citrate, Lactulose, Sorbitol, Polyethylene glycol.

4. **Stimulant purgatives**
   - Phenolphthalein, bisacodyl, castor oil, Anthraquinones - cascara sagrada, senna

Bulk laxatives

Bulk laxatives include indigestible vegetable fibre and hydrophilic colloids that increase the volume and lower the viscosity of intestinal contents forming a large, soft, solid stool. Dietary fibre consists of cell walls and other parts of fruits and vegetables that are unabsorbable. Adding fibre to the diet is a safe and natural way of treating constipation in persons on low-fibre diet. **Bran** is the residue left when flour is made from cereals and contains 40% fibre - but is unpalatable and can cause flatulence. Ispaghula and plantago seeds contain natural mucilage which absorbs water to form a gelatinous mass and are more palatable than bran. Methylcellulose is a semisynthetic derivative of cellulose. Adequate water intake should be stressed.

Faecal softeners

Docusate sodium (dioctyl sodium sulphosuccinate) softens faeces by lowering the surface tension of the intestinal contents which allows more water to be retained in the faeces.

Liquid paraffin is a chemically inert mineral oil that is not digested. It lubricates and softens faeces. It is unpalatable; aspiration may cause lipoid pneumonia; small amounts absorbed in intestines may cause paraffinomas; it may leak out of the anus causing discomfort. Long term use can result in deficiency of fat-soluble vitamins due to impaired absorption. Hence not preferred.

Osmotic purgatives

Osmotic purgatives are solutes that are not absorbed in the intestine, osmotically retain water and increase the bulk of intestinal contents. They increase peristalsis to evacuate a fluid stool. They produce soft liquid stools in 1-3 hours. Osmotic purgatives include

- Nonabsorbable salts (saline purgatives)
- Nonabsorbable sugars - Lactulose
- Polyethylene glycol

Nonabsorbable salts

Magnesium hydroxide, magnesium sulphate, sodium potassium tartrate (Rochelle's salt), sodium sulphate and phosphate are some inorganic salts used as osmotic or **saline purgatives.** They are used to prepare the bowel before surgery and in food poisoning.

Nonabsorbable sugars

Lactulose is a synthetic disaccharide that is not absorbed, holds water and acts as an osmotic purgative. Flatulence and cramps may be accompanied. In the colon, lactulose is fermented to lactic and acetic acids which inhibit the growth of colonic ammonia - producing bacteria. It also

TABLE 46.1 Choice of purgatives	
Conditions	*Preferred laxative*
1. Functional constipation	Increasing dietary fibre and adequate fluid intake
2. Elderly patients	Increasing dietary fibre and adequate fluid intake
3. Pregnancy	Dietary fibre
4. To avoid straining at stools - as in hernia, piles, fissure, cardiovascular diseases like myocardial infarction	Bulk laxatives or faecal softeners
5. Irritable bowel syndrome - chronic constipation	Bulk laxatives
6. Food or drug poisoning	Osmotic purgatives
7. Bowel preparation before surgery, endoscopy and radiological examination	Bisacodyl, osmotic purgatives

inhibits the absorption of ammonia by lowering pH and lowers blood ammonia levels. It is used in hepatic coma for this effect (hepatic coma is worsened by ammonia).

Sorbitol is similar to lactulose.

Glycerine is used as rectal suppository or as enema (with an oil). By an osmotic effect, it softens and lubricates the stools.

Polyethylene glycol (PEG) is a nonabsorbable sugar. Balanced isotonic solution containing PEG with sodium sulphate, sodium chloride, sodium bicarbonate and potassium chloride is given orally. The solution is balanced in such a way that it avoids electrolyte imbalance or fluid shift into the gut. Large volumes are rapidly ingested -3-4 litres over 2 hours - for cleaning the bowel before endoscopic examination of the bowel before endoscopic examination of the bowel. PEG powder may be taken with water for chronic constipation. It has the advantage that there is no associated flatulence or abdominal cramps.

Stimulant purgatives

Stimulant purgatives increase intestinal motility and increase secretion of water and electrolytes by the mucosa. They may cause abdominal cramps.

When anthraquinones like **Cascara sagrada** and **senna** (source: plants) are given orally, active anthraquinones are liberated in the intestines and stimulate the myenteric plexes in the colon. Evacuation takes 6-8 hr. Long-term use causes melanotic pigmentation of the colon.

Phenolphthalein an indicator, acts on the colon after 6 to 8 hours to produce soft, semiliquid stools with some griping. It undergoes enterohepatic circulation which prolongs its actions. Allergic reactions including pink coloured skin eruptions, other severe forms of allergy and risk of cardiac toxicity and colic limit its use.

Bisacodyl related to phenolphthalein is converted to active metabolite in the intestines. It can be given orally (5 mg) but usually is used as rectal suppositories (10 mg) which results in defecation in 15-30 minutes. It is safe except that prolonged use may cause local inflammation.

Castor oil is hydrolysed in the upper small intestine to ricinoleic acid, a local irritant that increases intestinal motility. It is a powerful and one of the oldest purgatives. Stool is semiliquid and is accompanied by griping. It is not preferred.

Enema

Enema produces defecation by softening stools and distending the bowel. Evacuant enema is used to prepare the gut for surgery, endoscopy and radiological examination (See page 13).

Use of laxatives in constipation

Fibre rich diet, adequate fluid intake and physical activity are the best measures to prevent and treat constipation in the otherwise normal subjects. If these measures are inadequate, a laxative may be given (see Table 46.1).

Drug induced constipation

Drugs like anticholinergics, NSAIDs, opioids, clonidine, iron, calcium channel blockers; antihistamines and tricyclic antidepressants (due to anticholinergic effect) can cause constipation. When withdrawal of the causative agent is not possible, a laxative may be used.

Laxative abuse

Habitual use of laxatives, especially stimulant laxatives may lead to various gastrointestinal disturbances like irritable bowel syndrome, loss of electrolytes, loss of calcium in the stool and malabsorption. Misconceptions regarding bowel habits should be cleared. The patient should be convinced that normal bowel habits may vary between 3 motions daily and 2 motions per week.

DRUGS USED IN THE TREATMENT OF DIARRHOEA

Diarrhoea is the frequent passage of liquid stools. It can be due to a variety of causes like infection, toxins, anxiety and drugs. Acute diarrhoea is one of the major causes of death in infants specially in the developing countries.

In diarrhoea, there is an increase in motility and secretions in the gut with absorption of water and electrolytes. Hence the approaches in the treatment of diarrhoea include

1. Replacement of fluid and electrolytes
2. Treatment of the cause
3. Antidiarrhoeal agents.

Replacement of fluid and electrolytes

Correction of fluid and electrolyte disturbances can be life saving in most cases especially infants. Oral rehydration with sodium chloride, glucose and water is useful. In the ileum, glucose and sodium citrate enhance sodium absorption and water follows. Oral rehydration powders are available (Table 46.2) to be mixed with water for mild to moderate cases. ORS with sodium bicarbonate and with sodium citrate are available. Trisodium citrate is used in place of bicarbonate because use of citrate makes ORS more stable, absorption of glucose is better and stool output is lower. If the ORS powder is not available, a mixture of 5g table salt with 20g sugar dissolved in one litre of boiled and cooled water may be used till regular ORS is available. In severe degrees of dehydration, prompt intravenous rehydration is vital (See page 156).

Treatment of the cause

Acute diarrhoea could often be due to viral, bacterial or protozoal infection. The pathogen should be identified whenever possible and treated accordingly. Gastroenteritis is often due to virus and does not require antibiotics. Mild bacterial gastro enteritis is also self-limiting but some infections like typhoid, cholera and amoebic dysentery need chemotherapy.

TABLE 46.2: Composition of oral rehydration salt/solution (ORS)

Sodium Chloride	—	3.5 g
Potassium chloride	—	1.5 g
Sodium citrate	—	2.9 g
Glucose	—	20 g

To be dissolved in 1 litre of boiled and cooled water

Antidiarrhoeal drugs

Antidiarrhoeal drugs afford symptomatic relief and include **adsorbents** and **antimotility drugs.**

Adsorbents

Adsorbents include kaolin, pectin, chalk and activated charcoal. Kaolin is a natural compound containing hydrated magnesium and aluminium silicate while pectin is the sugar obtained from apples. These adsorb intestinal toxins and microorganisms by coating them. They are not absorbed and have no prominent side effects. They bind to and interfere with the absorption of other drugs because of which a 2 hour interval is required after administration of other drugs.

Keybox 46.1
Pathogens commonly causing diarrhoea

Virus	*Bacteria*
Rotavirus	*E. coli*
Astrovirus	*Salmonella*
Adenovirus	*Shigella*
Coronavirus	*V. cholerae*
Enterovirus	*C. jejuni*

Others

E. histolytica
Giardia lamblia
Intestinal worms

Antimotility Drugs

Codeine an opium alkaloid, stimulates the opioid receptors on the gastrointestinal smooth muscles to reduce peristalsis. This delays passage of intestinal contents and facilitates absorption of water. Nausea and vomiting may occur.

Diphenoxylate is an opioid related to pethidine. It is given with a small dose of atropine in order to discourage abuse. In therapeutic doses CNS effects are not prominent and is used only in diarrhoeas. Nausea, drowsiness and abdominal pain may occur. (Table 46.3)

Loperamide is an opiate. It has selective action on GI tract with additional antisecretory activity. CNS effects are negligible. It is less sedating, less addicting and is the most commonly used antimotility drug. Its low solubility in water discourages abuse by injection. Loperamide may cause nausea, vomiting and abdominal cramps.

Uses

Antimotility drugs are used for symptomatic treatment of non-infective diarrhoeas and traveller's diarrhoea (as adjuvant). Antimotility drugs should be avoided in infective diarrhoeas due to invasive pathogens for the following reasons -

- They ↑ the risk of systemic invasion by the pathogen.
- Risk of intestinal perforation.
- Delayed clearance of the infecting organisms.
- Risk of megacolon

Keybox 46.2
Some drugs that produce diarrhoea
- Ampicillin
- Erythromycin
- Colchicine
- Prostaglandins and their analogs
- Emetine
- Lithium
- Magnesium sulphate (oral)
- Cisapride
- Digitalis

Other Drugs

Lactobacillus preparations
Lactobacillus acidophilus and *Lactobacillus sporogenes* are available as powders and tablets and are useful in some diarrhoeas. They colonise the intestines and promote the growth of saccharolytic flora and alter the gut pH so that the growth of pathogenic organisms is inhibited. They are called **probiotics** and are found to be useful in reducing the incidence of antibiotic induced diarrhoea. (See page 345)

Glucocorticoids

In active IBD, treatment is initiated with prednisolone 40 - 60 mg/day and the dose tapered after about 2 weeks. If the part involved is rectum or sigmoid colon, prednisolone retention enema or other rectal preparations may be used. Budesonide controlled - release oral formulations which release the drug in the distal bowel are now being tried.

TABLE 46.3: Antimotility drugs—some preparations and dosage

Drugs	Trade names	Doses
Diphenoxylate 2.5 mg + Atropine 0.025 mg	LOMOTIL	2-4 tablets stat; 1 every 6 hr
Loperamide	LOPESTAL	4 mg stat; 2 mg every 6 hr

Antispasmodics: Atropine derivatives like propantheline and dicyclomine relax gastrointestinal smooth muscles and relieve abdominal colics.

Octreotide is a synthetic analog of somatostatin. Somatostatin has the following actions on the gut.

- Reduces g.i. motility and fluid secretion.

- Inhibits the secretion of various hormones like gastrin, secretin, cholecystokinin, growth hormone, insulin, glucagon, 5HT, pancreatic polypeptide and vasoactive intestinal peptide.

Octreotide is a longer acting analog and can be given subcutaneously. It is used in gastrointestinal secretory tumors causing diarrhoea and in diarrhoea due to vagotomy, dumping syndrome and AIDS.

Traveller's diarrhoea

Infection is the most common cause of traveller's diarrhoea and should be treated with suitable antimicrobials like doxycycline or ciprofloxacin. Oral rehydration salts may also be used.

IRRITABLE BOWEL SYNDROME

Irritable bowel syndrome (IBS) is a common condition characterised by abnormal bowel functions with no specific organic cause. Diarrhoea or constipation with abdominal pain are seen. Causes could be stress, lack of dietary fibre, food allergy or emotional disturbances. When constipation is prominent, soluble dietary fiber like ispaghula is recommended while loperamide is preferred for diarrhoea. Benzodiazepines are given for the treatment of anxiety and other appropriate measures are taken depending on the symptoms and probable cause. Newer antidepressants have shown good response in several studies.

Newer drugs like aloesetron and tegaserod have been found to be useful in IBS.

Aloesetron is a selective $5HT_3$ receptor antagonist. Blocking the $5HT_3$ receptors in the gut can influence intestinal motility and afferent pain impulses from the gastrointestinal tract. Aloesetron inhibits reflex activation of the g.i. smooth muscle and thus reduces colonic motility. It is longer acting than other $5HT_3$ antagonists like ondansetron used in vomiting.

Aloesetron is approved for use in women having IBS with prominent diarrhoea - not responding to other drugs. Adverse effects include constipation and colitis.

Tegaserod is a partial agonist at $5HT_4$ receptors. It promotes gastric emptying and increases chloride secretion in the colon resulting in soft stools. It is approved for use in patients with IBS with predominent constipation. Adverse effects are uncommon - rarely diarrhoea and headache can occur.

INFLAMMATORY BOWEL DISEASES (IBD)

IBD like ulcerative colitis and Crohn's disease are treated with glucocortcoids, sulphasalazine and immunosuppresants.

Glucocorticoids

In active IBD, treatment is initiated with prednisolone 40-60mg per day and the dose is tapered after 2 weeks. If the part involved is rectum or sigmoid colon, prednisolone retention enema or other rectal preparations may be used. Budesonide controlled-release oral formulations which release the drug in the distal bowel are now being tried.

Sulphasalazine is split by flora in the colon to 5-aminosalicylate (5ASA) and sulfapyridine.

Adverse effects are common and are mostly due to sulfapyridine. Nausea, vomiting, fever, headache, diarrhoea, megaloblastic anaemia and various allergic manifestations ranging from skin rashes to Steven Johnson's Syndrome can occur.

Mesalamine is 5-ASA which is better tolerated with minor side effects. Mesalamine retention enema and suppositories are used. Other compounds in this group are *olsalazine* and *balsalazide*. Balsalazide contains mesalamine linked to an inert carrier which is split by colonic bacteria and 5-ASA is released in the colon. It provides remission in mild to moderate IBD (1.5-4 g - daily)

Immunosuppressants - like azathioprine and 6-mercaptopurine are used for induction and maintenance of remission in patients with active IBD.

CHEMOTHERAPY

47 *General Considerations*

CHAPTER

- Introduction
- Classification
- Antibacterial spectrum
- Resistance to antimicrobial agents
- Selection of an antibacterial agent
- Dose of the antimicrobials
- Combination of antimicrobials
- Chemoprophylaxis
- Superinfection
- Misuse of antibiotics

INTRODUCTION

Chemotherapy can be defined as the use of chemicals in infectious diseases to destroy microorganisms without damaging the host tissues.

Antibiotics are substances produced by microorganisms which suppress the growth of or destroy other microorganisms.

Pasteur and Joubert were the first to identify that microorganisms could destroy other microorganisms. Paul Ehrlich 'The father of Modern Chemotherapy' coined the term 'chemotherapy'. He showed that certain dyes can destroy microbes and demonstrated that methylene blue can be used in malaria. He synthesized many arsenical compounds for the treatment of syphilis and sleeping sickness. Paul Ehrlich was awarded Nobel prize for his work on chemotherapy. The evolution of chemotherapy can be studied in three periods

i. Pre Ehrlich era - before 1891

ii. The period of Paul Ehrlich

iii. Post Ehrlich era - after 1935

Domagk in 1935 demonstrated that prontosil, a sulfonamide dye, is effective in some infections. Domagk was awarded Nobel prize for his work. Sir. Alexander Fleming discovered penicillin in 1928. He was studying different varints of staphylococci and found that a fungus was contaminating one of the culture plates. This fungus, *Pencillium notatum* produced a substance which inhibited the growth of a variety of micro organisms The substance was named Penicillin. It needed extensive research and purification for clinical use. In 1941 penicillin was first used therapeutically on a policeman. The discovery of Pencillin is described as the beginning of the 'golden era' of antibiotics. In the last 60 years, several powerful antibiotics and their semisynthetic derivatives have been produced.

Many infectious diseases, which were earlier incurable can now be treated with just a few doses of antimicrobial drugs. Thus the development of antimicrobial drugs is one of the important advances of modern medicine. In fact antimocrobials are one of the most commonly prescribed drugs but are often the most over used or misused drugs.

CLASSIFICATION

Antimicrobials may be classified (Fig 47.1) as drugs that:

1. *Inhibit cell wall synthesis-*

    Penicillins, cephalosporins, carbapenems, monobactam, vancomycin, bacitracin, cycloserine.

2. *Damage cell membranes -*
    (causing leakage of cell contents)

    Polymyxins, amphotericin B, nystatin.

3. *Bind to ribosomes and inhibit protein synthesis -*

    Chloramphenicol, tetracyclines, erythromycin, aminoglycosides, clindamycin.

4. *Inhibit DNA gyrase -*
    Fluoroquinolones

5. *Inhibit DNA function -*
    (↓DNA dependent RNA polymerase)
    Rifampicin

6. *Interfere with metabolic steps -*
    (Antimetabolite action)

    Sulfonamides, sulfones, trimethoprim, pyrimethamine

Antimicrobials may also be classified as -

1. Bacteriostatic - agents that suppress the growth of bacteria.

    E.g. Sulfonamides, tetracyclines, linezolid chloramphenicol, clindamycin

2. Bactericidal - agents that kill the bacteria.

    E.g. Penicillins, cephalosporins, aminoglycosides, fluoroquinolones, rifampicin, metronidazole, vancomycin

However, some drugs may be bacteriostatic at low doses and bactericidal at higher doses.*e.g.*erythromycin; also, some drugs may be bacteriostatic to some microorganisms and 'cidal' to others. *e.g.* chloramphenicol is bactericidal to *H. influenzae, S. pneumoniae* and *N. menigitidis,* while it is bacteriostatic to other microorganisms.

Factors that influence the successful chemotherapy of an infection are:

- Site   The drug should reach the site of infection.

- Concentration   It should attain adequate concentration at the site.

- Host defence   Active host defences reduce the antibiotic requirement.

- Sensitivity   The microorganism should be sensitive to the antimicrobial agent.

Antibacterial spectrum

An antimicrobial may have a narrow or broad spectrum of activity.

- *Narrow spectrum -*
    e.g. Penicillin G   - gram positive organisms

    Aminoglycosides   - gram negative organisms

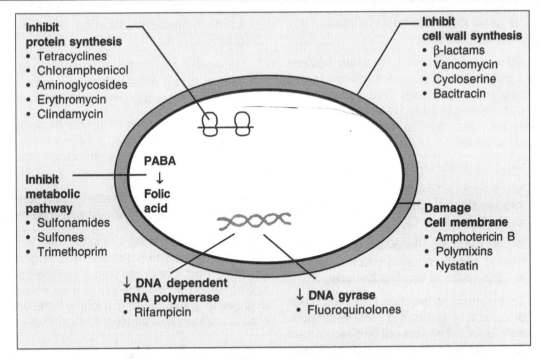

Fig. 47.1: Classification of antimicrobials based on their mechanisms of action

- *Broad spectrum -*

Tetracyclines
Chloramphenicol } - gram positive & gram negative organisms, ricketssiae, chlamydiae, mycoplasma.

Broad spectrum antibiotics are so called because in addition to suppression of gram positive and gram negative bacteria, they also inhibit the growth of other microorganisms like rickettsiae, chlamydiae, mycoplasma and some protozoa. But in practice the term 'broad spectrum' is often used to include all antimicrobials with a wide spectrum of activity *i.e.* those effective against both gram positive and gram negative organisms *e.g.* ampicillin.

Resistance to antimicrobial agents

Resistance is the unresponsiveness of a microorganism to the antimicrobial agent. The resistance may be natural or acquired.

Natural resistance In natural resistance, the organisms have never responded to the antimicrobial - may be due to the absence of the particular enzyme or target site affected by the drug, *e.g.* gram - negative bacilli are not sensitive to Pencillin G. But this type of resistance is clinically not a problem as alternative drugs are available.

Acquired resistance Here, the microbes which were previously sensitive to the antimicrobial agents become resistant to it. Clinically this poses a problem.

Bacteria acquire resistance by a change in their DNA. Such DNA changes may occur by:

(i) **mutation**
(ii) **transfer of genes.**

- *Mutation* Mutation is a genetic change that occurs spontaneously. In any population of bacteria, a few resistant mutants may be present. When the sensitive organisms are destroyed by the antibiotic, the resistant mutants freely multiply. Mutation may take place in a single step (e.g *Staph. aureus* to rifampicin) or multiple steps where several gene modifications are made, *e.g.* gonococci to penicillin G.

• Transfer of genetic material Many bacteria contain extrachromosomal genetic material called **plasmids** in the cytoplasm. These carry genes coding for resistance (called R-factors). These R-factors are transferred to other bacteria and spread resistance (Fig. 47.2).

This may take place by:

1. Transduction Plasmid DNA is transferred through bacteriophage, i.e. virus which infects bacteria.

2. Transformation Resistant bacteria may release genetic material into the medium which is taken up by other bacteria.

3. Conjugation is the most important mode of spread of resistance. The R-factor is transferred from cell to cell by direct contact through a sex pilus or bridge and the process is known as conjugation.

The resistance acquired by the bacteria may be exhibited in the following ways:

• Production of enzymes that inactivate the drug, *e.g.* β-lactamase by staphylococci; aminoglycoside inactivating enzymes by *E.coli.*

• Decreased accumulation of the drug in the bacterium, *e.g.* resistance to tetracyclines by gram-positive and gram-negative bacteria.

• Altered target for the drug - the binding site may be altered, *e.g.* binding sites for aminoglycosides on the ribosomes may be altered.

• Altered metabolic pathway - bacteria may produce folic acid by an alternative pathway.

Cross resistance is the resistance seen among chemically related drugs. When a microorganism develops resistance to one drug, it is also resistant to other drugs of the same group, even when not exposed to it, *e.g.* resistance to one tetracycline means resistance to all other tetracyclines.

Prevention of Resistance to antimicrobials

Development of resistance to drugs can be avoided to some extent by the following measures:

• Antibiotics should be used only when

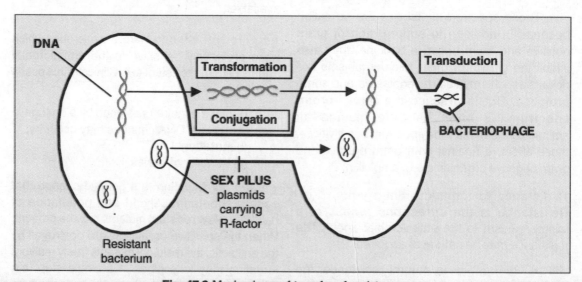

Fig. 47.2 Mechanisms of transfer of resistance

necessary

- Selection of the appropriate antibiotic is absolutely important
- Correct dose and duration of treatment should be followed
- Combination of drugs should be used as in tuberculosis to delay the development of resistance.

Selection of an Antibacterial Agent

Various factors should be considered in selection of an antibiotic like, the patient factors, the microbe factors, the properties of the drug and the clinical assessment. Site of infection is the prime factor that guides the choice of the drug and its route of administration. Age of the patient, host defence status, renal and hepatic functions should be considered. Whenever possible, bacteriological culture report should guide the drug selection. When not available, empirical therapy should be started to cover all the likely organisms. Drug toxicity and cost should be borne in mind. With proper clinical judgement - considering the above factors, most infections can be successfully treated.

Antibiotics are used in 2 ways

1. **Empiric therapy:** The antibiotic must cover all the likely pathogens. A combination or a broad spectrum agent may be used. This therapy should be employed only in some situations. But when the culture report is available, antimicrobial agents should be changed accordingly.

2. **Definitive therapy:** When the micro organism is identified, specific antibacterial agents are given.

Dose of the antimicrobials

The dose of the antimicrobial should be adequate enough for the drug to attain plasma concentrations above the **minimum inhibitory concentration** (MIC). MIC is the lowest concentration of the antimicrobial agent that prevents visible growth of the microorganism after 18 to 24 hours of incubation. The bactericidal effect with many drugs is dose-dependent i.e. higher the concentration, greater is the bactericidal effect *e.g.* aminoglycosides.

Postantibiotic effect

Some antibiotics have a postantibiotic effect i.e., they continue to suppress the bacterial multiplication even after their plasma concentration falls below the MIC. Aminoglycosides and fluoroquinolones have such effect against gram negative bacteria.

COMBINATION OF ANTIMICROBIALS

Use of a combination of antimicrobials may have synergistic, antagonistic or indifferent (no change) effects. Hence appropriate drugs should be used for combination.

Two bactericidal drugs given together (*e.g.* penicillin + aminoglycosides) are generally synergistic.

Combination of a bacteriostatic with a bactericidal drug is not useful because bacteriostatic drugs inhibit the multiplication of bacteria and thereby antagonize the effect of bactericidal drugs (as bactericidal drugs act on actively multiplying bacteria). Hence such combinations should be avoided.

A combination of antimicrobial agents is indicated in certain specific situations. The combination serves one of the following purposes.

1. **To obtain synergism:** Combination of antibiotics to attain synergism is recommended in -

   - Bacterial endocarditis
     Penicillin + streptomycin/gentamicin is synergistic.

   - Pseudomonas infections
     Carbenicillin + gentamicin

   - *Pneumocystis carinii* pneumonia
     Trimethoprim + sulfamethoxazole

- β-lactamase producing organisms like *H. influenzae*
  Amoxicillin + clavulinic acid
- Tuberculosis - INH + rifampicin.

2. **Treatment of mixed infections:** Intra-abdominal infections, brain abscesses, genitourinary infections are often mixed infections. Aerobic and anaerobic organisms may be involved. Two or more antimicrobials can be used depending on the culture and sensitivity report.

3. **Initial treatment of severe infections** Drugs covering both gram-positive and gram-negative pathogens may be used initially till the culture report is available, *e.g.* penicillin + aminoglycoside; cephalosporin + aminoglycoside. If anaerobes are likely to be present, metronidazole may be added. Samples for culture should however be taken before starting the antibiotics.

4. **To prevent the emergence of resistance** In the treatment of tuberculosis and leprosy, combination of drugs is used to prevent the development of resistance.

5. **To reduce the adverse effects** The doses needed may be lower when a combination is used. This may reduce the incidence and severity of adverse effects, *e.g.* Amphotericin B + flucytosine in cryptococcal meningitis.

Disadvantages of antimicrobial combination

1. Risk of toxicity from each agent - especially if toxicity is overlapping - may get added up *e.g.* many antitubercular drugs are hepatotoxic.

   Toxicity of one drug may be enhanced by another - *e.g.*,

   Vancomycin + aminoglycoside → more severe renal toxicity

2. Selection of resistant strains → The few resistant mutants that remain may multiply unchecked.

3. Emergence of organisms resistant to multiple drugs.

4. Increased cost of therapy.

CHEMOPROPHYLAXIS

Chemoprophylaxis is the use of antimicrobial agents to prevent infection. This is recommended in the following situations:

1. To protect healthy persons

- Penicillin G is given for prevention of gonorrhoea or syphilis in patients after contact with infected persons - postexposure prophylaxis.

- For preventing meningococcal infection in healthy children during an epidemic - rifampicin or sulfonamides may be used.

- Malaria - in healthy individuals visiting an endemic area. Chemoprophylaxis with chloroquine or pyrimethamine + sulfadoxine is given. (Page 417).

2. To prevent infection in high risk patients

- In neutropenic patients - like patients receiving anticancer drugs, immunosuppressive agents and patients with AIDS penicillin or fluoroquinolones or cotrimoxazole may reduce the incidence of bacterial infection.

- In patients with valvular heart diseases even minor procedures like dental extraction, tonsillectomy or endoscopies may result in bacterial endocarditis (damage to mucosa results in bacteremia). Penicillin is used for prophylaxis.

- In patients with contaminated or exposed wounds as in road traffic accidents.

- Catheterisation of urinary tract - norfloxacin is used.

- In burns - to prevent colonisation by bacteria.

3. Surgical prophylaxis

Certain guidelines are to be followed:

- Adequate antibacterial activity should be present during surgery. Hence the drug should be started parenterally 30-60 minutes before surgery.
- The drug should be effective against all organisms that are likely to contaminate the wound.
- A single dose of 1 g IV cefazolin injection is the most commonly used.
- The drug should not be continued beyond 24 hours after surgery (due to the risk of resistance development).

4. In close contacts

Chemoprophylaxis is recommended particularly in children when infectious (open) cases of leprosy or tuberculosis are in close contact.

SUPERINFECTIONS

Superinfection/suprainfection is the appearance of a new infection resulting from the use of antimicrobials. Antibacterials alter the normal microbial flora of the intestinal, respiratory and genitourinary tracts. The normal flora contribute to host defence mechanisms as follows - they inhibit colonisation of pathogenic organisms by producing antibacterial substances called bacteriocins and by competing for nutrients. When the normal flora are destroyed by antibacterials, there can be dangerous infections due to various organisms especially the normal commensals which become pathogenic. The broader the antibacterial spectrum of a drug, the more are the chances of superinfection, as the alteration of the normal flora is greater (Table 47.1).

Sites involved - intestinal, respiratory and genitourinary tracts.

Misuse of Antibiotics

Antibiotics are one of the most overused or misused drugs. Faulty practices like the use of antibacterials in viral infections which are self-limiting, using too low doses or unnecessarily prolonged treatment, using antibiotics in all fever cases - are all irrational and can do more harm than any benefit. Since most of the vulnerable sites in the microorganisms have already been targeted by various antibiotics, we are left with very few / no targets for development of antibiotics in future. Hence it is absolutely necessary that we do not encourage the development of resistance by microbes due to inappropriate use of the available antimicrobials. Successful treatment of infections will then be beyond imagination, considering the methods and speed with which bacteria are developing resistance to antimicrobials at present.

Probiotics

Probiotics are products containing viable, non pathogenic micro-organisms administered orally to alter the intestinal microflora. *Lactobacillus, Bifido bacterium, Streptococcus salivarius,* some *enterococci* and *Saccharomyces boulardii* are some of the presently tried probiotics. Studies have shown them to be useful in acute infectious diarrhoea and diarrhoea following antibiotic administration. Probiotics have also been tried in ulcerative colitis and irritable bowel syndrome.

TABLE 47.1 Common microorganisms causing superinfection		
Microorganisms	*Manifestations*	*Treatment*
Candida albicans	Oral thrush, diarrohea, vaginitis	Clotrimazole
Staphylococci	Enteritis	Cloxacillin
Clostridium difficile	Pseudomembranous colitis	Metronidazole, Vancomycin
E.coli	UTI	Norfloxacin
Pseudomonas	UTI	Carbenicillin

TABLE 47.2: Choice of antibiotics recommended in the treatment of some common infections

Microorganisms	Clinical diagnosis	Drug of first choice	Alternative drugs
Gram-positive organisms			
Group A Streptococcus	Pharyngitis, Otitis media, Sinusitis, Cellulitis, Erysipelas, Impetigo, Bacteraemia	Penicillin or amoxicillin	Erythromycin, A first generation cephalosporin
Group B Streptococcus	Bacteraemia, Endocarditis, Meningitis	Ampicillin or penicillin + an aminoglycoside	A first generation cephalosporin
Staphylococcus aureus	Furuncle, Cellulitis, Bacteraemia, Osteo-myelitis, Pneumonia		
• *Methicillin sensitive*		Cloxacillin or dicloxacillin	A first generation cephalosporin or vancomycin
• *Methicillin resistant*		Vancomycin	Ciprofloxacin + rifampicin Quinupristine-dalfopristine, Linezolid
Pneumococcus	Pneumonia, Sinusitis, Otitis, Endocarditis Meningitis	Penicillin	A first generation cephalosporin Amoxicilln
Penicillin resistant		Ceftriaxone Cefotaxime Vancomycin	Clindamycin Cotrimoxazole
Enterococcus	Endocarditis	Penicillin G + gentamicin	Vancomycin + gentamicin
Corynebacterium diphtheriae	Diphtheria	Erythromycin	A first generation cephalosporin Clindamycin
Clostridium tetani	Tetanus	Penicillin G Doxycycline	Clindamycin
Clostridium difficile	Pseudomembranous colitis	Metronidazole	Vancomycin
Clostridium perfringens	Gas gangrene	Penicillin G	Ceftizoxime Cefoxitine Chloramphenicol Doxycycline
Bacillus anthracis	Malignant pustule, pneumonia	Penicillin G	Erythromycin Doxycycline A first generation cephalosporin

Microorganisms	Clinical diagnosis	Drug of first choice	Alternative drugs
Gram-negative organisms			
Gonococcus	Gonorrhoea, Pelvic inflammatory disease	Ceftriaxone	Ampicillin Amoxicillin Doxycycline Erythromycin
Meningococcus	Meningitis	Ceftriaxone Cefotaxime	Penicillin G Chloramphenicol Minocycline
	Carrier state	Rifampicin	
Escherichia coli	Urinary tract infection	Norfloxacin Ciprofloxacin Cotrimoxazole	Ampicillin + gentamicin; Amoxicillin + clavulinic acid; Aztreonam
Proteus mirabilis	Urinary tract infection Bacteraemia and other infections	Ampicillin or Ciprofloxacin Amoxicillin	Cephalosporin I or II Generation A cephalosporin Gentamicin
Pseudomonas aeruginosa	Urinary tract infection	A broad spectrum pencillin + Ciprofloxacin	Gentamicin Ceftazidime A cephalosporin Imipenem Aztreonam
Klebsiella pneumoniae	Urinary tract infection Pneumonia	A cephalosporin	Mezlocillin/ Piperacillin An aminoglycoside
		A cephalosporin + gentamicin	Mezlocillin/ Piperacillin Aztreonam Amoxicillin + clavulinic acid
Salmonella	Typhoid fever, Bacteraemia	Ciprofloxacin Ceftriaxone	Chloramphenicol Ampicillin Cotrimoxazole
Shigella	Gastroenteritis	Ciprofloxacin or norfloxacin	Cotrimoxazole Ampicillin
Haemophillus influenzae	Sinusitis, Pneumonia, Otitis media	Amoxicillin + clavulinic acid Cotrimoxazole	Amoxicillin Ciprofloxacin Azithromycin A cephalosporin
	Meningitis	Ceftriaxone	Chloramphenicol Ampicillin + sulbactam
Haemophillus ducreyi	Chancroid	Ceftriaxone Cotrimoxazole	Ciprofloxacin Erythromycin Doxycycline

Microorganisms	Clinical diagnosis	Drug of first choice	Alternative drugs
Brucella	Brucellosis	Doxycycline + rifampicin	Cotrimoxazole Gentamicin
Yersenia pestis	Plague	A tetracycline + streptomycin	Doxycycline Chloramphenicol Ciprofloxacin
Vibrio cholerae	Cholera	Doxycycline Ciprofloxacin	Cotrimoxazole Chloramphenicol
Campylobacter jejuni	Enteritis	Ciprofloxacin	Erythromycin
Treponema pallidum	Syphilis	Penicillin G	Ceftriaxone Doxycycline
Leptospira	Weil's disease Meningitis	Penicillin G	Doxycycline
Helicobacter pylori	Peptic ulcer	Metronidazole + amoxicillin + Bismuth/omeprazole	Omeprazole+ amoxicillin+ clarithromycin
Legionella	Pneumonia	Azithromycin + rifampicin	Erythromycin Clarithromycin Doxycycline Ciprofloxacin + rifampicin
Other agents			
Mycoplasma pneumoniae	Atypical pneumonia	Erythromycin Doxycycline	Azithromycin
Rickettsiae	Typhus fever, Q fever, Rocky mountain spotted fever	Doxycycline	Chloramphenicol
Chlamydia trachomatis	Lymphogranuloma venereum, Trachoma, Inclusion conjunctivitis, Urethritis	Doxycycline	Erythromycin Azithromycin
Chlamydia psittaci	Psittacosis	Doxycycline	Chloramphenicol
Chlamydia pneumoniae	Pneumonia	Doxycycline	Erythromycin Azithromycin
Pneumocystis jiroveci *Pneumocystis carinii*	Pneumonia	Cotrimoxazole	Atovaquone Trimethoprim + dapsone Pentamidine

48 Sulfonamides And Cotrimoxazole

SULFONAMIDES

Sulfonamides were the first effective antibacterial agents to be used systemically in man. They were introduced by Domagk in 1935 and in the next few years several of them were synthesized and widely used. Currently, their role in therapeutics is limited because of their toxicity, development of resistance and availability of safer drugs.

Chemistry

Para

Sulfonamides are structural analogs of p- amino benzoic acid (PABA). They are synthetic agents that contain a sulfonamide group.

CLASSIFICATION

1. **Short-acting**
   - Sulfisoxazole, sulfadiazine

2. **Intermediate-acting**
   - Sulfamethoxazole

3. **Long-acting**
   - Sulfamethoxypyridazine, Sulfadoxine

4. **Poorly absorbed**
   - Sulfasalazine

5. Topical

- Sulfacetamide, Mafenide,
  Silver suphadiazine

Antibacterial spectrum

Sulfonamides inhibit many gram-positive and some gram-negative bacteria including *streptococci, H. influenzae, H. ducreyi, nocardia, E. coli, proteus, V. cholerae,* few strains of *staphylococci, gonococci, meningococci* and *pneumococci.* They are also effective against *chlamydiae, Pl. falciparum and Toxoplasma gondii.*

Mechanism of action

PABA

$\quad$|Folic acid synthetase ◄- - - Sulfonamides

Dihydrofolic acid

Folic acid is essential for the synthesis of nucleic acids. Bacteria synthesize their own folic acid from PABA with the help of the enzyme folic acid synthetase. Sulfonamides are structurally similar to PABA and competitively inhibit the enzyme folic acid synthetase. This results in folic acid deficiency and thereby inhibition of bacterial growth as well as injury to the bacterial cell.

Human cells are not affected because they require preformed folic acid supplied from the diet and cannot synthesize folic acid by themselves. Sulfonamides are bacteriostatic.

Presence of pus, blood and tissue breakdown products make sulfonamides ineffective because these are rich in PABA.

Resistance Bacteria acquire resistance to sulfonamides by:

1. Mutations - resulting in over production of PABA.

2. Using alternative metabolic pathway for folic acid synthesis.

3. Low permeability to sulfonamides.

Pharmacokinetics

Sulfonamides are well-absorbed, extensively bound to plasma proteins and are well distributed to all tissues. They are metabolized in the liver by acetylation.

Preparations of Sulfonamides

Drug	Route of administration	Dose
Sulfisoxazole	oral	0.5-2g 12 hrly
Sulfadiazine	oral/IM	1-2 g 4-6 hrly
Sulfasalazine	oral	0.5 - 1g 12 hrly
Mafenide	Topical (cream/ointment)	

Adverse effects

1. Renal irritation, haematuria, albuminuria and crystalluria - due to precipitation of the drug in acidic urine. This can be avoided by intake of large volumes of fluids and by alkalinising the urine with sodium bicarbonate.

2. Sulfonamides can produce a range of hypersensitivity reactions like rashes, fever, anaphylactoid reactions, urticaria, photosensitivity and rarely, Steven-Johnsons syndrome (SJS) and exfoliative dermatitis. SJS can be fatal and should be watched for. Nephritis may also be of allergic etiology.

3. Anorexia, nausea, stomatitis and abdominal pain.

4. Sulfonamides can cause haemolytic anaemia and decreased granulocyte and thrombocyte count. Haemolytic anaemia may be precipitated in patients with G_6PD deficiency.

5. Kernicterus - sulfonamides displace bilirubin from the binding sites which crosses the BBB and may cause kernicterus in the newborn. Hence sulfonamides are contraindicated in pregnancy and in infants.

Uses

Because of the development of resistance and availability of better antimicrobials which are more effective and less toxic, sulfonamides are not commonly used now except in a few cases.

1. Urinary tract infections Uncomplicated acute UT I can be treated with sulfonamides in areas where resistance is not high.

2. Nocardiosis High doses of sulfonamides can be used as alternatives.

3. Toxoplasmosis Sulfonamides with pyrimethamine is the treatment of choice in *T. gondii* infection. Sulfadoxine is given in the dose of 4 g/day while pyrimethamine is given as a bolus dose of 200 mg followed by 50 mg daily. The treatment is continued for 4-6 weeks. Such doses require leucovorin rescue (10 mg folinic acid daily) to prevent severe folic acid deficiency. (See page 419)

4. Trachoma and inclusion conjunctivitis Tetracylines are the drugs of choice, sulfonamides are used as alternatives.

5. Lymphogranuloma venereum and chancroid Sulfonamides are used as alternatives to tetracyclines.

6. Malaria Sulfadoxine is used with pyrimethamine in chloroquine resistant malaria.

7. Prophylactic use In patients allergic to penicillins, sulfonamides may be used for prophylaxis of streptococcal pharyngitis in rheumatic fever.

8. Topical Sulfacetamide eye drops are used in bacterial conjunctivitis - Sulphacetamide also readily penetrates into the aqueous humor; mafenide and silver sulfadiazine ointment is used in burns to prevent infection.

9. Ulcerative colitis Sulfasalazine is useful in ulcerative colitis (See page 335) and rheumatoid arthritis.

COTRIMOXAZOLE

The combination of trimethoprim and sulfamethoxazole is cotrimoxazole. Trimethoprim is effective against several gram-positive and gram-negative organisms. But when used as a sole agent, resistance develops rapidly.

Mechanism of action

Sulfonamides inhibit the conversion of PABA to dihydrofolic acid (DHF) and trimethoprim (Fig 48.1) inhibits dihydrofolate reductase (DHFR) and thus prevents the reduction of DHF to tetrahydrofolic acid (THF). The two drugs thus block sequential steps in folic acid synthesis and the combination is *synergistic*. Given alone, both

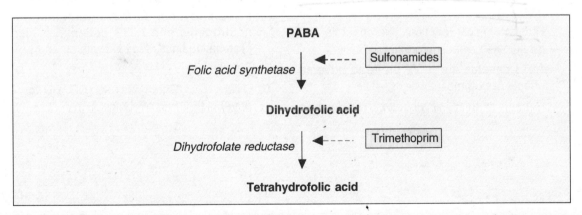

Fig. 48.1 Sequential blockade by sulfonamides and trimethoprim in folic acid synthesis

trimethoprim and sulfonamides are bacteriostatic but the combination is bactericidal.

The ratio of 'trimethoprim : sulfamethoxazole' used is 1:5 to attain the right plasma concentration. Among sulfonamides, sulfamethoxazole is chosen since its pharmacokinetic properties closely match with that of trimethoprim.

Antibacterial spectrum

Cotrimoxazole is effective against several gram-positive and gram-negative organisms like *Staph. aureus, streptococci, meningococci, C. diphtheriae, E. coli, Proteus, H. influenzae, Salmonella and Shigella.*

Resistance

Development of resistance to the combination is slower when compared to either drugs given alone. Bacteria may acquire resistance by mutation or by acquisition of a plasmid coding for an altered DHFR.

Adverse effects

- Nausea, vomiting, headache, glossitis, stomatitis and allergic skin rashes are relatively common.
- In patients with folate deficiency, cotrimoxazole may precipitate megaloblastic anaemia.
- Haematological reactions like anaemia and granulocytopenia are rare.
- AIDS patients are more prone to adverse effects of cotrimoxazole.
- Patients with renal disease may develop uraemia.

Preparations

Trimethoprim	Sulfamethoxazole (SEPTRAN, CIPLIN)
80 mg	400 mg
160 mg	800 mg - double strength (DS)

Uses

1. Urinary tract infection
   - *Uncomplicated acute UTI* - is treated for 7-10 days with cotrimoxazole (DS, twice a day).
   - *Chronic and recurrent UTI* - small doses are given for prophylaxis.
   - *Bacterial prostatitis* - Trimethoprim attains high concentration in prostatic fluid.

2. Respiratory tract infections Upper and lower respiratory infections including bronchitis, sinusitis and otitis media respond.

3. Bacterial gastroenteritis due to *Shigella* and *E. coli* respond to cotrimoxazole.

4. Typhoid Cotrimoxazole is used as an alternative to fluoroquinolones.

5. *Pneumocystis carinii* infection (now identified as *Pneumocystis jiroveci*) Cotrimoxazole is used for the prophylaxis and high doses for the treatment of *Pneumocystis carinii* pneumonia in neutropenic and AIDS patients. It also protects against infections with other gram-negative bacteria.

6. Chancroid Cotrimoxazole (DS, BD for 7 days) is the drug of choice.

49 *Quinolones*

- Nalidixic Acid
- Fluoroquinolones
  - Mechanism of action
  - Antibacterial spectrum
  - Pharmacokinetics
  - Adverse reactions
  - Uses

The quinolones are a group of synthetic antimicrobial agents. Nalidixic acid is the older agent in the group. Oxalinic acid and cinoxacin are other quinolones.

NALIDIXIC ACID

Nalidixic acid is bactericidal against various gram-negative organisms like *E. coli, Shigella, Proteus and Klebsiella.* Its mechanism of action is the same as that of fluoroquinolones (see below). Nalidixic acid is well absorbed orally. However, the plasma concentration of the drug is inadequate to produce systemic effects because it is too rapidly excreted; but it attains high concentrations in the urine.

Adverse effects

Adverse effects are uncommon; haemolytic anaemia, particularly in G_6PD deficient individuals, allergic reactions and CNS effects like headache, myalgia, drowsiness visual disturbances may be encountered.

Uses

Nalidixic acid is used in uncomplicated UTI and diarrhoea due to *E.coli, Shigella* and *Proteus* (0.5-1g 3-4 times a day).

Oxalinic acid and cinoxacin have properties and uses similar to nalidixic acid.

FLUOROQUINOLONES

The fluorinated quinolones were derived with wider spectrum of activity, fewer side effects, lesser chances of resistance and better tissue penetration when compared to quinolones. The fluoroquinolones (FQs) include *norfloxacin, ciprofloxacin, pefloxacin, ofloxacin, lomefloxacin and sparfloxacin* - many more are being added. The newer agents include *levofloxacin, trovafloxacin, gatifloxacin, moxifloxacin,* and *clinafloxacin.*

Mechanism of action

Fluoroquinolones are bactericidal. They inhibit the bacterial enzymes DNA gyrase and topoisomerase IV which are required for DNA replication and transcription.

During DNA replication there is positive supercoiling of the DNA. This is corrected by the enzyme DNA gyrase by introducing negative supercoils and therefore this enzyme is necessary for DNA replication. By inhibiting the enzyme DNA gyrase, fluoroquinolones inhibit DNA replication. Instead of DNA gyrase, human cells have topoisomerase II which functions as DNA gyrase. Topoisomerase II is also inhibited by FQs but only

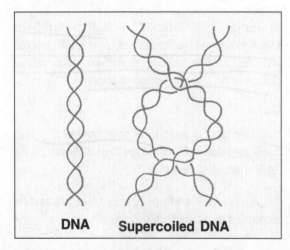

DNA   **Supercoiled DNA**

Fig 49.1. Schematic diagram showing DNA and supercoiled DNA.

at 500-1000 times higher concentration. Hence FQs are reasonably safe drugs.

Topoisomerase IV is essential for separation of the daughter cells following replication. FQs also inhibit topoisomerase IV and block this separation of daughter cells. This activity of FQs is primarily responsible for inhibiting the gram positive bacteria while DNA - gyrase inhibition suppresses gram-negative bacteria.

Bacteria with damaged DNA are formed which are degraded by nuclease enzymes. Thus FQs are *bactericidal* (Fig 49.1).

Resistance is not very frequent due to the unique mechanism of action. Resistance is due to mutations in the target enzyme or a change in the permeability of the organism. Several strains of *E.coli, Staphylococci, Pseudomonas* and *Serratia* have now developed resistance.

Antibacterial spectrum

Gram-negative organisms like *gonococci, meningococci, H. influenzae, E. coli, Salmonella, Shigella, enterobacteria, H. pylorii* and gram-positive organisms like *staphylococci* are susceptible; *chlamydiae, mycoplasma and mycobacterium* also respond to FQs. Some of the newer fluoroquinolones are effective against some anaerobic organisms and *Streptococcus pneumoniae.*

Pharmacokinetics

On oral administration, fluoroquinolones are well-absorbed and widely distributed. Food and antacids interfere with absorption; Pefloxacin and ofloxacin cross the BBB. All FQs are metabolised by hepatic microsomal enzymes and FQs are *microsomal enzyme inhibitors* – can result in related drug interactions. These drugs are excreted by the kidneys. Hence dose should be reduced in renal failure. Plasma $t_{1/2}$ varies from 3 hrs (norfloxacin) 10 hrs (pefloxacin) to 18-20 hrs (sparfloxacin given once daily). Dose - Table 49.1.

Adverse reactions

Fluoroquinolones are well-tolerated. Nausea, vomiting, abdominal discomfort, diarrhoea and rashes may be seen. Tendinitis with associated risk of tendon rupture has been reported. Fluoroquinolones damage the growing cartilage resulting in arthropathy and are therefore contraindicated upto 18 years of age. CNS effects include headache and dizziness. In patients receiving NSAIDs and other epileptogenic drugs like theophylline, fluoroquinolones can sometimes precipitate seizures. Grepafloxacin was found to cause cardiac arrhythemias due to which it has already been withdrawn from the market. Calcium in antacids and iron chelate FQs - hence they should not be administered together.

Uses

1. **Urinary tract infections:** Very effective in UTI even when caused by multi-drug resistant bacteria - norfloxacin is generally used (400 mg - BD for 5-10 days).

2. **Typhoid:** Ciprofloxacin is the drug of choice (500 mg BD - 10 days) - it also eradicates the carrier state.

3. **Diarrhoea:** due to *Shigella, E.coli* and *Campylobacter* respond.

4. **Gonorrhoea:** Single dose 250 mg ciprofloxacin is curative.

5. **Chancroid:** As an alternative to cotrimoxazole, ciprofloxacin is used for 3 days. In chlamydial urethritis and cervicitis, ciprofloxacin or sparfloxacin can be used

TABLE 49.1: Dose and route of administration of some fluoroquinolones

Drug	Dose and route	Remarks
Norfloxacin (NORFLOX)	Oral: 400 mg BD	Preferred in urinary and genital infections; Does not achieve adequate plasma concentration
Ciprofloxacin (CIPLOX)	Oral: 250-750 mg BD IV: 100-200 mg 12 h	Most widely used fluoroquinolone
Pefloxacin (PEFLOX)	Oral: 400 mg BD IV: 400 mg q 12 h	Penetration into CSF is good
Ofloxacin (TARIVID)	Oral: 200-400 mg OD IV: 200-400 mg q 12-24 h	Indicated in urinary and respiratory tract infections and gonorrhoea; Effective in chlamydial infections
Lomefloxacin (LOMEF)	Oral: 400 mg OD	Has a long t½
Sparfloxacin (SPARLOX)	Oral: 200-400 mg OD	Enhanced activity against gram +ve organisms and in atypical pneumonia; also useful in chlamydial infections.
Gatifloxacin	Oral : 400 mg OD	Better activity against gram positive organisms and atypical pneumonia pathogens.
Levofloxacin	Oral : 500 mg OD	Better activity against gram positive organisms and atypical pneumonia pathogens; excreted mainly through kidneys.
Trovafloxacin	Oral : 200 mg	Excreted by nonrenal mechanisms.

as alternatives to tetracyclines.

6. Respiratory tract infections - due to *H. influenzae, Legionella and Mycoplasma* can be treated with fluoroquinolones.

7. Bone, joint, soft tissue and intra abdominal infections - osteomyelitis and joint infections require prolonged treatment. Soft tissue infections due to sensitive bacteria can be treated with fluoroquinolones.

8. Tuberculosis Ciprofloxacin is one of the drugs in multi-drug regimens used for resistant tuberculosis. It is also useful in atypical mycobacterial infections.

9. Bacterial prostatitis and cervicitis FQs are useful.

10. Eye infections - Ciprofloxacin and ofloxacin may be used topically in the treatment of eye infections.

11. Anthrax- also responds to fluoroquinolones.

12. Neutropenic patients - FQs may be used for prophylaxis of infection in neutropenic patients.

Contraindications

1. Fluoroquinolones are contraindicated in pregnancy.

2. To be avoided in boys and girls less than 18 years of age.

3. To be avoided in patients with prolonged QTc interval, in patients receiving other drugs that prolong QTc interval (Eg. mefloquine, erythromycin) and class I and II antiarrhythmics.

4. Concurrent use of theophylline (and other epileptogenic drugs) is contraindicated because theophylline toxicity can be precipitated.

5. Concurrent use of calcium, iron and other preparations containing divalent cations should be avoided.

50 | *Beta-Lactam Antibiotics*

- **Penicillins**
- **Natural pencillins**
- **Semisynthetic penicillins**
    - **- Acid resistant penicillins**
    - **- Penicillinase resistant penicillins**
    - **- Extended spectrum penicillins**
    - **- Antipseudomonal penicillins**
    - **- Beta-Lactamase inhibitors**
- **Cephalosporins**
- **Carbapenems**
- **Monobactams**

The β-lactam antibiotics have a β-lactam ring. Penicillins, cephalosporins, monobactams and carbapenems are β-lactams.

PENICILLINS

Sir Alexander Fleming discovered penicillin in 1928 from *Penicillium notatum*. In 1941 penicillin became available for therapeutic use. Penicillins are one of the most important groups of antibiotics. Penicillin is now obtained from the fungus *Penicillium chrysogenum* for therapeutic use.

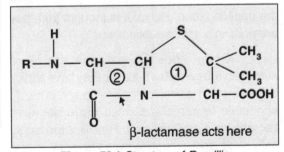

β-lactamase acts here

Figure 50.1 Structure of Pencillin

Mechanism of action

The rigid cell wall of the bacteria protects it from lysis. Peptidoglycan - a complex polymer, is an important component of the cell wall. It consists of glycan chains which are cross-linked by peptide chains. The synthesis of this peptidoglycan requires enzymes called transpeptidases. The last step in the synthesis

357

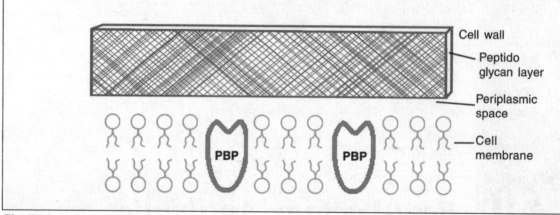

Fig 50.2 In gram positive bacteria; the thick peptidoglycan layer provides mechanical strength to the cell wall. Penicillins inhibit the synthesis of the peptidoglycan layer. PBP - Penicillin Binding Protein.

of peptidoglycan chain is the process of crosslinking with the help of the enzymes transpeptidáses. β-lactam antibiotics inhibit these transpeptidases and thus inhibit the synthesis of peptidoglycan, resulting in the formation of cell wall deficient bacteria. These undergo lysis. Thus penicillins are bactericidal. Pencillin binding proteins (PBPs) are proteins present in the cell membrane which take part in cross - linking of the peptidoglycan. Hence it is thought that they are nothing but transpeptidases.

Gram - positive bacteria are more susceptible to pencillins because they have a thick cell wall which is vital for their living and is easily accesible to penicillins while gram negative bacteria have a thin cell wall. Pencillins are highly safe because the peptidoglycan layer is unique to bacteria and is absent in higher animals.

Classification

A. Natural — *Penicillin G*

B. Semisynthetic

1. **Acid resistant** — *Penicillin V*

2. **Penicillinase resistant** -

   Methicillin, oxacillin

   Cloxacillin, nafcillin

3. **Aminopenicillins** -

   Ampicillin, Bacampicillin
   Amoxicillin

4. **Antipseudomonal penicillins**

   • *Carboxypenicillins* -

   Carbenicillin
   Carbenicillin-indanyl
   Ticarcillin

   • *Ureidopenicillins* -

   Azocillin
   Mezlocillin
   Piperacillin.

NATURAL PENICILLINS

Penicillin G (Benzyl Penicillin)

Antibacterial spectrum

Penicillin G (PnG) has a narrow antibacterial spectrum and is effective against gram-positive cocci and bacilli and a few gram-negative cocci. Thus streptococci, pneumococci, gonococci, meningococci, B. anthracis, C. diphtheriae, clostridia, listeria and spirochetes are highly sensitive. Penicillins are also effective against some anaerobes.

TABLE 50.1 Preparations, dose and route of administration of penicillins

Drug	Dose	Route	Trade name
NATURAL PENICILLINS			
Sodium penicillin G (Crystalline penicillin)	0.5-5 MU q 4-6 hr	IM/IV	CRYSTAPEN
Procaine penicillin G	0.5-1 MU q 12-24 hr	IM	PROCAINE PENICILLIN G
Benzathine penicillin G	1.2-2.4 MU every 3-4 weeks	Deep IM	PENIDURE LA
SEMISYNTHETIC PENICILLINS			
Penicillin v	250-500 mg QID	Oral	CRYSTAPEN-V
Cloxacillin	250-500 mg QID	Oral	KLOX
Dicloxacillin	250-500 mg QID	Oral	BIOCLOX
Nafcillin	1-2 gm q 4-6 hr	IV	UNIPEN
Ampicillin	250 mg to 1 gm QID	Oral IM/IV	AMPILLIN ROSCILLIN
Ampicillin + sulbactum	1 gm Ampi + 0.5 gm sulb q 6-8 hr	IV	SULBACIN
Amoxicillin	250-500 mg TID	Oral	NOVAMOX SYNAMOX
Amoxicillin + clavulanic acid	250 mg Amox + 125 mg Clav TID	Oral	AUGMENTIN
Piperacillin	3-4 gm q 4-6 hr	IV	PIPRAPEN
Piperacillin + tazobactam		IV	ZOSYN
Ticarcillin	3 gm q 4-6 hr	IV	TICAR

q4-6hr — every 4 to 6 hours. MV - Mega units or Million units

Resistance

Many organisms like staphylococci produce a penicillinase which is a beta-lactamase - which opens the β-lactam ring and inactivates penicillins. Altered target proteins on the bacterial cell which reduces affinity for penicillins also lead to resistance.

Pharmacokinetics

PnG is destroyed by gastric juice; food interferes with its absorption - hence it is to be given 2 hr after food. It has a short t½ of 30 min. Though generally it does not readily cross the BBB, in presence of inflammation, therapeutic concentration is attained in the CSF because inflammation weakens the BBB and allows penicillins to reach the brain. Pencillin G is excreted by the kidneys. Probenecid blocks the renal tubular secretion of penicillin and thereby prolongs its duration of action.

Preparations and dose (Table 50.1)

PnG is mainly given parenterally though orally effective form - potassium PnG is also available.

Oral penicillin is used only in minor infections. Since benzyl penicillin is short-acting, repository forms like procaine penicillin and benzathine penicillin, which are longer-acting are made available. Given deep IM they release penicillin slowly from the site. Procaine penicillin is given 12-24 hourly while a single injection of benzathine penicillin is effective for 3-4 weeks. For preparation and dose see Table 50.1.

Penicillins are highly safe because this peptidoglycon layer is unique to bacteria and is absent in higher animals.

Adverse effects

Hypersensitivity PnG is the most common cause of drug allergy. Manifestations range from skin rashes, urticaria, fever, bronchospasm, serum sickness and rarely, exfoliative dermatitis and anaphylaxis. Though all forms of penicillins can cause allergy, anaphylaxis is more common following parenteral than oral preparations. Topical penicillins are highly sensitizing and their use is banned. The highest incidence is with procaine penicillin where allergy is most often due to the procaine component. There is cross-sensitivity among different penicillins.

History of allergy to penicillins should be taken before prescribing; incidence is higher among atopic individuals. A scratch test or intradermal sensitivity test with 2-10 units should be done. Even if this is negative, it does not completely rule out allergy. Penicillin should be given cautiously and a syringe loaded with adrenaline to treat anaphylaxis should be kept ready.

Other adverse effects

Local Pain at the site of injection, thrombophlebitis on IV injection.

CNS Large doses of PnG may produce confusion, muscle twitchings, convulsions and coma.

Suprainfections are rare because of narrow spectrum of activity of penicillins.

Jarisch-Herxheimer reaction When penicillin is injected to a patient with syphilis, there is sudden destruction of spirochetes and release of their lytic products. This triggers a reaction with fever, myalgia, shivering, exacerbation of syphilitic lesions and vascular collapse.

Uses

Penicillin G is the antibiotic of choice for several infections unless the patient is allergic to it.

1. **Pneumococcal infections** For infections like pneumonia, meningitis and osteomyelitis due to penicillin-sensitive pneumococci, PnG is the **drug of choice**.

2. **Streptococcal infections** Pharyngitis, sinusitis, pneumonia, meningitis and endocarditis are all treated with penicillin. Infective endocarditis due to *Strep. viridans* is treated with high dose PnG in combination with an aminoglycoside.

3. **Meningococcal infections** PnG is the drug of choice for all meningococcal infections.

4. **Staphylococcal infections** Since most staphylococci produce penicillinase, a penicillinase resistant penicillin should be used.

5. **Syphilis** is treated with procaine penicillin for 10 days or with benzathine penicillin.

6. **Diphtheria** Antitoxin is the only effective treatment. PnG eliminates carrier state - PP$_6$ given for 10-12 days.

7. **Anaerobic infections** Pulmonary, periodontal and brain abscesses due to anaerobes respond to PnG.

8. **Actinomycosis** PnG is the drug of choice for all forms of actinomycosis. 12 to 20 MU should be given for 6 weeks.

9. **Tetanus and gas gangrene** Antitoxin is the treatment for tetanus - but PnG has adjuvant value.
   Gas gangrene - PnG is the **drug of choice**.

10. **Other infections** PnG is the **agent of choice** for infections like anthrax, trench

mouth, rat bite fever and listeria infections.

11. Prophylactic uses:

- Rheumatic fever Benzathine penicillin 1.2 MU every month prevents colonisation by streptococci and thereby decreases the recurrences of rheumatic fever. It is to be continued for several years.

- Gonorrhoea and syphilis Sexual contacts are effectively protected against these diseases when treated with penicillin within 12 hours of exposure.

- Valvular heart diseases - 25% cases of bacterial endocarditis are seen following dental extractions. Patients with valvular heart diseases undergoing dental extractions, endoscopies and other minor surgical procedures that may cause bacteraemia should be given penicillin prophylaxis.

Disadvantages of natural pencillins

Natural penicillins have the following disadvantages

- Narrow spectrum of activity
- Not effective orally - acid labile
- Susceptible to penicillinase
- Risk of hypersensitivity

Hence semisynthetic pencillins were obtained to overcome these disadvantages

SEMISYNTHETIC PENICILLINS

Acid resistant penicillins

Penicillin V (Phenoxymethyl penicillin) is acid stable and can be given orally. It is used only in mild streptococcal pharyngitis, sinusitis and trench mouth. **Dose** 250-500 mg 6 hourly.

Penicillinase resistant penicillins

Penicillianase resistant penicillins are resistant to hydrolysis by penicillinase produced by bacteria. However, against other microorganisms

they are less effective than PnG. **Methicillin** is destroyed by gastric juice - hence given parenterally. **Cloxacillin** is given orally. **Nafcillin** is highly resistant to penicillinase and also has useful activity against non penicillinase producing organisms. It requires parenteral administration because of its unreliable absorption from the gut.

Uses

Penicillinase resistant penicillins are the drugs of choice for infections with penicillinase producing staphylococci. Methicillin resistant strains have now emerged and are treated with vancomycin.

Extended Spectrum Penicillins

Aminopenicillins

These agents cover a wider antibacterial spectrum including many gram-negative bacilli. They are orally effective but are sensitive to beta lactamases.

Antibacterial spectrum Both gram-positive and gram-negative organisms including streptococci, meningococci, pneumococci, *H. influenzae, E. Coli, Proteus, Salmonella, Shigella* and *Klebsiella* are sensitive. Many strains are now resistant.

Ampicillin

Ampicillin is well-absorbed orally; food interferes with its absorption. It is excreted mainly through kidneys.

Adverse effects Diarrhoea due to irritation of the gut by the unabsorbed drug is the most common adverse effect with ampicillin. Skin rashes are also fairly frequent.

Uses

1. Respiratory tract infections like bronchitis, sinusitis and otitis media respond to ampicillin.
2. Urinary tract infections Though ampicillin was the drug of choice earlier, many

organisms have now become resistant.

3. **Meningitis** Ampicillin is given with a cephalosporin.

4. **Typhoid** Ampicillin is an alternative to ciprofloxacin.

5. **Septicaemia due to gram-negative organisms.** Intravenous ampicillin may be used with an aminoglycoside.

Bacampicillin is an ester of ampicillin. It is a prodrug that is better absorbed (hence diarrhoea is less common) and longer-acting than ampicillin.

Amoxicillin Differs from ampicillin in the following:

1. Amoxicillin is better absorbed orally

2. Food does not interfere with its absorption

3. Diarrhoea is rare (because it is well absorbed).

4. Given thrice daily

Amoxicillin is used in similar infections as ampicillin like respiratory infections, salmonella gastroenteritis and urinary tract infections. Amoxicillin is a component of the various regimens to eradicate H. pylori. Amoxicillin is preferred over ampicillin by many.

Antipseudomonal Penicillins

Carboxypenicillins

Carbenicillin in addition to activity against gram positive and gram negative organisms, carbenicillin is also effective against *Pseudomonas aeruginosa* and *Proteus* infections. Carbenicillin is given parenterally in the dose of 2-5 grams 6 hourly IM or IV while **carbenicillin indanyl** is effective orally. **Ticarcillin**, an analog of carbenicillin has better activity than carbenicillin against *P. aeruginosa*. It is often combined with an aminoglycoside for synergistic activity against pseudomonas. It may be given both IM and IV. Ticarcillin is used in severe urinary tract infections especially due to

P.aeruginosa. All three are susceptible to penicillinase.

Adverse effects Carbenicillin is used as a sodium salt and in higher doses this excess sodium may cause oedema and CCF; may also cause bleeding due to abnormal platelet aggregation.

Ureidopenicillins

Ureidopenicillins have a wider antibacterial spectrum and are effective against a variety of gram negative organisms including *pseudomonas, klebsiella, proteus* and *H.influenzae.* Ureidopenicillins have greater activity against pseudomonas than ticarcillin. Moreover, their sodium content is low. Hence ureidopenicillins have almost replaced carboxypenicillins. It crosses the BBB and is therefore useful in meningitis.

Azlocillin, mezlocillin and **piperacillin** are all administered intravenously. When combined with a beta lactamase inhibitor, piperacillin can be considered to have the broadest antibacterial spectrum among the penicillins. It crosses the BBB and is therefore useful in meningitis. Dose 3-4 grams 4-6 hourly. Piperacillin is indicated in severe infections particularly due to pseudomonas.

BETA-LACTAMASE INHIBITORS

β-lactamases are enzymes produced by bacteria that open up the β- lactam ring and inactivate the β-lactam antibiotics. β-lactamase inhibitors bind to and inactivate β-lactamases thereby preventing the destruction of the β-lactam antibiotics. They broaden the antibacterial spectrum of penicillins to include penicillinase producing *staephylococci, gonococci, E.coli, H.influenzae* and others. The antibacterial spectrum depends on the penicillin used. There are several types of β-lactamases.

Some of them are inhibited by these β-lactamase inhibitors. β lactamase inhibitors are **clavulanic acid, sulbactam** and **tazobactam**. These are themselves β-lactam compounds but have no significant antibacterial activity.

Clavulanic acid is obtained from *Streptomyces clavuligerus*. It binds to the enzyme β-lactamase, inactivates it and itself gets inactivated in this process. Such a compound is called a 'suicide' inhibitor. Clavulanic acid is combined with amoxicillin for both oral and parenteral administration. It extends the antibacterial spectrum of amoxicillin and the combination inhibits organisms like beta lactamase producing *staphylococci, gonococci, E.coli* and *H.influenzae.* The combination is used for cellulitis, diabetic foot, in neutropenic patients and for mixed aerobic-anaerobic and nosocomial infections. Clavulanic acid is also combined with ticarcillin for parenteral use. It is useful in treating mixed infections and nosocomial infections.

Sulbactam is combined with ampicillin. It is given parenterally for mixed pelvic and other infections.

Tazobactam is combined with piperacillin for parenteral administration.

They are available in fixed combinations.

Drugs	Route
Clavulanic acid + amoxicillin	oral, IV
Clavulinic acid + ticarcillin	IV
Sulbactam + ampicillin	IV
Tazobactam + piperacillin	IV

CEPHALOSPORINS

Cephalosporins are semisynthetic antibiotics with a beta-lactam ring related to penicillins. They are derived from cephalosporin-C and have a wider spectrum of activity than penicillins (Table 50.1).

Mechanism of action

Cephalosporins inhibit the bacterial cell wall synthesis similar to penicillins (see page 357).

They are bactericidal.

Resistance

As in the case of penicillins, beta-lactamases and altered target proteins determine resistance to cephalosporins.

Classification

	Parenteral	Oral
First generation	Cephalothin	Cephalexin
	Cefazolin	Cefadroxil
		Cefradine
Second generation	Cefamandole	Cefaclor
	Cefuroxime	Cefuroxime axetil
	Cefotetan	Ceftibuten, Cefdinir
	Cefoxitin	
Third generation	Cefotaxime	Cefixime
	Ceftrioxone	Cefpodoxime proxetil
	Cefoperazone	Ceftibuten
	Ceftizoxime	Cefdinir
	Ceftazidime	
Fourth generation	Cefepime	
	Cefpirome	

Cephalosporins are classified into 4 generations based on their antibacterial spectrum and stability to beta-lactamases as follows:

First Generation Cephalosporins

First generation cephalosporins are very effective against gram-positive organisms. Cephalothin is resistant to penicillinase, hence can be used in staphylococcal infections. Cefazolin has a longer t½ and its tissue penetrability is good - therefore used for surgical prophylaxis. Streptococci, staphylococci, *E.coli* and klebsiella are inhibited. Cephalexin is used orally for minor infections like abscesses or cellulitis.

Second Generation Cephalosporins

Second generation cephalosporins are more active against some gram-negative organisms compared to first generation ones, and are also active against some anaerobes. They are more resistant to beta-lactamases and *H. influenzae, E. coli, Proteus* and *Klebsiella* are inhibited. Cefuroxime is resistant to β-lactamases; attains good CSF concentration and is useful in meningitis. Cefoxitin and cefotetan are effective against *B.fragilis* and are used in mixed infections like in intra-abdominal infections.

Third Generation Cephalosporins

Third generation cephalosporins are highly resistant to β-lactamases; have good activity against gram-negative organisms and anaerobes. Antibacterial spectrum includes *Citrobacter, serratia, enterobacteriaceae, Pseudomonas aeruginosa, N.gonorrhoeae* and beta lactamase producing *H.influenzae*; but these have weak activity against some gram positive cocci though they are highly effective against streptococci. Many cross BBB and are useful in meningitis. Ceftriaxone has a long t½ and can be given once daily. It is excreted mainly through biliary tract and no dosage adjustment is needed in renal insufficiency. Ceftazidime is effective against *P.aeruginosa*.

Fourth Generation Cephalosporins

Fourth generation cephalosporins - cefepime and cefpirome are active against a variety of gram positive and gram negative organisms including streptococci, staphylococci, meningococci, gonococci, some enterococci, enterobacteriaecae, *H.influenzae and Pseudomonas aeruginosa*. They are more resistant to β lactamases. Both cefepime and cefpirome are administered parenterally. Cefepime attains good CSF levels while cefpirome has good tissue penetrability. Both are excreted almost completely through the kidneys.

The fourth generation agents are used in septicaemia, nosocomial and other serious infections of the skin, respiratory and urinary tract and infections in immunocompromised patients.

Adverse reactions

Cephalosporins are generally well-tolerated.

1. **Hypersensitivity reactions** like skin rashes, fever, serum sickness and rarely anaphylaxis are seen. 20% of patients allergic to penicillin show cross-reactivity to cephalosporins. There are no reliable skin tests for testing allergy.

2. **Nephrotoxicity** Mild nephrotoxicity is noted with some cephalosporins. Combination with other nephrotoxic drugs should be avoided.

3. **Diarrhoea** can result from some of the cephalosporins.

4. **Bleeding** is due to hypoprothrombinaemia which is more common in malnourished patients.

5. **Low WBC count** may be seen though rarely.

6. **Pain** at the injection site may occur.

7. **Disulfiram-like reaction** with alcohol is reported with some cephalosporins.

Uses of cephalosporins

1. **Gram-negative infections** Urinary, respiratory and soft tissue infections due to gram-negative organisms respond - a third generation agent is used.

2. **Surgical prophylaxis** Cefazolin is preferred due to its longer $t^1/_2$ and better tissue penetrability.

3. **Gonorrhoea** Ceftriaxone (single dose 250 mg) is the drug of choice.

4. **Meningitis** Due to *H. influenzae. N.meningitidis* and *S.Pneumoniae* - 3rd generation agents are useful- cefotaxime or ceftriaxone may be used. Pseudomonas meningitis → ceftazidime + an aminoglycoside very effective.

Drugs	Doses	Routes
Cephalothin (KAFLIN)	1-2 g q 6 h	IV
Cefazolin (ALCIZON)	0.5-1g q8h	IM/IV
Cephalexin (SPORIDEX)	0.25-1 g qid	Oral
Cefadroxil (DROXYL)	0.5-1 g bid	Oral
Cefamandole (KEFADOL)	0.5-2 g q 4-8 h	IM/IV
Cefuroxime (SUPACEF)	0.75-1.5 g q 8 h	IM/IV
Cefuroxime axetil (CEFTUM)	0.25-0.5 g bid	Oral
Cefachlor (KEFLOR)	0.25-0.5 g q 8 h	Oral
Cefotaxime (OMNATAX)	1-2 g q 8 h	IM/IV
Ceftriaxone (OFRAMAX)	1-2 g q 8h	IM/IV
Cefoperazone (CEFOBID)	1-2 g q 8-12 h	IM/IV
Cefixime (CEFSPAN)	0.2-0.4 g q 12h	Oral
Cefpodoxime proxetil (CEPODEM)	200-400 mg q 12h	Oral
Cefpirome (CEFROM)	1-2 gm q 12 h	IV

5. **Mixed aerobic-anaerobic infections** - common following pelvic surgeries - a 3rd generation agent is used.

6. **Typhoid** As alternative to ciprofloxacin.

7. **Nosocomial infections** can be treated with 3rd generation cephalosporins.

CARBAPENEMS

Carbapenems contain a β-lactam ring fused with a five-membered penem ring. Carbapenems include **imipenem, meropenem** and **ertapenem.**

Antibacterial Spectrum

Carbapenems have a wide antibacterial spectrum and inhibit various gram positive, gram negative organisms and anaerobes including *streptococci, staphylococci, enterococci, listeria, enterobacteriaeceae, pseudomonas* and *B.fragilis.*

Mechanism of action

Carbapenems inhibit bacterial cell wall synthesis similar to penicillins (see page 357).

Imipenem

Imipenem is not absorbed orally and is administered intravenously (250-500 mg every 6-8 hours); it has good tissue penetrability. Imipenem is inactivated quickly by a dehydropeptidase in the renal tubules. Hence it is always combined with **cilastatin**, an inhibitor of dehydropeptidase in order to prolong its plasma half life.

Adverse effects to imipenem include nausea, vomiting, diarrhoea and allergic reactions especially in patients allergic to other β-lactam antibiotics. High doses can occasionally cause seizures.

Uses

Imipenem-cilastatin is used in UTI, respiratory, skin, bone, soft tissue, intra-abdominal and gynaecological infections due to susceptible microorganisms. It is particularly useful in enterobacter, penicillin-resistant pneumococci and other nosocomial infections resistant to other antibiotics. It is used with an aminoglycoside in pseudomonas infections.

Meropenem has the following advantages over imipenem -

- Meropenem is not destroyed by renal dipeptidase and therefore does not require to be combined with cilastatin.

- Risk of seizures is less than with imipenem.

Indications of meropenem are similar to imipenem.

Ertapenem is similar to meropenem except that it is not useful against *P.aeruginosa*.

CARBACEPHEMS

Loracarbef is a carbacephem. It is a synthetic beta-lactam antibiotic with properties similar to second generation cephalosporins - and is therefore included by some under second generation cephalosporins. It is orally effective and is largely excreted by the kidneys.

MONOBACTAMS

Monobactams are monocyclic betalactams i.e they contain a single ring – the beta lactam ring.

Aztreonam is the monobactam available. It is active against gram-negative bacilli including *Pseudomonas aeruginosa* but is not effective against gram-positive organisms and anaerobes. Aztreonam acts by inhibiting cell wall synthesis like penicillins. It is given parenterally (IM / IV 1-2G every 6-8hrs).

Aztreonam can be used in patients allergic to pencillins as there is no cross allergenicity with other β lactams. The only reported adverse effects are occasional skin rashes. Aztreonam is used in pseudomonas infections especially nosocomial and in other gram-negative infections.

- **Tetracyclines**
  - **- Mechanism of action**
  - **- Antibacterial spectrum**
  - **- Pharmacokinetics**
  - **- Adverse effects**
  - **- Uses**
- **Chloramphenicol**
  - **- Mechanism of action**
  - **- Antibacterial spectrum**
  - **- Pharmacokinetics**
  - **- Adverse effects**
  - **- Uses**

TETRACYCLINES

Tetracyclines are antibiotics with four rings (hence the name) obtained from the soil actinomycetes. Chlortetracycline was the first tetracycline to be obtained from *'Streptomyces aureofaciens'* in 1948. Several semisynthetic derivatives were then produced. In addition to gram-positive and gram-negative bacteria, tetracyclines also inhibit the growth of other microorganisms like *Rickettsiae, Chlamydiae, Mycoplasma* and some protozoa. Therefore they are called *broad spectrum antibiotics.*

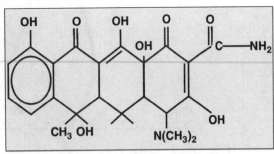

Fig 51.1 Structure of tetracycline

367

Classification

Short acting (t ½ 6 hrs)
Chlortetracycline
Tetracycline
Oxytetracycline

Intermediate acting (t ½ ~ 12 hrs)
Demeclocycline
Methacycline

Long acting (t ½~18 hrs)
Doxycycline
Minocycline

Intermediate and long acting agents are semisynthetic tetracyclines.

Mechanism of action

Tetracyclines are taken up by susceptible microorganisms by active transport. Since mammalian cells lack this active transport process, tetracyclines are selectively toxic to micro-organisms. The bacterial ribosome (Fig 51.2) consists of 50S and 30S subunits and tetracylines bind to 30S subunit. The tRNA carries amino acids to the ribosome for protein synthesis. The 50S ribosome has three binding sites viz. A, P and E sites. Tetracyclines bind to 'A' site and prevent the binding of tRNA to this site. Thus they prevent protein synthesis and are **bacteriostatic**.

Antibacterial spectrum

Antibacterial spectrum of tetracycline is broad including gram-positive and gram-negative organisms like *Streptococci, Staphylococci, Gonococci, Meningococci, H. influenza, Brucella, V. cholerae, Campylobacter, Y.pestis* and many anaerobes. They also inhibit rickettsiae, chlamydiae, *Mycoplasma, Actinomyces, E. histolytica* and Plasmodia. Many organisms have now become resistant.

Pharmacokinetics

Older tetracyclines are incompletely absorbed from the gut; bioavailability of chlortetracycline is 30% and that of tetracycline, oxytetracycline, demeclocycline and methacycline range between 60% - 70%. Food interferes with their absorption. Doxycycline - 95% and minocycline is 100% absorbed and food does not affect the absorption

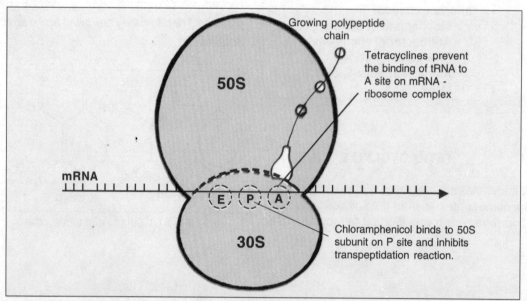

Fig. 51.2 Mechanism of action of tetracyclines and chloramphenicol

of these two agents. Tetracyclines chelate calcium and other metals which reduce their absorption. Hence tetracyclines should not be given with milk, iron preparations and antacids. Tetracyclines undergo enterohepatic circulation. Tetracyclines like oxytetracycline and doxycycline can be given intravenously but they cause irritation and thrombophlebitis. Intramuscular injections are painful due to local irritation and should therefore be avoided.

Tetracyclines except doxycycline and minocycline are excreted through kidneys. Doxycycline and minocycline are excreted through the gut and are therefore safe in renal insufficiency. Dose - Table 51.1.

Adverse effects

1. *GIT* Gastrointestinal irritation, nausea, vomiting and diarrhoea can occur - tetracyclines are to be given with food to minimize these effects.

2. *Hepatotoxicity* may result in jaundice. Acute hepatic necrosis may occur in pregnant women but is rare.

3. *Renal toxicity* Renal failure may be aggravated. Outdated tetracyclines cause a syndrome like Fanconi's syndrome with vomiting, polyuria, proteinuria, glycosuria and acidosis due to metabolites of the outdated tetracyclines.

4. *Phototoxicity* Skin reactions and dermatitis on exposure to sun are more likely with doxycycline and demeclocycline.

5. *Effect on teeth and bones* Tetracyclines chelate calcium. The calcium tetracycline orthophosphate complexes get deposited in the developing teeth and bones. The deformities depend on the time of tetracycline administration.

Period	Structure affected	Deformity
• Mid pregnancy to 5 months of postnatal life	Deciduous teeth	Brownish discolouration, ill formed and are more susceptible to caries
• 2 months to 5 years of age	Permanent teeth	Pigmentation, discolouration
• Pregnancy and childhood up to 8 yrs of age	Skeleton	Depressed bone growth

Tetracyclines are thus teratogenic.

6. *Suprainfections* Since the intestinal flora are extensively suppressed by tetracyclines, these are the most common antibiotics to cause suprainfections.

7. *Hypersensitivity reactions* are not very common.

8. *Local* IV injections can cause thrombophlebitis.

9. *Pseudotumor cerebrii* Tetracyclines may increase intracranial pressure specially in infants. This results in bulging of anterior fontanelle in infants giving a false

Table 51.1: Dosage of some tetracyclines	
Tetracyclines	*Doses*
Chlortetracycline (AUREOMYCIN)	250-500 mg QID
Tetracycline (HOSTACYCLINE)	250-500 mg QID
Doxycycline (DOXYCAPS)	200 mg initially then 100 mg OD
Minocycline (CYANOMYCIN)	200 mg initially then 100 mg OD

impression of tumor. This is described as pseudotumor cerebrii. In adults it can result in headache.

10. *Antianabolic effect* When large doses are given for long periods, tetracyclines can increase the urinary excretion of nitrogen by an antianabolic effect.

Uses

A. Tetracyclines are the drugs of choice in

1. Rickettsial infections All rickettsial infections respond to tetracyclines- fever subsides and clinical improvement is seen in 48 hours. Dose: 2grams 6 hourly initially and then reduced to 1gram 6 hourly.

2. Chlamydial infections:
   - Lymphogranuloma venereum - tetracyclines are given for 2 weeks
   - Trachoma - both topical and oral tetracyclines are needed - treatment should be continued upto 40 days
   - Inclusion conjunctivitis.
   - Chlamydia pneumoniae

3. Atypical pneumonia due to *Mycoplasma pneumoniae.*

4. Cholera Tetracyclines reduce the duration of illness and are of adjuvant value.

5. Brucellosis Doxycycline 200 mg + Rifampicin 600 mg daily for 6 weeks is the treatment of choice.

6. Plague Tetracyclines may be combined with an aminoglycoside.

B. Tetracyclines are useful in other infections like -

1. Traveller's diarrhoea - Doxycycline reduces the incidence of traveller's diarrhoea.

2. Sexually transmitted diseases - like syphilis, gonorrhea and chancroid also respond to tetracyclines - but are not preferred.

3. Acne - The propionibacteria in the sebaceous follicles metabolize lipids into irritating free fatty acids which trigger the development of acne. Tetracyclines inhibit these bacteria. Low doses are given for a long time (250 mg BD for 4 weeks).

4. Tularaemia - A combination of tetracycline with an aminoglycoside can be used in tularaemia.

5. Other infections - Tetracyclines are also useful in the treatment of Lyme disease, relapsing fever, leptospirosis and post exposure prophylaxis of anthrax.

6. Protozoal infections
   - Amoebiasis - Tetracyclines are useful in chronic intestinal amoebiasis (See page 424)
   - Malaria - Doxycycline is given with quinine in multi-drug resistant malaria.

C. Inappropriate secretion of ADH

Demeclocycline is used because it inhibits the action of ADH in the kidney.

Contraindications

1. Tetracyclines are contraindicated in pregnancy, lactation and in children up to 8 years of age for the following reasons:
   - Their effects on teeth and bones.
   - Risk of acute hepatic necrosis in pregnent women.
   - Risk of pseudotumor cerebrii in infants.

2. Should be used cautiously in renal and hepatic impairment.

Doxycycline and minocycline are semisynthetic tetracyclines.

- Given orally they are 95% and 100% absorbed respectively
- Food does not interfere with their absorption

- Both are highly lipid soluble
- Have long t½ - can be given once daily
- Excreted through gut - hence can be given in usual dose even in the presence of renal impairment
- Both can be given orally and parenterally (IV) though doxycycline is preferred for parentral use.
- Microsomal enzyme inducers can hasten the metabolism of doxycycline resulting in shorter t1/2 of doxycycline.
- Minocycline causes vestibular toxicity characterised by vertigo, dizziness, ataxia, nausea and vomiting.
- Minocycline can be used as an alternative to rifampicin to eradicate meningococcal carrier state.
- Doxycycline is preffered for post exposure prophylaxis of anthrax.

CHLORAMPHENICOL

Chloramphenicol is a broad spectrum antibiotic first obtained from *Streptomyces venezuelae* in 1947.

Mechanism of action

Chloramphenicol is bacteriostatic but to some organisms it is bactericidal. It binds to 50S ribosomal subunit and inhibits protein synthesis - by inhibiting transpeptidation reaction (Fig. 51.2).

Antibacterial spectrum

Antibacterial spectrum is broad and includes gram-negative organisms, some gram-positive organisms, anaerobic bacteria, *rickettsiae, chlamydiae* and *Mycoplasma*. Thus *H. influenzae, Salmonella, Shigella, Bordatella, Brucella, gonococci, meningococci, streptococci, staphylococci, Clostridium, E.coli* and *Klebsiella* - are inhibited apart from *Rickettsiae, Chlamydiae* and *Mycoplasma*.

Resistance is plasmid mediated and may be due to:

1. Inactivating enzymes
2. ↓permeability of the microorganisms to the antibiotic.
3. Ribosomal insensitivity.

Pharmacokinetics

Chloramphenicol is rapidly absorbed from the gut; penetration into tissues is excellent; attains high concentration in CSF. It is metabolised in the liver by reduction and glucuronide conjugation. The metabolites are excreted in the urine.

Adverse reactions

1. Gastrointestinal disturbances Nausea, vomiting and diarrhoea.
2. Bone marrow depression Chloramphenicol may cause bone marrow depression in two ways:
   - dose dependent anaemia, leukopenia and thrombocytopenia due to inhibition of protein synthesis. It is reversible.
   - idiosyncratic response - resulting in aplastic anaemia which may be fatal. It may be due to a toxic metabolite. Incidence is 1 in 30,000 patients and occurs in genetically predisposed individuals. This toxicity has limited the use of chloramphenicol.
3. Gray baby syndrome Newborn babies given high doses of chloramphenicol may show *'gray baby syndrome'* manifested as vomiting, refusal of feeds, hypotonia, hypothermia, abdominal distension, metabolic acidosis and ashen gray cyanosis. It may be fatal. As the newborn cannot metabolize (due to inadequate hepatic glucuronidation) and excrete chloramphenicol adequately, toxicity results.
4. Hypersensitivity reactions like rashes and fever are uncommon.
5. Superinfection can occur.

Drug interactions

Chloramphenicol inhibits hepatic microsomal enzymes and thereby prolongs the half-life of drugs metabolised by this system. This may result in enhanced toxicity of some drugs like phenytoin, tolbutamide and dicumarol.

Uses

Because of the risk of bone marrow toxicity and availability of safer drugs, chloramphenicol is not generally preferred. The indications are:

1. Typhoid fever Very effective in typhoid; given for 14 days (500 mg QID till fever subsides then 250 mg QID up to 14th day).

2. Bacterial meningitis In meningococcal and *H. influenzae* meningitis - chloramphenicol is an alternative to penicillin.

3. Anaerobic infections Chloramphenicol + penicillin + an aminoglycoside can be used in severe anaerobic infections as an alternative to metronidazole and clindamycin.

4. Rickettsial infections As an alternative when tetracyclines are contraindicated.

5. Eye infections Chloramphenicol is used topically because of the good penetration into aqueous humour.

52 *Aminoglycosides*

- **Common properties of aminoglycosides**
- **Antibacterial spectrum**
- **Mechanism of action**
- **Pharmacokinetics**
- **Adverse effects**
- **Precautions in using aminoglycosides**

Aminoglycosides are antibiotics with amino sugars in glycosidic linkages. They are derived from the soil actinomycetes of the genus streptomyces (streptomycin, kanamycin, tobramycin, neomycin) and the genus micromonospora (gentamicin and netilmicin) hence the difference in spelling. Amikacin and netilmicin are semisynthetic products.

Common Properties of Aminoglycosides

1. Aminoglycosides are polycationic carbohydrates containing aminosugars in glycosidic linkages.

2. They are highly water soluble.

3. Aminoglycosides are not absorbed orally (as they ionize in solution) therefore they are given parenterally.

4. They remain extracellularly and penetration into CSF is very poor.

5. They are excreted unchanged by the kidneys.

6. They are all bactericidal.

7. They act by inhibiting bacterial protein synthesis.

8. They are mainly effective against gram-negative organisms.

9. They produce variable degrees of ototoxicity and nephrotoxicity as adverse effects.

Antibacterial spectrum

Aminoglycosides have a narrow spectrum and are effective mainly against aerobic gram-negative

373

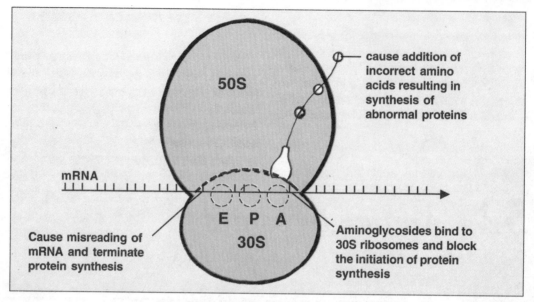

cause addition of incorrect amino acids resulting in synthesis of abnormal proteins

mRNA

50S

E P A
30S

Cause misreading of mRNA and terminate protein synthesis

Aminoglycosides bind to 30S ribosomes and block the initiation of protein synthesis

Fig. 52.1 Mechanism of action of aminoglycosides

bacilli like *E. coli, Proteus, Pseudomonas, Brucella, Salmonella, Shigella* and *Klebsiella*.

Mechanism of action

Aminoglycosides, being water-soluble, penetrate the bacterial cell membrane through aqueous pores. It is observed that aminoglycosides disrupt the bacterial cell membrane and this also allows penetration of the drug into the bacterium from the periplasmic space. They are taken up by an active transport process. Inside the cell, (Fig 52.1) aminoglycosides bind to 30S ribosomes and inhibit bacterial protein synthesis - block initiation of protein synthesis, cause termination of protein synthesis and cause addition of

incorrect amino acids resulting in the synthesis of abnormal proteins. Aminoglycosides are **bactericidal.** Higher the concentration, greater is the bactericidal effect (dose dependent killing). A residual bactericidal effect - **postantibiotic effect** - remains even after the plasma levels of aminoglycosides fall. Hence, even though they have a short t½, they can be given once a day (Table 52.1).

Low pH and anaerobic environment inhibit the uptake of aminoglycosides by active transport. Drugs acting on the cell wall like penicillins counter this negative effect of low pH and anaerobiasis - this is one of the reasons for synergism of the combination.

TABLE 52.1: Doses and routes of administration of aminoglycosides

Aminoglycosides	Doses	Routes
Streptomycin (STREPTONEX)	1-2 g/day	IM
Gentamicin (GARAMYCIN)	3-5 mg/kg/day in 3 divided doses	IM/IV
Tobramycin (TOBRANEG)	3-5 mg/kg/day in 3 divided doses	IM/IV
Amikacin (AMICIN)	15 mg/kg/day in 2-3 divided doses	IM/IV
Netilmicin (NETROMYCIN)	4-6 mg/kg/day in 2-3 divided doses	IM/IV

Resistance to aminoglycosides is acquired by

1. Aminoglycoside inactivating enzymes.

2. Low affinity of ribosomes - acquired by mutation.

3. Decrease in permeability to the antibiotic.

There is partial cross-resistance among various aminoglycosides.

Pharmacokinetics

Aminoglycosides are not absorbed from the gut but when instilled into body cavities or applied over large wounds, they may get rapidly absorbed. Following IM injection peak levels are seen in 60 minutes. They are not bound to plasma proteins and do not enter cells or cross barriers - mostly remain in the vasculature. In patients with severe infection, plasma concentration of aminoglycosides should be determined to guide the treatment. Aminoglycosides are excreted almost completely through the kidneys. Dose should be reduced in renal impairment.

Adverse effects

1. Ototoxicity is the most important toxicity. Both vestibular and auditory dysfunction can occur depending on the dose and duration. The aminoglycosides get concentrated in the labyrinthine fluid of the inner ear and damage both cochlear hair cells and vestibular sensory cells. As the cochlear cells cannot regenerate, there is progressive, **permanent deafness.** The auditory nerve degenerates. Tinnitus appears first, followed by deafness; elderly people are more susceptible. Stopping the drug can prevent further damage. Vestibular dysfunction is manifested by headache, nausea, vomiting, dizziness, vertigo, nystagmus and ataxia. Most symptoms subside in two weeks except ataxia which may persist for 1-2 years. Neomycin, amikacin and kanamycin are the aminoglycosides which are most likely to cause deafness, while streptomycin and gentamicin are most likely to cause vestibular toxicity.

2. Nephrotoxicity Aminoglycosides attain high concentration in the renal cortex and cause damage to the renal tubules. This results in loss of urine concentrating capacity, low GFR and albuminuria. These effects are reversible. Most symptoms subside in 2 weeks except ataxia which may persist for 1-2 years. Gentamicin, neomycin and tobramycin are the most nephrotoxic.

3. Neuromuscular blockade Aminoglycosides have curare-like effects and block neuromuscular transmission.

Precautions in using aminoglycosides

1. Avoid concurrent use of other ototoxic drugs like loop diuretics.

2. Avoid concurrent use of other nephrotoxic drugs like amphotericin B, cephalothin and cisplatin.

3. Avoid concurrent use of curarimimetic drugs.

4. To be used cautiously in elderly, in renal damage and in combination with skeletal muscle relaxants.

5. Contraindicated in pregnancy because of risk of deafness in the child.

6. Do not mix aminoglycosides with any other drug in the same syringe.

7. Determination of plasma levels of aminoglycosides may be needed in severe infections and in patients with renal dysfunction.

Uses

Aminoglycosides are used in the treatment of infections due to gram-negative bacteria.

Aminoglycosides are also used in streptococcal and enterococcal endocarditis in combination with a penicillin. The combination is synergistic due to the following reasons:

- Both are bactericidal
- Low pH and anaerobiasis reduce the uptake of aminoglycosides by active transport . This negative effect is reversed by penicillins. Some aminoglycosides - (streptomycin, kanamycin, amikacin) are also used in tuberculosis. Indications are discussed under individual aminoglycoside agents.

Streptomycin

Streptomycin obtained from *Streptomyces griseus* is mainly effective against aerobic gram-negative bacilli. When used alone, bacteria, especially the tubercle bacillus rapidly develops resistance to it. Streptomycin is the least nephrotoxic among aminoglycosides.

Uses

1. Tuberculosis

2. Subacute bacterial endocarditis (SBE) - Combination of streptomycin and penicillin is synergistic in this condition.

3. Plague, tularaemia and brucellosis - streptomycin is given with a tetracycline.

Gentamicin

Gentamicin obtained from *Micromonospora purpurea* is more potent and has a broader spectrum of action compared to streptomycin. Development of resistance has limited its use.

Uses

1. UTI   Gentamicin is effective in uncomplicated UTI as it is released for a long time from the renal cortex.

2. Pneumonia   due to gram-negative organisms may be treated with gentamicin + penicillin.

Keybox 52.1	
Antibiotics that inhibit protein synthesis by binding to ribosomes	
50S	**30S**
Erythromycin	Tetracyclines
Chloromphenicol	Aminoglycosides
Clindamycin	
Streptogramins	
Linezolid	

3. Osteomyelitis, peritonitis, septicaemia caused by gram-negative organisms can be treated with gentamicin.

4. Meningitis due to gram-negative bacilli . gentamicin is used with a third generation cephalosporin.

5. SBE Gentamicin may be used in place of streptomycin in SBE.

6. Topical Gentamicin cream is used topically in burns and other infected wounds.

Gentamicin eye drops are used in the prevention and treatment of bacterial conjunctivitis.

Tobramycin

Tobramycin has better activity against Pseudomonas and is used with an antipseudomonal penicillin in such infections.

Kanamycin

Due to its toxicity, its use is limited to multi-drug resistant tuberculosis.

Amikacin

Amikacin has widest antibacterial spectrum among the aminoglycosides. It is resistant to aminoglycoside inactivating enzymes.

Uses

1. Nosocomial infections due to gram-negative organisms

2. Tuberculosis - Amikacin is useful in multidrug

resistant tuberculosis in combination with other drugs. It is also used in infections due to atypical mycobacteria in patients with AIDS.

Netilmicin Like amikacin, netilmicin is resistant to aminoglycoside inactivating enzymes. It is used in serious infections due to gram-negative bacilli.

Sisomicin has actions, toxicity and uses similar to gentamicin.

Neomycin has a wide antibacterial spectrum. As it is highly ototoxic, it is not given systemically. It is used topically as ointments, creams and powder.

Adverse effects

Neomycin can cause skin rashes on topical use. Oral use can cause diarrhoea, steatorrhoea and malabsorption due to damage to the intestinal villi.

Superinfection with Candida can also occur.

Uses

1. Neomycin is used topically in skin infections, burns, ulcers and wounds; eye and ear infections.

2. Orally - neomycin is not absorbed when given orally. It is used to prepare the bowel for surgery, i.e. for preoperative gut sterilization.

3. Hepatic coma - ammonia produced by colonic bacteria is absorbed and converted to urea by the liver. In severe hepatic failure, as liver is unable to handle this NH_3, blood NH_3 levels rise resulting in encephalopathy. As neomycin inhibits intestinal flora, NH_3 production falls. Neomycin is given orally for this purpose.

53

Macrolides, Other Antibacterial Agents & Chemotherapy of Urinary Tract Infection

CHAPTER

- **Erythromycin**
- **Roxithromycin**
- **Clarithromycin**
- **Azithromycin**
- **Ketolides**
- **Miscellaneous antibiotics**
  - **Spectinomycin**
  - **Lincosamides**
  - **Glycopeptides**
  - **Polypeptide antibiotics**
  - **Other antimicrobial agents**
- **Newer agents**
  - **Streptogramins**
  - **Oxazolidinones**

Macrolides are antibiotics with a large (macrocyclic) lactone ring to which sugars are attached. Erythromycin and its semisynthetic derivatives roxithromycin, clarithromycin and azithromycin are macrolides (Table 53.1).

ERYTHROMYCIN

Erythromycin is obtained from *Streptomyces erythreus.*

Antibacterial spectrum

Erythromycin has a narrow spectrum and is effective against aerobic gram-positive bacteria and a few gram-negative organisms.

Streptococci, pneumococci, staphylococci, gonococci, legionella, *C. diphtheriae, C. jejuni, Mycoplasma, Chlamydiae* and some atypical mycobacteria are sensitive.

Mechanism of action

Erythromycin is bacteriostatic at low and cidal at high concentrations. It is more effective in the alkaline pH. It binds to 50 S ribosomes (Fig 53.1) and inhibits bacterial protein synthesis. Macrolides inhibit the translocation of the growing

378

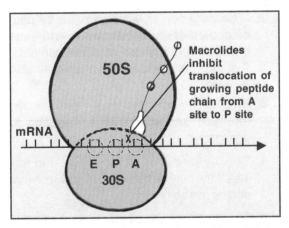

Fig 53.1 Mechanism of action of Macrolide antibiotics

peptide chain from A site to P site. Hence A site is not available for binding of next aminoacid (brought by tRNA). Hence protien synthesis stops. Chloramphenicol and clindamycin also bind to 50 S ribosomes and the three may antagonise each others activity because they compete for the binding site. Hence the combination should be avoided (Fig 53.1).

Resistance

Resistance to macrolides is acquired through plasmids. The mechanism involved may be:

- Low permeability of the bacteria to the antibiotic
- Production of inactivating enzymes
- Low affinity of ribosomes to macrolides.

Pharmacokinetics

Erythromycin is destroyed by gastric acid and is therefore given as enteric coated tablets. Good concentration is attained in most fluids except brain and CSF. It is mainly excreted through bile; dose adjustment is not needed in renal failure. Dose and duration - Table 53.1.

Adverse effects

1. Hepatitis with cholestatic jaundice starts after 2-3 weeks of treatment and clinical incident is more common with the estolate salt. The symptoms - nausea, vomiting and abdominal cramps, mimic acute cholecystitis and may be wrongly treated. These are followed by jaundice and fever. It may be an allergic response to the estolate salt. Hepatitis is self- limiting but erythromycin should be avoided in such patients as they are likely as to get hepatitis again.

2. Epigastric distress, nausea, vomiting and diarrhoea are often reported. Erythromycin is a motilin receptor agonist due to which it causes increased intestinal motility.

3. Allergic reactions including fever and skin rashes can occur.

4. Cardiac arrhythmias are reported in patients with cardiac diseases or on other arrhythmogenic drugs.

Erythro - My - Sin

Mr. Raju a 42 year old man reported to a hospital with nausea, vomiting and abdominal cramps. After examination and investigations, a diagnosis of acute cholecystitis was made and the patient was taken for chloecystectomy. On opening the abdomen it was found that the gall bladder was normal. The patient developed jaundice (cholestatic) after 2 days. When history was re-elicited, the patient revealed that 2 weeks back he was treated with a long course of erythromycin estolate for respiratory infection. His present symptoms were a result of an adverse effect of erythromycin. The right treatment was just to do nothing - it is self limiting. Here the patient was subjected to unnecessary trauma of surgery because a proper history was not elicited.

5. Erythromycin can also cause reversible hearing impairment in some patients.

Drug Interactions

Erythromycin and clarithromycin inhibit the hepatic metabolism and thereby rise the plasma levels of carbamazepine, terfenadine, theophylline, valproate, digoxin and warfarin resulting in toxicity due to these drugs.

Uses

Erythromycin can be used as an alternative to penicillin in patients allergic to penicillin.

1. Atypical pneumonia may be caused by agents like mycoplasma, chlamydia and legionella. Atypical pneumonia due to *Mycoplasma pneumoniae* - erythromycin is the **drug of choice**- 500 mg 6 hrly oral or IV.

2. Legionnaires' pneumonia - is treated for 10-14 days with erythromycin IV erythromycin is preferred. Azithromycin is now considered the drug of choice.

3. Whooping cough - erythromycin is the drug of choice for the treatment and post exposure prophylaxis of close contacts. Clarithromycin and azithromycin may also be used.

4. Streptococcal infections - pharyngitis, tonsillitis and scarlet fever respond to erythromycin.

5. Staphylococcal infections - minor infections may be treated. But now resistant strains are common.

6. Diphtheria - erythromycin is very effective in acute stage though antitoxin is life saving. Erythromycin also eradicates carrier state.

7. Syphilis and gonorrhoea - erythromycin is used as an alternative to penicillins.

8. Campylobacter gastroenteritis - as an alternative to fluoroquinolones.

9. Tetanus - erythromycin eradicates carrier state.

10. Anthrax - erythromycin is an alternative to penicillin.

TABLE 53.1: Adult dose and duration of treatment with macrolide antibiotics	
Drug	**Dose (oral) and duration**
Erythromycin stearate (ERYTHROCIN)	250-500 mg QID 7-14 days
Erythromycin estolate (ALTHROCIN)	250-500 mg QID 7-14 days
Erythromycin base (ERYSAFE)	250-1000 mg 6 hrly for 7-14 days
Erythromycin - ointment (2-4%)	To be applied twice daily.
Roxithromycin (ROXID)	150 mg BD for 7-10 days (to be taken 30 minutes before food)
Clarithromycin (CLARIBID)	250-500 mg BD 7-14 days
Azithromycin (AZITHRAL)	Ist day 500 mg OD 250 mg OD for next 3-4 days (to be taken 1 hr before or 2 hrs after food)

11. Topical - erythromycin ointment (2-4%) is used for skin infections and boils, lotion for acne vulgaris.

Roxithromycin

Roxithromycin is longer-acting, acid stable, more potent, better absorbed and has better tissue penetrability compared to erythromycin. It does not inhibit the metabolism of other drugs - hence no risk of related drug interactions. Roxithromycin should be taken 30 min before food.

It can be used as an alternative to erythromycin but is more expensive.

Clarithromycin

Compared to erythromycin, clarithromycin is longer-acting, acid stable and better absorbed; it is more effective against *H.influenzae, legionella, atypical mycobacteria, H. pylori* and some protozoa. Clarithromycin is structurally similar to erythromycin and therefore its drug interactions are also similar to erythromycin.

Clarithromycin is used

1. As a component of triple regimen for *H. pylori* infections in peptic ulcer patients.
2. Atypical mycobacterial infections for the prevention and treatment in AIDS patients.

Though clarithromycin is effective in other indications of erythromycin, its higher cost makes it less preferable.

Azithromycin

Azithromycin an azalide, is a derivative of erythromycin with activity similar to clarithromycin. Antibacterial spectrum is similar to erythromycin except that it is also effective against Mycobacterium avium complex (MAC). It has excellent activity against *H.influenzae*. It is acid stable, rapidly absorbed, has better tissue penetrability, is longer acting and better tolerated than erythromycin. It is given as a single loading dose of 500 mg followed by 250 mg for the next 4 days. Azithromycin is free of drug interactions as it does not suppress hepatic metabolism of other drugs.

It is used in the prophylaxis and treatment of atypical mycobacterial infections in AIDs patients. Like erythromycin it can also be used in respiratory, genital and skin infections and in pneumonias.

KETOLIDES

Ketolides are modified macrolides that are similar to newer macrolides except that they are effective against macrolide - resistant pneumococci. **Telithromycin** is a ketolide.

MISCELLANEOUS ANTIBIOTICS

Spectinomycin is related to aminoglycosides and is effective against gram-negative bacteria. It is used only in gonorrhoea (2 g IM) in patients allergic to penicillin and quinolones.

LINCOSAMIDES

Lincomycin and clindamycin are lincosamides.Lincomycin is no longer used clinically.

Clindamycin

Clindamycin is a congener of lincomycin. It binds to 50S ribosomal subunit and suppresses protein synthesis. Streptococci, staphylococci, pneumococci and many anaerobes are inhibited by clindamycin. Clindamycin is well-absorbed on oral administration. It attains good concentration in the bone and many other tissues. It is metabolised in the liver.

Adverse effects include diarrhoea due to pseudomembranous colitis, skin rashes and neuromuscular blockade. Intravenous use can cause thrombophlebitis.

Uses Anaerobic infections - abdominal, pelvic, bone and joints infections due to anaerobes are treated with clindamycin. It may be combined with an aminoglycoside or a cephalosporin.

Clindamycin is also useful in *Pneumocystis carinii* pneumonia and toxoplasmosis in AIDS patients.

GLYCOPEPTIDES

Vancomycin and teicoplanin are glycopeptides.

Vancomycin produced by Streptococcus orientalis is active against gram-positive bacteria particularly staphylococci including those resistant to methicillin. It acts by inhibiting cell wall synthesis and is bactericidal. Vancomycin is not absorbed orally - given IV. It is widely distributed and excreted through kidneys.

Adverse effects are skin rashes, pain at the site of injection, thrombophlebitis, ototoxicity and nephrotoxicity. Concurrent use of other ototoxic and nephrotoxic drugs should be avoided; dose should be adjusted in renal dysfunction.

Uses

1. Pseudomembranous colitis - oral vancomycin is used.
2. Methicillin resistant staphylococci - vancomycin is given IV for serious infections like osteomyelitis, endocarditis and soft-tissue abscesses.
3. Enterococcal endocarditis - as an alternative to penicillin.
4. Penicillin resistant pneumococcal infections - vancomycin is recommended with a cephalosporin.

Teicoplanin has mechanism of action and antibacterial spectrum similar to vancomycin, but teicoplanin can be safely given intramuscularly. It is also less toxic. Occasionally causes allergic reactions. It is used in osteomyelitis and endocarditis due to methicillin resistant staphylococci and enterococci. TARGOCID 200-400 mg/day.

POLYPEPTIDE ANTIBIOTICS

Polymyxin and Colistin are too toxic to be given systemically. They are used topically. Polymyxin obtained from Bacillus polymyxa and colistin from Bacillus colistinus are effective against gram-negative bacteria.

Mechanism of action

Polymyxin and colistin alter the permeability of the cell membrane resulting in leakage of the cell contents. They are bactericidal.

Polypeptide antibiotics are not absorbed orally; applied topically, they may rarely cause skin rashes.

Uses

1. Used topically for skin infections, ear and eye infections.
2. Oral colistin is used in children for diarrhoea due to gram-negative bacilli.

OTHER ANTIMICROBIAL AGENTS

Bacitracin produced by Bacillus subtilis is effective against gram-positive bacteria. It inhibits the cell wall synthesis and is bactericidal. It is too toxic to be given systemically, not absorbed orally and is therefore used only for topical application - in skin infections, surgical wounds, ulcers and ocular infections (NEOSPORIN powder is bacitracin + neomycin).

Sodium Fusidate (Fusidic acid) obtained from Fusidium coccineum is effective against gram-positive organisms particularly staphylococci. It is bactericidal. It is mainly used topically as a 2% ointment (FUCIDIN). It may be given orally for resistant staphylococcal infections.

Mupirocin or pseudomonic acid is obtained from Pseudomonas fluorescens. It is bactericidal against gram-positive and some gram-negative organisms including MRSA. Mupirocin acts by inhibiting the enzyme tRNA synthetase. It is used as a 2% ointment (BACTROBAN) for minor skin infections particularly due to staphylococci and streptococci. It is also used intranasally as spray to eradicate staphylococcal carrier state.

Fosfomycin is an analog of phosphoenol pyruvate.Fosfomycin is effective against both gram positive and gram negative organisms. It acts by inhibiting the enzyme endopyruvate transferase. This enzyme is required for the first step in bacterial cell wall synthesis. Thus it inhibits bacterial cell wall synthesis. The salt used is fosfomycin tetrametol which is available for both oral and parenteral use. It is excreted by the kidneys and attains high concentration in the urine. Fosfomycin is approved for use in uncomplicated lower UTI in women - single ·3g dose is effective.

Cycloserine obtained from *Streptomyces orchidaceus* inhibits many gram positive and gram negative organisms including *M. tuberculosis*. It acts by inhibiting cell wall synthesis and is used as a second line drug in tuberculosis (See page 391).

Newer Agents

Streptogramins quinupristin and dalfopristin are obtained from *Streptomyces pristinaspiralis*. A combination of **quinupristin** and **dalfopristin** in the ratio 30:70 is bactericidal against gram-positive cocci including methicillin-resistant staphylococci.

Mechanism of action Streptogramins bind to 50S ribosomal subunit and inhibit protein synthesis.

Given intravenously, streptogramins are

Drugs used in MRSA*
• Vancomycin
• Teicoplanin
• Quinupristin-dalfopristin
• Linezolid
• Rifampicin

* Methicillin - Resistant *Staphylococcus aureus*

Pseudomonas aeruginosa
• Antipseudomonal penicilin + tobramycin
• Ceftazidime or cefepime
• Antipseudomonal pencillin + ciprofloxacin
• Imipenem/meropenem + tobramycin
• Aztreonam + tobramycin

Anaerobic infections
• Metronidazole
• Clindamycin
• Chloramphenicol
• Cefotaxime, ceftizoxime, cefotetan
• Imipenem
• Ampicillin + Sulbactam
• Piperacillin + Tazobactam

Atypical mycobacteria
• Clarithromycin + ethambutol
• Rifabutin + ethambutol + ciprofloxacin
• Amikacin

Toxoplasma gondii
• Pyrimethamine + Sulfadiazine + folinic acid
• Spiramycin
• Pyrimethamine + clindamycin

rapidly metabolised and excreted largely through faeces. Hence adjustment of dose is not required in renal insufficiency. Adverse effects include arthralgia, myalgia, nausea, vomiting, diarrhoea and pain at the site of injection. The combination is used intravenously in the treatment of infections due to streptococci, methicillin-resistant staphylococci and enterococci. Streptogramins are not effective orally as they are rapidly metabolised in the liver - undergo extensive first pass metabolism.

Oxazolidinones

Linezolid is an oxazolidinone effective against gram-positive bacteria including methicillin resistant staphylococci and gram positive anaerobic organisms. It acts by inhibiting protein synthesis on binding to 50S ribosomes. Adverse effects include nausea, diarrhoea, dizziness and thrombocytopenia. It can be given oral or IV. Linezolid is useful in the treatment of nosocomial infections resistant to other drugs.

CHEMOTHERAPY OF URINARY TRACT INFECTION

Infection of the urinary tract is quite common and may be acute or chronic. **Urinary antiseptics** are

ANTIMICROBIAL AGENTS			
β lactam antibiotics	**Quinolones**	**Sulphanomides**	**Macrolides**
• *Penicillins*			
Benzyl penicillin	Nalidixic acid	Sulfisoxazole	Erythromycin
Ampicillin	Cinoxacin	Sulfadiazine	Roxithromycin
Amoxicillin	Oxalinic acid	Sulfadoxine	Azithromycin
Methicillin	*Fluoroquinolones*	Sulfacetamide	Clarithromycin
Cloxacillin	Ciprofloxacin	Sulfasalazine	
Nafcillin	Norfloxacin		
Carbenicillin	Ofloxacin		
Ticarcillin	Sparfloxacin	**Cotrimoxazole**	**Aminoglycosides**
Azlocillin	Trovafloxacin	Trimethoprim	Gentamicin
Piperacillin		+	Streptomycin
• *Cephalosporins*		Sulfamethoxazole	Neomycin
Cephalexin			Amikacin
Cephazolin	**Newer agents**	**Miscellaneous**	Netilmicin
Cefuroxime	*Streptogramins*	• Glycopeptides	Sisomycin
Cefachlor	Quinupristin	- Vancomycin	
Ceftriaxone	+	- Teicoplanin	**Broad spectrum**
Ceftazidime	Dalfopristin	• Lincosamides	**Antibiotics**
Cefpirome	*Oxazolidinones*	- Clindamycin	Chloramphenicol
Cefepime	- Linezolid	• Polypeptides	Tetracycline
• *Carbapenems*		- Polymyxin	Oxytetracycline
Imipenem		- Colistin	Demeclocycline
Meropenem		• Others	Doxycycline
Ertapenem		- Bacitracin	Minocycline
• *Carbacephem*		- Sodium fusidate	Tetracycline
Loracarbef		- Mupirocin	
• *Monobactams*			
Aztreonam			

drugs which exert antibacterial activity only in the urinary tract (and no systemic activity). They include nitrofurantoin and methenamine mandelate.

Nitrofurantoin is bacteriostatic, but at higher concentrations it may be bactericidal. It is a synthetic compound, effective against many gram-positive and gram-negative bacteria.Mechanism of action is not exactly known. Nitrofurantoin is reduced to highly reactive derivatives which damage DNA and affect DNA and RNA synthesis. Since human cells require a long time to reduce nitrofurantoin, toxicity is not significant. It is rapidly and completely absorbed from the gut. It attains high concentration in urine and is used in acute UTI, long-term suppression of chronic UTI (single dose 100 mg at bed time) and for prophylaxis of UTI. It may cause nausea,vomiting, diarrhoea and allergic reactions.Development of resistance is rare. Dose 50 - 100 mg 6 hrly (FURADANTIN).

Methenamine mandelate

Methenamine mandelate a salt of mandelic acid and methenamine. It releases formaldehyde in acidic urine below pH 5.5. Formaldehyde is bactericidal and resistance does not develop to it.

High doses can cause nausea, epigastric distress, haematuria and painful micturition.

Drug interactions

Methenamine binds sulfonamides and neutralises their action. Also, sulfonamides are precipitated in the acidic urine. Hence the combination should be avoided.

Uses

Methenamine mandelate is used orally in chronic UTI that is resistant to other drugs.

Other drugs used in UTI are sulfonamides, cotrimoxazole, nalidixic acid, fluoroquinolones, ampicillin, cloxacillin, carbenicillin, aminoglycosides, tetracyclines and cephalosporins.

Urinary analgesic

Phenazopyridine has analgesic actions on the urinary tract and relieves burning symptoms of dysuria and urgency.

54 Chemotherapy of Tuberculosis and Leprosy

- **Drugs used in tuberculosis**
  - First line drugs
  - Second line drugs
  - Treatment of tuberculosis
  - Resistant tuberculosis
  - Chemoprophylaxis
  - Tuberculosis in AIDS patients
  - Drugs for Mycobacterium avium complex
- **Drugs used in leprosy**
  - Dapsone
  - Rifampicin
  - Clofazimine
  - Lepra reactions
  - Chemoprophylaxis

Tuberculosis is a chronic granulomatous disease caused by *Mycobacterium tuberculosis.* In developing countries, it is a major public health problem; 5 lakh people die in India every year due to this disease. After the spread of AIDS, the problem has become more complex, as tuberculosis and *Mycobacterium avium complex* (MAC) infections are more common and rapidly progress in these patients.

Drugs used in tuberculosis

First line drugs	Second line drugs
• Isoniazid	• Ethionamide
• Rifampicin	• Thiacetazone
• Pyrazinamide	• Para aminosalicylic
• Ethambutol	acid (PAS)
• Streptomycin.	• Amikacin • Ciprofloxacin
	• Capreomycin • rifabutin
	• Cycloserine • Kanamycin

Based on antitubercular activity, drugs may be grouped as:

1. **Tuberculocidal agents -**

• Isoniazid	• Rifampicin
• Streptomycin	• Pyrazinamide
• Capreomycin	• Kanamycin
• Ciprofloxacin	

2. Tuberculostatic agents -

- Ethambutol • Ethionamide
- Thiacetazone • Cycloserine • PAS

FIRST LINE DRUGS

First line drugs are superior in efficacy to second line drugs. Most patients can be treated successfully with these drugs.

Isoniazid (INH) is the most effective and cheapest primary antitubercular drug. It is tuberculocidal for rapidly multiplying bacilli but static for resting bacilli. INH destroys:

i.   Intracellular bacilli as it freely penetrates into the cells, i.e. tubercle bacilli in macrophages, and

ii. Bacilli multiplying in the walls of the cavities. Thus it is effective against both intra and extracellular organisms. (Fig. 54.1, Table 54.2) If used alone, mycobacteria develop resistance to it. Hence it should be used in combination with other drugs.

Mechanism of action

INH inhibits the synthesis of mycolic acids which are important components of the mycobacterial cell wall.

INH

Myco-
bacterium

Enters myco bacteria

Active form
Covalent Bond

Binds enzymes

– cell wall

↓Mycolic acid synthesis

Weak cell wall

Tuberculocidal

The cell wall of mycobacteria differs from other bacteria in having large amounts of mycolic acids which form essential component of mycobacterial cell wall. INH freely enters the mycobacteria and is converted to an active form by an enzyme catalase - peroxidase present in the mycobacteria. This active form covalently binds certain enzymes and thereby inhibits mycolic acid synthesis.

Resistance to INH is seen when there is over production of the enzymes that are inhibited by INH.

Pharmacokinetics

INH is completely absorbed orally, penetrates all tissues, tubercular cavities, necrotic tissues and CSF. It is metabolised by acetylation and this is genetically determined. Patients can be fast or slow acetylators depending on the genetic inheritance - slow acetylators responding better. The t½ in slow acetylators is 3-5 hours while in fast acetylators it is 1 hour. Peripheral neuropathy is more common in slow acetylators while hepatotoxicity is more likely in fast acetylators. If INH is given once weekly in fast acetylators, adequate therapeutic concentrations may not be attained. Metabolites of INH are excreted in urine.

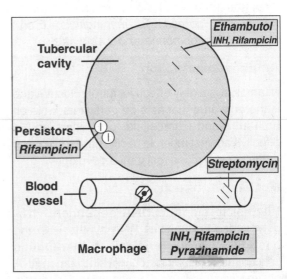

Fig 54.1 Sites of action of antitubercular drugs

Adverse effects

Peripheral neuritis (due to interference with utilization and increased excretion of pyridoxine) can be avoided by giving prophylactic pyridoxine (10-50mg) with INH. Hepatitis is another major adverse effect, more common in alcoholics and in elderly. If hepatitis is mild, INH may be continued, but in a small percentage of patients, INH can cause hepatic necrosis with anorexia, nausea, vomiting and jaundice - can sometimes be fatal. In such patients with signs of hepatic necrosis INH should be withdrawn. It can cause CNS toxicity including psychosis and seizures but are less common - epileptics are more prone to this effect. Other minor effects like anorexia, gastrointestinal discomfort, fever and allergic reactions can occur. Haemolysis can occur in patients with G_6PD deficiency.

RIFAMPICIN

Rifampicin (rifampin) is a semisynthetic derivative of rifamycin, an antibiotic obtained from *Streptomyces mediterranei*. The other rifamycins are rifabutin and rifapentine. Rifampicin is bactericidal to *M. tuberculosis, M. leprae* and atypical mycobacteria. It also inhibits most gram-positive and gram-negative bacteria like *Staph. aureus, N. meningitidis, E.coli, Proteus, Pseudomonas* and *Legionella.*

Antitubercular action

Rifampicin is highly effective, tuberculocidal and is the only drug that acts on persisters; acts on both intra and extracellular organisms and is effective against tubercle bacilli resistant to other drugs. If used alone resistance develops.

Mechanism of action

Rifampicin binds to DNA dependent RNA polymerase and inhibits RNA synthesis in the bacteria. It is bactericidal. In therapeutic concentrations, rifampicin cannot bind human RNA polymerase and it therefore selectively destroys the bacteria.

Pharmacokinetics

Rifampicin is well-absorbed and has good tissue penetrability - reaches caseous material, cavities, macrophages and CSF; it also appears in saliva, tears and sweat. It is a microsomal enzyme

TABLE 54.1 Recommended doses of antitubercular drugs

Drugs	Doses
Isoniazid (INH)	300-400 mg
Ethambutol (E)	800-1000 mg
Rifampicin (R)	450-600 mg
Streptomycin (S)	750-1000 mg
Pyrazinamide (Z)	1200-1500 mg
Thiacetazone (T)	150 mg

inducer - hence can result in many drug interactions. Dose - Table 54.1.

Adverse effects

1. **Hepatotoxicity** - rifampicin can cause hepatitis. Patients receiving other hepatotoxic drugs or those with any liver dysfunction should be carefully monitored - deaths have been reported in such patients.

2. Gastrointestinal disturbances - epigastric distress, nausea, vomiting, abdominal cramps and diarrhoea can occur.

3. Flu - like syndrome - characterised by fever, bodyache, chills and haemolytic anaemia is more common in intermittent dosing regimen.

4. CNS symptoms - including headache, drowsiness, dizziness, ataxia, confusion and peripheral neuropathy with pain and numbness in the extremities and muscle weakness have been reported.

5. Hypersensitivity reactions - with fever, skin rashes and urticaria, rarely renal manifestations with nephritis, hemolysis, haematuria and renal insufficiency can occur.

6. **Staining of secretions** - Rifampicin stains the secretions including tears, saliva and sweat - an orange red colour and the patient should be informed about this.

Drug interactions

1. Aminosalicylic acid may delay the absorption and reduce the bioavailability of rifampicin. When both are needed in a patient, there should be a gap of 8 - 12 hours between them.

2. Rifampicin is a microsomal enzyme inducer. It hastens the metabolism of many drugs including anticoagulants, hormonal contraceptives, ketoconazole, cyclosporine, some anticonvulsants and antiretroviral protease inhibitors. Oral contraceptive failures can be expected - a preparation with higher doses of estrogen should be used or alternative methods of contraception followed.

Uses

1. Tuberculosis and atypical mycobacterial infections.

2. Leprosy (See page 393).

3. Prophylaxis of *H. influenzae* and meningococcal meningitis in close contacts particularly children - 20mg/kg/day for 4 days.

4. Resistant staphylococcal infections - rifampicin may be given in combination with a beta lactam antibiotic or vancomycin.

5. Brucellosis - Rifampicin 600-900mg. + doxycycline 200mg daily for 6 weeks - drug of choice.

6. Pneumococcal meningitis - if resistant to penicillin can be treated with rifampicin + ceftriaxone.

7. To eradicate carrier state - rifampicin eradicates the nasal carrier state of *N.*

TABLE 54.2 Antitubercular actions and characteristic adverse effects of some antitubercular drugs

Drug	Antitubercular action	Serious toxicity
Isoniazid	Tuberculocidal; acts on intra and extracellular organisms including bacilli present in the walls of the cavities.	Peripheral neuritis, hepatitis, seizures, psychosis
Rifampicin	Tuberculocidal; Acts on intra and extracellular organisms, persisters and drug resistant organisms	Hepatotoxicity, flu-like syndrome, nephritis; urine and secretions are coloured orange-red
Pyrazinamide	Tuberculocidal, kills intracellular organisms; more active in acidic pH	Hepatotoxicity, arthralgia, hyperuricaemia
Streptomycin	Tuberculocidal, acts on extracellular organisms	Ototoxicity, nephrotoxicity
Ethambutol	Tuberculostatic; inhibits tubercle bacilli in the walls of cavities	Optic neuritis with ↓ visual acuity and red-green colour blindness
Thiacetazone	Tuberculostatic; low efficacy; delays development of resistance to other drugs	Hepatotoxicity, dermatitis

meningitidis, *H. influenzae* and *S. aureus* - 600mg B.D. for 2 days.

Rifabutin is similar to rifampicin except that it causes milder enzyme induction and is more active against atypical mycobacteria. Rifabutin may be used in place of rifampicin in tuberculosis patients with AIDS who are receiving antiretroviral drugs. These antiviral drugs are also metabolised by microsomal enzymes and rifampicin being a powerful enzyme inducer, can result in many drug interactions.

Rifapentine is an analog of rifampicin and is similar to it.

PYRAZINAMIDE

Pyrazinamide, an analog of nicotinamide was introduced in 1952 - it is tuberculocidal. It requires an acidic pH for its tuberculocidal activity. This is infact advantageous because tubercle bacilli reside in the phagosomes of the macrophages where the pH is acidic.

Mechanism of action is not exactly known. Pyrazinamide is converted to its active metabolite pyrazinoic acid by an enzyme pyrazinamidase present in the mycobacteria. This metabolite may inhibit the synthesis of mycolic acids by the mycobacteria. If used alone resistance develops.

Pyrazinamide is well-absorbed (achieves good concentration in CSF). Hepatotoxicity is the most common adverse effect. It is dose dependent - can result initially in raised serum transaminases and later jaundice and rarely hepatic necrosis. Deaths due to hepatic necrosis have been reported. Liver function tests should be done before starting pyrazinamide and it should be avoided in patients with hepatic impairment. Patient should be monitored for signs and symptoms of hepatotoxicity and if present, pyrazinamide should be stopped. Hyperuricaemia due to decreased excretion of uric acid may result in gouty arthritis; other effects like arthralgia, anorexia, vomiting, fever and rashes may be seen.

STREPTOMYCIN (See page 376) is tuberculocidal, acts only against extracellular organisms due to poor penetrating power. It has to be given IM. When used alone resistance develops because of these disadvantages and its toxicity (oto and nephrotoxicity), streptomycin is the least preferred of the first line drugs.

ETHAMBUTOL

Ethambutol is tuberculostatic and acts on fast multiplying bacilli in the cavities. It is also effective against atypical mycobacteria. It inhibits the incorporation of mycolic acids into the mycobacterial cell wall.

Optic neuritis resulting in decreased visual activity and inability to differentiate red from green is an important adverse effect which needs withdrawal of the drug. Colour vision should be monitored during treatment. Ethambutol is to be avoided in children because their ability to differentiate red from green cannot be reliably tested. Other adverse effects include nausea, anorexia, headache, fever and allergic reactions.

Drug interactions

Ethambutol decreases the renal excretion of uric acid and thereby enhances plasma urate levels.

SECOND LINE DRUGS

Second line drugs are generally less effective and more toxic when compared to first line drugs. They are used only if the organism is resistant to first line drugs.

THIACETAZONE

Thiacetazone is tuberculostatic with low efficacy; it delays the development of resistance to other drugs and its low cost makes it a suitable drug in combination regimens. Hepatotoxicity, dermatitis, allergic reactions and GI side effects may occur.

ETHIONAMIDE

This tuberculostatic drug is effective against both

intra and extracellular organisms. It is also effective in atypical mycobacteria.

Anorexia, nausea, vomiting and metallic taste in the mouth are the most common adverse effects. It can also cause hepatitis, skin rashes and peripheral neuritis (needs prophylactic pyridoxine).

Ethionamide is a second line agent used only when primary drugs are ineffective.

PARA-AMINOSALICYLIC ACID (PAS)

Para-aminosalicylic acid (PAS) related to sulfonamides is tuberculostatic. Gastrointestinal effects like nausea, anorexia, epigastric pain and diarrhoea make it a poorly tolerated drug. Allergic reactions and hepatitis are also seen. It is rarely used.

Other Second Line Drugs

Amikacin, kanamycin and capreomycin are second line drugs that need parenteral administration. They are oto and nephrotoxic and are used only in resistant cases. Amikacin is also effective against atypical mycobacteria.

Cycloserine is an antibiotic that inhibits cell wall synthesis, is tuberculostatic and is also effective against some gram-positive organisms. It causes CNS toxicity including headache, tremors, psychosis and sometimes seizures. It is used only in resistant tuberculosis.

Fluoroquinolones Ciprofloxacin, ofloxacin and sparfloxacin inhibit tubercle bacilli and atypical mycobacteria. They are useful in multi-drug resistant tuberculosis in combination with other drugs.

Treatment of Tuberculosis

Tuberculosis is one of the most difficult infections to cure. The properties of the mycobacteria like slow division, development of resistance, ability to remain as persisters for years and intracellular location of the bacilli have enhanced the problem. Moreover, the caseous material makes it difficult for the drugs

to reach. The need for long-term treatment, drug toxicity, cost and thereby poor patient compliance have all added to further complicate the problem. But with the availability of effective drugs, most patients can now be treated as outpatients.

The aim of treatment is to kill the dividing bacilli thus making the patient sputum negative and to destroy the persisters in order to prevent relapse and ensure complete cure.

A combination of drugs is used in tuberculosis to -

1. delay the development of resistance
2. reduce toxicity
3. shorten the course of treatment.

Majority of cases are sensitive to first line drugs. Initial treatment should be intensive and include drugs that have maximum effect. Good patient compliance and cost of therapy should also be considered.

Chemotherapy is given in two phases-

- First phase - initial, intensive phase of 1-3 months duration aimed at killing as many bacilli as possible.
- Second phase - continuation phase to destroy the dormant or persisters- duration 6-9 months.

Short-term regimens

1. INH + R + Z + E/S daily for 2 months followed by

   INH + R daily for 4 months.
2. INH + R + Z daily for 2 months followed by

   INH + R daily for 7 months.

Advantages

Short-term therapy has rapid response, lower failure rates, lesser chances of resistance and better patient compliance.

Conventional regimen

- INH + S + T daily for 2 months
- INH + T daily for 10 months

Failure rates are high and compliance is poor.

TABLE 54.3 Treatment categories of DOTS chemotherapy in India				
Category	Patients	Initial phase daily/ 3 per week	Continuation Phase	Total Duration (months)
I	• New sputum smear - positive • Sputum negative with extensive pulmonary Tb. • Severe extrapulmonary Tb.	HRZE for 2 m	HR daily for 4 or HE twice weekly for 6 m	6
				8
II	Sputum +ve relapse Sputum +ve failure Sputum +ve interrupted Sputum +ve treatment	HRZES 2 m HRZE 1 m	HRE 5 m	8
III	Sputum negative extrapulmonary	HRZ 2 m.	HR 4 m	6

H - INH R = rifampin, Z = pyrazinamide, E = ethambutol, S = streptomycin, m =months

Directly Observed Treatment Short course Chemotherapy (DOTS)

Though many effective antitubercular drugs are available, the success of chemotherapy depends on regular intake of appropriate drugs by the patients. Directly Observed Treatment, Short course chemotherapy (DOTS) is a strategy that is found to be effective and is recommended throughout the world. It involves providing most effective medicine and confirming that it is taken - a health worker ensures that the drug is taken by the patient. Patients are grouped into 3 categories for treatment (Table 54.3).

Resistant tuberculosis

If sputum remains positive even after 6 months of treatment, organisms are likely to be resistant. Such patients should be treated with 4-5 drugs, of which 3 are first line drugs and treatment is continued for at least 1 year after the sputum becomes negative. Fluoroquinolones (Ofloxacin 300 - 800mg daily) and amikacin may be considered for multidrug resistant strains.
Role of glucocorticoids

As steroids depress host defense mechanisms, they should be used only in conditions like tubercular meningitis, miliary tuberculosis, pleural effusion, renal tuberculosis and rapidly progressing pulmonary tuberculosis. Steroids suppress inflammatory reaction which can lead to extensive fibrosis and damage.

Chemoprophylaxis is given only in:

i. Contacts of open cases especially children

ii. Patients with old inactive disease who have not been adequately treated. INH is used daily (5 mg/kg) for 6-12 months. Rifampicin can be used as an alternative to INH

iii. HIV infected patients exposed to multi-drug resistant tuberculosis - rifampicin and pyrazinamide are given daily for 2 months.

Tuberculosis in AIDS patients

Due to depressed immunity, AIDS patients are at a higher risk (25-30 times). AIDS patients are likely to have more severe and rapidly progressing tuberculosis. Adverse effects to antitubercular drugs are more common in them. They should be given more vigorous and supervised chemotherapy as the guidelines of DOTS. INH + R + S + Z for 2 months followed by INH + R for 7 months.

DRUGS FOR MYCOBACTERIUM AVIUM COMPLEX (MAC)

Infection with MAC is more common in HIV patients and is more severe in them. With the use of prophylactic regimens, the incidence of MAC infections has greatly decreased. In non-HIV patients MAC infection causes milder disease with chronic productive cough. The drugs effective are rifabutin, clarithromycin, azithromycin, fluoroquinolones, ethambutol, clofazimine, amikacin and ethionamide. The macrolides clarithromycin and azithromycin are highly effective - and are the first choice drugs in MAC therapy. Clarithromycin (500mg twice a day) or azithromycin (500mg once daily) with ethambutol is the preferred regimen (rifabutin may be added) for MAC infection and needs life long treatment. Fluoroquinolones like ciprofloxacin, ofloxacin and sparfloxacin have useful activity against M. tuberculosis and MAC bacteria. Ciprofloxacin 1500mg in two or three divided doses is used in combination therapy in HIV patients with MAC infections (4 drug regimen with ciprifloxacin + clarithromycin + rifabutin + amikacin). Rifabutin, clarithromycin or azithromycin are used for prophylaxis.

LEPROSY

Leprosy caused by *Mycobacterium leprae* is a chronic infectious disease affecting skin, mucous membranes and nerves. Hansen discovered lepra bacillus in 1873. As lepra bacillus does not grow on artificial media and cannot be transmitted to all animals, it is difficult to culture this organism and study the effect of drugs.

In India leprosy (kusta roga) is a major public health problem affecting millions of people. Drugs used in leprosy

- Sulfones: Dapsone
- Rifampicin
- Clofazimine
- Ethionamide and Protionamide

DAPSONE

Dapsone is diaminodiphenylsulfone (DDS) and is related to sulfonamides.

Mechanism of action

Like sulfonamides, dapsone inhibits the incorporation of PABA into folic acid.

Actions

Dapsone is leprostatic. Though it inhibits the growth of many other bacteria, the dose needed is high and is therefore not used. The lepra bacillus develops resistance to dapsone on prolonged use.

Dapsone is completely absorbed on oral administration and reaches high concentrations in skin. It is metabolised in the liver and excreted in bile.

Adverse effects

Dapsone is well-tolerated - anorexia, nausea and vomiting are common. Fever, pruritus, rashes and dermatitis can occur. Haemolytic anaemia is the most important dose-related toxicity (more common in patients with G_6PD deficiency). Iron preparations should be given to prevent anaemia. Hepatitis and agranulocytosis are seen. Patients with lepromatous leprosy may develop lepra reactions.

RIFAMPICIN

Rifampicin is rapidly bactericidal to *M. leprae* and is highly effective - a single dose of 1500 mg can kill 99% of the lepra bacilli. It can be conveniently given once monthly. Used in combination with dapsone, it shortens the duration of treatment. Given alone - resistance develops.

CLOFAZIMINE

Clofazimine a dye, has weak bactericidal actions against *M. leprae.* It also has anti-inflammatory properties which is useful in suppressing lepra reactions. It is used orally in multi-drug regimens.

Clofazimine imparts a reddish-black discolouration to the skin specially on the exposed parts which remains for several months. It can also cause dryness of skin, itching and phototoxicity.

ETHIONAMIDE

Ethionamide is bactericidal to lepra bacilli but is more expensive and more toxic than dapsone. It can cause gastric irritation, peripheral neuritis and hepatotoxicity. Ethionamide can be used in multidrug regimen in patients who canot tolerate clofazimine. **Protionamide** is similar to ethionamide.

OTHER DRUGS

Fluoroquinolones

Ofloxacin is lepricidal and is suitable for use in multidrug regimens in leprosy along with rifampicin.

Minocycline

Minocycline a tetracycline has been found to have useful activity against M. leprae and is being tried in combination regimens to shorten the duration of treatment.

Clarithromycin

Clarithromycin a macrolide antibiotic has

bactericidel activity against M.leprae. Given 500mg daily for 28 days can kill 99% of viable bacilli.

TREATMENT OF LEPROSY

For the sake of treatment, leprosy is divided into paucibacillary (non-infectious) and multibacillary (infectious) leprosy. (Table 54.4) Several atlernative and short term regimens including drugs like ofloxacin, minocycline and clarithromycin are under evaluation.

WHO has recommended a combination of drugs in leprosy to:
1. eliminate persisters
2. prevent drug resistance
3. reduce the duration of therapy.

LEPRA REACTIONS

Lepra reactions are the acute exacerbations that occur in leprosy. They are triggered by acute infections, stress, anxiety and treatment with dapsone.

Type I reactions seen in tuberculoid leprosy are cell mediated, delayed hypersensitivity reaction (Cell-mediated hypersensitivity) to the antigens of M. leprae. Cutaneous ulcerations

TABLE 54.4 Multi-drug regimen for leprosy		
Drugs	**Multibacillary leprosy (for 24 months)**	**Paucibacillary leprosy (for 6 months)**
Rifampicin	600 mg once monthly supervised	600 mg once monthly supervised
Dapsone	100 mg daily self-administered	100 mg daily self-administered
Clofazimine	300 mg once monthly supervised 50 mg daily self-administered	— —
Single-lesion paucibacillary leprosy		
Rifampicin	600 mg ⎫ given as a	
Ofloxacin	400 mg ⎬ single dose.	
Minocycline	100 mg ⎭	
All drugs are given orally		

occur and existing lesions show more erythema; nerves may be painful and tender. They are treated with corticosteroids or clofazimine while in mild cases aspirin suffices.

Type II reactions are seen in lepromatous leprosy (are known as **erythema nodosum leprosum** or ENL). New lesions appear and the existing lesions become worse. Fever, lymphadenitis, myositis. and neuralgia may occur. It is a hypersensitivity reaction to the antigens of *M. leprae* - an arthus type reaction . Type II reactions can be treated with clofazimine which is effective due to its anti-inflammatory properties. Chloroquine, corticosteroids or thalidomide are also effective. Aspirin is effective in mild cases. Dapsone should be continued throughout.

Chemoprophylaxis

Only about 1% of contacts develop clinical disease. Dapsone 100 mg daily and rifampicin 600 mg once a month for 6 months or till the contact case becomes noninfectious are recommended for child contacts. Acedapsone is found to be advantageous for chemopro-phylaxis as a single IM injection every 10 weeks. All contacts should be examined every 6 months.

55 *Antifungal Drugs*

- Antifungal antibiotics
- Antimetabolites
- Azoles
- Terbinafine
- Pneumocandins or echinocandins

There has been an increase in the incidence and severity of fungal infections in the recent years. Several unusual and drug-resistant organisms have emerged. This may be consequent to the use of broad spectrum antibiotics, anticancer drugs and HIV infections all of which impair host defense mechanisms. Fungal infections may be systemic or superficial. Superficial fungal infections include infections of the skin, mucous membrane, hair and nails. They required prolonged treatment. Some of the systemic fungal infections may be life threatening, particularly in immunocompromised. patients.

Antifungal drugs may be classified into:

Classification

1. Antifungal antibiotics
- *Polyene antibiotics -*
  Amphotericin B, nystatin, hamycin, natamycin
- *Others*
  Griseofulvin

2. Antimetabolites
- Flucytosine (5-FC)

3. Azoles
- *Imidazoles*
  Clotrimazole, econazole, miconazole, ketoconazole, butaconazole, oxiconazole, sulconazole, isoconazole.
- *Triazoles*
  Fluconazole, itraconazole, terconazole.

4. Miscellaneous
- Terbinafine, pneumocandins

5. Other topical agents

- Tolnaftate, undecylenic acid, benzoic acid, salicylic acid, selenium sulfide, ciclopirox olamine.

Sites of action

Antifungal drugs may act (Fig. 55.1) on the fungal cell wall (pneumocandins), cell membrane (polyenes, azoles) or on the nucleus (griseofulvin, flucytosine).

ANTIFUNGAL ANTIBIOTICS

Amphotericin B

Amphotericin B obtained from *Streptomyces nodosus* is a polyene antibiotic containing many double bonds.

Antifungal spectrum

Amphotericin B has a wide antifungal spectrum. It inhibits the growth of *Candida albicans, Histoplasma capsulatum, Cryptococcus neoformans, Coccidioides, Aspergillus* and *Blastomyces dermatitidis*. It is fungistatic at low and fungicidal at high concentrations. Amphoterecin B also has activity against leishmania.

Mechanism of action

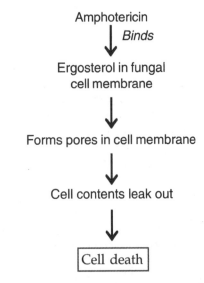

Amphotericin B binds to ergosterol present in fungal cell membrane and forms pores in the

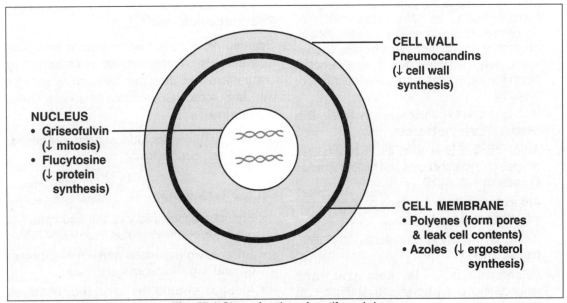

Fig. 55.1 Sites of action of antifungal drugs.

cell membrane. Through these pores, cell contents leak out resulting in cell death. Since amphotericin has greater affinity for the fungal membrane sterol *i.e.,* ergosterol, its action is selective for the fungi.

Pharmacokinetics

Amphotericin is not absorbed orally. It is insoluble in water. Given IV, it is widely distributed in the body and has a long t½ of 15 days.

Adverse effects

Fever, chills, muscle spasms, vomiting, dyspnoea, headache and hypotension can be encountered on IV infusion. Amphotericin should be injected slow IV, cautiously - to avoid arrhythmias. Pain and thrombophlebitis at the site of injection are common. Dose should be gradually increased. Renal impairment, neurotoxicity and anaemia due to decreased production of erythropoietin and bone marrow depression can also occur. Concurrent administration of other nephrotoxic drugs should be avoided.

Uses

- Amphotericin B is the drug of choice for all life-threatening mycotic infections. 0.5 mg/Kg in 5% dextrose infused over 4 hrs is the usual therapeutic dose. Amphotericin B is given intravenously in the treatment of mucormycosis, invasive aspergillosis, cryptococcosis, sporotrichosis, trichosporanosis, blastomycosis, histoplasmosis, coccidioidomycosis and paracoccidioidomycosis.

- In cystitis due to candida, amphotericin B is used to irrigate the bladder.

- Amphotericin B is also used to prevent relapse of cryptococcosis and histoplasmosis in patients with AIDS.

- Amphotericin B can be given orally in fungal infections of the gut.

- It is used topically in candidiasis (3% lotion, cream, ointment).

- Leishmaniasis: In kala-azar and mucocutaneous leishmaniasis, amphotericin is used as an alternative.

Nystatin

Nystatin obtained from *Streptomyces noursei* has actions similar to amphotericin B. But as it is too toxic for systemic use, it is used topically. It is used for local candidial infections like oral thrush and vaginal candidiasis. 5ml oral nystatin suspension should be swished in the mouth and then swallowed 4 times a day to treat the candida in the oesophagus.

Hamycin is similar to nystatin. It is used topically for cutaneous candidiasis and otomycosis.

Griseofulvin

Griseofulvin is a fungistatic derived from *Penicillium griseofulvum*. It is effective in superficial dermatophytosis (caused by *Trichophyton, Microsporum and Epidermophyton).* Griseofulvin is the antifungal given orally for superficial dermatophytosis.

Mechanism of action

Griseofulvin binds to microtubular protein in the nucleus, disrupts the mitotic spindle and inhibits mitosis in the fungus. It gets deposited in the newly forming skin, binds to keratin and protects the skin from getting newly infected.

Pharmacokinetics

Griseofulvin is poorly water soluble with poor bioavailability. Absorption can be enhanced by using microfined drug particles and by giving it with fatty food. Griseofulvin is a microsomal enzyme inducer.

Adverse effects include allergic reactions, hepatitis and neurotoxicity.

Drug interactions

- Phenobarbitone reduces the absorption of griseofulvin - may result in therapeutic failure

- Griseofulvin enhances warfarin metabolism by inducing microsomal enzymes.

- Alcohol should be avoided because griseofulvin can cause intolerance to alcohol.

Uses

Griseofulvin is used orally in superficial dermatophytosis. Dose : 1g daily. It is particularly preferred when a larger area is involved when topical antifungals are not suitable. Duration of treatment varies from 3 weeks to 1 year depending on the site of infection. Nail infections require 6-12 months of treatment.

ANTIMETABOLITES

Flucytosine is a fluorinated pyrimidine effective against *Cryptococcus neoformans* and some strains of *Candida*. It is taken up by the fungal cells and converted to 5-fluorouracil which inhibits DNA synthesis.

Bone marrow depression and gastrointestinal disturbances are the most common adverse effects. It is used with amphotericin B (used alone, resistance develops rapidly) in cryptococcal meningitis and systemic candidiasis.

AZOLES

Imidazoles and Triazoles

The older antifungals need to be given intravenously and are quite toxic. Azoles are newer synthetic antifungals that are effective orally and are less toxic. Imidazoles and triazoles are azoles; the triazoles have more selective effect on fungal sterol synthesis than imidazoles.Triazoles are also longer acting.

Antifungal spectrum

Azoles have a broad spectrum antifungal activity. They inhibit *dermatophytes, candida, cryptococcus neoformans, H.capsulatum* and other deep mycoses.

Mechanism of action

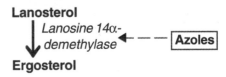

Azoles inhibit the synthesis of ergosterol, an important component of the fungal cell membrane. Azoles inhibit the fungal cytochrome P450 enzyme lanosine 14a - demethylase which catalyses the convertion of lanosterol to ergosterol. Thus it results in ergosterol deficiency which alters enzyme activity and fungal replication. They also interfere with the function of some fungal enzymes and inhibit the growth of the fungi.

Of the azoles, clotrimazole and miconazole are used only topically.

Ketoconazole (KTZ)

Ketoconazole is the first oral azole to be available. It is well-absorbed from the gut. Food and low gastric pH enhance absorption.

Adverse reactions include gastric irritation, nausea, vomiting, headache, allergic reactions, and rarely fatal hepatotoxicity. In large doses KTZ inhibits the biosynthesis of adrenal and gonadal steroids in humans - resulting in gynaecomastia, infertility, decreased libido, azoospermia, menstrual irregularities and hypertension.

Preparations

FUNGICIDE, NIZRAL - ointment, shampoo, 20 mg tablets are available.

Drug interactions

- Antacids, H_2 receptor blockers, and proton pump inhibitors reduce the bioavailability of KTZ because acidic medium is necessary for KTZ dissolution.
- Rifampicin and phenytoin induce KTZ metabolism and decrease its efficacy.
- Ketoconazole increases arrhythmogenic effects of terfenadine and astemizole by

TABLE 55.1 Drugs used in fungal infections

Fungal infection	Drug of Choice	Alternative Drugs
Systemic		
Invasive aspergillosis	Amphotericin	Itraconazole
Blastomycosis	Amphotericin	Itraconazole Ketoconazole
Candidiasis	Fluconazole	Amphotericin Flucytosine
Coccidiodomycosis	Amphotericin Itraconazole Fluconazole	Ketoconazole
Cryptococcosis	Amphotericin ± Flucytosine Fluconazole	Itraconazole
Histoplasmosis	Amphotericin Itraconazole	Flucanazole
Mucormycosis	Amphotericin Flucytosine	Itraconazole
Paracoccidiodomycosis	Fluconazole Itraconazole	Amphetericin
Sporotrichosis	Amphotericin	Itraconazole

increasing their blood levels.

Uses (Table 55.1)

Mucocutaneous candidiasis and dermatophytosis can be treated with ketoconazole. It is also useful in Cushing's syndrome. KTZ is also useful in deep mycoses but is not preferred in them because of slow response, toxicity and long duration of treatment (6 to 12 months) required.

Clotrimazole and miconazole

Clotrimazole and miconazole are used topically in dermatophytic infections (ringworm) and mucocutaneous candidiasis. (Table 55.2) Miconazole penetrates the cutaneous layer - stratum corneum and remains at this site for 3-4 days. It has better efficacy. Clotrimazole troche is available for oral thrush. Both can cause mild irritation at the site of application - particularly on mucous membrane. Skin preparations can rarely cause rashes, edema and pruritus.

Preparations

- Clotrimazole (CANDID, CLODERM) Lotion, cream, vaginal pessary 100mg inserted into the vagina at bed time for 7 days or 200mg daily for 3 days or 500mg single dose.
- Miconazole (DAKTARIN, ZOLE) 2%-4% ointment, gel, cream, lotion and vaginal suppository (100, 200mg)

Fluconazole

Fluconazole is water soluble, well-absorbed orally and attains good CSF concentration. Hence it is useful even in fungal meningitis. Fluconazole is available for oral and IV use.

Adverse effects are mild gastrointestinal disturbances, headache and rashes. Since it has very little effect on hepatic microsomal enzymes, drug interactions are less common.

Uses

Fluconazole is used in cryptococcal meningitis after initial treatment with amphotericin B and is the drug of choice in coccidial meningitis. It is also useful in systemic candidiasis and other systemic fungal infections. Though it is also effective in tinea infections and mucocutaneous candidiasis, its higher cost makes it less preferable.

Itraconazole

Itraconazole is the most potent azole. Given orally, its absorption is increased by food and gastric acid. It does not have much effect on hepatic microsomal enzymes and does not affect steroid synthesis. Thus it is preferred over ketoconazole. It has a t½ of 36 hours. It is available both for oral and IV use. Adverse effects include headache, dizziness, g.i. disturbances and allergic reactions. It can rarely cause hepatitis and hypokalemia.

Itraconazole is the drug of choice in most systemic mycoses (without meningitis) (Table 55.1) 100mg BD with food. It can be given IV in severe infections.

Itraconazole can also be used in onychomycosis, candidiasis and dermatophytoses but is expensive. (ITASPOR, SPORANOX 100 mg cap).

Econazole, terconazole, tioconazole, butaconazole, oxiconazole and sulconazole are all azoles available for topical use as creams and lotions for use in dermatophytoses and mucocutaneous candidiasis.

Terbinafine

Terbinafine is a synthetic antifungal that is effective against dermatophytes and Candida. It is orally effective and is fungicidal. It gets concentrated in the keratin like griseofulvin. Terbinafine inhibits an enzyme needed for biosynthesis of ergosterol by fungi.

Adverse effects are rare - gastrointestinal disturbances, rashes and headache can occur.

Terbinafine is used in dermatophytosis, pityriasis, onychomycosis and candidiasis. It is particularly preferred in onychomycosis - 250 mg OD for 12 weeks - where it is superior to azoles and griseofulvin.

Dose SEBIFIN - 250 mg daily ; 1% cream is also available.

Table 55.2 Drugs used in Superficial mycosis

	Topical	Oral
Ringworm	An azole	Terbinafine
		Itraconazole
Candidiasis		
• *Cutaneous*	Amphotericin	
	An azole	
	Ciclopirox	
	Nystatin	
• *Oropharyn-geal*	Amphotericin	Itraconazole
	An azole	
	Nystatin	
	Fluconazole	
• *Vaginal*	An azole	
	Nystatin	Fluconazole

Pneumocandins or echinocandins

Pneumocandins inhibit the formation of the fungal cell wall. They inhibit the synthesis of an important component of the fungal cell wall - a glucose polymer, as a result of which the fungal cell lysis occurs.

Echinocandins include caspofungin, micafungin and amorolfine. Caspofungin has activity in candidiasis, aspergillosis and in *P.carinii* infections. Micafungin is effective against candida and aspergillus while amorolfine is useful in fungal infections of the nail.

Other topical antifungal agents

Apart from nystatin, clotrimazole, miconazole and terbinafine, some drugs like salicyclic acid, benzoic acid, tolnaftate, naftifine and ciclopirox olamine are used topically for dermatophytosis and pityriasis versicolor.

Selenium sulfide

Selenium sulfide is useful in tinea versicolor caused by *Malassezia furfur*, and also in dandruff. SELSUN is 2.5% suspension of selenium sulfide in a shampoo base. It is an irritant to the eyes and the odour is unpleasant.

56 *Antiviral Drugs*

- **Classification**
- **Anti-herpes virus agents**
- **Anti-influenza virus agents**
- **Other Antiviral Agents**
- **Anti-retroviral Agents**
    - **Nucleoside reverse transcriptase inhibitors**
    - **Nonnucleoside reverse transcriptase inhibitors**
    - **Protease inhibitors**
    - **Nucleotide reverse transcriptase inhibitors**

Viruses are intracellular parasites and depend on the host cells for their food, growth and multiplication. The virus attaches (Fig 56.1) itself to the host cell membrane and penetrates it (entry), DNA/RNA is released in the host cell (uncoating) where it is duplicated. The viral components are assembled (assembly) and the mature viral particle is then released from the host cell (budding and release). Chemotherapy can interfere with any of these steps. But drugs that interfere with viral replication may also interfere with host cell function. Currently, efforts are being made to develop drugs that selectively inhibit the virus without affecting the host cell function.

There are two types of viruses - DNA and RNA viruses and there are minor differences in their replicative cycles. The DNA virus depends on host cell enzymes (mRNA polymerase) to synthesize mRNA while RNA viruses use their own enzymes for mRNA synthesis.

Retroviruses

Retroviruses a type of RNA viruses are known to cause AIDS. In retroviruses a viral enzyme reverse transcriptase is involved in replication. Two groups of antiviral drugs inhibit this enzyme. The immature virion formed undergoes maturation with the help of the enzyme protease. Inhibitors of this protease prevent maturation of the virions.

Antiviral drugs may be classified as follows:

CLASSIFICATION

1. **Anti-herpes virus agents**

   Acyclovir, ganciclovir, famciclovir, penciclovir, valaciclovir, idoxuridine, trifluridine, vidarabine, foscarnet, fomivirsen, cidofovir

2. **Anti-influenza virus agents**

   Amantadine, rimantadine, oseltamivir, zanamivir,

3. **Others**   Ribavirin, interferons, lamivudine, palivizumab, adefovir

4. **Anti-retroviral agents**
   - *Nucleoside Reverse Transcriptase inhibitors (NRTIs)*

     Zidovudine, didanosine, stavudine
     zalcitabine, lamivudine, abacavir
   - *Nonnuclease Reverse Transcriptase inhibitors (NNRTIs)*

     Nevirapine, efavirenz, delavirdine
   - *Protease inhibitors (PIs)*

     Saquinavir, indinavir, ritonavir, nelfinavir,
     amprenavir, lopinavir
   - *Nucleotide Reverse Transcriptase inhibitors (NTRTIs)*

     Tenofovir

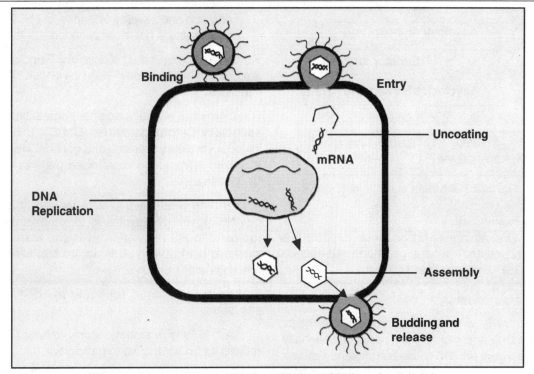

Fig 56.1 Stages of viral replication and sites of action of antiviral drugs

ANTI-HERPES VIRUS AGENTS

Acyclovir

Acyclovir is effective against Herpes simplex virus (HSV) type 1 and type 2, Varicella zoster virus (VZV) and Epstein-Barr virus (EBV).

Mechanism of action

Acyclovir (Fig.56.2) is taken up by the virus infected cell, converted to acyclovir triphosphate and this inhibits viral DNA synthesis by inhibiting viral DNA polymerases and causing DNA chain termination.

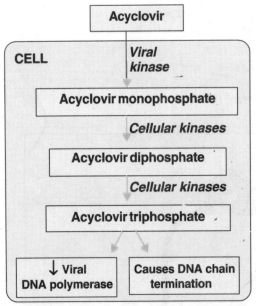

Fig. 56.2 Mechanism of action of acyclovir

Pharmacokinetics

Oral absorption of acyclovir is poor; it is well distributed - attains good concentration in the CSF and aqueous humour.

Adverse effects

Acyclovir is well-tolerated; nausea, diarrhoea, headache and rashes may occur occasionally. Topical acyclovir can cause burning and irritation. Given IV, it may cause renal and neurotoxicity but are uncommon.

Uses

1. *HSV infections* Infection with HSV-1 causes diseases of the mouth, face, skin, oesophagus or brain. HSV-2 usually causes infections of the genitals, rectum, skin, hands or meninges.

   - Oral acyclovir is effective in primary and recurrent genital and labial herpes. In mild cases, topical acyclovir can be tried. In recurring genital herpes - oral acyclovir is given for 1 year.
   - *HSV* encephalitis and other severe HSV infections - IV acyclovir is the drug of choice.
   - *HSV* keratoconjunctivitis Acyclovir eye drops are effective.

2. *Herpes zoster* Acyclovir shortens the duration of illness. In immunodeficient patients - IV acyclovir is used.

3. *Chickenpox* In adults and in immunodeficient patients, acyclovir reduces duration and severity of illness. In children, routine use is not recommended.

Valacyclovir is a prodrug of acyclovir. Famciclovir is a prodrug of penciclovir - used in HSV and VZV infections.

Ganciclovir is effective against herpes viruses especially Cytomegalovirus (CMV). Toxicity includes myelosuppression and gonadal toxicity. It is used in immunocompromised patients with CMV retinitis.

Idoxuridine is effective in DNA viruses. It acts by inhibiting viral DNA synthesis. Idoxuridin is used topically in HSV keratitis (it is too toxic for systemic use). Eyelid oedema, itching, allergic reactions may occur.

Trifluridine is used topically in HSV eye infections.

Foscarnet is given intravenously to treat CMV retinitis as an alternative to ganciclovir.

Vidarabine was used earlier for HSV and VZV infections but is now replaced by acyclovir.

Fomivirsen is effective against cytomegalo virus. It is given by intravitreal injection in severe cases of CMV retinitis which do not respond to other drugs.

Cidofovir is a cytidine analog effective against herpes viruses, VZV, CMV, EBV, human papilloma virus (HPV) and adenoviruses – has a broad spectrum of activity. Cidofovir acts by inhibiting viral DNA synthesis. It is given intravenously to prevent the progression of CMV retinitis in AIDS patients. It can also be used topically in HPV skin infections.

ANTI-INFLUENZA VIRUS AGENTS

Amantadine and Rimantadine

Amantadine and rimantadine inhibit the replication of influenza A viruses. They are generally well-tolerated; nausea, vomiting, diarrhoea, dizziness, insomnia and ankle oedema are reported. Rimantadine is longer-acting and has fewer adverse effects.

Uses (Table 56.2)

1. **Treatment of influenza A** during an epidemic- they reduce the duration and severity; dose: 200 mg/day for 5 days.

2. **Prophylaxis of influenza A** during an epidemic especially in high-risk patients.

Also for seasonal prophylaxis in high-risk patients.

3. **Parkinsonism:** Amantadine enhances the release of dopamine and is beneficial in parkinsonism.

Oseltamivir and Zanamivir

Oseltamivir and zanamivir inhibit viral replication. They act by inhibiting the neuraminidase activity which is essential for the release of daughter virions. Oseltamivir is given orally, can cause nausea and vomiting while zanamivir is given by inhalation which can occasionally cause respiratory distress.

Oseltamivir and zanamivir are indicated in the prevention and treatment of influenza.

Docosanol suppresses viral replication by inhibiting the viral entry into the cell. It is used topically in the treatment of orolabial herpes. It should be used early at the onset of lesion.

OTHER ANTIVIRAL AGENTS

Ribavirin has broad spectrum antiviral activity. It is effective against influenza A and B, respiratory syncytial virus (RSV) and many DNA and RNA viruses. It is used as an aerosol in RSV bronchiolitis in children. Also it can be used in severe influenza and measles in immunocompromised patients.

Table 56.1 Drugs acting on viral replication steps

Viral replication steps	Drugs effective
Uncoating	Amantadine, Rimantadine
Transcription	Interferons
Translation of viral proteins	Fomivirsen, interferons
DNA & RNA replication	Acyclovir, cidofovir, famciclovir, ganciclovir, foscarnet, idoxuridin, ribavirin sorivudine
Assembly	Interferons
Budding and release	Zanamivir, oseltamivir

Interferons are cytokines produced by host cells in response to viral infections. There are three types - α, β and γ interferons in man. They also have immunomodulating and antiproliferative properties. They inhibit the multiplication of many DNA and RNA viruses.

Adverse effects include myelosuppression, hypotension, arrhythmias, alopecia, headache and arthralgia. It can also cause neurotoxicity resulting in confusion, sedation and, rarely, seizures.

Uses

1. Chronic hepatitis B and C.
2. Kaposi's sarcoma in AIDS patients.
3. Genital warts caused by Papilloma virus - interferons are injected into the lesion.
4. Hairy cell leukaemia.
5. HSV, herpes zoster and CMV infections in immunocompromised patients.
6. Rhinovirus cold - interferon a is given intranasally for prophylaxis.

Lamivudine is a cytidine analog. Apart from HIV (See page 408) lamivudine is also effective against hepatitis B virus. But discontinuation of lamivudine can result in recurrence.

Palivizumab is a monoclonal antibody effective against respiratory syncytial virus. It is used in high risk children < 2 years of age who also have chronic lung disease.

Adefovir is effective against hepatitis B virus. It is a nucleotide analog - an adenosine analog. It is incorporated into viral DNA and causes chain termination. It is orally effective and used in the treatment of HBV infection not responding to lamivudine.

ANTI-RETROVIRAL AGENTS

Acquired Immunodeficiency Syndrome (AIDS) results from infection with Human Immunodeficiency Virus (HIV) - a retrovirus. The spread of HIV infection is alarmingly high with around 20 million deaths. Two types of HIV have been identified - HIV-1 and HIV-2.

Drugs used in the treatment of AIDS are of two groups- the reverse transcriptase inhibitors

TABLE 56.2: Indications of some antiviral drugs

Drugs	Routes	Indications
Acyclovir	Topical	Herpes genitalis, HSV eye infections
	Oral	Herpes genitalis, mucocutaneous HSV, chickenpox
	IV	HSV encephalitis, severe herpes genitalis, chickenpox/herpes zoster in immunocompromised patients
Idoxuridine, Trifluridine	Topical	HSV keratitis
Ganciclovir	IV/oral	CMV infections
Foscarnet	IV	CMV retinitis, acyclovir resistant HSV infections
Amantadine, Rimantadine	Oral	Influenza A
Ribavirin	Aerosol	RSV bronchiolitis
	Oral/IV	Severe influenza and measles
Interferon α	IV	Chronic hepatitis B and C, genital warts, Kaposi's sarcoma
Zidovudine	Oral	HIV infection

and protease inhibitors. A combination of drugs is used in AIDS to improve prognosis - known as **Highly Active Antiretroviral Therapy** (HAART). A HAART regimen includes two NRT inhibitors with either NNRT or protease inhibitors. Using a HAART regimen supresses HIV replication, plasma HIV RNA levels are greatly reduced and prolongs patient survival. HAART also has some disadvantages of being difficult to follow and is associated with adverse effects from drugs and with relapse.

HIV has a high mutation rate and therefore easily develops resistance to the drugs. Multi-drug resistant strains have emerged and further complicate treatment.

NUCLEOSIDE REVERSE TRANSRIPTASE INHIBITORS

Zidovudine is the first drug to be used in the treatment of HIV infection. Others including didanosine, stavudine, zalcitabine, lamivudine and abacavir were developed later (Table 56.3).

Mechanism of action

NRT inhibitors are converted to their corresponding triphosphate derivatives which have a high affinity for reverse transcriptase, an enzyme specific to HIV and required for DNA synthesis. The NRT inhibitors are nucleoside analogs. They competitively inhibit reverse transcriptase and terminate DNA chain elongation.

Pharmacokinetics The NRT inhibitors are well absorbed when given orally. Their plasma t ½ varies from 1–4 hours. All NRT inhibitors (except abacavir) are excreted in the urine.

Zidovudine (Azidothymidine, AZT)

Zidovudine is a thymidine analog, active against

TABLE 56.3 Nucleoside reverse transciptase inhibitors – common features

Drug	Analog of	Dose	Adverse effects
Zidovudine	Thymidine	200 mg b.i.d	Myelosuppression headache, nausea, insomnia
Didanosine	Adenosine	125 – 200 mg b.i.d	Pancreatitis, peripheral neuropathy, diarrhoea, hyperuricaemia
Stavudine	Thymidine	20-40 mg b.i.d.	Peripheral neuropathy, stomatitis
Zalcitabine	Cytidine	0.75 mg t.i.d	Peripheral neuropathy, stomatitis, pancreatitis
Lamivudine	Cytidine	150 mg b.i.d	Headache, nausea
Abacavir	Guanosine	300 mg b.i.d	Hypersensitivity syndrome

Keybox 56.1

NNRT inhibitors

- Nevirapine, delavirdine, efavirenz.

- Bind reverse transcriptase of HIV - 1 and inactivate it.

- They are well absorbed and extensively bound to plasma proteins.

- Metabolised by microsomal enzymes. Nevirapine and efavirenz are enzyme inducers; delavirdine is an enzyme inhibitor - drug interactions are common.

- Allergic reactions, headache and nausea are common.

- Used in HIV-1 infections in combination with other antiretroviral drugs.

HIV infections and other retroviruses.

Adverse effects

Bone marrow suppression in the most prominent adverse effect of zidovudine. Myelosuppression is more common in patients with advanced AIDS. Anaemia can be treated with erythropoietin while neutropenia needs G-CSF or GM-CSF. Headache, nausea, myalgia, fatigue and insomnia can occur. High doses cause myopathy and neurotoxicity.

Uses

AZT is the drug of choice in AIDS. Treatment with AZT results in prolonged survival, decreased opportunistic infections, weight gain and, in early cases, it delays disease progression.

Given during pregnancy and continued in the new born for 6 weeks, AZT reduces the risk of transmission to the baby. But it has **no** prophylactic value in those who are accidentally exposed to HIV infection (e.g. following blood transfusion). Combination therapy of AZT with other antiretroviral drugs gives better results.

Didanosine, Zalcitabine, Stavudine Lamivudine and Abacavir are other reverse transcriptase inhibitors effective against AZT resistant HIV infections. They are used as alternatives to AZT or with AZT in patients with advanced HIV who are intolerant of AZT or are not responding to AZT.

Lamivudine is well tolerated with no serious adverse effects in therapeutic doses. It can cause insomnia, fever, headache and diarrhoea. Abacavir can cause a hypersensitivity syndrome with fever, rash and bronchitis, which can be fatal. Hence abacavir should be withdrawn at the onset of such symptoms. Peripheral neuropathy, pancreatitis, rash, fever and headache can occur.

Drug interactions of NRT inhibitors

- Since AZT causes myelosuppression, it should not be combined with other myelosuppressants.

- Stavudine competes with zidovudine for activation pathway. Zidovudine decreases efficacy of stavudine. Hence the combination should be avoided.

- Combination of zalcitabine and didanosine should be avoided due to overlapping toxicity i.e. pancreatitis and peripheral neuropathy.

- Zalcitabine and lamivudine may antagonise each other - combination should be avoided.

- Plasma levels of abacavir is increased by alcohol.

NONNUCLEOSIDE REVERSE TRANS-CRIPTASE INHIBITORS

The NNRT inhibitors nevirapine, delavirdine and efavirenz are synthetic compounds.

Mechanism of action

The NNRT inhibitors bind to reverse transciptase, (are not converted to triphosphate derivatives) and bring about a change in the enzyme thereby inactivating the enzyme. NNRT inhibitors are effective only against HIV -1 (not against HIV-2 and other retroviruses)

Nevirapine is well absorbed orally and metabolised by the microsomal enzymes in the liver. Allergic reactions ranging from skin rashes, pruritus to Steven Johnson syndrome and toxic epidermal necrolysis can occur. Fever, nausea, headache, drowsiness are common. Occasionally fulminant hepatitis can occur.

Nevirapine is used in the treatment of HIV – 1 infections in combination with other drugs. Nevirapine can be tried in pregnant women during labour and in new born to prevent vertical transmission to the newborn.

Delavirdine is well absorbed, extensively bound to plasma proteins and metabolised mainly by the hepatic microsomal enzymes. The most common adverse effect is skin rash. Other occasional effects include headache, nausea and diarrhoea.

Delavirdine is used in combination with other antiretroviral drugs in the treatment of HIV - 1 infection.

Efavirenz has an oral bioavailability of 50% , it is 99% bound to plasma proteins, is long acting and can be given once daily. It is metabolised by the microsomal enzymes.

Side effects include headache, dizziness, drowsiness, nightmares, confusion, vomiting diarrhoea and skin rashes. Efavirenz has teratogenic effects in monkeys and is contraindicated in pregnant women.

Efavirenz is used in the treatment of HIV - I infection in combination with other antiretroviral drugs.

Drug interactions of NNRT inhibitors

• Nevirapine is a microsomal enzyme inducer.

Drug	Recommended dose	Adverse effects
Saquinavir	120 mg t.i.d.	Gastrointestinal disturbance
Ritonavir	600 mg b.i.d.	Gastrointestinal disturbance, taste perversion , perioral and peripheral paresthesias, ↑ Serum cholesterol, ↑ TG
Indinavir	800 mg t.i.d.	Crystalluria, nephrolithiasis (advise lot of fluid intake) ↑ serum bilirubin, alopecia, dry skin, gastrointestinal disturbances
Nelfinavir	750 mg t.i.d.	Diarrhoea ↑ Blood glucose ↑ Serum lipids
Amprenavir	1200 mg bid.	Gastrointestinal disturbances, rash, ↑ blood glucose, avoid high - fat meals
Lopinavir	400 mg bid.	Gastrointestinal disturbances ↑ Serum lipids

TABLE 56.4 Protease inhibitors

Concurrent administration of rifampicin and ketoconazole should be avoided. Oral contraceptives can fail, hence alternative methods of contraception should be followed.

- Delavirdine is a microsomal enzyme inhibitor. It also increases plasma levels of protease inhibitors like saquinavir and indinavir.
- Efavirenz is a microsomal enzyme inducer.

PROTEASE INHIBITORS (PI)

Saquinavir is the first agent in this group to be used (Table 56.4) therapeutically.

Mechanism of action

HIV protease activity is essential for the activation of viral enzymes and HIV replication. It is needed for the production of mature virion and for viral infectivity. The protease inhibitors bind competitively to HIV protease and block viral maturation. This makes the daughter viral particles immature and noninfectious.

Pharmacokinetics

Saquinavir has poor oral bioavailability (4-10%) while others are well absorbed. All PIs are extensively bound to plasma proteins. They are all metabolised by hepatic microsomal enzymes (cytochrome P 450) and are also microsomal inhibitors. Hence many drug interactions can occur.

Adverse effects Protease inhibitors are well tolerated. Gastrointestinal symptoms like nausea, vomiting and diarrhoea can occur. For other adverse effects see Table 56.4.

Uses

Protease inhibitors are used in combination with other antiretroviral drugs in the treatment of HIV infections. Ritonavir inhibits microsomal enzymes and thereby prolongs the plasma half-life of other protease inhibitors. This beneficial

---

Keybox 56.2

Protease inhibitors

- Bind HIV protease and prevent viral maturation
- All except saquinavir all well absorbed
- All are metabolised by microsomal enzymes and inhibit these enzymes - drug interactions are common.
- Gastrointestinal disturbances are the common side effects
- Used in combination with other antiretroviral drugs in HIV infections.

---

drug interaction permits use of lower doses of other PIs with ritonavir.

NUCLEOTIDE REVERSE TRANSCRIPTASE INHIBITORS (NTRTIs)

Tenofovir- is an adenosine analog. It is converted to tenofovir diphosphate which is incorporated into reverse transcriptase and causes termination of the chain. Tenofovir is used as an alternative in the treatment of HIV infections in combination with other drugs.

Tenofovir is orally effective and well tolerated with occasional nausea, vomiting and diarrhea. It is contraindicated in renal failure.

OTHER DRUGS

Enfuvirtide is a recent introduction for use in AIDS. It inhibits the binding of the virus to the host cell membrane (fusion inhibitor) and thereby blocks the entry of the virus. It is tried as an add-on drug in patients not responding to other antiretroviral drugs in HIV-1 infected patients.

Many new antiretroviral agents are under evaluation.

57 *Chemotherapy of Malaria*

- **Life cycle of the malaria parasite**
- **Classification**
- **Chloroquine**
- **Quinine**
- **Mefloquine**
- **Halofantrine**
- **Primaquine**
- **Folate antagonists**
- **Atovaquone**
- **Artimisinin and derivatives**
- **Newer antimalarials**
- **Immunity in malaria**

Malaria is caused by protozoa of the genus Plasmodium. It is most commonly transmitted through the bite of a female Anopheles mosquito though malaria can also be transmitted by blood transfusion and vertically from mother to the foetus across the placenta. It is a major public health problem in most of the developing countries including India. Every year about 200-500 million cases of malaria occur throughout the world with 2 million deaths.

The 4 species of the malarial parasite include:

- *P. falciparum* – causes the most severe form of malaria (malignant tertian) which can be fatal. 90% of deaths due to malaria is due to *P.falciparum*. The parasite in the RBCs requires about 48 hours to complete its lifecycle and ruptures every 3rd day (hence the name tertian) and this results in fever. In later stages of the erythrocytic cycle of the parasite, the infected erythrocytes get sequestered in capillaries of various tissues resulting in tissue anoxia . But relapses do not occur because *P.falciparum* has no exoerythrocytic stage in its life cycle.

- *P. vivax* - causes less severe malaria (benign tertian) with a lower mortality rate. Relapses can occur because of the exoerythrocytic forms or hypnozoites.

- *P.ovale* - is mostly seen in Africa, causes milder form of malaria similar to *P.vivax* - but relapses can occur.

- *P. malariae* - also causes malaria of milder

type similar to *P.vivax* (benign quartan) with no exoerythrocytic cycle. Febrile attack is seen every fourth day because 72 hours are needed for the maturation of the parasite in the RBCs and it is therefore called quartan malaria.

Life cycle of the malaria parasite

The bite of an infected female anopheles mosquito introduces sporozoites into the blood stream of man (Fig 57.1). These sporozoites enter the liver cells where they develop and multiply and the cells rupture to release merozoites (pre-erythrocytic stage). The merozoites enter red blood cells to develop and mature (erythrocytic stage/ erythrocytic schizogony) for which it needs 48 hours (72 hours in *P. malariae*) and then the RBCs rupture releasing merozoites which invade fresh RBCs and continue to multiply. The material that is released when the RBCs rupture induces the release of cytokines and other mediators of inflammation which is responsible for fever and other symptoms of malaria. In *P. vivax* and *P.*

ovale species, some sporozoites in the liver cells enter a dormant stage (hypnozoites or sleeping forms) which can multiply later (even after several months) resulting in relapse (exoerythrocytic stage). Some merozoites entering the RBCs, differentiate into male and female sexual forms or gametocytes. These forms enter the mosquito when they suck the blood and undergo sexual cycle in the mosquito.

Clinical features

Signs and symptoms of malaria include fever with chills, myalgia, arthralgia, headache, vomiting and fatigue - these symptoms mimic viral fever and malaria may often go undiagnosed for sometime and by this time it could assume a more severe form. Diarrhoea, abdominal pain, dizziness, hypotension and in more severe forms convulsions may occur. Mild anaemia and splenomegaly and in some of them mild hepatomegaly are the expected findings.

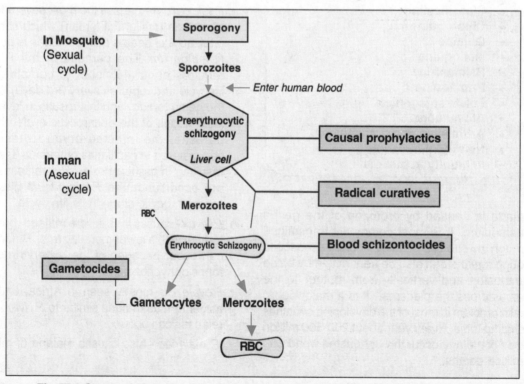

Fig 57.1 Stages of life cycle of the malaria parasite and drugs acting on these stages.

Antimalarial drugs can be classified therapeutically and chemically as follows -

A. Therapeutic Classification

1. *Causal Prophylactics* (primary tissue schizontocides) - (destroy parasite in liver cells and prevent invasion of erythrocytes)	Primaquine, pyrimethamine
2. *Blood schizontocides* (suppressives) (destroy parasites in the RBCs and terminate clinical attacks of malaria.)	Chloroquine, quinine, mefloquine, halofantrine, pyrimethamine, atovaquone chloroguanide, artemisinin.
3. *Tissue schizontocides used to prevent relapse* (hypnozoitocidal drugs) - (act on hypnozoites of P. vivax and P. ovale that produce relapses).	Primaquine
Radical curatives- (eradicate all forms of P.Vivax & P.ovale from the body)	Blood schizontocides+ hypnozoitocidal drugs
4. *Gametocidal drugs* (destroy gametocytes and prevent transmission).	Primaquine, chloroquine, quinine.

B. Chemical Classification

1. 4-aminoquinolines
   Chloroquine, amodiaquine

2. 8 – aminoquinolines
   Primaquine, bulaquine

3. Quinoline methanols
   Quinine, quinidine, mefloquine

4. Acridine
   Mepacrine

5. Folate antagonists
   Proguanil, sulfadoxine, pyrimethamine

6. Phenanthrene Methanol
   Halofantrine, lumefantrine, atovaquone

7. Sesquiterpine lactones
   Artesunate, artemether, arteether

CHLOROQUINE

Chloroquine is a synthetic 4-aminoquinoline.

Antimalarial actions

Chloroquine is a highly effective blood schizontocide with activity against all 4 species of plasmodia. It completely cures falciparum malaria. It is rapidly acting - patients become afebrile in 24-48 hr. Chloroquine also destroys gametocytes of P. vivax, P. ovale and P. malariae. Chloroquine is safe in pregnancy.

Mechanism of action is not clear. Chlorquine is specifically taken up by the parasite in the erythrocytes by a specific uptake mechanism. Chloroquine is a base. It concentrates in acidic food vacuoles of the parasite. Malarial parasites digest the host haemoglobin (which is their source of aminoacids) and transport it into their acidic food vacuoles In this process a toxic product 'haeme' is formed. This haeme is converted to

---

Keybox 57.1

Some points of clinical relevance

- *P. falciparum* attacks all stages of RBCs resulting in severe malaria and severe anaemia which can be fatal.
- Most antimalarials including chloroquine and quinine do not destroy gametocytes of *P. falciparum*. Hence patients with *P. falciparum* malaria also should be treated with primaquine (45 mg single dose) to destroy the gametocytes and thereby prevent the spread of malaria.
- The rupture of RBCs and the release of the parasite lytic products result in chills and fever.
- *P. falciparum* and *P. malariae* hepatic forms rupture simultaneously and do not remain in the liver.
- Both mefloquine and halofantrine are effective only orally and not parenterally – which becomes a problem in severely ill patients.
- In endemic areas, for the prevention of relapse in *P. vivax* and *P. ovale,* WHO recommends just 5 days of primaquine (15mg/day).

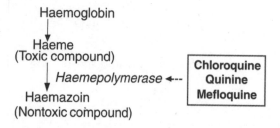

Haemoglobin

↓

Haeme
(Toxic compound)

↓ *Haemepolymerase* ← --- | Chloroquine Quinine Mefloquine |

Haemazoin
(Nontoxic compound)

nontoxic 'haemazoin' a malarial pigment, by the enzyme haeme polymerase. Chloroquine, quinine and mefloquine inhibit the enzyme haeme polymerase resulting in accumulation of haeme which causes lysis of the parasite membrane and thereby death of the parasite. Chloroquine also prevents the digestion of haemoglobin by the parasite thereby disrupting the parasite's aminoacid supply.

Chloroquine resistant strains of *P.falciparum* are now common throughout the world. Chloroquine is rapidly transported out of the food vacuole by the resistant strains. Chloroquine resistant *P. vivax* strains are also increasing and posing a problem in controlling malaria. Several studies have shown that resistance to chloroquine can be reversed by using drugs like verapamil, chlorpheniramine and desipramine. These drugs prevent the efflux of chloroquine from the parasite. But the benefits of their clinical application need to be established.

Chloroquine also has anti-inflammatory properties and is used in rheumatoid arthritis as a disease - modifying antirheumatic drug. It has activity against *Giardia lamblia* and *Entamoeba histolytica*.

Pharmacokinetics

Chloroquine is rapidly and almost completely absorbed from the gut. It is widely distributed in the tissues. It has a high affinity for melanin rich tissues and nuclear chromatin. Chloroquine has a half-life of six to seven days. It is metabolized by hepatic microsomal enzymes and is largely excreted in the urine.

Adverse effects

Though chloroquine is considered a reasonably safe drug, doses used for the treatment of malaria are often poorly tolerated as compared to prophylactic doses. Nausea and vomiting may be quite severe in some patients. Prior treatment with an antiemetic 30 minutes before chloroquine is generally practiced. Anorexia, pruritus, headache, dizziness, visual disturbances, insomnia and skin rashes may occur. IV chloroquine may cause hypotension, widening of QRS complex and arrhythmias. High doses can also cause cardiomyopathy, peripheral neuropathy and psychiatric problems. Long term suppressive therapy can cause blurring of vision, confusion, bleaching of hair and rarely blood dyscrasias. Prolonged treatment with high doses can cause irreversible retinopathy - as chloroquine accumulates in retina and can result in blindness.

Uses (Table 57.1)

1. Malaria Chloroquine is highly effective in the treatment of malaria due to sensitive strains of all 4 species - Chloroquine phosphate 250mg tab contains 150mg base; Dose 600 mg (base) stat, 300 mg after 6 hours and 300 mg for the next 2 days. It is also used for prophylaxis - 300 mg base per week.

2. Extraintestinal amoebiasis (See page 424)

3. Rheumatoid arthritis

4. Photogenic reactions

5. Lepra reactions (See page 394)

Precautions and contraindications

- Chloroquine should be avoided or used carefully in patients with myopathy and hepatic, gastrointestinal or neurological disorders, psoriasis and porphyria.

- Parenteral administration of chloroquine should be avoided but when required, it should be given as a slow infusion.

- Concurrent use of gold or d-penicillamine with chloroquine can cause more severe dermatitis.

- Chloroquine, quinine and mefloquine should not be given concurrently because they compete for accumulation in the parasite and may result in therapeutic failure. Also, chloroquine + mefloquine → increased risk of seizures.

- Chloroquine + halofantrine → increased risk of arrhythmias. Hence a gap of atleast 12 hours should be given if patients have to be switched over from chloroquine to quinine/ mefloquine/halofantrine.

- Chloroquine should be avoided in patients with retinal diseases. When chloroquine is given in high doses for a long time, regular neurological and eye examination should be done.

- Magnesium containing antacids and kaolin interfere with the absorption of chloroquine - hence concurrent use should be avoided.

QUININE

Quinine is an alkaloid obtained from the bark of the cinchona tree. It destroys erythrocytic forms of the parasite similar to chloroquine and is useful as a suppressive. It is rapidly acting and is often effective even in chloroquine resistant strains of *P.falciparum*. It is also gametocidal for three species of the malarial parasite except for *P. falciparum*. Mechanism of action is not exactly known - it may act like chloroquine by inhibiting the enzyme haeme polymerase.

Other actions

- Quinine also has mild analgesic and antipyretic activity.
- Like quinidine it is also a myocardiac depressant. IV administration can cause significant hypotension.
- It acts as a local anaesthetic (sodium channel blocker) and has skeletal muscle relaxant properties.
- Quinine stimulates the uterus and is an abortifacient.

Pharmacokinetics

Quinine is rapidly and well absorbed orally, with peak plasma levels in 1to 4 hrs widely distributed in the body, metabolized in the liver and excreted in the urine.

Adverse effects are high.

- Quinine is highly bitter and is a gastric irritant - causes nausea, vomiting and epigastric pain - hence poorly tolerated.
- Hypoglycaemia can be quite profound to result

in coma. Hypoglycemic coma should be distinguished from cerebral maleria. Hypoglycaemia may be because

   i. Quinine stimulates the insulin release.

   ii. Parasite consumes glucose.

- Cinchonism with ringing in the ears, headache, nausea, visual disturbances and vertigo may be encountered.
- Quinine produces neurotoxicity particularly in higher doses.
- Quinine can cause hypotension, (this can be profound if injected rapidly) widening of QRS complex, AV block and arrhythmias. Hence constant monitoring of cardiovascular function is a must while administering quinine intravenously.
- In more severe poisoning, hypoglycaemia, fever, delirium, confusion, hypotension, cardiac arrhythmias and coma may develop. Death is due to respiratory arrest.
- Black water fever - quinine can precipitate acute haemolytic anaemia with renal failure, haemoglobiniria and fever, which can be fatal. Fortunately this complication is uncommon and is thought to be a hypersensitivity reaction.
- Quinine can also cause skin rashes, urticaria and angioedema. Idiosyncratic reactions where the patient develops symptoms of cinchonism with a single dose of quinine is not very common.

Precautions and contraindications

1. Intravenous quinine should be injected as slow infusion and cardiac function should be monitored.

2. Hypoglycaemia should be watched for - adequate glucose supplementation should be given.

3. Quinine should never be combined with mefloquine for the risk of cardiotoxicity. If the patient has received mefloquine earlier (even upto 20-30 days) and if quinine is needed, it should be used with great caution.

Uses

- Quinine is used in the treatment of resistant falciparum malaria and cerebral malaria. Dose-Table 57.1. Quinidine can be used in the place of quinine.
- Nocturnal muscle cramps.

MEFLOQUINE

In a single dose given orally mefloquine is highly effective against erythrocytic forms of the malaria parasite including the multi-drug resistant (MDR) strains of *P. falciparum.*

Mefloquine gets concentrated in the acidic vacuoles of the parasite. Mechanism of action is not exactly known but it is thought to act like chloroquine by inhibiting haeme polymerase in the parasite. Some strains of *P. falciparum* have developed resistance to mefloquine in parts of Asia.

It is well absorbed orally and has a long t½ of nearly 20-30 days as it undergoes extensive enterohepatic circulation.

Nausea, vomiting, dizziness, confusion, abdominal pain and bradycardia are common. CNS effects like ataxia, disorientation, seizures, encephalopathy and psychotic manifestations are rare and reversible, particularly when given IV. It is contraindicated in pregnant women because its safety in them is not proved.

Uses

Mefloquine is indicated only in MDR strains of falciparum malaria - 20 mg/ kg, single dose or in two divided doses. Mefloquine can also be used in the prophylaxis of multidrug resistant malaria in travellers (250mg/week).

HALOFANTRINE

Halofantrine is schizonticidal against erythrocytic forms of all Plasmodium species including MDR strains of *P. falciparum*. Actions are similar to mefloquine. It is given orally, absorption is erratic, it is excreted in the stools.

Adverse effects

Halofantrine can cause gastrointestinal disturbances including vomiting, diarrhoea and abdominal pain. Headache and pruritus can occur. Halofantrine can also cause cardiotoxicity including prolongation of QT interval and arrhythmias. It should therefore not be given with other arrhythmogenic drugs including mefloquine.

Halofantrine has the following disadvantages:

- Mechanism of action is not known.
- The response to oral dosage is unpredictable due to variable absorption. Toxicity due to good absorption or therapeutic failure due to poor absorption may result. Absorption is enhanced by food particularly fatty food.
- Cannot be given parenterally- a disadvantage in emergencies.
- Can cause cardiotoxicity.

TABLE 57.1 Preferred antimalarials in the treatment and prophylaxis of malaria

Malaria	Drug therapy
• Chloroquine sensitive strains	
Treatment	Chloroquine Oral - 600 mg base stat, 300 mg after 6 hrs, 300 mg/day for next 2 days or 600mg (4 tabs) *stat.* 600mg (4 tabs) after 24hrs, 300mg (2 tabs) after 48hrs.
Prophylaxis	Chloroquine 2 tabs/week; start 1 week before and continue for 4 weeks after leaving the endemic area
• Chloroquine resistant and MDR strains	

Treatment	Choices are:
	1. Quinine Oral - 600 mg TDS for 3 days
	Severe cases IV 10 mg/kg 8 hourly
	followed by one of the following
	  • Doxycycline 100 mg BD for 7 days
	     or
	  • Pyrimethamine + sulfadoxine 3 tabs as a single dose on the last day of quinine therapy.
	
	2. Mefloquine 15 mg/kg single dose (Max 1500 mg)
	3. Artemisinin 100 mg BD on first day, 50 mg BD for next 5 days
	4. Atovaquone 250 mg + proguanil 100 mg daily for 3 days

Prophylaxis	1. Mefloquine 250 mg weekly; start 1 week before and continue for 4 weeks after leaving the area 2. Doxycycline 100 mg daily; start 2 days before and continue for 4 weeks after leaving the area

Keybox 57.2	
Recrudescence	- Symptoms resume after a period of remission- i.e. the disease becomes active again.
Relapse	- A new attack of the disease after a period of improvement.
Recurrence	- Same as relapse

Uses

- Halofantrine is used as an alternative in MDR strains of falciparum malaria. Dose 1500mg in three divided doses.

Lumefantrine is related to halofantrine but is not known to cause cardiotoxicity. It is combined with artemisinin/ mefloquine in the treatment of MDR falciparum malaria.

PRIMAQUINE

Primaquine is effective against all forms of the malarial parasite except erythrocytic forms.

- It destroys the parasite in the liver cells and prevents the invasion of erythrocytes - causal prophylactic. But it is generally not used for this purpose.
- Primaquine destroys the hypnozoites (exoerythrocytic form) in the liver and thereby prevents relapse of P. vivax and P. ovale malaria.
- It is also effective against the gametocytes of all four species of the malarial parasite.
- It has weak and insignificant activity against the erythrocytic forms.

Mechanism of action of primaquine is not known. It is completely absorbed orally. It is well tolerated in therapeutic doses. Epigastric distress can occur. It may cause haemolysis in patients with G_6PD deficiency.

Uses

1. Primaquine is used for radical cure along with a blood schizontocide in *P. vivax* and *ovale* - it also destroys gametocytes.

   Dose: 15mg /day for 14 days.

2. Gametocidal agent   Primaquine is used for its gametocidal effect in *P. falciparum* malaria - 45 mg single dose.

Bulaquine is an analog of primaquine developed in India (CDRI, Lucknow). It is claimed that patients require fewer days (5 days) of antirelapse therapy when compared to primaquine. But further extensive clinical trials are required to prove its clinical benefits.

Etaquine and tafenoquine are other longer acting analogs of primaquine under trial.

FOLATE ANTAGONISTS

Pyrimethamine

Pyrimethamine is effective against the erythrocytic forms of all 4 species of plasmodia but it is slow acting when given alone. Pyrimethamine is combined with sulfadoxine, a sulfonamide and the combination acts faster.

Mechanism of Action

Pyrimethamine is a dihydrofolate reductase inhibitor. Pyrimethamine preferentially binds plasmodial dihydrofolate reductase (Fig 57.2). When pyrimethamine is given with sulfadoxine, together they produce sequential blockade resulting in inhibition of nuclear division. This mode of action makes it slow acting. The combination is synergistic and the development of resistance is slower. (However, given alone sulfadoxine has no significant activity aganist erythrocytic forms of P.vivax). Pyrimethamine can also be combined with dapsone.

Pyrimethamine is quite safe; the

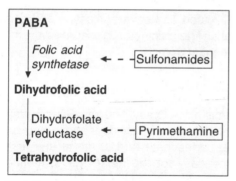

Fig. 57.2 Sequential blockade in folic acid synthesis

combination may cause nausea, rashes and in high doses megaloblastic anaemia. Sulfadoxine may cause serious allergic reactions including Steven Johnsons syndrome.

Preparations

Tablets

- Pyrimethamine 25mg + Sulfadoxine 500mg
- Pyrimethamine 25mg + Dapsone 100mg.

Uses

1. Malaria

   i. Acute attacks - Pyrimethamine + sulfadoxine combination is used as an alternative in uncomplicated, chloroquine resistant falciparum malaria. It is also used as an adjunct to quinine in acute attacks of malaria. Dose: 3 tablets as a single dose.

   ii. Prophylaxis - 1-2 tablets once weekly for prophylaxis against MDR falciparum malaria - when a person is visiting an endemic area - generally not preferred.

2. Toxoplasmosis - Pyrimethamine + sulfadoxine combination is the treatment of choice for *Toxoplasma gondii* infection. Pyrimethamine is given as 200mg bolus dose followed by 50mg daily for 4 to 6 weeks along with sulfadoxine 4g/day. Leucovorin (folinic acid) should be given 10mg daily to prevent severe folate deficiency.

Chloroguanide (Proguanil)

Chloroguanide is an erythrocytic schizontocide which also has causal prophylactic activity against the pre-erythrocytic forms of the malaria parasite.

Mechanism of action Proguanil, a prodrug, is converted to cycloguanil in the body. This metabolite is an inhibitor of dihydrofolate reductase in the plasmodium.

Adverse effects are minor including nausea, vomiting, diarrhoea, abdominal pain and rarely haematuria.

Uses

- With atovaquone in the treatment of MDR falciparum malaria.(see atovaquone).
- For causal prophylaxis of falciparum malaria.
- As an alternative to pyrimethamine-sulfadoxine for prophylaxis of MDR falciparum malaria.

ATOVAQUONE

Atovaquone is a naphthaquinone, effective against the erythrocytic forms of plasmodia. When combined with proguanil, the activity is synergistic and development of resistance is less common.

Mechanism of action

Atovaquone inhibits the mitochondrial electron transport leading to the collapse of the mitochondrial membrane potential in the malarial parasite. Proguanil potentiates this action. Atovaquone also interferes with pyrimidine synthesis in the parasite because pyrimidine (and ATP) synthesis in the parasite are dependent on mitochondrial electron transport.

Atovaquone is also effective against *T. gondii* and *P. carinii* infections.

Adverse effects include vomiting, headache and abdominal pain. Atovaquone is contraindicated in pregnancy.

Uses

Atovaquone + Proguanil can be used in the treatment of chloroquine resistant and multi drug – resistant falciparum malaria. Atovaquone 250 mg + proguanil 100 mg daily for three days. Atovaquone may also be used in *P. carinii* infection as an alternative to cotrimoxazole.

ARTEMISININ AND DERIVATIVES

Artemisinin

Artemisinin a highly bitter compound is a sesquiterpene lactone obtained from the plant Artemisia annua which has been used in Chinese traditional medicine 'Quinghaosu' for almost 2000 years

Mechanism of action

Artemisinin interacts with heme resulting in the generation of free radicals that bind to the membrane protein and damages the parasite membrane.

Artemisinin is a potent, rapidly acting, erythrocytic schizontocide effective against all the 4 plasmodial species, including MDR *P. falciparum*. It is also effective against gametocytes. It is useful in cerebral malaria. No resistant strains are known so far. Recrudescence is common due to its short t½. Combining with mefloquine avoids this. Though it is thought to be safe in pregnancy it has been shown to be teratogenic in animals.

Artesunate (oral, IM, IV, rectal) and artemether (IM, oral) artemisinin (oral) and arteether (IM) are the compounds used. Arteether is longer acting - given 150mg (IM) for 3 days. Artemisinin and its derivatives are the best tolerated antimalarials - mild GI symptoms, fever, itching and bradycardia are reported.

Uses

Acute attacks of MDR falciparum malaria including complicated and severe infection and cerebral malaria. Artemisinin can be used in severe malaria in pregnant women.

Dose

Artemisinin - Orally 100 mg BD on first day, 50 mg BD for the next 4 days and in more severe cases, artesunate IV 120 mg on the first day, 60 mg daily for the next 4 days; mefloquine (25mg/kg)is given on the second day.

NEWER ANTIMALARIALS

Pyronaridine was synthesized in China. It is effective against erythrocytic forms of the malaria parasite.

Lumefantrine is related to halofantrine but is not known to cause cardiotoxicity.

IMMUNITY IN MALARIA

People residing in an endemic area can develop antibodies to erythrocytic forms of the malaria parasite. Immunity infact can be both humoral and cell mediated. The immunity is specific to the species and strain prevalent in that particular area. Immunity could be the reason why many people do not suffer from malaria though they live in an endemic area. Passive immunity with IgG antibodies has shown to be effective in children. The transfer of maternal antibodies protects the infants from the disease upto a few months of life. If an immune person is away from the endemic area for a period of 6-12 months, his immunity is lost.

Malaria vaccine

Vaccines have been developed against the different stages of the parasite *viz* sporozoite vaccine, merozoite vaccine and gametocyte vaccine. Studies are on to evaluate the efficacy of vaccines in malaria. Pesence of multiple strains of the malaria parasite has been a major problem in the development of an effective vaccine for malaria.

58

Antiamoebic Drugs and Drugs used in Pneumocystosis, Leishmaniasis and Trypanosomiasis

- **Antiamoebic drugs**
  - **Metronidazole**
  - **Tinidazole**
  - **Secnidazole**
  - **Emetine and dehydroemetine**
  - **Diloxanide furoate**
  - **Chloroquine**
  - **Iodoquinol and quiniodochlor**
  - **Tetracylines**
  - **Treatment of different forms of amoebiasis**
- **Treatment of Pneumocystosis**
- **Treatment of Leishmaniasis**
- **Treatment of Trypanosomiasis**

ANTIAMOEBIC DRUGS

Amoebiasis caused by the protozoan Entamoeba histolytica is a tropical disease common in developing countries. It spreads by faecal contamination of food and water. Though it primarily affects colon, other organs like liver, lungs and brain are the secondary sites. Acute amoebiasis is characterised by bloody mucoid stools and abdominal pain. Chronic amoebiasis manifests as anorexia, abdominal pain, intermittent diarrhoea and constipation. Cyst passers or carriers are symptom free - they are asymptomatic carriers.

Classification

1. Drugs effective in both intestinal and extraintestinal amoebiasis

   Metronidazole, Tinidazole, Secnidazole, Ornidazole, Satranidazole, Emetine, Dehydroemetine.

2. Drugs effective only in intestinal amoebiasis (Luminal amoebicides)
   Diloxanide furoate, Quiniodochlor, Iodoquinol, Tetracylines, Paromomycin.

3. Drugs effective only in extraintestinal amoebiasis
   Chloroquine.

Ulcerative Gingivitis 200-400mg TDS is disleusum used to treat Oro dental inf

METRONIDAZOLE

Metronidazole a nitroimidazole, is a powerful amoebicide. Apart from this it also inhibits *Trichomonas vaginalis, Giardia lamblia* and *Balantidium coli.* Anaerobic bacteria are also sensitive.

Mechanism of action

Metronidazole is a prodrug. Susceptible microorganisms including anaerobic bacteria and certain protozoa reduce the nitro group of metronidazole by a nitroreductase and convert it to a cytotoxic derivative. This derivative binds to DNA and inhibits protein synthesis. Aerobic bacteria lack this nitroreductase and are therefore not susceptible to metronidazole.

Metronidazole

↓ *Nitroreductase*

Active metabolite
(Cytotoxic)

↓

Binds to DNA

↓

Inhibits protein synthesis

Pharmacokinetics

← 4m small Intestine.

Metronidazole is well-absorbed and reaches adequate concentrations in the CSF. It has a plasma t½ of 8 hrs. It is metabolised in the liver by oxidation and glucuronide conjugation.

Adverse effects

Gastrointestinal effects like nausea, anorexia, abdominal pain and metallic taste in the mouth are the most frequent. Headache, stomatitis, glossitis, furry tongue; dizziness, insomnia, ataxia, vertigo and rarely, on IV use, peripheral neuropathy can occur. Pruritus, urticaria and skin rashes can also occur. High doses given IV can cause convulsions. Hence metronidazole should be cautiously used in patients with neurological

diseases and severe hepatic dysfunction. On long term administration metronidazole is carcinogenic in mice though such an effect is not yet seen in human beings. However it is contraindicated in pregnancy. (1st trimester

Drug interactions

- Metronidazole can produce a disulfiram - like reaction in patients taking alcohol. (See page 192). Hence patients should be advised to avoid alcohol while on metronidazole.

- Drugs like cimetidine which are microsomal enzyme inhibitors, enhance plasma levels of metronidazole resulting in toxicity.

Preparations

Metronidazole is available as 200, 400 mg tablets; 200 mg /5 ml suspension; 500 mg /100 ml inj and 1% gel and ointment.

Uses

1. *Amoebiasis* - Metronidazole is the drug of choice in all forms of amoebiasis in the dose of 400-800 mg TDS for 7-10 days. But it does not eradicate the cysts.

2. *Trichomonas vaginitis* - Metronidazole 200mg TDS for 7 days or a single 2 g dose is the drug of choice.

3. *Giardiasis* - Metronidazole given 200 mg TDS for 7 days is the treatment of choice.

4. *Anaerobic infections* - Metronidazole is given intravenously for serious anaerobic infections. It is also useful for surgical prophylaxis of abdominal and pelvic infections. It is particularly useful in *C. difficile* enteritis.

5. *H. pylori infections* in peptic ulcer patients can be treated with a combination of metronidazole, clarithromycin and omeprazole/ranitidine.

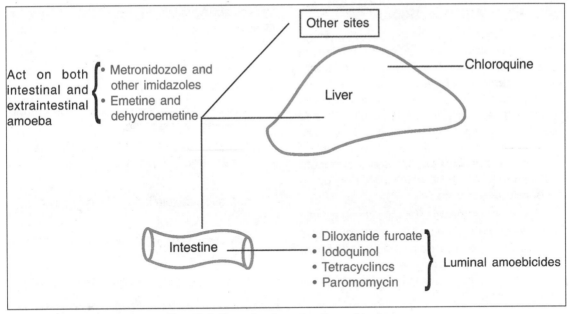

Fig. 58.1 Sites of action of antiamoebic drugs.

6. *Pseudomembranous colitis* due to *Clostridium difficile* - responds to metronidazole.

7. *Acute ulcerative gingivitis*-metronidozole can be used as an alternative to penicillin G.

8. *Dracunculosis* Metronidazole facilitates extraction of the guinea worm.

9. *Topical preparations* - 1% Gel is used in skin infections and acne.

Tinidazole is longer-acting and is better tolerated than metronidazole due to lesser side effects. It can be given 2 g once daily for 3 days in amoebiasis and as a single dose for most other indications of metronidazole.

Secnidazole is longer-acting and can be given as a single 2 g dose for most indications of metronidazole.

EMETINE AND DEHYDROEMETINE

Emetine is an alkaloid, derived from Ipecac (Brazil root) while dehydroemetine is a semisynthetic analog. They directly affect the trophozoites but not the cysts. As oral absorption is improper, they are given parenterally (SC or IM but not IV). Emetine or dehydroemetine can be used only in severe amoebiasis for 3-5 days in patients in whom metronidazole cannot be used but are generally not preferred due to toxicity. Adverse effects include pain at the injection site, thrombophlebitis, nausea, vomiting and diarrhoea. Cardiotoxicity including arrythmias, hypotension and cardiac failure can occur. These drugs should be avoided in patients with cardiac dysfunction. Dehydroemetine is preferred over emetine as adverse effects are milder.

DILOXANIDE FUROATE

Diloxanide furoate is directly amoebicidal. Flatulence, nausea and occasionally abdominal cramps and rashes can occur. It is used alone in asymptomatic cyst passers, mild intestinal amoebiasis and along with a nitroimidazole - for the cure of amoebiasis, as diloxanide eradicates cysts. It is given orally - 500 mg TDS for 10 days. It is also available in combination with metronidazole (DYRADE-M).

IODOQUINOL AND QUINIODOCHLOR

These 8-hydroxyquinolines are directly acting luminal amoebicides. The exact mechanism of action is not known. They are effective orally. Adverse effects include headache, nausea, vomiting, abdominal pain and diarrhoea. Iodine present in these componds may result in thyroid enlargement, pruritus and skin rashes. Prolonged used of some of these compounds like clioquinol can produce neurotoxicity including subacute myelooptic neuropathy in which there may be an irreversible loss of vision.

Iodoquinol appears to be safe at therapeutic doses and is often used for asymptomatic amoebiasis - requires treatment for 20 days. However diloxanide furoate which is safer and needs shorter duration of administration (10 days) is now preferred.

PAROMOMYCIN

Paromomycin is an aminoglycoside antibiotic given orally. It is poorly absorbed from the gut and acts as an intestinal amoebicide. Adverse effects are mild and include diarrhoea and abdominal discomfort. Paromomycin is used as a luminal amoebicide.

TETRACYLINES

The older tetracylines like chlortetracycline are not well-absorbed and large amounts reach the colon - hence these are useful in intestinal amoebiasis. They inhibit the intestinal flora and break the symbiosis between them and the amoebae. Tetracyclines are used as adjuvants in chronic cases.

CHLOROQUINE

Chloroquine attains high concentration in the liver, is directly toxic against trophozoites and is therefore useful in hepatic amoebiasis. As chloroquine is completely absorbed from the small intestines, it is not effective against amoebae in the colon. It is used (300 mg base/day for 21 days) as an alternative to metronidazole in hepatic

amoebiasis. A luminal amoebicide should also be given.

Treatment of different forms of amoebiasis

1. **Acute intestinal amoebiasis** - one of the following can be given.
   - Metronidazole 400-800 mg TDS for 5-7 days (METROGYL)

     or
   - Metronidazole 2.4 g OD for 3 days

     or
   - Tinidazole 2 g OD for 3 days (TINIBA)

     or
   - Secnidazole 2 g single dose (SECZOL).

   All of the above should be followed by diloxanide furoate 500 mg TDS for 10 days to eradicate the cysts.

2. **Chronic amoebiasis and asymptomatic cyst passers** - Diloxanide furoate 500 mg TDS for 10 days or tetracycline 250 mg qid for 10 days. The alternatives are iodoquinol (650 mg TDS for 21 days) or paromomycin (10 mg/kg TDS for 7 days).

3. **Hepatic amoebiasis** - requires intensive treatment for the complete eradication of the parasite from the liver in order to avoid relapses. A course of metronidazole 600-800 mg TDS for 10 days or tinidazole are the first line drugs. In addition chloroquine may be given to ensure complete destruction of the liver forms. A course of diloxanide furoate 500 mg TDS for 10 days should follow in order to eradicate the cysts.

TREATMENT OF PNEUMOCYSTOSIS

Pneumocystis carinii is a micro organism having features of both protozoa and fungi though now considered by most to be a fungus. Recent studies have shown that pneumocystosis in human beings is caused by *Pneumcystis jiroveri* while *P.carinii* causes pneumocystosis in animals.

It is now known to cause opportunistic infections particularly pneumonia in patients with AIDS which can often be fatal.

Drugs used in the treatment of pneumocystosis include

- Cotrimoxazole - high oral dose of Trimethoprim 20 mg/kg + sulphamethoxazole 100 mg/kg daily.
- Pentamidine - 4 mg/kg daily for 14 days parenterally.
- Atovaquone - as an alternative to cotrimoxazole.

TREATMENT OF LEISHMANIASIS

Leishmaniasis is caused by protozoa of the genus leishmania kala-azar or visceral leishmaniasis is caused by Leishmania donovani; oriental sore by L. tropica and mucocutaneous leishmaniasis by L. braziliensis. The infection is transmitted by the bite of the female sandfly phlebotomus. It is endemic in Bihar.

Drugs used in leishmaniasis include

Antimony compounds -Sodium stibogluconate
Meglumine antimonate

Diamidines - Pentamidine

Other drugs - Amphotericin B, Ketoconazole, Allopurinol, Paramomycin.

ANTIMONY COMPOUNDS

Sodium stibogluconate

Sodium stibogluconate a pentavalent antimonial is the most effective drug in kala-azar. It is also effective in mucocutaneous and cutaneous leishmaniasis. It is given as a 4% solution in the dose of 10-20 mg/kg IM (gluteal region) or IV for 20 days. Mechanism of action is unknown.

Adverse effects include a metallic taste in the mouth, nausea, vomiting, diarrhoea, headache, myalgia, arthralgia, pain at the injection site, bradycardia, skin rashes, haematuria and jaundice. Some cases of sudden death due to shock have occurred. ECG should be monitored as arrhythmias can occur during the later days of therapy.

Though sodium stibogluconate is quite effective, resistance has been encountered in endemic areas like Bihar.

Meglumine antimonate and ethyl stibamine can also be used in all forms of leishmaniasis.

Pentamidine

Pentamidine is an aromatic diamidine effective against *Leishmania donovani,* trypanosomes, *Pneumocystis carinii* and some fungi. Given intramuscularly the drug is rapidly absorbed but very little reaches the CNS. Dose 4 mg/kg deep IM/slow IV on alternate days for 5-25 weeks.

Adverse effects Pentamidine liberates histamine which is responsible for vomiting, diarrhoea, flushing, pruritis, rashes, tachycardia and hypotension apart from pain at the injection site. Other effects include hepatotoxicity, renal impairment, ECG changes and in some patients diabetes mellitus may be precipitated.

Uses

1. Leishmaniasis Pentamidine can be used in visceral leishmaniasis as an alternative to sodium stibogluconate.

2. Trypanosomiasis (sleeping sickness) Pentamidine can be used as an alternative to suramin or along with suramin in trypanosomiasis. It can also be used for chemoprophylaxis against African trypanosomiasis.

3. Pneumocystosis Pentamidine is an alternative in Pneumocystis jiroveci infections in patients unable to tolerate

cotrimoxazole.

OTHER DRUGS

Amphotericin B (See page 397) has been tried in leishmaniasis in the endemic areas where antimonials may be ineffective.

Ketoconazole inhibits ergosterol synthesis in the leishmania and is effective in cutaneous leishmaniasis.

Allopurinol (See page 240) In leishmania, allopurinol is converted to a metabolite which inhibits protein synthesis. It may be used along with antimonials.
Dose 300 mg 3-4 times a day for 2-4 weeks.

Paromomycin (aminosidine) is an amoebicidal drug which is also found to be effective in leishmaniasis. It is useful in all forms of leishmaniasis. It can be used alone or in combination with antimonials.

TREATMENT OF TRYPANOSOMIASIS

Trypanosomiasis is caused by protozoa of the genus Trypanosoma. African trypanosomiasis or sleeping sickness is caused by *T. gambiense* and *T. rhodesiense* while South American trypanosomiasis is caused by *T. Cruzi*. Drugs used in trypanosomiasis are suramin, pentamidine, melarsoprol, eflornithine, nifurtimox and benznidazole.

Suramin sodium

Suramin sodium is the drug of choice for early stage of trypanosomiasis but it does not cross the BBB and therefore cannot be used in later stages of the disease. It is also useful for the prophylaxis but pentamidine is preferable. Suramin is given IV; it is extensively bound to plasma proteins and may be traced for nearly 3 months in the plasma. Suramin is also effective in eradicating adult forms of Onchocerca volvulus.

Toxicity is high; vomiting, shock and loss of consciousness may follow IV injections. Rash, neuropathies, haemolytic anaemia and agranulocytosis may also occur.

Melarsoprol

Melarsoprol is the preferred drug in later stages of trypanosomiasis which is associated with encephalitis and meningitis.

Eflornithine

Eflornithine is used as an alternative in CNS trypanosomiasis. Nifurtimox and benznidazole are useful in Chaga's disease (American trypanosomiasis).

59

Anthelmintics & Drugs used in Scabies & Pediculosis

- • **Benzimidazoles**
- • **Pyrantel pamoate**
- • **Piperazine citrate**
- • **Levamisole**
- • **Niclosamide**
- • **Praziquantel**
- • **Diethylcarbamazine**
- • **Ivermectin**
- • **Metrifonate**

Worm infestations are more common in the developing countries. It is seen in people with poor hygiene. Anthelmintics are deworming agents. A **vermicidal** kills while a **vermifuge** promotes expulsion of worms. Several deworming agents are now available and it is possible to successfully treat many worm infestations.

BENZIMIDAZOLES

Benzimidazoles include thiabendazole, mebendazole and albendazole. Thiabendazole the first agent of this group was discovered in 1961 but now the newer ones, mebendazole and albendazole are more commonly used due to lesser toxicity and better anthelmintic effect.

MEBENDAZOLE

Mebendazole a broad spectrum anthelmintic cures roundworm, hookworm, pinworm and strongyloides infestations. The eggs and larvae are also destroyed. The dead parasites are slowly expelled from the gut over several days.

Mechanism of action

Benzimadazoles bind to β- tubulin of the parasite with high affinity and inhibit the synthesis of microtubules these microtubules are essential for several metabolic process in the parasite. Benzimidazoles also inhibit glucose uptake in the parasite.

Pharmacokinetics

Mebendazole is poorly absorbed from the gut and also undergoes first pass metabolism -

bioavailability around 20%. Fatty food enhances absorption. Mebendazole is extensively bound to plasma proteins and is metabolised by the liver.

Mebendazole is given orally 100mg twice a day for 3 days.

Adverse effects

Mebendazole is well-tolerated; nausea, abdominal pain and diarrhoea may be seen in heavy infestations. Large doses may cause headache, dizziness, loss of hair and granulocytopenia. Rarely it may provoke abnormal migration of the roundworms which may come out through the mouth or nose.

Uses

Mebendazole is used in the treatment of roundworm, hookworm, pinworm, tapeworm, trichuriasis and hydatid disease. It is of special value in multiple worm infestations (Table 59.1).

ALBENDAZOLE

Albendazole is a congener of mebendazole with actions and mechanism of action similar to mebendazole but it has several advantages over it. It is also a broad spectrum anthelmintic with many advantages over mebendazole.

Advantages over mebendazole

* Albendazole is better tolerated
* Effective in single dose in most infections
* Superior to mebendazole in hook worm and thread worm infections, hydatid disease and neurocysticercosis

TABLE 59.1 Preferred drugs for helminthiasis infections		
Worms	*Drugs of choice*	*Alternative drugs*
1. Roundworm (*Ascaris lumbricoides*)	Mebendazole/albendazole/ pyrantel	Piperazine
2. Hookworms (*Ancylostoma duodenale, Necator americanus*)	Mebendazole/ albendazole	Pyrantel
3. Pinworm (*Enterobius vermicularis*)	Mebendazole/albendazole/ pyrantel	Piperazine
4. Whipworm (*Trichuris trichura*)	Mebendazole	Albendazole
5. Strongyloides stercoralis	Albendazole	Thiabendazole
6. Guineaworm (*Dracunculous medinensis*)	Metronidazole	Mebendazole
7. Tapeworms (*Taenia saginata, Taenia solium, H. nana, D. latum*)	Niclosamide/ praziquantel	Albendazole
Neurocysticercosis	Albendazole	Praziquantel
8. Hydatid disease (*E. granulosus, E. multilocularis*)	Albendazole	Mebendazole
9. Filaria (*Wuchareria bancrofti, Brugia malayi*)	Diethylcarbamazine + albendazole	Ivermection albendazole
10. Schistosomes	Praziquantel	—
11. Onchocerca volvulus	Ivermectin	—
12. Fasciola hepatica (Sheep liver fluke)	Bithionol	—

- Albendazole also has some activity against *Trichomonas vaginalis*, *Giardia lamblia* and *W.bancrofti*.

- The active metabolite of albendazole achieves a higher concentration (100 times more) than mebendazole.

Pharmacokinetics

Albendazole is rapidly absorbed from the gut and fatty food enhances its absorption. Hence it should be given on an empty stomach for treating intestinal worms while for parasites in the tissues, albendazole is given with a fatty meal. It penetrates well into tissues including hydatid cyst. It is rapidly metabolised in the liver and excreted in urine.

Adverse effects - are minor similar to mebendazole. Nausea, diarrhoea, abdominal pain, headache and dizziness can occur. High doses used over a long time can cause jaundice, fever, weakness, alopecia and graunlocytopenia. Albendazole is teratogenic in animals and therefore should not be given in pregnancy.

Uses

1. Albendazole is the drug of choice in roundworm, hookworm, pinworm, trichuriasis infestations in a single 400 mg dose. Dose should be repeated after 2 weeks in pinworm infestation to prevent reinfection from ova that have matured later.

2. Trichinosis, tapeworms and strongyloidosis require 400mg daily for 3 days.

3. Neurocysticercosis - Albendazole is the drug of choice in a dose of 400mg twice daily but the duration depends on the number of cysts and may vary from 3 to 28 days. Glucocorticoids should be given before starting albendazole to prevent immunological reactions to the dead parasite.

4. Hydatid disease - Albendazole is the drug of choice; 400mg twice daily is given for 4 weeks. If needed, the course may be repeated after 2 weeks. When the cysts are removed by surgery, albendazole is more effective in providing cure.

5. Filariasis - Combination of albendazole (400mg) with DEC (6mg/kg) or ivermectin (0.3mg/kg) given as a single dose is found to be effective in *W. bancrofti* in suppressing microfilariae for one year. This also prevents the spread of filariasis and may be continued once a year for 5-6 years.

THIABENDAZOLE

Thiabendazole a benzimidazole, acts like mebendazole. But due to frequent side effects, it is not preferred. Dizziness, anorexia, vomiting, diarrhoea, drowsiness, paraesthesia, bradycardia, hypotension, convulsions and liver damage can occur. It is used as an alternative to albendazole in strongyloidosis and cutaneous larva migrans.

PYRANTEL PAMOATE

Pyrantel pamoate is effective against roundworm, hookworm and pinworms. It stimulates the nicotinic cholinergic receptor in the worm leading to persistent depolarisation and spastic paralysis (depolarising neuromuscular blocker). The paralysed worms are expelled.

It is well-tolerated; occasional abdominal pain, headache, rashes, weakness and dizziness may occur. Dose: 10-15 mg/kg single dose.

Uses

Pyrantel is used in the treatment of roundworm, hookworm and pinworm infestations.

OXANTEL PAMOATE

Oxantel pamoate an analog of pyrantel pamoate is effective in the treatment of trichuriasis infection.

PIPERAZINE CITRATE

Piperazine citrate is effective in roundworm and pinworm infestations. It competitively blocks the action of acetylcholine and thereby contractions in the worms. Flaccid paralysis results and the worms are expelled.

Adverse effects are mild - gastrointestinal symptoms, headache and dizziness are seen occasionally. Piperazine citrate is indicated for roundworm and pinworm infestations. It is also safe in pregnancy.

LEVAMISOLE

Levamisole is effective against roundworms and hookworms and can be used as an alternative drug in these infestations. It is well-tolerated and is effective in a single dose. It is also an immunomodulator.

NICLOSAMIDE

Niclosamide is effective against most tapeworms. The segments of the dead tapeworms are partly digested and in case of *T. solium*, the ova released from these segments may develop into larvae and reach various organs resulting in visceral cysticercosis. Purge may be given 2 hours after niclosamide to wash off the worms and avoid cysticercosis. The scolex detected in the stool ensures eradication.

Niclosamide is well-tolerated. Abdominal discomfort and rarely pruritus and rashes may occur.

Uses

Niclosamide is the drug of choice in infestations by tapeworms like *T. solium, T. saginata, H. nana* and *D. latum*. It is also an alternative drug in intestinal fluke infestation.

PRAZIQUANTEL

Praziquantel is effective against schistosomes of all species, most other trematodes and cestodes including cysticercosis. It is effective as a single oral dose in most infestations. It increases cell membrane permeability to calcium resulting in contraction followed by paralysis and the worms are expelled.

Adverse effects are mild and include GI disturbances, headache, dizziness, drowsiness, rashes and myalgia.

Uses

1. Schistosomiasis: Praziquantel is the drug of choice in all forms of schistosomiasis.

2. Tapeworms: Single dose (10 mg/kg) of praziquantel is effective in all tapeworm infestations. In *T. solium* it has the advantage that it kills the larvae and therefore visceral cysticercosis is avoided.

3. Neurocysticercosis: Praziquantel is an alternative to albendazole.

DIETHYLCARBAMAZINE (DEC)

Diethylcarbamazine is the drug of choice in filariasis. It immobilizes the microfilariae resulting in their displacement in the tissues and also alters their surface structure making them more susceptible to the host defense mechanisms. Microfilariae rapidly disappear from the blood except those present in hydrocele and nodules.

Adverse effects are mild; anorexia, nausea, vomiting, dizziness and headache; allergic reactions with itching, rashes and fever due to release of antigens from the dying worms may occur. Antihistamines are given with DEC to minimize these reactions. DEC can be given during pregnancy.

Uses

- Filariasis DEC is the drug of choice (2 mg/kg TDS for 21 days). In 7 days patients are rendered non-infective to mosquitoes as microfilariae rapidly disappear. But adult worms may need repeated courses.

- Tropical eosinophilia (2 mg/kg TDS for 7 days). Symptoms rapidly disappear.

IVERMECTIN

Ivermectin is a semisynthetic analog of

avermectin B obtained from *Streptomyces avermitilis*. Ivermectin is effective against many nematodes, arthropods and filariae that infect animals and human beings. Ivermectin is very effective against the microfilaria of *Onchocerca volvulus*. It is microfilaricidal and also blocks the release of microfilariae from the uterus of adult worms. There is a rapid decrease in the microfilarial count in the skin and eyes.

Ivermectin is believed to act by paralysing the worms by binding to GABA - gated chloride channels and enhancing GABA activity.

Ivermectin is as effective as DEC against *W. bancrofti* and *B.malayi*. It is also effective against *Strongyloidis stercoralis, Ascaris lumbricoides, cutaneous larva migrans, Sarcoptis scabii* and lice.

Adverse effects

Ivermectin is well tolerated. Apart from nausea and vomiting, allergic reactions can result due to hypersensitivity to the dying microfilarial proteins (mazotti reaction).

Ivermectin should not be used with other drugs that influence GABA activity (eg. benzodiazepines, valproic acid) in patients with meningitis and sleeping sickness as these conditions impair the BBB.

Uses

1. Ivermectin is the preferred drug in the treatment of onchocerciasis.

2. Ivermectin is also useful in the treatment of lymphatic filariasis.

3. A single dose of 400 mg/kg ivermectin with 400 mg albendazole is given once a year for mass chemotherapy of lymphatic filariasis.

4. Strongyloidiasis - A single dose of 200 mg/kg is curative in strongyloidiasis. However the dose is to be repeated on the second day.

5. Ivermectin is also useful in cutaneous larva migrans, ascariasis, in scabies and lice

infestations.

METRIFONATE

Metrifonate is a prodrug that is converted to dichlorovas – an organophosphorus insecticide. Metrifonate is used as an alternative to praziquantel in the treatment of *Schistosoma haematobium* infections.

OXAMNIQUINE is effective against *S. mansoni* and is used as an alternative to praziquantel in the treatment of *S. mansoni* infections.

BITHIONOL is the drug of choice in the treatment of *Fasciola hepatica* infections.

DRUGS USED IN SCABIES AND PEDICULOSIS

Scabies is caused by *Sarcoptes scabiei* or *Acarus scabiei* (itch mite). Scabies is more common in people with poor hygiene. It is transmitted by close body contact with an infected person and spreads easily in overcrowded housing conditions. Drugs used in scabies are as follows

Benzyl Benzoate

Benzyl Benzoate is a liquid applied in the form of 25% emulsion. After a hot scrub bath, the emulsion should be applied over the entire body below the chin including the soles of the feet. The application should be repeated after 12 hours and after the next 12 hours the hot scrub bath should be repeated. Benzyl benzoate can cause irritation, specially when repeated frequently.

Permethrin

Permethrin a synthetic pyrethroid, is an insecticide effective against scabies and lice. The insects are paralysed and a single application is sufficient in most patients. 5% cream is applied all over the body below the chin and washed after 12 hours. It is safe, effective, convenient to use and well tolerated with nearly 100% cure rates. It has therefore now been preferred by many over benzyl benzoate for the treatment of scabies and pediculosis. For pediculosis 1% cream is rubbed over the scalp, allowed to remain for 10 minutes and then washed off.

Lindane or Gamma benzene hexachloride (Gammexane, BHC)

1% of lindane in a vegetable oil/cream is applied over the body and the treatment repeated after 2-3 days. It is found to be an effective scabicide as well as pediculocide and causes milder irritation when compared to other drugs. But resistance to lindane is common this can be prevented by combining it with benzyl benzoate which improves efficacy. Another disadvantage is that lindane is highly lipid soluble because of which it can be absorbed through intact skin resulting in systemic toxicity. Lindane can cause arrhythmias and seizures - it is a CNS stimulant. It can rarely cause aplastic anaemia.

OTHER DRUGS

Crotamiton

Crotamiton is effective against both lice and scabies. It needs to be applied as 10% cream 2-3 times at an interval of 24 hours followed by a wash. It is unlikely to cause irritation because of which it may be preferred in children.

Ivermectin

Ivermectin an anthelmintic, is also found to be effective in scabies and pediculosis. It differs from all other scabicides in that it is given orally. A single dose of 200 mcg/kg is highly effective and cure rates have been 91 – 95%. It is well tolerated but should be avoided in pregnant and lactating women and in children.

Sulfur

10% sulfur ointment was used earlier but it is now not preferred because it is inconvenient to use, has an unpleasant smell and needs to be applied repeatedly.

DDT

DDT is applied as a 2% lotion for pediculosis and scabies. It paralyses the insects. It is now not preferred because of the availability of better scabicides and pediculocides.

Tetmosol (monosulphiram)

Tetmosol is related to disulfiram. 5% solution is applied three times in 24 hours for scabies. It is an effective sarcopticide. It can cause mild irritation. Alcohol consumption should be avoided and tetmosol should not be used in children below 5 years of age.

PEDICULOSIS

Pediculosis is caused by the louse *Pediculus humanus.* Lice can infest scalp, body or pubic region. Drugs used in lice infestations include permethrin 1% lotion (left for 10 minutes), DDT 2% lotion, gammaxane 2% shampoo, malathion 0.5% lotion or any of the other drugs for scabies including benzyl benzoate (not preferred because of weak ovicidal action). Permethrin is the preferred drug for topical use while ivermectin may be used orally as a single dose.

60 Cancer Chemotherapy

- Phases of cell cycle
- Classification
- General adverse effects to anticancer drugs
- Alkylating Agents
- Antimetabolites
- Natural products
- Miscellaneous
- Hormones in cancer chemotherapy
- Radio active isotopes
- Bioloical Response Modifiers
- General principles in the treatment of cancers

Cancer is one of the major causes of death. The treatment of cancers after so many years of research and experience is still unsatisfactory due to certain characteristics of the cancer cells - like capacity for uncontrolled proliferation, invasiveness and metastasis. Moreover the cancer cells are our own cells unlike microbes, which means that, drugs which destroy these cancer cells also can affect normal cells. The host defence mechanisms which help us in infections are not doing so in cancers as these cancer cells are also host cells. To further complicate the problem, the cancer cells can be in a resting phase during which they are not sensitive to anticancer drugs but can start multiplying later - resulting in recurrence. These features have made treatment of cancers quite difficult.

Phases of cell cycle

Four phases of the cell cycle are G_1, S, G_2, and M (Fig 60.1). G_1 is the presynthetic phase and the duration is variable. During the S phase the synthesis of DNA occurs and hence the activity of replicating enzymes like DNA and RNA polymerases, topoisomerases, thymidine kinases and dihydrofolate reductases are maximum at this

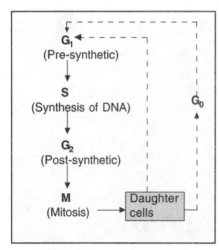

Fig 60.1 Phases of Cell Cycle

phase of 12 to 18 hrs duration. G_2 is the postsynthetic phase (1 to 8 hrs) and in the M phase (1 to 2 hrs) the mitosis takes place. The daughter cells may start dividing or may enter into a dormant phase called G_0. The knowledge of cell cycle may be used for staging and scheduling treatment because different drugs act at different stages of the cell cycle. However, some drugs are cell cycle non specific (Table 60.1).

GENERAL ADVERSE EFFECTS TO ANTICANCER DRUGS

Since most anticancer drugs act on the rapidly multiplying cells, they are also toxic to the normal rapidly multiplying cells in the bone marrow, epithelial cells of skin and mucous membranes lymphoid organs and gonads. Thus the common adverse effects are:

1. **Bone marrow depression** resulting in leukopenia, anaemia, thrombocytopenia and in higher doses - aplastic anaemia. In such patients, infections and bleeding are common.

2. **Other proliferating cells**
   - GIT - stomatitis, oesophagitis, glossitis and proctitis can be painful. Diarrhoea and ulcers along the gut are common.
   - Alopecia (loss of hair)- partial to total alopecia is seen following treatment with most anticancer drugs but it is reversible and the hair grows after the chemotherapy is completed.
   - Reduced spermatogenesis in men and amenorrhoea in women (due to damage to the germinal epithelium) can occur. For example: men treated with mechlorethamine for 6 months can become infertile.

3. **Immediate adverse effects** Nausea and vomiting are very common with most cytotoxic drugs. They result from the stimulation of the CTZ and starts about 4 to 6 hrs after treatment and may continue for 1 to 2 days. Prior treatment with powerful antiemetics is required. (Table 60.2)

4. **Hyperuricaemia** Rapid tumor cell lysis can result in an increased plasma uric acid levels and may precipitate gout.

5. **Teratogenicity** All cytotoxic drugs are teratogenic and are therefore contraindicated in pregnancy.

6. **Carcinogenicity** Cytotoxic drugs themselves may cause secondary cancers, e.g. leukaemias may follow the treatment of Hodgkin's lymphoma.

Measures to prevent adverse effects to antica cer drugs - See table 60.2. Apart from the above, the adverse effects unique to some drugs are discussed under individual drugs and listed in Table 60.3.

Drugs used in cancers may be classified as follows:

CLASSIFICATION	
1. Alkylating agents	
Nitrogen mustards	Mechlorethamine, cyclophosphamide, ifosfamide, chlorambucil, melphalan
Ethylenimines	Thio-TEPA
Alkyl sulfonate	Busulfan
Nitrosoureas	Carmustine, streptozocin
Triazine	Dacarbazine
2. Antimetabolites	
Folate antagonist	Methotrexate
Purine analogues	6-Mercaptopurine, thioguanine, pentostatin, fludarabin,cladribin.
Pyrimidine analogues	5-Fluorouracil, floxuridine, capecitabine, cytarabine (cytosine arabinoside) gemcitabine
3. NATURAL PRODUCTS	
• **Antibiotics**	Actinomycin-D (Dactinomycin), daunorubicin, doxorubicin, bleomycin, mitomycin-C, mithramycin
• **Epipodophyllotoxins**	Etoposide, teniposide
• **Camptothecins**	Topotecan, irinotecan
• **Taxanes**	Paclitaxel, docetaxel
• **Vinca alkaloids**	Vincristine, vinblastine, vinorelbine
4. Miscellaneous	Hydroxyurea, procarbazine, mitotane, l-asparaginase, cisplatin, interferon alpha, imatinib.
5. Hormones and their antagonists	Glucocorticoids, androgens, antiandrogens, oestrogens, antioestrogens, progestins, aromatase inhibitors.

ALKYLATING AGENTS

Alkylating agents are drugs that alkylate (donate an alkyl group to) other molecules by covalent bonds. They also alkylate DNA, RNA and various enzymes and there is interstand cross linking of DNA.

Actions

Alkylating agents exert -

1. Cytotoxic effects - Alkylating agents destroy the rapidly multiplying cells - both cancer cells and normal host cells.

2. Immunosuppresant effects- Alkylating agents are good immunosuppressants for which they are used in rheumatoid arthritis and other autoimmune disorders.

3. Radiomimetic effects- the actions of alkylating agents resemble that of radiotherapy.

Mechanism of action

On administration, alkylating agents form highly reactive derivatives (carbonium ions) which transfer alkyl groups to various (nucleophilic) cellular constituents and bind them with covalent bonds. Thus such constituents are not available for normal metabolic reactions. Moreover, alkylation of DNA results in breakage of the DNA strand. Thus they produce cytotoxicity.

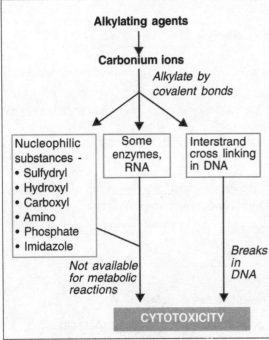

Mechanism of action of alkylating agents

NITROGEN MUSTARDS

Mechlorethamine

Mechlorethamine is given IV as it is a highly irritant compound. It is used in Hodgkin's lymphoma (MOPP regimen). Adverse effects are those discussed under general adverse effects including bone marrow suppression, nausea, vomiting, diarrhoea, alopecia, gut ulcerations, amenorrhoea in women and reduced spermatogenesis in men. Since it is an irritant it can cause severe pain and irritation at the site of injection. mechlorethamine is not preferred nowadays and mechlorethamine is now generally replaced by cyclophosphamide in MOPP regimen for Hodgkin's lymphoma.

Cyclophosphamide

Cyclophosphamide is a prodrug it is converted to its active metabolite aldophosphamide in the body. It can be given orally, IM or IV.

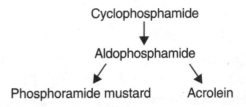

Cyclophosphamide causes cystitis due to a metabolite acrolein. This can be prevented by giving IV **Mesna,** irrigating the bladder with acetylcysteine, and by giving large amounts of fluids. Mesna (sodium-2-mercaptoethane sulfonate) and acetylcysteine contain SH groups which bind the toxic metabolites and inactivate them.

Uses

- Cyclophosphamide can be used in Hodgkin's lymphoma in place of mechlorethamine in MOPP regimen.
- In non Hodgkin's lymphomas (NHL) it can be

TABLE 60.1 Cell cycle specific and non-specific drugs	
Cell cycle specific drugs	*Cell cycle non-specific drugs*
S phase- Antimetabolites, Doxorubicin, Epipodophyllotoxins, Vinca alkaloids.	Alkylating agents
	Anticancer antibiotics
G₂ and M Phases - Bleomycin	Cisplatin
M phase - Taxanes, Vinca alkaloids.	Procarbazine, Camptothecins.

TABLE 60.2 Measures to prevent the adverse effects of anticancer drugs.

	Toxity	Measures
1.	Nausea, vomiting	Antiemetics - Ondanseteron, Granisetron, Metoclopramide.
2.	Hyperuricaemia	Allopurinol
3.	Methotrexate toxicity	Folinic acid (10mg). Dose as per blood methotrexate levels.
4.	Cystitis due to cyclophosphamide & Ifosphamide	Mesna -IV; n-acetyl cysteine- bladder wash; Plenty of oral fluids.
5.	Myelosuppression	Iron, blood transfusion,
	- Anaemia	Erythropoietin
	- Leukopenia	G-CSF, GM- CSF
	- Thrombocytopenia	Thrombopoietin
6.	• Nephrotoxicity due to cisplatin • Xerostomia due to radiation	Amifostin

used with Doxorubicin (hydroxydaunomycin), Vincristine (oncovin) and Prednisolone (CHOP regimen). Cyclophosphamide is also useful in Burkitt's lymphoma in children, leukemias and myeloma.

- Cyclophosphamide is an immunosuppressive agent.

Ifosfamide an analog of cyclophosphamide has actions and toxicities similar to cyclophosphamide except that it is longer acting. It causes cystitis like cyclophosphamide but it is less myelotoxic than cyclophosphamide. Mesna is given with ifosfamide.

Chlorambucil (LEUKERAN) is very effective against lymphoid series. It was the drug of choice in chronic lymphocytic leukaemia. Chlorambucil is also used in lymphomas. Alopecia, nausea and vomiting are milder than many other alkylating agents.

Melphalan is given orally in multiple myeloma. Its actions and toxicities are similar to other nitrogen mustards but alopecia, nausea and vomiting are comparatively milder.

Busulfan (MYLERAN) an alkyl sulfonate has selective activity against cells of the myeloid series and was used in chronic myeloid leukaemia- but now other drugs are preferred - (Table 60.4). Busulfan can cause skin pigmentation, gynaecomastia and pulmonary fibrosis.

NITROSOUREAS

Carmustine

Carmustine is effective in meningeal leukaemias and brain tumours because it crosses the blood-brain barrier. It causes profound bone marrow depression. It is also used in lymphomas and malignant melanoma.

Streptozocin is an antibiotic. It is used in pancreatic islet cell tumors. It can cause nephrotoxicity apart from the other adverse effects common to most anticancer drugs.

Dacarbazine is useful in malignant melanoma and Hodgkin's lymphoma.

Temozolamide is a new introduction used in gliomas and melanoma.

TABLE 60.3 Specific adverse effects of some anticancer drugs		
Drugs	**Specific adverse effects**	**Other prominent adverse effects**
Cyclo-phosphamide	Cystitis stomatitis,	Bone marrow depression, alopecia, vomiting, amenorrhoea, teratogenicity
Busulfan	Pulmonary fibrosis stomatitis,	Bone marrow depression, alopecia, vomiting, amenorrhoea, teratogenicity
Cisplatin	Ototoxicity	Renal dysfunction
Bleomycin	Pulmonary fibrosis, oedema of hands	Stomatitis, alopecia
Daunorubicin	Cardiotoxicity, red coloured urine	Bone marrow depression, alopecia
Doxorubicin	Cardiotoxicity	Bone marrow depression, aiopecia
Mithramycin (Plicamycin)	Hepatotoxicity	Thrombocytopenia
Vincristine	Neurotoxicity, Peripheral neuritis, mental depression	Muscle weakness, alopecia
Asparaginase Mitotane	Pancreatitis, hepatotoxicity, Dermatitis, mental depression	Allergic reactions Diarrhoea

ANTIMETABOLITES

FOLATE ANTAGONIST

Methotrexate is a folic acid antagonist. It binds to dihydrofolate reductase and prevents the formation of tetrahydrofolate (THF). This THF is a coenzyme essential in several reactions in DNA, RNA and protein synthesis. The deficiency results in inhibition of protein synthesis. Thus rapidly multiplying cells are the most affected. Methotrexate is most effective on cells in the 'S' phase of cell cycle.

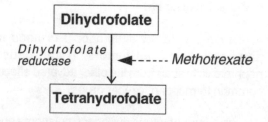

Actions

Cytotoxic actions - methotrexate mainly affects the bone marrow, skin and gastrointestinal mucosa and other rapidly dividing cells.

It also has immunosuppresant and some anti-inflammatory properties.

Pharmacokinetics

Methotrexate is well absorbed when given orally. It can be given parenterally (IM, IV, intrathecal). It poorly crosses the BBB due to low lipid solubility. Methotrexate is taken up into the cells by the same active transport process as that of folic acid. It is metabolised in the liver to polyglutamates. These polyglutamates are inhibitors of DHFR. Methotrexate is excreted largely by the kidneys.

Adverse effects to methotrexate include the general adverse effects to most anticancer drugs - bone marrow suppression, nausea, vomiting, diarrhoea, alopecia and dermatitis.

Methotrexate can cause nephrotoxicity because the drug may be precipitated in the renal tubules and it is contraindicated in patients with renal impairment. Allergic pneumonitis can sometimes be fatal. When injected intrathecally methotrexate can cause myelopathy and encephalopathy.

Methotrexate toxicity can be largely prevented by administering folinic acid. This folinic acid (also called leucovorin or citrovorum factor) gets converted to a form of THF that can be utilised by the cells.

When high doses are needed, **folinic acid** 'rescue' is recommended to avoid severe toxicity.

Drug interactions

Salicylate, sulfonamides and probenecid inhibit the renal tubular secretion of methotrexate. They also displace methotrexate from plasma protein binding sites.

Uses Methotrexate is curative in choriocarcinoma and is useful in acute leukaemias, breast cancer and soft tissue sarcomas. It is also used in rheumatoid arthritis and psoriasis.

PURINE ANALOGS

6 Mercaptopurine, thioguanine, fludarabine, pentostatin and cladribine are purine analogs or purine antagonists. They are structurally similar to purines.

Mechanism of action

Purine analogs enter the cells and get converted to active metabolites (triphosphates in most compounds) which are incorporated into DNA. They cause breakages in DNA strands and inhibit protein synthesis. Fludarabine triphosphate inhibits DNA polymerase while pentostatin inhibits adenosine deaminase.

Purine analogs

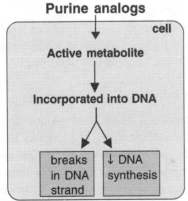

Mechanism of action of Purine analogs

Mercaptopurine

Mercaptopurinte (6-MP) is converted to an active metabolite which gets incorporated into the DNA and inhibits purine synthesis and thereby protein synthesis.

Mercaptopurine undergoes extensive first pass metabolism. It is metabolised by xanthine oxidase.

Adverse effects include bone marrow depression, anorexia, nausea, vomiting, stomatitis, jaundice and dermatitis.

Uses

6-MP is used in acute leukaemias in children, choriocarcinoma and some solid tumours.

Drug interaction

6-Mercaptopurine is metabolised by xanthine oxidase. Allopurinol inhibits xanthine oxidase and thus prolongs the action of 6-MP. When both drugs are given concurrently, the dose of 6-MP should be reduced.

Thioguanine is an analogue of guanine, is effective orally and is used in acute leukemias particularly acute granulocytic leukemia.

Fludarabine an analog of vidarabine (antiviral drug) is converted to an active triphosphate

---

Keybox 60.1

Purine analogs

- Purine analogs get incorporated into DNA and inhibit protein synthesis.

- Mercaptopurine and thioguanine are used in acute leukemias, fludarabine and pentostatin in CLL and non-Hodgkins lymphomas; cladribin is the drug of choice in hairy cell leukemia.

- Purine analogs share the general adverse effects of anticancer drugs. Fludarabine and pentostatin combination can cause fatal lung toxicity.

derivative which inhibits DNA polymerase. It is also incorporated into DNA and causes breakage and termination of the DNA chain.

Adverse effects include nausea, vomiting, anorexia, bone marrow depression, and neurotoxicity.

Fludarabine is used in the treatment of chronic lymphocytic leukemia (CLL) and non Hodgkins lymphomas.

Pentostatin

Pentostatin obtained from *Streptomyces antibioticus* inhibits the enzyme adenosine deaminase. This results in accumulation of adenosine in the cells and other nucleotides which inhibit DNA synthesis.

Pentostatin can cause nausea, vomiting, diarrhoea, skin rashes and bone marrow suppression.

Pentostatin is used intravenously in the treatment of hairy cell leukemia and other chronic leukemias and non-Hodgkins lymphomas.

Cladribine

Cladribine is another purine analog. It gets activated intracellularly to cladribine triphosphate - which gets incorporated into DNA causing breakages in the DNA strands and also inhibits protein synthesis. Cladribine causes mild bone marrow suppression, nausea, vomiting, weakness and skin rashes.

Cladribine is the drug of choice in hairly cell leukemia. It is also useful in CLL, AML and some lymphomas.

PYRIMIDINE ANALOGS

Pyrimidine analogs are converted to active metabolites which resemble natural nucleotides. They compete with natural nucleotides, are incorporated into DNA in place of natural nucleotides and inhibit DNA synthesis.

5-Fluorouracil

5-Fluorouracil is a pyrimidine analog. It inhibits the enzyme thymidylate synthetase due to which it inhibits the synthesis of thymine and thereby inhibits DNA synthesis. It is used in carcinoma of the stomach, colon, rectum, breast and ovaries.

Capecitabine

Capecitabine is an orally effective fluoropyrimidine. It is a prodrug which is converted to an intermediate metabolite in the liver. This metabolite is then converted to the active metabolite fluorouracil in the tumor cells. The convertion to fluorouracil is much more in the tumor cells (due to presence of a specific enzyme) than normal cells. This is therefore like achieving some drug targeting. Toxicity is milder than with fluorouracil. Nausea, vomiting and myelosuppression are milder. Capecitabine is used in breast cancer and colorectal cancer.

Cytosine arabinoside Cytosine arabinoside or cytarabine is the most effective agent in acute myeloblastic leukemia. It enters the cells and is converted to an active metabolite. The active metabolite cytosine arabinoside triphosphate is incorporated into the DNA and inhibits DNA polymerase and thereby inhibits DNA synthesis.

It causes nausea, vomiting and bone marrow depression.

Cytarabine is useful in acute leukemias particularly myeloid leukemia and in relapsed cases of acute lymphocytic leukemia.

Gemcitabine

Gemcitabine is a recently developed analog of cytarabine with mechanism of action similar to cytarabine. Adverse effects are milder with flu-like syndrome and mild bone marrow depression. Gemcitabine is used in pancreatic, lung, cervical, ovarian and breast cancers.

Drugs which cause least/no bone marrow depression	Curable cancers	Tumors resistant to treatment
• Hormones • Vincristine • Bleomycin • L-asparaginase • Cisplatin	• Hodgkin's disease • Choriocarcinoma • Burkitt's lymphoma • Testicular tumours • Wilms' tumour • Acute leukaemias in children • Ewing's sarcoma	• Melanomas • Pancreatic tumors, • Renal cancers • Some lung cancers.

NATURAL PRODUCTS

ANTIBIOTICS

Actinomycin D

Actinomycin D (Dactinomycin) is obtained from Streptomyces species. It acts by inhibiting DNA-dependent RNA synthesis. It is one of the most potent anticancer drugs and is used in Wilms' tumour, rhabdomyosarcoma, choriocarcinoma and some soft tissue sarcomas.

Daunorubicin and doxorubicin

Daunorubicin and doxorubicin (Adriamycin, Doxorubin, Cardia) are anthracyclines. They are converted to active metabolites which inhibit DNA synthesis. They act on the 'S' phase of the cell cycle. Cardiotoxicity with hypotension, arrhythmias and CCF, is unique to both these drugs. They also cause vomiting, stomatitis, alopecia and bone marrow depression.

Daunorubicin is used in acute leukaemias while doxorubicn is useful in solid tumours and in acute leukaemias and non Hodgkin's lymphomas.

Epirubicin and mitoxantrone are analogs of doxorubicin which are less cardiotoxic.

Mitomycin C is converted to an alkylating agent in the body. It is used in cancers of the stomach, lungs and cervix.

Bleomycin

Bleomycin is obtained from *Streptomyces verticillus.* It binds with iron and generates free radicals and causes breakage in DNA strand. It has the advantages of the unique mechanism of action and is less toxic to the bone marrow - these are advantageous in combination regimens.

Bleomycin is used in solid tumours - testicular tumours, squamous cell carcinoma of the head, neck and oesophagus.

It's most serious toxicity includes pulmonary fibrosis and cutaneous toxicity but does not cause significant bone marrow depression.

Mithramycin

Mithramycin (Plicamycin) is highly toxic, used in disseminated testicular tumours and in severe hypercalcaemia due to bone cancers. It reduces plasma calcium levels by its action on the osteoclasts.

EPIPODOPHYLLOTOXINS

Podophyllotoxin is obtained from the root of mandrake plant or May apple. **Etoposide** (VP-16) and **teniposide** (VM-26) are semisynthetic derivatives of podophyllotoxin. Etoposide is available for both oral and parentral use.

Mechanism of action Epipodophyllotoxins bind to topoisomerase II as well as DNA and result in DNA strand breakages. The cells in S and G_2 phase of cell cycle are susceptible to these drugs.

Adverse effects include thrombophlebitis at the site of injection, nausea, alopecia, allergic reactions and myelosuppression.

Uses

• Etoposide is useful in germ cell cancers (testicular and ovarian), lung and stomach cancers, leukemias and lymphomas.

• Teniposide is used in acute lymphoblastic leukemia.

CAMPTOTHECINS

Camptothecin was the first anticancer agent in this group but was found to be too toxic. Its analogs, topotican and irinotecan are less toxic and useful. They inhibit topoisomerase I resulting in DNA strand breakages leading to cell death. They act on the S phase of the cell cycle. Both are given intravenously.

Toxicity is mild and includes diarrhoea and reversible bone marrow suppression, nausea, weakness and skin rash. Irinotecan inhibits the enzyme acetylcholinestrase resulting in accumulation of acetylcholine causing excessive salivation, abdominal cramps, miosis, bradycardia and sweating which respond to treatment with atropine.

TAXANES

Paclitaxel is obtained from the bark of the western yew tree. It binds to beta-tubulin of microtubules and arrests mitosis- mitotic spindle poison.

Paclitaxel is given intravenously; it is metabolised by the liver microsomal enzymes. Adverse effects include myelosuppression, myalgia, allergic reactions, hypotension, arrhythmias and peripheral neuropathy. Docetaxel is more potent and orally effective.

Taxanes are useful in breast cancers and ovarian cancers. They are also found to be effective in the cancers of head and neck, oesophagus and lungs.

VINCA ALKALOIDS

Vincristine and vinblastine are obtained from the leaves of *Vinca rosea*, the periwinkle plant.

Mechanism of action Vinca alkaloids bind to microtubules in the mitotic apparatus and arrest cell division in metaphase. They are spindle poisons. They are cell- cycle specific - act on the 'M' phase of the cell cycle.

Though the structure and mechanism of action of vinca alkaloids are similar they differ in toxicity and therapeutic uses.

Vincristine (Oncovin) is neurotoxic while bone marrow depression is less. Peripheral neuropathy and mental depression can occur. Other adverse effects include nausea, vomiting, alopecia and inappropriate secretion of ADH. It is used in leukaemias, Hodgkin's lymphoma (MOPP regimen), breast, lung and cervical tumors. It is also used in many paediatric solid tumors like Wilm's tumor, Ewing's sarcoma, brain tumor and rhabdomyosarcoma.

Vinblastine causes bone marrow depression, alopecia and vomiting. It is used with bleomycin and cisplatin (VBC) in testicular tumours; it is also useful in Hodgkin's lymphoma.

Vinorelbine is a semisynthetic vinca alkaloid used intravenously in lung cancers (on-small cell type). It can cause bone marrow suppression, (granulocytopenia), nausea, vomiting and neurotoxicity (paraesthesias).

MISCELLANEOUS

Hydroxyurea is an analogue of urea and acts by inhibiting the enzyme ribonucleotide reductase and thereby inhibits DNA synthesis. It acts on the 'S' phase of the cell cycle. It is orally effective, almost completely and rapidly absorbed. Adverse effects are myelosuppression, nausea, vomiting and skin pigmentation. Hydroxyurea is the most useful drug in chronic myeloid leukemia and is now considered the first line drug in it.

Procarbazine is effective orally in Hodgkin's lymphoma (MOPP regimen component). It damages DNA. This may make it carcinogenic.

Cisplatin, Carboplatin and oxaliplatin are platinum containing compounds. They get converted to the active form in the cell, inhibit

DNA synthesis and cause cytotoxicity. Cisplatin causes ototoxicity, nephrotoxicity, peripheral neuropathy, nausea, vomiting and anaemia. Anaphylactoid reactions can follow its use. It is relatively less toxic to bone marrow. Cisplatin is used in ovarian and testicular tumours and cancers of the head and neck.

Carboplatin is a less toxic derivative of cisplatin and is better tolerated than cisplatin. Nausea, vomiting, ototoxicity, nephrotoxicity and neurotoxicity are milder but it causes myelosuppression.

Oxaliplatin is effective in advanced colorectal cancer and in other cancers like ovarian and cervical cancers.

L-asparaginase

The amino acid asparagine is synthesized by the normal cells but malignant cells are unable to synthesize asparagine and depend on the host for the supply. Asparaginase is an enzyme that converts asparagine to aspartic acid and deprives the malignant cells of asparagine supplies resulting in inhibition of protein synthesis. For therapeutic purpose it is obtained from *E. coli*. It is used in acute leukaemias. Hypersensitivity reactions are common as it is a foreign protein. Haemorrhage due to inhibition of clotting factors, hepatotoxicity with raised serum transaminases and pancreatitis can occur. Inhibition of insulin synthesis may result in hyperglycaemia. It also causes nausea, vomiting and CNS depression. Bone marrow suppression and effect on GI epithelium are mild and it does not cause alopecia. (Crisantaspase is the preparation of L asparaginase used)

Imatinib is a recent introduction in cancer chemotherapy. It acts by inhibiting some selective tyrosine kinases (taking part in signal transduction) which are considered to be involved in the pathogenesis of chronic myeloid leukemia.

Imatinib is almost completely absorbed when given orally and is metabolised by microsomal enzymes. It can cause skin rashes and elevated serum transaminases. Imatinib is now the drug of choice in chronic myeloid leukemia.

HORMONES IN CANCER CHEMOTHERAPY

Glucocorticoids Due to their lympholytic action, glucocorticoids are used in acute leukaemias and lymphomas. Rapid clinical improvement is seen but duration can vary from 2 weeks to 9 months. They are used for initiation of therapy due to their rapid action.

Glucocorticoids are also of value in the following.
1. With radiation therapy to reduce radiation oedema

2. In intracranial tumours to reduce cerebral oedema

3. For symptomatic relief in critically ill patients.

Prednisolone or dexamethasone are commonly used.

Estrogens are useful in (i) prostatic carcinoma as it is an androgen dependent tumour, (ii) breast cancer in males and in postmenopausal women - oestrogens are used in advanced cases where surgery or radiotherapy cannot be employed.

Progestins are useful in the palliative management of endometrial carcinoma.

Androgens are used in the palliative treatment of breast cancer in postmenopausal women along with oophorectomy.

HORMONE ANTAGONISTS

Aromatase inhibitors

The enzyme aromatase catalyzes the convertion of androgens to estrogens. Inhibitors of aromatase have been found to be effective in breast cancers. Formestane, exemestane, anastrozole, vorozole and letrozole are the aromatase inhibitors used.

Aminoglutethimide and trilastane inhibit the convertion of cholesterol to pregnenolone (the first step in corticosteroid synthesis) and thereby inhibit the synthesis of adrenocorticoids. Aminoglutethimide is useful in advanced breast cancers when cancer cells contain estrogen receptors.

Octreotide a somatostatin analog is useful to reduce the secretion of growth hormone, insulin, glucagon and peptide hormones in carcinoid tumors and islet cell carcinomas of the pancreas.

Antiestrogens

Tamoxifen is an estrogen receptor antagonist used in oestrogen receptor containing breast cancer (See page 474).

GnRH analogs

Long term administration of leuprolide, goserelin and buserelin are useful in prostatic and breast cancers. They may be combined with tamoxifen in breast cancers.

Estramustine is a molecule containing both estradiol and nitrogen mustard. It is useful in prostatic cancers which are not responding to estrogens. Adverse effects are similar to that of estrogen administration.

Antiandrogen

Flutamide is used in prostatic cancer.

RADIO ACTIVE ISOTOPES

Some radioactive isotopes can be used in the treatment of certain specific cancers.

Radiophosphorus P^{32} is used in polycythemia vera. It is taken up by the bone where it emits β rays and has a half-life of about 14 days.

Strontium chloride emits β rays and has a longer $t\frac{1}{2}$ in the bony metastases. It is used to alleviate pain in painful bony metastases.

Radio active iodine I^{131} is used in the treatment of thyroid cancers (See page 461).

BIOLOGICAL RESPONSE MODIFIERS

Several agents are used to beneficially influence the patients' response to treatment and to overcome some adverse effects. These have also been termed **biological response modifiers.** They are as follows:

1. Haematopoietic growth factors like erythropoietin and myeloid growth factors like GM-CSF, G-CSF, M-CSF and thrombopoietin (See page 299) are used to treat bone marrow suppression.

2. Interferons (See page 406) like interferon alpha is used in hairy cell leukemia, Kaposi's sarcoma and condylomata acuminata.

3. Monoclonal antibodies are immunoglobulins that react specifically with antigens present on the cancer cells. Allergic reactions are common. **Trastuzumab** also enhances hostimmune responses and is useful in breast cancers. **Rituximab** attaches to antigens on the B cells causing lysis of these cells. It is used in B cell lymphomas.

4. Aldesleukin is recombinant interleukin -2. It enhances cytotoxic activity of T-cells , induces activity of natural killer cells and also induces interferon production. It is useful in inducing remission in renal cell carcinoma. Hypotension is the most troublesome side effect.

5. Tretinoin - (Alltransretinoic acid) induces differentiation in leukemic cells and the leukemic promyelocytes loose their ability to proliferate. It is useful to induce remission in acute promyelocytic leukemia.

6. Amifostine - has been designed to offer selective cytoprotection to normal tissues from the effects of cytotoxic drugs. Amifostine activates an enzyme in the normal tissues which can inactivate the active form of cisplatin and radiation. It has also been shown to stimulate the bone marrow in some bone marrow disorders. Amifostine is used to prevent toxicity due to cisplatin and radiation induced xerostomia.

TABLE 60.4: Choice of drugs in some malignancies	
Malignancy	**Preferred drugs**
Acute lymphatic leukaemia	Vincristine + prednisolone + L- asparaginase Maintanence - Mercaptopurine/Methotrexate, Cyclophosphamide
Acute myeloid leukaemia	Cytosine arabinoside + daunorubicin
Chronic lymphatic leukaemia	Fludarabine / Chlorambucil + Prednisolone
Chronic myeloid leukaemia	Hydroxyurea, busulfan Imatinib; interferons
Hodgkin's disease	MOPP ABVD M-Mechlorethamine A-Adriamycin O-Oncovin (Vincristine) (doxorubicin) P-Procarbazine OR B-Bleomycin P-Prednisolone - V-Vinblastin D-Dacarbazine
Non-Hodgkins lymphoma	Cyclophosphamide + Doxorubicin + vincristine (Oncovin) + Prednisolone (CHOP)*
Carcinoma of stomach Carcinoma of colon Multiple myeloma	Fluorouracil + cisplatin Fluorouracil + irinotecan, oxaliplatin Melphalan + Prednisolone / Vincristine + Doxorubicin + Dexamethasone
Choriocarcinoma	Methotrexate
Carcinoma of testis	Etoposide + bleomycin + cisplatin
Osteogenic sarcoma	Methotrexate or doxorubicin, vincristine
Wilms' tumour	Vincristine + actinomycin-D after surgery
Carcinoma of the head and neck	Fluorouracil + cisplatin
Carcinoma of lung	Cisplatin + paclitaxel, Gemcitabine

In CHOP, 'H' stands for doxorubicin formerly called hydroxydaunomycin.

General Principles in the Treatment of cancers (Table 60.4)

Chemotherapy in most cancers (except the curable cancers) is generally palliative and suppressive. Because of the ability of cancers for recurrence i.e even if a few cells are spared during treatment, these cells can multipy and result in (the regrowth of a tumor of earlier dimensions) recurrence. To avoid this it is essential to kill all the cells or as many cells as possible during treatment - to achieve what is known as 'Total Cell Kill'. Chemotherapy is just one of the modes in the treatment of cancer. Other modes like radiotherapy and surgery are also employed to ensure 'total cell kill'. Combination of drugs is preferred for synergistic effect, to reduce adverse effects and to prevent rapid development of resistance. Drugs which do not depress bone marrow are useful in combination regimens to avoid overlapping of adverse effects. With appropriate treatment, cure can now be achieved in a few cancers. Maintenance of good nutrition, treatment of anemia, protection against infections, adequate relief of pain and anxiety and good emotional support - all go a long way in the appropriate management of these dreaded diseases.

61 | *Immunopharmacology*

- **Immunosuppressants**
  - T-cell inhibitors
  - Cytotoxic drugs
  - Adrenocorticosteroids
  - Antibody reagents.

- **Immunostimulants**
  - Interferons

Drugs influencing the immune system include immunosuppressants, immunostimulants and immunomodulators. Vaccines and antisera are discussed in chap 72.

IMMUNOSUPPRESSANTS

Immunosuppressants are drugs which inhibit immunity. They may suppress cell mediated or humoral immunity or both. It is necessary to suppress immune reaction in organ transplantation (to prevent graft rejection) and in autoimmune disorders. Immunosuppressants are classified as-

CLASSIFICATION

1. T-cell inhibitors
Cyclosporine, tacrolimus, sirolimus, mycophenolate mofetil

2. Cytotoxic drugs
Azathioprine, methotrexate, cyclophospha-mide, chlorambucil

3. Glucocorticoids

4. Antibody reagents
Muromonab CD3, Antithymocyte globulin

T-CELL INHIBITORS

Cyclosporine

Cyclosporine is a cyclic peptide produced by a fungus *Beauveria nivea*.

Actions Cyclosporine acts at an early stage, selectively inhibits T cell-proliferation and suppresses cell mediated immunity. It can be given orally and intravenously.

Mechanism of action

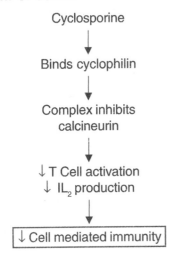

Cyclosporine

↓

Binds cyclophilin

↓

Complex inhibits
calcineurin

↓

↓ T Cell activation
↓ IL$_2$ production

↓

| ↓ Cell mediated immunity |

Cyclosporine binds to cyclophilin (an immunophilin) and this complex binds to and inhibits phosphatase calcineurin. This results in inhibition of T cell activation and IL-2 production. T cells do not respond to specific antigenic stimulation. Cyclosporine also suppresses the proliferation of cytoxic T cells. Tacrolimus binds to another immunophilin and then the complex inhibits calcineurin.

Pharmacokinetics Cyclosporine is metabolised by microsomal enzymes cytochrome P450 in the liver. It can therefore interact with many drugs given concurrently.

Adverse effects include nephrotoxicity, hepatotoxicity, anorexia, gum hypertrophy and increased susceptibility to infections, hypertension, hyperglycaemia, hyperlipidaemia and hirsutism.

Uses

- **In organ transplantation** Cyclosporine is very effective for the prophylaxis and treatment of graft rejection in organ transplantation surgeries - like kidney, liver, bone marrow and other transplants.

- **Autoimmune disorders** Cyclosporine is also useful in some autoimmune disorders like rheumatoid arthritis as an alternative in patients who do not respond to methotrexate. Cyclosporin is also tried in severe psoriasis, atopic dermatitis, inflammatory bowel disease and nephrotic syndrome.

Tacrolimus

Tacrolimus is a macrolide antibiotic obtained from *Streptomyces tsukubaensis*. Its mechanism of action is similar to cyclosporine. Tacrolimus can be given both orally and parenterally but absorption from the gut is incomplete. It is extensively bound to plasma proteins.

Adverse effects include nephrotoxicity, gastrointestinal disturbances, hypertension, hyperglycaemia, tremors and seizures.

Sirolimus

Sirolimus obtained from *Stretomyces hygroscopicus,* acts by inhibiting the activation of T-cells. Sirolimus may be used in combination with other drugs for the prophylaxis of organ transplant rejection and in psoriasis and uveoretinitis.

Toxicity includes hyperlipidaemia, gastrointestinal disturbances and an increased risk of infections and lymphomas.

Mycophenolate mofetil

Mycophenolate mofetil a prodrug is converted to mycophenolic acid, which inhibits guanine nucleotide synthesis and inhibits the proliferation and functions of lymphocytes.

Mycophenolate mofetil is indicated as an adjunct to other immunosuppressive drugs in the prophylaxis of transplant rejection.

CYTOTOXIC DRUGS

Cytotoxic drugs like azathioprine, cyclophosphamide and methotrexate inhibit cell mediated immunity (while cyclophosphamide predominantly suppresses humoural immunity).

They are used in the prevention of graft rejection and in autoimmune disorders.

GLUCOCORTICOIDS

Glucocorticoids have potent immunosuppresant activity and are used in the prevention of organ transplant rejection and in autoimmune disorders.

ANTIBODY REAGENTS

Muromonab CD3 is a monoclonal antibody to CD3 antigens on T lymphocytes. On intravenous administration, T cells disappear from the circulation within minutes. It is used with other immunosuppressants in organ transplantation. Fever, chills and pulmonary oedema may occur.

Antithymocyte globulin (ATG) binds to T lymphocytes and deplete them thereby suppressing immune response. It is used in the management of organ transplantation.

Infliximab is a monoclonal antibody and etanercept is a protein that blocks TNFα. They are useful in rheumatoid arthritis and Crohn's disease.

Anti Rh (D) Immuneglobin is human IgG with a high titer of antibodies to Rh(D) antigen of the red blood cell. When Rh negative mother delivers a Rh positive baby (or aborts) the Rh positive antigens from the red cels of foetus enters into the maternal blood stream. This sensitizes the mother to produce antibodies against Rh positive cells. In subsequent pregnancies the maternal antibodies against Rh positive cells reach the foetus and may result in hemolytic disease of the new born.
Injection of anti Rh(D) immuneglobulin to the mother at the time of child birth (or after abortion) will bind the antigens on the RBCs of the baby which have entered the maternal circulation. This will prevent the formation of antibodies in the Rh negative mother against the Rh positive RBCs. Thus subsequent pregnancies would not be affected. The immuneglobulin should be given within 24-72 hours of child birth. Dose: 300 mcg intramuscularly.

IMMUNOSTIMULANTS

Immunostimulants and immunomodulaters are drugs that modulate the immune response and can be used to increase the immune responsiveness of patients with immunode-ficiency as in AIDS, chronic illness and cancers. This is still a developing field of pharmacology. The drugs currently used for this purpose are:

- BCG
- Cytokines
- Thymosin
- Others
- Levamisole
- Inosiplex
- interferons

BCG has been tried in cancers. Levamisole, used in helminthiasis, is also found to enhance cell-mediated immunity in humans. It has been tried in some cancers.

Cytokines

Interferons are cytokines with antiviral and immunomodulatory properties. Recombinant interferons α, β and γ are available for clinical use. They bind to specific receptors and bring about immune activation and increase host defences. There is an increase in the number and activity of cytotoxic and helper T cells and killer cells (See chap. 60) Interferons α and β are mainly used for antiviral effects while interferon γ for its immuno modulating actions.

Interferons are indicated in several tumors including malignant melanoma, hairy cell leukemia, lymphomas, kaposi's sarcoma, condylomata acuminata and in viral infections.

Other Cytokines like IL - 2 are being tried as adjuvants to vaccines. Cytokine inhibitors are also under investigation as immunomodulators.

Thymosin is synthesized in the thymus and purified from bovine and human thymus glands for therapeutic use. It induces the maturation of precursor T cells and is tried in hepatitis B and C.

HORMONES

- Hypothalamus and anterior pituitary hormones
- Thyroid hormones and antithyroid drugs
- Corticosteroids
- Estrogens, progestins and hormonal contraceptives
- Androgens and anabolic steroids
- Insulin and oral hypoglycaemics
- Oxytocin and drugs acting on the uterus
- Agents affecting bone mineral turnover

Hypothalamus & Anterior Pituitary Hormones

- **Hypothalamic Hormones**
  - **Growth hormone releasing hormone**
  - **Somatostatin**
  - **Octreotide**
  - **Thyrotrophin releasing hormone**
  - **Corticotrophin releasing factor (CRF)**
  - **Gonadotrophin - releasing hormone**

- **Anterior Pituitary Hormones**
  - **Growth hormone**
  - **Corticotrophin**
  - **Thyroid-stimulating hormone**
  - **Gonadotrophins**
  - **Prolactin**
  - **Bromocriptine**

The pituitary gland, under the influence of the hypothalamus secretes many hormones which either control the secretion of other glands or directly act on the target tissues. These are peptides and act by binding to specific receptors present on the target cells (Table 62.1).

HYPOTHALAMIC HORMONES

Growth hormone releasing hormone (sermorelin) stimulates anterior pituitary to secrete growth hormone. Sermorelin is an analog of GHRH used in diagnostic tests of growth hormone deficiency (Table 62.3).

Somatostatin

Somatostatin is growth hormone release-inhibiting hormone present in the hypothalamus, parts of the CNS, pancreas and in gastrointestinal tract. It inhibits secretion of GH, TSH, PRL, insulin, glucagon and gastrointestinal secretions. But it is very short-acting. **Octreotide** is the synthetic analog of somatostatin which is longer-acting and useful in acromegaly, some hormone secreting tumours and in bleeding esophageal varices.

TABLE 62.1 Hormones secreted by the hypothalamus and anterior pituitary and their chief functions

Hypothalamic hormone	Anterior pituitary hormone	Chief actions
1. a. Growth hormone releasing hormone (GHRH)	Growth hormone (GH)	Regulates growth
b. Growth hormone release-inhibiting hormone (soma-tostatin) (GHRIH)	Inhibits GH release	
2. Corticotropin releasing factor (CRF)	Corticotrophin (ACTH)	Stimulates adrenal cortex to secrete glucocorticoids, mineralocorticoids and androgens
3. Thyrotropin–releasing hormone (TRH)	Thyroid-stimulating hormone (TSH) (Thyrotrophin)	Stimulates release of T_3 and T_4
4. Gonadotrophin releasing hormone (GnRH, somatorelin)	• Follicle stimulating hormone (FSH)	Stimulates growth of ovum and graafian follicle in the female and gametogenesis in the male
	• Luteinising hormone (LH) or (ICSH)	Stimulates ovulation in females and regulates testosterone secretion in males
5. Prolactin–releasing factor	Prolactin (PRL)	Development of breast and lactation
6. Prolactin-release inhibiting factor	-	Inhibits prolactin-release
7. Melanocyte stimulating hormone - releasing factor	Melanocyte stimulating hormone	Promotes melanine synthesis causing darkening of skin; regulates feeding

Pegvisomant is a recently developed growth hormone receptor antagonist. It is useful in the treatment of acromegaly.

Thyrotrophin releasing hormone (TRH) secreted by the hypothalamus stimulates the release of TSH from the anterior pituitary.

Protirelin is a synthetic analog of TSH used in the diagnosis of thyroid disorders.

Corticotrophin releasing factor (CRF) releases ACTH and β-endorphins from the anterior pituitary. It is used in diagnostic tests in Cushing's disease.

Gonadotrophin-releasing hormone - secreted in a pulsatile manner, regulates the secretion of gonadotrophins - FSH and LH. It is used in

diagnostic tests in hypogonadism. Therapeutically pulsatile administration is used in infertility and delayed puberty. Continuous administration inhibits gonadotrophin secretion and is used in prostatic cancers. GnRH analogue **leuprolide** is more potent and is used for pharmacological orchiectomy/oophorectomy in prostatic cancer and some gynaecological conditions like uterine fibroids and endometriosis.

GnRH antagonist

Cetrorelix is a synthetic compound that binds to and blocks pituitary GnRH receptors. It therefore suppresses the secretion of LH, FSH and delays ovulation. When used for *in vitro* fertilization. GnRH antagonists produce less ovarian hyperstimulation when compared to GnRH analogs. Hence

TABLE 62.2 : Analogs of antertior pituitary hormones	
Hormones	**Analogs**
Growth hormone	Sermorelin
Somatostatin	Octreotide
Thyrotrophin (TSH)	Protirelin
GnRH	Buserelin
	Leuprorelin
	Goserelin
	Nafarelin
ADH	Desmopressin
	Terlipressin
	Felypressin

cetrorelix is used for *in vitro* fertilization. It is also useful in reducing uterine fibroids and endometriosis.

ANTERIOR PITUITARY HORMONES

Growth hormone (GH) a peptide, which stimulates the growth of all organs except brain and eye. It increases the uptake of amino acids by the tissues, promotes protein synthesis and positive nitrogen balance. It causes lipolysis and reduces glucose uptake by skeletal muscles. It brings about linear growth. These anabolic actions are mediated by **somatomedins or insulin-like growth factors** (IGF) produced in the liver.

The secretion of growth hormone is regulated by GHRH and somatostatin (GHRIH).

GH deficiency in children results in **dwarfism** while excessive production results in **gigantism** in children and **acromegaly** in adults.

Uses (Table 62.4)

- GH deficiency Replacement therapy with GH in deficient children brings about normal growth. It can also be used in GH deficient adults.
- Other conditions GH has been tried in chronic renal failure and in catabolic states -- like severe burns and AIDS. It is liable for abuse by athletes to promote growth.

Corticotrophin

Corticotrophin (Adrenocorticotrophic hormone, ACTH) controls the synthesis and release of glucocorticoids, mineralocorticoids, and androgens from the adrenal cortex (Fig. 64.1). It is used in the diagnosis of adrenocortical insufficiency.

Thyroid-stimulating hormone (TSH, Thyrotrophin)

Thyrotrophin stimulates the production and secretion of thyroid hormones and thus regulates

TABLE 62.3 Uses of Hypothalamic hormones	
Hypothalamic hormone	*Uses*
1. Sermorelin	Diagnosis of GH deficiency
2. Octreotide	Acromegaly, hormone secreting tumors, bleeding oesophageal varices.
3. TRH	Diagnosis of thyroid disorders
4. CRF	Diagnostic tests in Cushing's disease, tests of hypothalamic and pituitary function
5. GnRH (gonadorelin)	Diagnostic tests of hypogonadism
6. Leuprolide	Prostatic cancer, uterine fibroids

TABLE 62.4 Uses of anterior pituitary hormones	
Anterior pituitary hormones	**Uses**
1. Growth hormone	GH deficiency, chronic renal failure, burns, diagnosis of GH deficiency
2. Corticotrophin	Diagnosis of adrenocortical insufficiency
3. Thyrotrophin	To test thyroid function
4. Gonadotrophins	FSH-LH deficiency, undescended testes, amenorrhea, infertility

thyroid function. It is used to test thyroid function and to increase the uptake of radioactive iodine in thyroid carcinoma.

Gonadotrophins

Follicle stimulating hormone (FSH) and luteinising hormone (LH) - produced by the anterior pituitary regulate gonadal function. They stimulate follicular development in women and also stimulate ovarian steroidogenesis (oestrogens and progesterone synthesis). In men they promote spermatogenesis.

Uses

Menotropins is the combination of FSH-LH obtained from the urine of postmenopausal women. It is used in:

1. Gonadotrophin deficiency in males.
2. Undescended testes.
3. Amenorrhoea and infertility.
4. *In vitro* fertilization - to time the ovulation.

Prolactin

This peptide hormone promotes the growth and development of breast during pregnancy. It stimulates milk production along with other hormones like oestrogens and progestins. Deficiency results in lactation failure while excess prolactin results in galactorrhoea.

Regulation of secretion Suckling is the principal stimulus for prolactin secretion. Suckling stimulates the release of prolactin-releasing factor from hypothalamus. Oestrogens and dopamine antagonists also stimulate prolactin-release. Prolactin is not used clinically.

Dopamine agonists like bromocriptine cabergoline, pergolide and quinagolide inhibit prolactin release from the pituitary by acting directly on dopamine receptors.

Bromocriptine is an ergot derivative with dopamine agonistic properties.

Bromocriptine is used -

1. To suppress lactation - Bromocriptine and other dopamine agonists stimulate the dopamine receptors in the pituitary to inhibit the release of prolactin. Bromocriptine is used to suppress lactation and breast engorgement after delivery (like in still birth) and following abortion.

2. In galactorrhea - due to excess prolactin.

3. Prolactin secreting tumours or prolactinomas.

4. Parkinsonism - bromocriptine is used with levodopa.

5. Acromegaly - In normal subjects, dopamine agonists stimulate the release of growth hormone by the pituitary but in patients with acromegaly, they supress growth hormone release by a paradoxical effect. Bromocriptine is therefore used in acromegaly. Bromocriptine may also help to reduce prolactin release.

HORMONES AND RELATED DRUGS

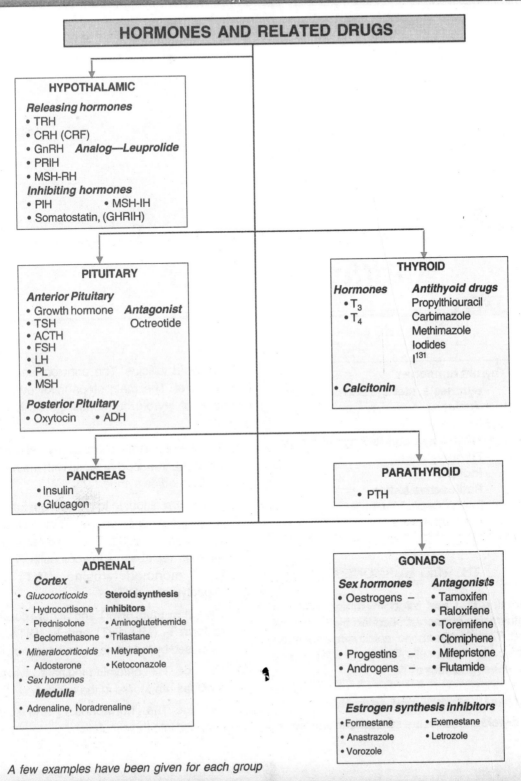

HYPOTHALAMIC

Releasing hormones
- TRH
- CRH (CRF)
- GnRH *Analog—Leuprolide*
- PRIH
- MSH-RH

Inhibiting hormones
- PIH   • MSH-IH
- Somatostatin, (GHRIH)

PITUITARY

Anterior Pituitary
- Growth hormone *Antagonist*
- TSH   Octreotide
- ACTH
- FSH
- LH
- PL
- MSH

Posterior Pituitary
- Oxytocin   • ADH

THYROID

Hormones	Antithyoid drugs
• T_3	Propylthiouracil
• T_4	Carbimazole
	Methimazole
	Iodides
	I^{131}

• *Calcitonin*

PANCREAS
- Insulin
- Glucagon

PARATHYROID

• PTH

ADRENAL

Cortex
- *Glucocorticoids*   **Steroid synthesis**
  - Hydrocortisone   **inhibitors**
  - Prednisolone   • Aminoglutethemide
  - Beclomethasone • Trilastane
- *Mineralocorticoids* • Metyrapone
  - Aldosterone   • Ketoconazole
- *Sex hormones*
    Medulla
- Adrenaline, Noradrenaline

GONADS

Sex hormones	Antagonists
• Oestrogens –	• Tamoxifen
	• Raloxifene
	• Toremifene
	• Clomiphene
• Progestins –	• Mifepristone
• Androgens –	• Flutamide

Estrogen synthesis inhibitors
- Formestane   • Exemestane
- Anastrazole   • Letrozole
- Vorozole

A few examples have been given for each group

63

Thyroid Hormones &
Antithyroid Drugs

CHAPTER

- **Thyroid hormones**
  - Synthesis, storage and secretion
  - Actions
  - Uses
- **Hyperthyroidism and Antithyroid Drugs**
  - Thioureylenes
  - Iodides
  - Radioactive iodine
  - β-adrenergic blockers
  - Ionic inhibitors

THYROID HORMONES

Thyroxine (T_4) and triiodothyronine (T_3) are iodothyronine hormones secreted by the thyroid gland. The other hormone, calcitonin is secreted by the parafollicular cells (See page 504). T_4 is a less active precursor of T_3.

Synthesis, storage and secretion

The thyroid hormones are synthesized and stored in the thyroid follicles. The principal source of iodine is diet. The main steps involved in the synthesis of thyroid hormones are as follows: (Fig. 63.1)

1. Uptake of plasma iodide by thyroid cells by an active transport process with the help of sodium iodide symporter.

2. Oxidation of iodide to I^+ (iodinium ions) by a thyroperoxidase enzyme with the help of hydrogen peroxide. These combine with tyrosine residues of thyroglobulin (TG) to form monoiodotyrosine (MIT) and diiodotyrosine (DIT).

3. Coupling Pairs of MIT and DIT are coupled to form T_3 (MIT+DIT) and T_4 (DIT+DIT) catalysed by the same peroxidase enzyme.

4. Storage TG containing iodinated tyrosine residues are stored in the follicles.

5. Release The hormones T_4 and T_3 are released into the circulation.

456

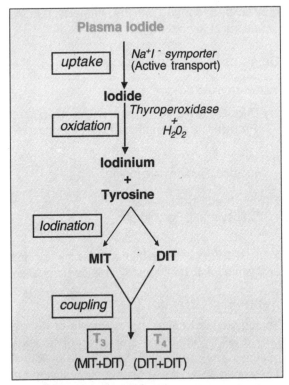

Fig. 63.1 Steps in thyroid hormone synthesis

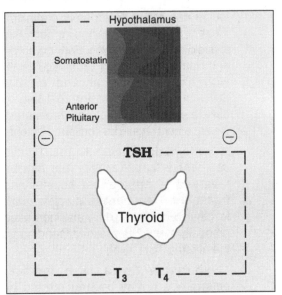

Fig. 63.2 Regulation of thyroid hormone secretion

Regulation

The thyroid secretion is regulated by TSH secreted by the anterior pituitary and TRH from the hypothalamus (Fig. 63.2). Normally about 70-90mcg of T_4 and 15-30mcg of T_3 are secreted daily. In the peripheral tissues, most of the secreted T_4 is converted to T_3 which is the active hormone. Both T_4 and T_3 are extensively bound to plasma proteins. The free hormone is metabolised in the liver and excreted in the bile. The t½ of T_4 is 6-7 days and that of T_3 is 1-2 days. T_3 is 3-5 times more potent than T_4 and acts faster.

Actions

Thyroid hormones are essential for normal growth, development, function and maintenance of all body tissues. Congenital deficiency results in cretinism. Thyroid hormones have important metabolic functions - they increase metabolic rate, enhance carbohydrate and protein metabolism and stimulate lipolysis. They facilitate erythropoiesis, are essential for normal functioning of the CNS (mental retardation is seen in cretinism), skeletal muscles, cardiovascular system, reproductive system and gastrointestinal system (hypothyroid patients are constipated while hyperthyroid have diarrhoea).

Mechanism of action

Thyroid hormones act on specific receptors. Thyroid receptors are nuclear receptors like the steroid receptors. T_3 enters into the cells, bind to the receptor and the T_3 - receptor complex moves to the nucleus where it binds to DNA, activates gene transcription and regulates protein synthesis (Fig. 64.3).

Uses

Both thyroxine and triiodothyronine are available. Levothyroxine is a synthetic T_4 and leothyronine is a synthetic T_3 and are given orally.

1. Replacement therapy
   - Cretinism may be sporadic or endemic. Congenital absence of thyroid or defective thyroid hormone synthesis cause sporadic cretinism. Extreme deficiency of

iodine can result in endemic cretinism. Treatment should be started immediately to avoid mental retardation. Early detection and treatment produce dramatic results with normal physical and mental development. Levothyroxine 10-15mg/kg daily is started and treatment monitored. Replacement should be continued lifelong.

- Hypothyroidism in adults results from decreased thyroid activity and can be reversed by appropriate activity and treatment. Treatment is started with levothyroxine 50 mg daily and increased gradually every 2-3 weeks, depending on the plasma TSH levels.

- Myxoedema coma is a medical emergency. It may be precipitated by infection, trauma, inadequate treatment or exposure to cold. Hypothermia, brady-cardia, hypotension,hypoglycaemia, hypoventilation, lactic acidosis and coma are the usual features.IV thyroxine 500 mg or liothyronine 100 mg should be given with prophylactic corticosteroids to avoid adrenal insufficiency. Gradual warming, prophylactic antibiotics, ventilatory support, correction of fluid and electrolyte balance are all important.

2. Non-toxic goitre T_4 suppresses TSH production and the goitre regresses.

3. Thyroid carcinoma T_4 induces temporary remission. It is used after surgery.

4. Miscellaneous Thyroxine is tried in refractory anaemias, infertility and non-healing ulcers.

HYPERTHYROIDISM AND ANTITHYROID DRUGS

Hyperthyroidism is due to an excess of circulating thyroid hormones and could be due to various causes. Graves' disease, an autoimmune discrder, is the most common cause. It is characterised by hyperthyroidism, diffuse goitre and IgG antibodies that activate TSH receptors. Antithyroid drugs may act by interfering with the synthesis, release or actions of thyroid hormones.

Drugs used in hyperthyroidism are-

1. Antithyroid drugs

   Thioureylenes -
   Propylthiouracil, methimazole, carbimazole

2.Iodine
   Iodides, Radioactive iodine.

3.Ionic Inhibitors
   Thiocyanate, Perchlorate.

THIOUREYLENES are thionamides and include propylthiouracil, methimazole and carbimazole.

Actions

Thioureylenes reduce the synthesis of thyroid hormones by inhibiting iodination of tyrosine residues and coupling of iodotyrosine residues. They bring about these effects by inhibiting the peroxidase enzyme. Propylthiouracil also inhibits peripheral conversion of T_4 to T_3. T_3 and T_4 levels fall. Large doses may stimulate the release of TSH resulting in thyroid enlargement. Over 3-4 weeks of treatment, the signs and symptoms of hyperthyroidism subside. Propylthiouracil is faster acting while carbimazole is longer acting. Carbimazole is a prodrug of methimazole. See Table 63.1

Pharmacokinetics

Thiourelyenes are effective orally; about 75% propylthiouracil is firmly bound to plasma proteins - hence very little crosses the placenta and a negligible fraction reaches the milk; but carbimazole and methimazole cross the the placenta and are secreted in the milk (table 63.1). Thioureylenes are concentrated in the thyroid. They are metabolised in the liver.

Adverse effects

Adverse effects include allergic reactions,

jaundice and headache. Agranulocytosis is a rare but serious adverse effect which occurs in about 0.1% of patients. It is reversible on stopping the antithyroid drug but patient should be monitored with frequent WBC counts. Thioureylenes can also cause arthralgia, myalgia, lymphadenopathy and rarely, psychosis.

Uses

Antithyroid drugs are used in hyperthyroid states like-

a. **Graves' disease** or diffuse toxic goitre needs long term (1-15 yrs) treatment with antithyroid drugs. Patients are usually euthyroid after 8-12 weeks of treatment. Smaller maintenance doses (Table 63.2) are then sufficient.

b. **Toxic nodular goitre** As an alternative - when surgery cannot be done as in the elderly - antithyroid drugs are used .

c. **Preoperatively** - hyperthyroid patients are made euthyroid with antithyroid drugs and then operated.

d. **Hyperthyroidism in pregnancy** - is rare but when severe, requires treatment. Propylthiouracil in the preferred drug as it poorly crosses the placental barrier. It is also

Keybox 63.1
Drugs that influence thyroid function

Amiodarone	Phenytoin
Sulfonamides	Carbamazepine
Lithium	Sodium nitroprusside

preferred in thyrotoxicosis in lactating mothers as only a negligible amount of propylthiouracil is secreted in the milk.

e. **Thyroid storm** or thyrotoxic crisis is sudden, severe exacerbation of thyrotoxicosis and can be life threatening. It is precipitated by factors like stress, infections, trauma, surgery etc. Inadequately treated thyrotoxic patients may go into thyroid storm. Symptoms include fever, tachycardia, nausea, vomiting, diarrhea, profuse sweating, confusion, restlessness, pulmonary edema, CCF and may lead on to coma and death. Propylthiouracil, oral/rectal potassium iodide, IV hydrocortisone, tepid sponging, sedation, IV fluids and supportive therapy are needed immediately. Propranolol may be used to rapidly control the symptoms. It also impairs conversion of T_4 to T_3 which may be of value.

TABLE 63.1 Differentiating features between Propylthiouracil & Methimazole (and Carbimazole)		
Features	**Propylthiouracil**	**Methimazole**
Onset of action	Faster acting	Slower acting
t½	1-2 hours	6 hours
Additional action	Prevents peripheral convertion of $T_4 \rightarrow T_3$	No such effect
Protein binding	75%, Firmly protein bound	Nil
Placental transfer	Negligible amount crosses placenta	Easily crosses
Secretion in milk	Negligible	Significant
Pregnancy	Preferred	Not Preferred
Lactating mothers	Drug of choice	Not used
Dose frequency	t.i.d.- q.i.d.	o.d.- b.i.d.
(Carbimazole is a prodrug, converted to methimazole in the body)		

IODIDES

Iodides inhibit the release of thyroid hormones and in thyrotoxic patients the symptoms subside in 1-2 days. The gland becomes firm, less vascular and shrinks in size over a period of 10-14 days. These effects are transient and decrease after 15 days. Iodides are administered orally as Lugol's iodine or as potassium iodide solution - 3 drops 3 times a day. Lugol's iodine is 5% iodine in 10% potassium iodide. Iodine is converted into iodides in the intestine which is then absorbed.

Uses

1. **Preoperative preparation for thyroidectomy** Iodine is started just 10 days prior to surgery to make the thyroid gland firm and less vascular.
2. **Thyroid storm** Iodides act rapidly to reduce the release of thyroid hormones.
3. **Prophylaxis** Iodide or iodate is added to common salt to prevent endemic goitre.
4. **Antiseptic** (See page 513).
5. **Expectorant** Potassium Iodide is used in cough.

Preparations

- Lugols iodine (5% iodine with 10% potassium iodide)
- Povidone iodine (5-10% solution)
- Tincture of iodine (2% iodine with 2.4% sodium iodide)

Adverse effects

Adverse effects include allergic reactions like skin rashes, conjunctivitis, rhinitis, vasculitis swelling of the lips, and salivary glands, fever and lymphadenopathy. Chronic overdose can cause **iodism** with metallic taste, excessive salivation, lacrimation, burning sensation in oral cavity and throat, running nose, sore throat, cough, headache and rashes.

Iodine overdosage

Acute toxicity with iodine can be fatal (3-4 grams is the fatal dose).

Signs and symptoms Iodine is a powerful irritant and vesicant.

- Nausea, vomiting, diarrhea, an unpleasant metallic taste.
- Vesication, desquamation and corrosion of skin and mucous membrane with brownish yellow stains.
- Corrosion and perforation of mouth, throat and GI tract can occur.
- Nephritis and renal failure.
- Delirium, stupor.
- Inhalation produces edema of glottis and pulmonary edema.
- Anaphylactic reactions can occur.

Treatment

- Induction of vomiting or stomach wash are contraindicated.
- Administer starch or flour solution (30g per litre of water). Milk is also helpful.
- Sodium thiosulphate is the antidote. A solution of 1 to 5% sodium thiosulphate is given orally. This will convert iodine to iodide which is relatively harmless.
- Skin lesions can be treated with 20% alcohol.
- Supportive therapy.

Iodism is a term used to denote chronic poisoning with iodide salts and is characterized by erythema, urticaria, acne, stomatitis, conjunctivitis, rhinorrhea, parotid swelling, lymphadenopathy, anorexia and insomnia. Treatment involves liberal intake of sodium chloride which promotes excretion of iodides. This is because chloride competes with iodide for excretion at the level of the renal tubules.

RADIOACTIVE IODINE

^{131}I given orally as a solution is rapidly absorbed and is concentrated by the thyroid in the follicles. It emits both γ and β rays. The γ rays pass

TABLE 63.2 Dosage of antithyroid drugs

Drug	Daily dose
Carbimazole	Start with 15-45 mg Maintenance 5-10mg
Methimazole	Start 15- 30 mg Maintenance 5-15 mg
Propylthiouracil	Start 150-300 mg Maintenance 40-100 mg
Lugol's Iodine (5% iodine in 10% potassium iodide solution)	5-15 drops

through the tissue while β particles penetrate only 0.5 mm to 2 mm of the tissue due to which it destroys only the thyroid tissue without damaging the surrounding structures. Iodides also inhibit the synthesis of thyroid hormone for 1-2 days (known as Wolff-Chaikoff effect). ^{131}I has a half-life of 8 days but the radioactivity is present upto 2 months. It is given as a single dose; clinically the effect is seen after 1-2 months.

Radioactive Iodine is used in the treatment of hyperthyroidism and in thyroid carcinoma. Small dose is used for diagnostic purpose in thyroid function tests.

Advantages of ^{131}I are that

i. Administration is simple
ii. Convenient
iii. Surgery and its associated risks can be avoided.
iv. Less expensive when compared to surgery.

The disadvantages are

i. The long time (3 months) taken for maximum response
ii. The risk of hypothyroidism which may develop

after months and years. The patient should be followed up for the symptoms of hypothyroidism and replacement therapy with thyroid hormones should be promptly given.

β-adrenergic blockers

Many of the symptoms of hyperthyroidism are of sympathetic overactivity as there is increased tissue sensitivity to catecholamines in hyperthyroidism. β adrenergic blockers like propranolol relieve symptoms like palpitation, tremors, nervousness, sweating and myopathy. They only afford symptomatic relief and are used as adjuvants.

Ionic inhibitors

Ionic inhibitors interfere with the concentration of iodine by the thyroid gland. Thiocyanate and perchlorate inhibit the organification of iodine but are not used now due to the adverse effects. Food like cabbage; cigarette smoking and drugs like sodium nitroprusside, increase the concentration of thiocyanate in the blood and may result in hypothyroidism.

Drugs that influence thyroid function

Apart from antithyroid drugs, amiodarone, lithium, sulfonamides, phenytoin, carbamazepine and sodium nitroprusside can influence thyroid function. Amiodarone, an antiarrhythmic drug contains iodine. It can cause hypothyroidism, hyperthyroidism or chemical thyroiditis and thyrotoxicosis. Treatment is to stop amiodarone if possible. Hypothyroidism is treated with thyroxine while hyperthyroidism is treated with a thioureylene and prednisolone.

Corticosteroid ⟨ Glucocorticoid — Cortisol-hydrocortis
Mineralo corticoid - aldosterone

ACTH - Adreno corticotrophin hormone.
CRF = Corticotrophin releasing factor.

64 Corticosteroids

CHAPTER

- Structure and synthesis
- Glucocorticoids
- Actions
- Mechanism of action
- Preparations
- Pharmacokinetics
- Adverse effects
- Uses
- Mineralocorticoids
- Inhibitors of Adrenal steriods synthesis

Corticosteroids are hormones produced in the cortex of the adrenal gland. They are glucocorticoids, mineralocorticoids and a small amount of androgens. Cortisol is the major glucocorticoid while aldosterone is the major mineralocorticoid. The secretion of adrenal cortex is under the control of ACTH, secreted by the anterior pituitary and this is in turn regulated by CRF and plasma corticosterone levels (Fig. 64.1). This is termed hypothalamic-pituitary-adrenal axis.

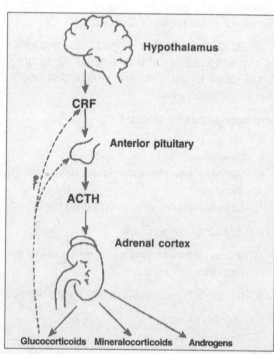

Fig. 64.1 Hypothalamo-pituitary-adrenal axis. Regulation of synthesis and secretion of adrenal corticosteroids

462

Structure and synthesis

The corticosteroids have a cyclopentanoperhydrophenanthrene (steroid) ring. (Fig 64.2) They are synthesized in the adrenal cortex from cholesterol (Fig. 64.3) under the influence of ACTH.

Every day about 10-20 mg of hydrocortisone (maximum in the early morning) and 0.125 mg of aldosterone are secreted. They are also released in response to stress.

GLUCOCORTICOIDS

Hydrocortisone is the natural glucocorticoid while prednisolone, triamcinolone, dexamethasone, paramethasone and betamethasone are synthetic derivatives. Hydrocortisone has both gluco-corticoid and mineralocorticoid activity.

ACTIONS

A. Glucocorticoid actions

1. Metabolic effects

Carbohydrate, protein and fat metabolism - Glucocorticoids promote gluconeogenesis and

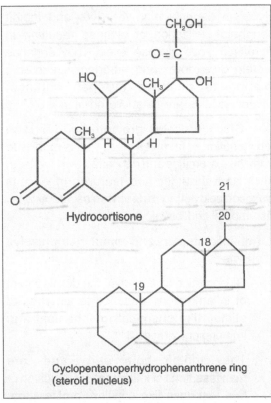

Fig 64.2: Structure of Hydrocortisone and the steroid nucleus

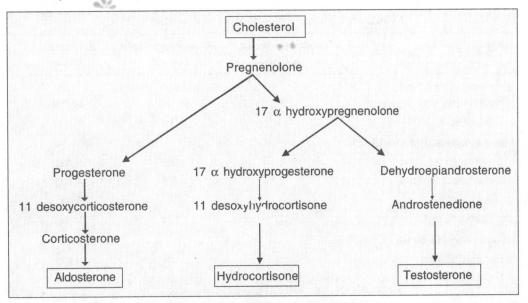

Fig. 64.3 Synthesis of adrenal steroids

glycogen deposition in the liver and inhibit peripheral utilization of glucose resulting in increased blood glucose levels. They enhance protein breakdown and nitrogen is excreted leading to negative nitrogen balance. Glucocorticoids are catabolic hormones.

Glucocorticoids promote lipolysis and redistribution of fat takes place - fat is mobilised from the extremities and deposited over the face, neck and shoulder and features of excess glucocorticoid activity is described as 'moon face', 'fish mouth' and 'buffalo hump'.

2. Anti-inflammatory and immunosuppressive effects

- Glucocorticoids suppress the development of inflammatory response to all types of stimuli like chemical, mechanical and immunological stimuli.

- They inhibit both early and late manifestations of inflammation. Inhibition of late response like capillary proliferation, collagen deposition, fibroblastic activity and scar formation may delay wound healing.

- They inhibit migration and depress the function of the leukocytes and macrophages and inhibit the release of chemical mediators. The ability of these cells to respond to antigens is decreased.

- Glucocorticoids - even a single dose bring about a decrease in the number of WBCs - lymphocytes, monocytes, eosinophils and basophils decline.

- Metabolites of arachidonic acid like prostaglandins and leukotrienes are important mediators of inflammation.

- Glucocorticoids induce the synthesis of a protein - lipocortin, which inhibits phospholipase A_2 thereby decreasing the production of prostaglandins and leukotrienes. Glucocorticoids also suppress the production of cyclooxygenase-2 (COX-2) in the inflammatory cells.

- They also suppress the production of cytokines (IL-6 and ILb) which play a key role in inflammation.

TABLE 64.1 Relative potency of some corticosteroids			
Drug	**Glucocorticoid activity**	**Mineralocorticoid activity**	**Equivalent dose**
Short-acting (8-12 hr)			
Hydrocortisone	1	1	20 mg
Cortisone	0.8	0.8	25 mg
Intermediate-acting (18-36 hr)			
Prednisolone	4	0.8	5 mg
Methylprednisolone	5	0.5	4 mg
Triamcinolone	5	0	4 mg
Fludrocortisone	10	125	2 mg
Long-acting (36-54 hr)			
Paramethasone	10	0	2 mg
Dexamethasone	25	0	0.75 mg
Betamethasone	30	0	0.6 mg

Glucocorticoids thus suppress cell-mediated immunity, prevent manifestations of allergy and inflammation and prevent homograft rejection. Large doses also inhibit antibody production.

3.Other actions

- Glucocorticoids reduce capillary permeability, thereby reducing fluid exudation and maintain the tone of arterioles. They have a positive inotropic effect on the heart. Prolonged use can cause hypertension.

- They are essential for normal muscular activity.

- They are required for normal functioning of the central nervous system. Deficiency results in apathy and depression while large doses result in restlessness, anxiety and sometimes, psychosis.

- GIT - Glucocorticoids enhance the secretion of gastric acid and pepsin in the stomach.

- Calcium metabolism - Glucocorticoids inhibit absorption and enhance the renal excretion of calcium - they antagonise the effect of vitamin D on calcium absorption. Bone resorption takes place.

- Formed elements of blood - glucocorticoids have a lympholytic effect which is very prominent in lymphomas; but they increase the number of platelets and RBCs.

- They are essential for maintaining normal GFR.

TABLE 64.2 Preparations and dose of some commonly used glucocorticoids			
Glucocorticoid	**Trade name**	**Dosage form**	**Daily dose**
Hydrocortisone hemisuccinate	EFCORLIN	10 mg tablet 50 mg/ml inj IM, IV Also available for retention enema, intraarticular inj and topical use	30-100 mg
Prednisolone	WYSOLONE	5,10, 20 mg tab 20 mg/ml inj pediatric and topical preparations also available	5-60 mg 10-40 mg IM
Methylprednisolone acetate	SOLVMEDROL	4 mg tab 20 mg/ml inj Retention enema	4-32 mg
Triamcinolone	KENACORT	4 mg tab 10 mg/ml inj 5- 40 mg inj IM/IA	4-20 mg
Dexamethasone	DEXONA	0.5 mg tab 4 mg/ml inj	0.5-5 mg oral 4-20 mg IV/IM
Betamethasone	BETNESOL	0.5 mg tab 4 mg/ml inj	0.5-5 mg oral 4-20 mg IM/IV
IM = intramuscular, IV = intravenous, IA = intra-articular			

B. Mineralocorticoid action

Glucocorticoids have a weak mineralocorticoid action - cause some salt and water retention and potassium excretion. Some synthetic glucocorticoids are devoid of this activity.

MECHANISM OF ACTION

Corticosteroids enter the cells by simple diffusion, bind to specific receptors in the cytoplasm (Fig. 64.4) and activate them. The drug-receptor complex is then transported into the nucleus where it binds to specific sites on DNA and induce the synthesis of specific mRNA. By this they regulate the synthesis of new proteins that bring about the hormone effects.

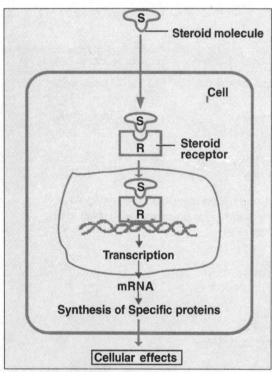

Fig. 64.4 Mechanism of action of Corticosteroids

PHARMACOKINETICS

Most glucocorticoids are well-absorbed orally. Hydrocortisone undergoes high first pass metabolism. It is 95% bound to plasma proteins -

corticosteroid binding globulin (CBG) or transcortin. Glucocorticoids are metabolised by microsomal enzymes in the liver. They first undergo oxidation and reduction followed by conjugation. Sulphate and glucuronide conjugation produce inactive water-soluble compounds which are excreted by the kidneys. The t½ varies with each agent and we have short, intermediate and long-acting agents (Table 64.1).

PREPARATIONS

Glucocorticoids are given by many routes - orally, parenterally, topically, by inhalation and nasal spray. They may also be injected intra-articularly. The synthetic analogs are more potent than hydrocortisone and have less or no mineralocorticoid activity - (Table 64.2).

- Hydrocortisone, the chief natural glucocorticoid is used orally and parenterally; in emergencies it is used intravenously.

- Prednisolone has potent glucocorticoid with mild mineralocorticoid activity. It is the most commonly used preparation.

- Prednisone is a prodrug converted to prednisolone in the liver.

- Methylprednisolone is similar to prednisolone and is used as retention enema and for high dose pulse therapy.

- Triamcinolone, dexamethasone and betamethasone have no mineralocorticoid activity and have selective, potent glucocorticoid effects.

Topical Preparations

Several glucocorticoid preparations are available for topical use as creams, ointments, nasal and eye drops. Some of them also contain antibiotics (Table 64.3). Glucocorticoids are also available for inhalation (Table 64.4)

TABLE 64.3 Some topical glucocorticoid preparations

Hydrocortisone acetate (LYCORTIN Oint)	1%
Triamcinolone (LEDERCORT Oint)	0.1%
Dexamethasone (DECADRON Cream)	0.1%
Flucinolone acetonide (FLUCORT Oint)	0.025%
Betamethasone dipropionate/valerate (BETNOVATE Oint, Cream)	0.025%
Beclomethasone dipropionate (BECLATE Cream)	0.025%
Clobetasol propionate (TOPIFORT CREAM)	0.05%

Table 64.4 Steroids for inhalation

Beclomethasone (BECLATE INHALER)	50 μg, 100 μg 200 μg / metered dose
Budesonide (BUDECORT)	200 μg / metered dose
Fluticasone (FLOHALE)	25, 50, 150 μg / metered dose

ADVERSE EFFECTS OF GLUCOCORTICOIDS

Adverse effects of glucocorticoids (Fig. 64.5) are dependent on dose, duration of therapy and the relative potency of additional mineralocorticoid effects. Whenever possible, they should be used topically to avoid systemic effects. Single doses are harmless while short courses are well-tolerated. Prolonged use is associated with toxicity. Adverse effects include:

1. **Cushing's syndrome** with characteristic appearance of moon face, supraclavicular hump (buffalo hump), truncal obesity, muscle wasting, thinning of the limbs and skin, easy bruising, purple striae and acne.

2. **Hyperglycaemia** and sometimes diabetes mellitus may be precipitated.

3. **Susceptibility to infections** is increased and the severity of any infection may be more because of immunosuppression. Opportunistic infections may occur. Previously dormant tuberculosis may become active.

4. **Osteoporosis** especially of the vertebrae is more common in the elderly.

5. **Avascular necrosis** of the bone due to restriction of blood flow through bone capillaries may cause joint pain, stiffness and restriction of movement. Head of the femur, humerus and distal part of fermur may be affected. Growth in children may be suppressed.

6. **Peptic ulceration** may sometimes occur on prolonged therapy especially when other ulcergenic drugs (e.g. NSAIDs) are used concurrently.

7. **Mental disturbances** Alterations in behaviour can occur with high doses of steriods. Symptoms may range from insomnia, anxiety, nervousness, mood changes, euphoria, psychosis or depression.

8. **Cataract** and glaucoma may follow long-term use of glucocorticoids even as eye drops. Patients receiving long term steroids should undergo eye examinations for these.

9. **Delayed wound healing** Steroids may delay wound healing.

10. **Other effects** include raised intracranial pressure, convulsions, hypercoagulability of the blood and menstrual disorders.

11. **HPA axis suppression** depends on the dose, duration and time of administration. After prolonged steroid therapy, adrenal cortex gradually atrophies due to feedback inhibition. If steroid administration is suddenly stopped, acute adrenal

insufficiency results. Hence after prolonged administration, steroids should be tapered before withdrawal to allow HPA axis to recover. Prior to surgery or general anaesthesia, it is advisable to elicit proper drug history. If the patient has received long-term steroids within previous six months, it is prudent to administer prophylactic hydrocortisone to avoid shock. Two weeks of use of > 20 mg hydrocortisone/day needs tapering of the dose.

In order to minimize HPA axis suppression, **lowest effective** dose of a glucocorticoid for the **shortest possible period** should be used. The drug should be given in a **single morning dose.** Administration on **alternate days** is found to be associated with least/no HPA axis suppression and whenever possible this measure should be followed, especially when long-term steroids are needed.

12. Mineralocorticoid effects including salt and water retention, oedema, hypokalaemia and hypertension are rare with selective glucocorticoids.

USES

I. Replacement therapy

1. Acute adrenal insufficiency is an emergency condition that could be precipitated by an infection or sudden withdrawal of steroids. Symptoms include

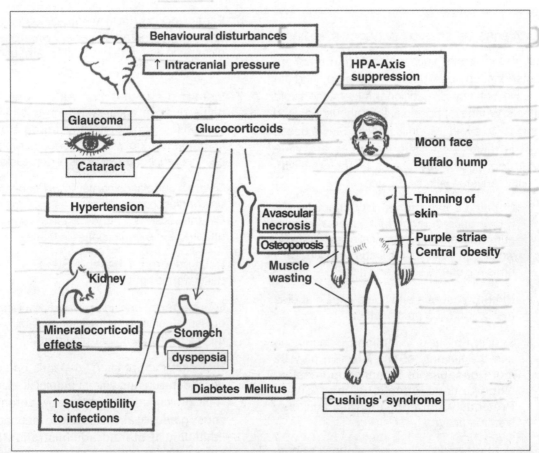

Fig. 54.5 Adverse effects of glucocorticoids

0946322 6299

nausea, vomiting, weakness, hypotension, dehydration, hyponatremia and hyperkalemia. Intravenous hydrocortisone hemisuccinate 100 mg bolus followed by infusion 100mg every 4-6 hours is given immediately. The dose may be repeated depending on the patient's condition. Once the patient recovers, switch over to oral preparations. Immediate correction of fluid and electrolyte balance is important. When acute adrenal insufficiency is not confirmed, dexamethasone (4mg IV) should be used in place of hydrocortisone because dexamethasone does not interfere in the estimation of hydrocortisone levels for diagnosis.

2. **Chronic adrenal insufficiency** (Addison's disease). Oral hydrocortisone 20-40 mg daily is given. Some patients may need additional fludrocortisone (a mineralocorticoid)

3. **Congenital adrenal hyperplasia** is characterised by impaired synthesis of corticosteroids due to deficiency of some enzymes involved in synthesis. As a result ACTH levels rise resulting in adrenal hyperplasia. Hydrocortisone is given daily and if mineralocorticoids are also deficient, fludrocortisone may be added.

II. Pharmacotherapy

Glucocorticoids have been used in a variety of nonendocrine conditions where they are of palliative value, but may even be life saving.

1. **Rheumatoid arthritis** In progressive disease steroids are given with NSAIDs. If 1-2 joints are involved, intra-articular injections are preferred.

2. **Osteoarthritis** Steroids are given as intra-articular injections with strict aseptic precautions. A minimum of 3 months interval should be given between two injections of steroids into the joint. Repeated injections can result in joint destruction.

3. **Rheumatic carditis** Severely ill-patients with fever and not responding adequately to NSAIDs require glucocorticoids.

4. **Acute gout** When treatment with NSAIDs has not been successful, prednisolone is used as an adjuvant.

5. **Allergic diseases** like angioneurotic oedema, hay fever, serum sickness, contact dermatitis, urticaria, drug reactions and anaphylaxis - steroids are indicated. Steroids are slow acting and in less severe cases, antihistamines should be preferred.

6. **Shock** Severe inflammatory reaction may be the cause for septic shock. An infusion of high dose of glucocorticoids may be life saving in such patients. Glucocorticoids act directly on the vascular smooth muscle and indirectly by sensitizing the adrenergic receptors to the effect of sympathomimetics.

7. **Bronchial asthma**

   - Acute exacerbations - a short course of prednisolone

   - Status asthmaticus - intravenous hydrocortisone hemisuccinate 100-200mg repeated after 8 hrs or methylprednisolone 60mg every 6 hours followed by oral prednisolone 40-60mg per day for 5 days till the patient recovers. Prednisolone should then be tapered.

   - Chronic asthma - steroids are used as supplement to bronchodilators. Inhalational steroids are used and in more severe cases low dose oral prednisolone is indicated. COPD - exacerbation may be treated with short courses of prednisolone.

8. **Collagen diseases** like polyarthritis nodosa, lupus erythematosus, polymyositis, Wegener's granulomatosis and other rheumatoid disorders respond to glucocorticoids. Glucocorticoids are the first-line drugs. Prednisolone is given for 6 weeks and tapered over another 6 weeks.

9. **Eye diseases** Allergic conjunctivitis, uveitis, optic neuritis and other inflammatory

TABLE 64.5 : Contraindications to glucocorticoid therapy

Steroids should be used with caution in:

1. Peptic ulcer	6. Osteoporosis
2. Hypertension	7. Psychoses
3. Infections	8. Epilepsy
4. Diabetes mellitus	9. CCF
5. Ocular infections particularly viral infections	10. Glaucoma
	11. Renal failure

conditions are treated with steroid eye drops. Long term steriods administration can increase IOP which should be monitored. In ocular infections, steroids are contraindicated.

10. **Renal diseases** like nephrotic syndrome are treated with steroids. Glucocorticoids are the first line drugs. Prednisolone is given for 6 weeks and tapered over another 6 weeks.

11. **Skin diseases** Atopic dermatitis, seborrhoeic dermatitis, inflammatory dermatoses and other local skin conditions are treated with topical steroids. Systemic steroids are **life saving** in pemphigus.

12. **Gastrointestinal diseases** Mild inflammatory bowel diseases like ulcerative colitis are treated with steroid retention enema while severe cases need oral prednisolone. Budesonide may be given as retention enema or as oral enteric coated capsule so that it is released in the ileum and colon. It causes fewer side effects when compared to other glucocorticoids.

13. **Liver diseases** Steroids are useful in conditions like autoimmune chronic active hepatitis and may be tried in alcoholic hepatitis.

14. **Haematologic disorders** like purpura and haemolytic anaemia having immunological aetiology respond to steroids.

15. **Cerebral oedema** Large doses of dexamethasone reduce cerebral edema occurring in some malignancies.

16. **Malignancies** Because of their lympholytic effects and inhibition of cell proliferation, steroids are used in the treatment of acute lymphocytic leukaemia and lymphomas - as a component of combination chemo-therapy. Steroids are used for rapid symptomatic relief in other malignancies like breast cancer.

17. **Lung diseases** Apart from bronchial asthma, steroids are used in other diseases like aspiration pneumonia and prevention of infant respiratory distress syndrome.

18. **Organ transplantation** For prevention and treatment of graft rejection, high doses of prednisolone are started at the time of surgery with immunosuppressive agents.

19. **Others** - Glucocorticoids are useful in

- *Sarcoidosis* to induce remission.

- *Pneumocystis carinii* - *pneumonia* in patients with AIDS - Glucocorticoids reduce the risk of respiratory failure and decrease mortality.

- *Haemolytic anaemia* - glucocorticoids reduce the autoimmune destruction of erythrocytes in haemolytic anaemia.

Contraindications

Glucocorticoids are contraindicated in several conditions - See table 64.5.

Drug interactions

- Drugs like erythromycin, ketoconazole, cyclosporin and isoniazid inhibit the metabolism of glucocorticoids resulting in an increase in the plasma levels of glucocorticoids.

- Microsomal enzyme inducers like

phenobarbitone and rifampicin enhance the rate of metabolism of glucocorticoids.

MINERALOCORTICOIDS

The most important natural mineralocorticoid is aldosterone synthesized in zona glomerulosa of the adrenal cortex. Small amounts of desoxycorticosterone is also released.

Actions

Mineralocorticoids promote sodium and water retention by distal renal tubules with loss of potassium. They act by binding to the mineralocorticoid receptor.

Adverse effects include weight gain, oedema, hypertension and hypokalaemia.

Fludrocortisone has predominantly mineralocorticoid properties and is used for replacement therapy in aldosterone deficiency as in Addison's disease. Although aldosterone is the principal natural mineralocorticoid, it is not used therapeutically since it is not effective orally.

INHIBITORS OF ADRENAL STEROIDS SYNTHESIS

Metyrapone, trilastane, aminoglutethimide and ketoconazole These drugs inhibit the synthesis of adrenal steroids by inhibiting certain enzymes involved in steroid synthesis. They are used in Cushing's syndrome and some prostatic and breast cancers.

65 Estrogens, Progestins & Hormonal Contraceptives

- • **Physiologic Consideration**
- • **Estrogens**
- • **Selective estrogen receptor modulators and antiestrogens**
- • **Estrogen synthesis inhibitors**
- • **Progestins**
- • **Antiprogestins**
- • **Hormonal contraceptives**
- • **Drugs used in the treatment of menopausal symptoms**
- • **Hormonal Contraceptives**
  - **- Mechanism of action of oral contraceptives**
  - **- Adverse effects**
  - **- Benefits of combined pills**
  - **- Contraindications to combined pills**
- • **Centchroman**

Physiologic Consideration

At puberty, the ovary begins its cyclic function which stretches over 30-40 years characterised by regular episodes of uterine bleeding.

The hypothalamus releases the GnRH in pulses which stimulates the release of FSH and LH from the anterior pituitary (Fig. 65.1). At the beginning of each cycle, a number of follicles begin to enlarge in response to FSH. After 5-6 days, one of the follicles begin to develop more rapidly. The granulosa cells of this follicle multiply and under the influence of LH and FSH, synthesize oestrogens. This oestrogen inhibits FSH release, resulting in regression of the smaller follicles. The ovarian follicle consists of an ovum surrounded by a fluid filled antrum, lined by granulosa and theca cells. Just before the midcycle, the oestrogen secretion reaches a peak, stimulating a brief surge in FSH and LH levels which results in **ovulation** by around the 14th day of the cycle (Fig 65.1).

ESTROGENS

The estrogens are produced by the ovaries, placenta and in small amounts by the adrenals,

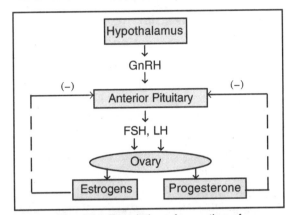

Fig. 65.1 Regulation of secretion of gonadal hormones

testes and by peripheral aromatisation of androgens. During the first part of the menstrual cycle, estrogens are produced by the granulosa cells by aromatisation of androgens derived from theca cells in the ovarian follicle. The major estrogens are estradiol, estrone and estriol. estradiol is converted to estrone and estriol by the liver and other tissues. Some chemical alterations have been made in the natural estrogens to produce synthetic estrogens. Some non steroidal compounds with estrogenic activity have also been synthesized - like diethyl stilbestrol, dienestrol and hexestrol.

Estrogens include -

Natural estrogens
- Estradiol, Estrone, Estriol.

Synthetic estrogens
- Oral   -   Ethinyl estradiol, Stilboestrol, Mestranol.
- Topical - Dienestrol.

Estrogen receptors

Estrogen receptors are nuclear receptors and are of two types. ER α and ER β.

Distribution

ERα - Female reproductive tract, breast, blood vessels and hypothalamus

ERβ - Ovaries and prostate

Selective agonists of these receptor subtypes are being developed. Selective estrogen receptor modulators (SERMs) are now available for clinical use.

Actions

Estrogens are required for -

1. the normal maturation of the female reproductive tract.

2. development of secondary sexual characters in the female.

3. stimulation of preovulatory endometrium.

4. metabolic effects - estrogens inhibit the resorption of bone and maintain the bone mass. They promote the fusion of epiphyses.

5. estrogens are important for the maintenance of normal structure of the skin and blood vessels in women.

6. estrogens decrease plasma LDL cholesterol and raise HDL cholesterol and triglycerides.

7. effect on blood coagulation - estrogens enhance the coagulability of the blood.

Pharmacokinetics

Natural estrogens are metabolised rapidly in the gut - hence are not effective orally; they have a short t½. All estrogens get absorbed through the skin and mucous membrane. They are largely bound to plasma proteins. Synthetic oestrogens are orally effective and are long-acting.

Adverse effects

- Nausea, breast tenderness, migraine headaches, hyperpigmentation, hypertension and cholestasis (gallstones are common) may be seen. In men gynaecomastia and feminization can occur.

- *Cancers* Increased incidence of endometrial and breast cancers are reported on long-term use of only estrogens. Therefore it should be combined with progesterone.

- *Teratogenicity* When given to a pregnant lady oestrogens (diethyl stilbosterol) may cause:
  - In female child - increased risk of vaginal -and cervical cancers
  - In male child - genital abnormalities.

Preparations

Estrogens are available for oral and parenteral use. A transdermal patch for cyclic estrogen therapy is available. Estrogen vaginal cream and vaginal pessaries are also available. Conjugated estrogens (Premarin) are available as tablets, injections and vaginal cream. **Cenestin** is a synthetic conjugated estrogen available as tablets (0.625mg) for control of menopausal symptoms.

Uses

1. **Replacement therapy** In primary hypogonadism - estrogen started at 11-13 years of age stimulates the development of secondary sexual characters and menstruation. It requires supplementation with progestins.

2. **Postmenopausal syndrome** Due to decreased estrogen production at menopause, hot flushes, anxiety, fatigue, sweating, muscle and joints pain are common. Other longer-lasting changes including osteoporosis, genital atrophy, skin changes, increased risk of cardiovascular disease and psychological disturbances may be seen. Estrogens given in low doses are highly effective in reversing most of the changes.

3. **Senile vaginitis** is common in elderly women due to reduced oestrogen synthesis by the ovary. Estrogen cream is used topically.

4. **Osteoporosis** In postmenopausal osteoporosis, oestrogens restore calcium balance and need to be given for a long time.

5. **Oral contraceptives** estrogens are used.

6. **Dysmenorrhoea** estrogens combined with progestins suppress ovulation and such anovulatory cycles are painless. estrogens are used only in severe dysmenorrhoea.

7. **Dysfunctional uterine bleeding** Oestrogens are used as adjuvants to progesterone.

8. **Carcinoma prostate** is an androgen dependent tumour. Estrogens antagonise the action of androgens, suppress androgen production and are useful for palliative therapy.

Contraindications

Estrogen dependent tumours, liver disease, thromboembolic disorders.

SELECTIVE ESTROGEN RECEPTOR MODULATORS (SERMS) AND ANTI-ESTROGENS

Tamoxifen was earlier considered to be an estrogen antagonist. But now it is understood that it acts as an agonist, antagonist or partial agonist depending on the site. **Raloxifene, toremifene** and **ormeloxifene** have actions similar to tamoxifen and are all termed selective estrogen receptor modulators (SERMs). SERMs have tissue-selective estrogenic activities. i.e.,

- They have agonistic effects on bone, lipid metabolism, brain and liver.

- Antagonists at breast, pituitary and endometrium;

- Partial agonist at genitourinary epithelium, bone remodeling and cholesterol metabolism.

Tamoxifen

By its tissue selective activity on the estrogen receptor, tamoxifen -

- Inhibits the proliferation of tumor cells in the breast.
- Stimulates the proliferation of the endometrium.
- Reduces bone resorption.
- Decreases total cholesterol

Side effects include hot flushes, nausea, vomiting, vaginal dryness, cataract and skin rashes. Tamoxifen increases the risk of endometrial cancer and thromboembolism

Uses

Breast cancer - Tamoxifen is used in the palliation of advanced breast cancer in postmenopausal women with estrogen receptor positive tumors.

Raloxifene

Raloxifene, a nonsteriodal SERM - acts as an estrogen receptor agonist in the bone. In women with postmenopausal osteoporosis, raloxifene has antiresorptive effects on the bone. It reduces bone loss and may even help to gain bone mass. Raloxifene also lowers LDL. It acts as an estrogen antagonist in the breast due to which it reduces the incidence of breast cancer. Raloxifene does not stimulate the uterine endometrial proliferation.

Adverse effects include hot flushes, leg cramps and an increased risk of deep vein thrombosis and pulmonary embolism.

Raloxifene is indicated for the prevention of postmenopausal osteoporosis.

Toremifene

Toremifene has actions similar to tamoxifen and is indicated in the treatment of metastatic breast cancer in postmenopausal women.

Ormeloxifene

Ormeloxifene has antagonistic effects on the estrogen receptors in the uterus and breast tissue. It prevents the endometrial proliferation. It prevents excessive bleeding in anovulatory cycles at the time of menopause. Ormeloxifene can cause headache, nausea, weight gain and prolonged menstrual cycles. It has been tried in dysfunctional uterine bleeding.

Clomiphene citrate

Clomiphene citrate binds to the estrogen receptors and acts as a competitive inhibitor of endogenous oestrogens. Like tamoxifen, it is also a partial agonist. Clomiphene opposes the negative feedback of endogenous oestrogens on the hypothalamo - pituitary axis resulting in increased gonadotrophin secretion and thereby induces ovulation.

Side effects include ovarian hyperstimulation resulting in multiple pregnancy, ovarian cysts, hot flushes, headache and skin rashes.

Uses

1. Infertility: Clomiphene citrate is used in infertility due to ovarian disorders. It is given orally, 50 mg daily for 5 days starting from 2nd - 5th day of the cycle; course is repeated till ovulation occurs

2. In vitro fertilization: Clomiphene induced ovulation is also useful in *in vitro* fertilization.

ESTROGEN SYNTHESIS INHIBITORS

- GnRH agonists administered continuously suppress the biosynthesis of estrogens.
- Aminoglutethimide inhibits the synthesis of all steroids by inhibiting the activity of aromatase - an enzyme involved in steroidogenesis.
- Newer generation selective aromatase inhibitors like formestane, exemestane, anastrozole, letrozole and vorozole block the production of estrogens and are used in the treatment of breast cancer.

PROGESTINS

Progesterone is the natural progestin synthesized in the ovary and placenta. It is also synthesized by the testis and adrenals where it acts as a precursor of various steroid hormones (see under corticosteroids).

Progestins

- Natural

    Progesterone

- Synthetic

    Medroxyprogesterone acetate
    Allylestrenol, Megestrol
    Norethisterone acetate
    Lynestrenol

- Newer progestins
  (with no androgenic activity)
    Norgestimate, Desogestrol,
    Gestodene

Actions

1. Uterus The secretory changes in the endometrium like increased tortuosity of the glands are due to progesterone. In pregnancy, decidual changes in the endometrium take place under the influence of progesterone. Progesterone is very important for the maintenance of pregnancy (**Progestin** = favours pregnancy).

2. Cervix The watery cervical secretions are changed to a viscid scanty secretion by progesterone.

3. Vagina Vaginal epithelium changes to that seen in pregnancy.

4. Mammary gland Along with oestrogen, progesterone is responsible for the development of the secretory apparatus in the breast and prepares the gland for lactation.

5. Body temperature Increase in the body temperature by 1°C during luteal phase beginning at ovulation is due to progesterone.

Adverse effects

Headache, breast engorgement, rise in body temperature, oedema, acne and mood swings may be seen. Progesterone is teratogenic. Some progestins can cause virilisation of the female foetus.

Uses

1. Contraception (see below).

2. Hormone replacement therapy (HRT) Progestins are combined with estrogens in HRT of postmenopausal women (given cyclically). Estrogen administration

TABLE 65.1 Therapeutic uses of estrogens and progestins	
Estrogens	*Progestins*
1. HRT - Primary hypogonadism - Postmenopausal syndrome	1. HRT
2. Contraception	2. Contraception
3. Senile vaginitis	3. Dysmenorrhoea
4. Osteoporosis	4. DUB
5. Carcinoma prostate	5. Endometriosis
6. DUB	6. Premenstrual syndrome
7. Dysmenorrhoea	7. Endometrial cancer

increases the risk of endometrial cancer - supplementing it with progestin counters this risk.

3. Ovarian suppression Progestins are used to suppress ovulation in dysmenorrhoea, endometriosis, dysfunctional uterine bleeding (DUB) and premenstrual syndrome.

4. Threatened or habitual abortion Efficacy in such patients is not proved.

5. Endometrial carcinoma Progestins are used as a palliative measure in cases with metastasis.

6. Endometrial hypoplacias Progestins are also used in these.

Other progesterone derivatives

Danazol is a derivative of ethisterone (17α ethinyl testosterone). It has weak progestational, androgenic and glucocorticoid activities. It inhibits the midcycle surge (but not the basal secretion) of FSH and LH in women. This reduction of ovarian function results in atrophic changes in the endometrium.

Danazol is primarily used in the treatment of endometriosis. It is also used in menorrhagia, fibrocystic disease of the breast, gynaecomastia and is tried in some disorders of allergic etiology like idiopathic thrombocytopenic purpura, angioedema, haemophilia and Christmas disease.

Danazol can cause side effects like hot flushes, edema, weight gain, acne, headache, adrenal suppression and hepatotoxicity.

ANTIPROGESTINS

Mifepristone

Mifepristone (RU 486) binds to the progesterone receptor and blocks the actions of progesterone. When given in early pregnancy - abortion occurs.

Mechanisms of action - Mifepristone blocks the progesterone receptors in the uterus which causes decidual breakdown; blastocyst gets detached, HCG and progesterone secretions fall. This in turn increases prostaglandin levels and stimulate uterine contractions. It also softens the cervix and facilitates expulsion of the blastocyst.

If given during the follicular phase - mifepristone prevents the midcycle surge of gonadotrophins and delays ovulation.

Mifepristone also binds to glucocorticoid receptors.

Uses

1. Termination of pregnancy Early pregnancy up to 9 weeks can be terminated with a single oral dose - 600 mg of mifepristone (Mifegest, Mifeprin) followed 48 hr later by a prostaglandin to increase uterine contractions and facilitate expulsion of the blastocyst.

Adverse effects include heavy bleeding,

TABLE 65.2 Antagonists of sex hormones and their uses		
Hormone	*Receptor antagonist*	*Uses of antagonist*
Estrogen	Tamoxifen Clomiphene citrate	Breast cancer • Infertility • *In vitro* fertilization
Progesterone	Mifepristone	Termination of pregnancy
Androgen	Flutamide Cyproterone	• Carcinoma prostate • Hypersexuality in men • Female hirsutism

nausea and abdominal pain.

2. **Postcoital contraception** Mifepristone prevents implantation when given within 72 hours after coitus.

When mifepristone is used regularly in late luteal phase it acts as a contraceptive.

DRUGS USED IN THE TREATMENT OF MENOPAUSAL SYMPTOMS

Decreased production of estrogen at menopause results in symptoms like hot flushes, vaginitis, dryness, anxiety, fatigue, sweating, muscles and joints pain; longer lasting changes include osteoporosis, urogenital atrophy, dyspareunia, skin changes, increased risk of cardiovascular disease and psychological disturbances.

Drugs used include -

- Hormonal agents
  Estrogen
  Progesterone
  Tibolone
- Nonhormonal agents
  Clonidine
  Veralipride
  Propranolol

Hormonal agents

Hormone replacement therapy (HRT) with estrogen reverses the menopausal symptoms and reduces the risk of osteoporosis and cardiovascular disease, but using oestrogen alone can increase the risk of endometrial carcinoma and may stimulate the growth of uterine fibroids. Addition of a progestin counters these unwanted effects. Hence a combination of oestrogen and progestin is now recommended for HRT at menopause.Various regimens with cyclic oestrogens and progestins are being used. If withdrawal bleeding is undesirable, the hormones are given continuously. They may be given orally or as transdermal patches or subcutaneous implants.

Tibolone is a synthetic steroid, which has effects like both estrogen and progesterone. It is found

to reduce the symptoms of estrogen deficiency in menopause.

Non-hormonal agents

Clonidine, an α adrenergic agonist and veralipride, a dopamine antagonist can reduce hot flushes. Propranolol can be used to overcome palpitations.

HORMONAL CONTRACEPTIVES

Millions of women around the world use hormonal contraceptives making them one of the most widely prescribed drugs.When properly used, they are the most effective spacing methods of contraception. Hormonal contraceptives have greatly contributed to the control of population throughout the world.

Oral Pills

1. Combined-pill
2. Mini-pill
3. Postcoital pills

Depot preparations

1. Injectables- progesterone
2. Subcutaneous implants
3. Transdermal patches
4. Vaginal rings

ORAL PILLS

Combined pill

Combined pills contain low doses of an estrogen and a progestin. They are highly efficacious (success rate 98%).

Ethinylestradiol or mestranol (in the dose of 20-50 mcg) are the oestrogens used. Newer progestins like desogestrel and norgestimate cause least side effects. The pill is started on 5th day of the menstrual cycle, taken daily for 21 days followed by a gap of 7 days, during which, bleeding occurs. This is monophasic regimen.

Oral contraceptives are also available as biphasic or triphasic preparations (see Table 65.3). This reduces the amount of hormones needed and more closely mimics menstrual cycles. Biphasic pills consists of estrogens given for 10 days followed by a progestin for the next 11 days. Because of the risk of endometrial cancer following such biphasic use of the hormones, biphasic pills are not preferred.

Triphasic pills with low doses of an estrogen with a progestin are very effective.

If a woman misses a pill, she should take 2 pills the next day and continue the course. If more than 2 pills are missed, then that course should be withdrawn, should follow an alternative method of contraception for that particular cycle and restart the course on the 5th day of the next menstrual cycle. If the woman has conceived, the pregnancy should be terminated as these hormones are teratogenic. However recent studies have shown that in such low doses, the hormones are not teratogenic.

Mini-pill

A low dose progestin is taken daily without a gap.

Estrogen and its accompanied long-term adverse effects are also eliminated. But efficacy is lower, menstrual cycles may be irregular and is therefore not popular.

Postcoital contraceptives

- High dose of an estrogen (stilboestrol - 25 mg daily for 5 days) was used earlier but this may cause severe nausea and vomiting. If the pills are expelled in vomiting, they need to be repeated.

- Combination of estrogen and progestins is now preferred due to lower doses needed and lesser side effects reported. Two tablets with ethinyl estradiol (50mcg) and a progestin is given as soon as possible (within 72 hours of coitus) and has an efficacy of 90-98%. The dose is repeated after 12 hours.

TABLE 65.3 : Oral contraceptive preparations			
Regimen	*Estrogen*	*Progestin*	*Trade name*
1. Combined pills			
Monophasic (21 days from day 5 of the menst. cycle)	EE 50 µg EE 30 µg	Norgestrel 0.5 mg Levonorgestrel 0.15 mg	OVRAL-G OVRAL-L
Biphasic (10+11)	EE 35 µg	Norethindrone 0.5 mg (10 days) 1 mg (11 days)	—
Triphasic (6+5+10)	6 days EE 30 µg next 5 days EE 40 µg next 10 days EE 30 µg	Levonorgestrel 50 µg Levonorgestrel 75 µg Levonorgestrel 125 µg	TRIQUILAR
2.Mini-pill	—	Norgestrel 75 µg	OVRETTE
3.Postcoital pills	• Diethyl stilbosterol (25 mg/day for 5 days) Or	—	—
	• Combined pill - EE 50 µg + Levonorgestrel 0.25 mg (2 stat. and 2 after 12 hours) Or		OVRAL
	• Levonorgestrel (0.75 mg 1 pill stat and 1 after 12 hours)		ECEE 2
EE - Ethinyl estradiol			

- Levonorgestrol 0.75 mg 2 doses 12 hours apart have also been found to be effective.

- Mifepristone (RU486) 600mg prevents implantation when given within 72 hours after coitus.

- Postcoital pills act by preventing implantation. The earlier they are started the better is their efficacy.

- If postcoital pills fail, pregnancy should be terminated by other methods because oral contraceptives are likely to be teratogenic.

- Insertion of an intrauterine device (IUD) within 5 days of coitus can also prevent implantation and thereby prevent pregnancy.

- Postcoital contraception is advocated as an emergency method in situations following rape or contraceptive failure.

DEPOT PREPARATIONS

Progestin Injections

Depot preparations contain a progestin and are given as:

1. *Intramuscular injections* at 3 - 6 months intervals, e.g. depot medroxyprogesterone acetate (DMPA) (150-400 mg) or Norethisterone enanthate (NET EN) (200 mg). Long term use of DMPA reduces menstrual blood loss. The risk of endometrial carcinoma is also reduced.

2. *Subcutaneous Implants* - They are implanted under the skin. **Norplant** capsules implanted subcutaneously in the forearm or upper arm work for 5 years. It contains a progestin and acts like DMPA.

Disadvantages

i.   Amenorrhoea is common.

ii. Disruption of menstrual cycle.

iii Suppression of ovulation may sometimes continue upto 18 months after the last injection.

iv Suppression of estrogen secretion may result in a reduced bone density - but is reversible.

Combined injectable contraceptives containing an estrogen with a progestogen are injected at monthly intervals. They are highly effective with side effects similar to progesterone-only implants. They are better tolerated but further reports of long term effects on reversal of ovulation are yet to be available.

Transdermal contraceptives - A transdermal patch containing a progestin (norelgestromin) and ethinyl estradiol is available. It is to be applied once a week for 3 weeks and the next week withdrawal bleeding follows. It has the advantage of better compliance.

Vaginal rings - containing levonorgestrel are now available. They are placed in the vagina for 3 weeks of the cycle and then removed for one week. The hormone is absorbed gradually through the vaginal mucosa. The advantage is the need for a low dose of the hormone because the first pass metabolism is avoided.

Mechanism of action of oral contraceptives

Combined pills act by multiple mechanisms. (Fig 65.2)

1. They prevent ovulation - By a negative feedback on the hypothalamus, progesterone decreases GnRH pulses and thereby LH release which is essential for ovulation.

2. Estrogens suppress FSH release by negative feedback on the pituitary. As a result the ovarian follicle fails to develop.

3. Progesterone also inhibits estrogen-induced mid-cycle LH surge.

4. Progesterone renders the cervical mucous

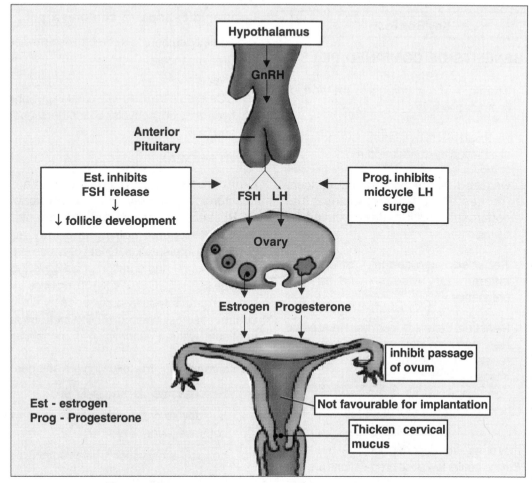

Fig. 65.2 Mechanism of action of hormonal contraceptives

thick and unfavourable for sperm penetration.

5. OCs alter the uterine endometrium making it unfavourable for implantation.

6. OCs also adversely influence the coordinated contractions of the cervix, uterus and fallopian tubes which are required for transport of ovum, sperm as well as fertilisation and implantation.

Adverse effects

- Headache, migraine headache in some women, nausea, vomiting, edema, breast tenderness, amenorrhoea and irregular menstrual cycles may commonly be seen.

- Weight gain, acne, mood swings and hirsuitism may occur.

More severe side effects include -

- Cardiovascular effects - in women above 35 years, OCs may increase the risk of MI and venous thromboembolism. OCs may also increase the coagulability of blood. But the newer low-dose preparations are found to be safer when used in healthy women with no

Key Box 65.1

BENEFITS OF COMBINED PILLS

1. Effective and convenient method of contraception.

2. Reduced risk of ovarian cancers (ovarian stimulation by gonadotropins)

3. Reduced risk of endometrial cancers (progesterone antagonises the endometrial proliferation induced by estrogens)

4. Reduced incidence of pelvic inflammatory disease and ectopic pregnancy.

5. Menstrual benefits - less menstrual blood loss, less iron - deficiency; premenstrual tension and dysmenorrhoea are less intense.

other risk factors for MI or thromboembolism.

- **Hypertension** - The high dose preparations may precipitate hypertension in some women. But the newer low dose preparations are safer.

- **Cancers** OCs may increase the incidence of cervical, breast and other cancers - but the risk is not significant.

- **Cholestatic jaundice and gallstones** Incidence may be higher in high dose preparations.

- **Impaired glucose tolerance** OCs may impair glucose tolerance - but the newer low dose preparations do not carry such risk.

Contraindications to combined pill

- Thromboembolic and cerebrovascular disease
- Breast cancers
- Liver disease
- OCs should be used with caution in diabetes, hypertension, convulsive disorders, oedema and CCF.

CENTCHROMAN

Centchroman a chroman derivative, is a nonsteroidal oral contraceptive developed by CDRI, Lucknow. It has antioestrogenic and antiprogestogenic activity and may act by preventing implantation. Onset of action is quick (< 60 minutes) and duration of action is 7 days. Dosage (SAHELI, CENTRON) 30 mg twice a week for 3 months followed by once a week till contraception is desired (The tablet should be continued without withdrawing for menstruation).

Centchroman has the following advantages

1. Success rate claimed is 97-99%

2. It is devoid of the side effects of hormonal contraceptives

3. Long $t\frac{1}{2}$ allows once a week administration

4. No teratogenicity, carcinogenicity or mutagenicity reported

5. It is well tolerated.

Centchroman may cause prolongation of menstrual cycles in 10% of women. It may cause ovarian enlargement and should be avoided in polycystic ovaries. It should also be avoided in renal and hepatic dysfunction, tuberculosis and in lactating mothers.

66 Androgens And Anabolic Steroids

- Physiological considerations
- Physiological actions
- Anabolic steroids
- Antiandrogens
- Male contraceptives
- Drugs used in male sexual impotence

Physiological Considerations

Androgens are produced chiefly in the testis and small amounts in the adrenal cortex. In the females, small amounts of androgens are produced in the ovary and adrenal cortex. Testosterone is the most important natural androgen. In the adult male, 8-10 mg of testosterone is produced daily. Secretion is regulated by gonadotrophins and GnRH.

Physiological actions

In the male, testosterone is essential for the development of secondary sexual characters and sex organs. It is necessary for normal spermatogenesis and is important for maintaining sexual function in men. Testosterone promotes bone growth, enhances the muscle mass, protein synthesis and positive nitrogen balance - has anabolic actions.

Mechanism of action

Mechanism of action of androgens is similar to other steroids. Androgens bind to androgen receptors on the target cells, the complex moves to the nucleus where it stimulates protein synthesis.

Adverse effects

Masculinization and acne in females; hepatotoxicity, increased libido and precocious puberty can occur in young boys. With large doses, salt and water retention, suppression of spermatogenesis resulting in infertility can be seen. Feminizing effects like gynaecomastia in men can occur as some androgens are converted to estrogens.

483

Uses

1. **Testicular failure:** Androgen replacement therapy in primary and secondary testicular failure.
2. **Other uses:** Androgens may be used in senile osteoporosis and carcinoma of the breast in premenopausal women.

ANABOLIC STEROIDS

Anabolic steroids are synthetic androgens with higher anabolic and low androgenic activity. These are believed to enhance protein synthesis and increase muscle mass. But with higher doses, the relative anabolic activity is lost (Table 66.1).

Adverse effects of anabolic steroids are similar to those caused by androgens.

Uses

1. **Catabolic states** Anabolic steroids may benefit patients following surgery, trauma, prolonged illness and debilitating conditions. Given during convalescence, the negative nitrogen balance is corrected, appetite improves and there is a feeling of well being.
2. **Senile osteoporosis** seen in elderly males respond by formation of new bone tissue.
3. **Growth stimulation in children** Anabolic steroids promote linear growth in prepubertal boys. They may be used only for short periods - but actual benefit on final height is not established.
4. **Other uses** Anabolic steroids are tried in chronic renal failure to reduce nitrogen load on the kidneys. They may benefit in refractory anaemias with bone marrow failure.
5. **Abuse in athletes** Anabolic steroids enjoy a reputation for improving athletic performance. When combined with adequate exercise, the muscle mass increases. But the dose used by athletes is very high and is associated with serious adverse effects like testicular atrophy, sterility and gynaecomastia in men and virilizing effects in women; increased aggressiveness, psychotic symptoms and increased risk of coronary heart disease in both sexes. Moreover, there is no evidence that athletic performance improves. Hence the use of anabolic steroids by athletes has been banned and is medically not recommended.

Contraindications for the use of androgens

1. Pregnancy
2. Carcinoma of prostate/breast in males
3. Infants and chlidren
4. Renal/cardiac/liver disease.

ANTIANDROGENS

Cyproterone acetate a derivative of progesterone competitively binds to androgen receptors and thus blocks the actions of androgens. It also has progestational activity.

Cyproterone is used to treat severe hypersexuality in males, in carcinoma prostate and in female hirsuitism.

Flutamide and **Bicalutamide** are potent competitive antagonists at androgen receptors. They are used with GnRH/leuprolide in the treatment of carcinoma prostate.

Finasteride inhibits the enzyme 5-alpha reductase and thus inhibits the convertion of testosterone to its active metabolite dihydrotestosterone which acts mainly in the male urogenital tract. Fenasteride is used in benign prostatic hypertrophy to reduce the prostate size.

Inhibitors of androgen synthesis

Gonadotrophin releasing hormone or its agonist like leuprolide when given continuously inhibit LH and testosterone secretion resulting in pharmacological castration - used in men with prostatic cancer.

Antifungal agent **ketoconazole** also inhibits steroid hormone synthesis and thereby inhibits androgen synthesis.

MALE CONTRACEPTIVES

The requirement of a safe and effective chemical contraceptive in men has not been fulfilled largely because it is difficult to totally suppress spermatogenesis. Various compounds including testosterone with progestin, oestrogens with progestins, antiandrogens like cypterone acetate have been tried, but are neither reliable nor safe.

GnRH agonists and antagonists along with testosterone inhibit gonadotrophin secretion and are being studied.

Gossypol, a cotton seed derivative has shown to produce oligozoospermia and impair sperm motility in Chinese studies. This effect is reversible in a few months. Hypokalaemia is the major adverse effect.

DRUGS USED IN MALE SEXUAL IMPOTENCE

Sexual impotence is the inability of a man to have satisfactory sexual intercourse due to inability to have and maintain an erection. Very often it is psychological while in some cases there could be an organic cause.

Several drugs have been tried including testosterone, yohimbine, papaverine and antidepressants. The recent introduction - Sildenafil (Viagra) has been a success in a large percentage of them.

Sildenafil (Viagra)

Sildenafil is the first agent to be effective orally for the treatment of erectile dysfunction. Sildenafil inhibits the enzyme phosphodiesterase in the penis and thus prolongs the life of cyclic GMP. This causes relaxation of smooth muscle in the corpus cavernosum and vasodilation - both resulting in cavernosal engorgement and penile erection.

Sildenafil is given orally (50-100 mg) 1 hour before sexual activity.

Adverse effects and precautions

Due to vasodilation - headache, dizziness and nasal stuffiness can occur. It potentiates the hypotensive action of nitrates and is contraindicated in patients on nitrates and in patients with coronary artery disease. Elderly men above 60 years need less dose (25 mg). Patients with liver disease, kidney disease, bleeding disorders and elderly people are at a higher risk of toxicity. Several deaths have been reported in such patients.

Two other derivatives tadalafil and vardanafil have properties similar to sildenafil. Tadalafil 10, 20mg tab (Zydalis).

TABLE 66.1 Preparations of anabolic steroids			
Anabolic steroid	*Route*	*Dose*	*Trade name*
Methandienone	Oral	2-10 µg/day	PRONABOL
Nandrolone phenylpropionate	IM	10-50 µg/week	DURABOLIN
Nandrolone decanoate	IM	25 -100 µg/3 weeks	DECADURABOLIN
Ethylestrenol	Oral	2-4 µg/day	ORABOLIN
Oxandrolone	Oral	5-10 µg/day	ANAVAR
Stanozolol	Oral	2-10 µg/day	STROMBA

67 *Insulin And Oral Hypoglycaemics*

CHAPTER

- **Diabetes mellitus**
- **Insulin**
- **Highly purified insulins**
- **Human insulins**
- **Insulin analogs**
- **Oral Hypoglycaemic Drugs**
  - Sulfonylureas
  - Biguanides
  - Meglitinides
  - Thiazolidinediones
  - α - Glucosidase inhibitors
- **Treatment of Diabetes Mellitus**
- **Glucagon**

Diabetes mellitus

Diabetes mellitus is a chronic metabolic disorder characterised by hyperglycaemia and altered metabolism of carbohydrates, lipids and proteins. It is a common condition affecting 1-2% of population with a strong hereditary tendency.

Diabetes mellitus can be of 2 types

Type I Insulin dependent diabetes mellitus (IDDM) is an autoimmune disorder where antibodies destroy the β cells of the islets of Langerhans. It usually occurs in the young children and adolescents (hence called juvenile onset diabetes mellitus).

Type II Non-insulin dependent diabetes mellitus (NIDDM) is of maturity onset. Most patients are obese. There is both reduced sensitivity of tissues to insulin and impaired regulation of insulin secretion.

Prolonged hyperglycaemia results in various complications including premature atherosclerosis, retinopathy, nephropathy and gangrene of the limbs. This is thought to be due to reduced blood supply to these structures - because of thickening of the capillary walls. Accumulation of glycosylated products in the vessel walls may be responsible for the thickening. Moreover, intracellular glucose is converted to sorbitol by the enzyme aldose reductase. This sorbitol exerts osmotic effect resulting in tissue damage

486

particularly in the retina and peripheral nerves. Hence, it is necessary to maintain normal blood glucose levels though diabetes mellitus as such does not cause significant troublesome symptoms. It helps to prevent or delay the onset of complications of diabetes.

INSULIN

In 1921 Banting and Best first obtained insulin in the form of pancreatic extract. In 1922 an extract containing insulin was first used on a 14 year old boy suffering from severe diabetes mellitus with excellent response. Insulin was then purified in a few years.

Chemistry, synthesis and secretion

The islets of Langerhans are composed of 4 types of cells - β (B) cells secrete insulin, α (A) cells glucagon, δ (D) cells somatostatin and P cells secrete pancreatic polypeptide. Glucose enters the pancreatic β cells with the help of glucose transporters. Insulin is released from the granules by a process of exocytosis. Natural insulin is a polypeptide synthesized from the precursor proinsulin. It has two peptide chains - A chain (21 amino acids) and B chain (30 amino acids) linked by disulphide bridges. Human insulin differs from bovine insulin by 3 amino acids and from porcine insulin by 1 amino acid. Hence porcine insulin is closer to human insulin. Insulin is stored in granules in the β islet cells of the pancreas. Normal pancreas releases about 40 to 50 units of insulin everyday. The secretion is regulated by factors like food, hormones and autonomic nervous system. Hypokalemia inhibits insulin release. Blood glucose concentration is the main factor.

Insulin is metabolised in the liver, kidney and muscle.

Glucose transporters - are proteins present in different tissues. They are of 5 subtypes - GLUT1 to GLUT5. They mediate various functions - for example- GLUT4 present in muscle and adipose tissues promotes the uptake of glucose.

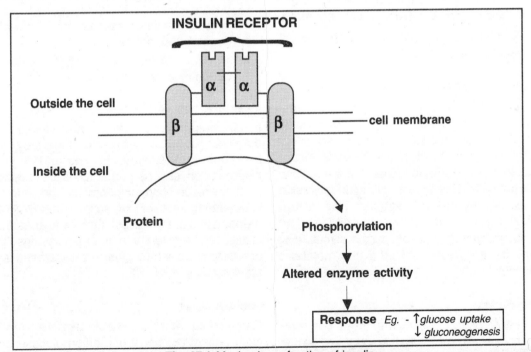

Fig. 67.1 Mechanism of action of insulin

Actions of Insulin

1. **Carbohydrate metabolism** Insulin stimulates the uptake and metabolism of glucose in the peripheral tissues especially skeletal muscles and adipose tissue. It inhibits glucose production in the liver by inhibiting gluconeogenesis and glycogenolysis.

   By the above actions, insulin lowers the blood glucose concentration.

2. **Lipid metabolism** Insulin inhibits lipolysis in adipose tissue and promotes the synthesis of triglycerides. In diabetes, large amounts of fat are broken down. The free fatty acids so formed are converted by the liver to acetyl CoA and then ketone bodies. This results in ketonaemia and ketonuria.

   Insulin indirectly enhances lipoprotein lipase activity resulting in increased clearance of VLDL and chylomicrons. In insulin deficiency, there is hypertriglyceridaemia.

3. **Protein metabolism** Insulin facilitates amino acid uptake and protein synthesis and inhibits protein break down - anabolic effect.

   In diabetes, there is increased catabolic effect and negative nitrogen balance.

Mechanism of action

Insulin acts by binding to specific receptors. (Fig 67.1) Insulin receptor is a glycoprotein made up of two α and two β subunits. Insulin receptors are present on almost all cells in the body. Insulin binds to these receptors present on the surface of target cells. This binding stimulates tyrosine kinase activity in the β subunit. This in turn activates a cascade of phosphorylation and dephosphorylation reactions which stimulate or inhibit the enzymes involved in the metabolic actions of insulin.

Side effects

1. **Hypoglycaemia** is the most common complication of insulin therapy. It may be due to too large a dose, inappropriate time of administration, unusually small meal or vigorous exercise. Symptoms - sweating, palpitation, tremors, blurred vision, weakness, hunger, confusion, difficulty in concentration and drowsiness. Severe hypoglycaemia may result in convulsion and coma.

Treatment

Oral glucose or fruit juice like orange juice or in severe cases IV glucose promptly reverse the symptoms.

2. **Allergy** This is due to the contaminating proteins. Urticaria, angiooedema and rarely anaphylaxis can occur. It is rare with purified preparations and human insulin.

3. **Lipodystrophy** Atrophy of the subcutaneous fat at the site of injection may be due to immune response to contaminating proteins.

   Lipohypertrophy *i.e.* enlargement of subcutaneous tissue can also occur due to the local action of insulin. Insulin absorption may be irregular from such areas. This can be prevented by frequently changing the sites of injection. Lipodystrophy is rare with purified preparations.

4. **Oedema** Some severe diabetics develop oedema which is self-limiting.

Preparations of Insulin (Table 67.1)

Insulin preparations differ in their source and duration of action. Based on the source they may be grouped as Bovine, Porcine and Human insulins. Conventional preparations are obtained from bovine and porcine pancreas. They may be short, intermediate or long-acting (Table 67.2) All preparations are given SC. Only regular (plane) insulin can be given IV in emergencies. Insulins are destroyed when given orally. Doses are expressed as units.

Insulin dose

Requirement of insulin should be calculated in each patient by monitoring blood glucose and *glycosylated haemoglobin* levels. Several regimens including mixtures of insulins are being used. Multiple doses of insulin offer better glycaemic control as compared to single bedtime dose. In an IDDM patient the daily requirement of insulin varies from 0.2 to 1 IU/kg. In obese patients the requirement is higher. Mixtures of short-acting and intermediate/long-acting preparations are given for a rapid onset and long duration of action.

Disadvantages of the conventional insulin preparations are that:

i. They are allergenic because of the impurities (1%) and their animal source.

ii. They are not very stable.

Hence highly purified preparations are now made available.

Highly purified insulins are mostly porcine insulins purified by more developed purification techniques including gel filtration and ion exchange chromatography. The contaminating protein content is negligible. They are available in short and long acting forms. Highly purified insulins have the following advantages over conventional insulins -

1. They are less antigenic
2. More stable
3. Lesser chances of resistance
4. Lesser chances of lipodystrophy.

Purified insulins are of two types based on the purification techniques used -

* *Single peak insulins*
* *Monocomponent insulins.*

They are available in regular and lente preparations but are expensive.

(ACTRAPID, LENTARD, MONOTARD MC, ACTRAPID MC)

TABLE 67.1 Preparations of insulin

CONVENTIONAL INSULINS	
• Short and Rapid acting	Regular
	Semilente
• Intermediate acting	Lente
	Isophane insulin (NPH)
• Long acting	Ultralente
	Protamine zinc insulin
HIGHLY PURIFIED INSULINS	
• Single peak insulin	Regular
	Lente
• Monocomponent insulins	Regular
	Lente
HUMAN INSULIN	Regular
	Lente
	Isophane
INSULIN ANALOGS	Insulin lispro
	Insulin aspart
	Insulin glargine
INSULIN MIXTURES	Combinations of 20 - 50% regular with 80 - 50% NPH Insulins

TABLE 67.2 Onset and duration of action of insulin preparations

Preparation	Onset (hrs)	Duration (hrs)
SHORT-ACTING		
Regular (plane, soluble)	0.5-1	8
Semilente (Insulin zinc suspension/amorphous)	1	14
INTERMEDIATE-ACTING		
Lente (Insulin zinc suspension)	2	24
NPH (Neutral protamine hagedorn) or Isophane insulin	2	24
LONG-ACTING		
Ultra lente (Insulin zinc suspension crystalline)	6	36
PZI (Protamine zinc insulin)	6	36

Human insulins are produced by recombinant DNA technology. Human proinsulin gene is introduced into *E.coli,* which is cultured and proinsulin is extracted. This is modified to get human insulin. It can also be obtained by enzymatic treatment of porcine insulin. Human insulin is available as regular, NPH, lente and ultralente preparations - but they are all expensive.

Human insulin is less immunogenic and is absorbed more rapidly; dose needed is lesser (10%). It is more expensive.

Indications for highly purified/human insulins

1. Allergy to conventional preparations
2. Insulin resistance
3. Lipodystrophy at the site of injection
4. Pregnancy

Insulin analogs

Insulin analogs with favourable pharmacokinetic properties have been synthesized.They are absorbed 3 times faster than human insulin - therefore can be given subcutaneously 10 minutes before food; have lesser chances of hypoglycemia. Blood glucose control is better than with regular insulin.

Insulin lispro and *insulin aspart* are genetically engineered recombinent insulin analogs. Insulin lispro differs from human insulin by the transposition of two aminoacids – proline and lysine in the β chain. Hence the name lispro. Insulin aspart is obtained by substituting aspartic acid in place of proline in the β chain.

Glargine is a long-acting analog which acts for 24 hr. The effect is peakless but attains a broad plasma concentration plateau. Insulin glargine should not be mixed with any other insulin in the syringe.

Insulin delivery devices have been designed which make insulin administration more convenient. Portable *pen injectors* are small pen-size devices containing multiple doses of insulin and retractable needles.They can be carried while travelling and to the place of work. Insulin pumps (also called continuous subcutaneous insulin infusion or CSII) deliver appropriate doses of insulin on the basis of self–monitored blood glucose results. The set is inserted subcutaneously.

Alternative routes of insulin delivery have been tried - by inhalation, nasal spray, orally, rectally and as subcutaneous pellet implants. Orally insulin is tried with liposomes as carriers, but results are not encouraging. Subcutaneous pellets deliver insulin over weeks. Inhaled insulin is absorbed through lungs.

Drug interactions

1. β adrenergic blockers mask tachycardia, the important warning symptom of hypoglycaemia. They also prolong hypoglycaemia by inhibiting compensatory mechanisms acting through β_2 receptors.

2. Salicylates precipitate hypoglycaemia by enhancing insulin secretion and β cell sensitivity to glucose.

Uses of insulin

1. Diabetes mellitus

2. Myocardial infarction – Insulin, glucose and potassium chloride drip have been tried in myocardial infarction with arrhythmias. In such patients, potassium deficiency may result in arrhythmias and the drugs combination often helps.

3. Schizophrenia – insulin coma induced for about 20 minutes followed by glucose administration was tried in some patients with schizophrenia.

4. Burns – In patients with severe burns, insulin may be administered with glucose to reduce nitrogen and potassium loss.

5. Hyperkalemia – Insulin–glucose drip may be tried.

6. Anorexia nervosa – Insulin increases the appetite and may benefit such patients. Patient should be warned of hypoglycemia.

ORAL HYPOGLYCAEMIC DRUGS

The main disadvantage of insulin is the need for injection. The advent of oral hypoglycaemics came as a boon to millions of NIDDM patients with early and mild diabetes. Sulfonylureas were the first oral antidiabetics (OAD) to be made available in 1950s. We now have 5 groups of oral hypoglycaemics - sulfonylureas, biguanides, meglitinides, alpha glucosidase inhibitors and thiazolidinediones.

Classification

1. Sulfonylureas

I generation

Tolbutamide, chlorpropamide, acetohexamide, tolazamide

II generation

Glibenclamide, glipizide, gliclazide, glimepiride

2. Biguanides

Phenformin, metformin

3. Meglitinides

Repaglinide, nateglinide

4. Thiazolidinediones

Troglitazone, rosiglitazone, pioglitazone

5. Alpha glucosidase inhibitors

Acarbose, miglitol

SULFONYLUREAS

A sulfonamide derivative used for its antibacterial effects in typhoid patients produced hypoglycaemia. This observation led to the development of sulfonylureas.

Mechanism of action

Sulfonylureas reduce the blood glucose level by:

1. Stimulating the release of insulin from the pancreatic β cells.

2. Increasing the sensitivity of peripheral tissues to insulin.

3. Increasing the number of insulin receptors.

4. Suppressing hepatic gluconeogenesis.

Sulfonylureas bind to the sulfonylurea receptors (SUR) which are nothing but the ATP sensitive K^+ channels (K_{ATP}) present on the cell membrane of the pancreatic beta cells . Sulfonylureas bind to the SUR1 subunit on the K_{ATP} and bring about closure of these K$^+$ channels causing depolarisation of the membrane. This inturn opens the voltage dependent calcium channels, thereby leading to calcium influx. This calcium brings about release of insulin that is stored in the granules of the beta cells.

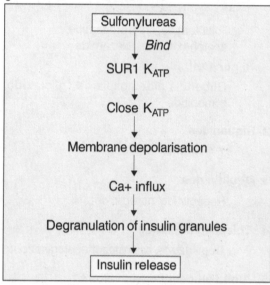

Sulfonylureas

Bind

SUR1 K$_{ATP}$

Close K$_{ATP}$

Membrane depolarisation

Ca+ influx

Degranulation of insulin granules

Insulin release

First generation agents

Tolbutamide is short acting and is therefore associated with lesser risk of hypoglycaemia - hence it is safer in the elderly diabetics.

Chlorpropamide is long acting (t ½ 32 hrs) and can cause prolonged hypoglycaemia particularly in the elderly.

Tolazamide has a slow onset of action. Use of first generation agents can result in several drug interactions.

Second generation agents

Second generation agents are more potent, have fewer side effects and drug interactions. But they can cause hypoglycaemia because of which they should be used cautiously particularly in the elderly. They are all contraindicated in renal and hepatic impairment.

Glibenclamide (Gliburide) is a commonly used sulfonylurea. It is longer acting - can be given once a day. It can cause hypoglycaemia and rarely, flushing after alcohol consumption.

Glipizide has a short t ½; food delays its absorption, it is less likely to cause hypoglycaemia.

Glimepiride is longer acting and can be given as a single morning dose.

Pharmacokinetics

Sulfonylureas are well-absorbed orally,

Drug	Dose	Duration of action
Tolbutamide (RASTINON)	500 mg q 8-12 h	6-8 hr
Chlorpropamide (DIABINESE)	250-500 mg OD	36-48 hr
Glibenclamide (DAONIL, EUGLUCON)	5 mg q 12-24 h	18-24 hr
Glipizide (D-GLIP, GLIBETIC)	5-15 mg OD-BD	12-18 hr
Gliclazide (D-GLIC, GLIX)	40-240 mg OD	12-24 hr
Glimepiride (GLYPRIDE, GLIMZ, AMRYL)	1-4 mg OD	12-24 hr
Metformin (GLYCIPHAGE, DIAFORMIN)	500 mg OD-BD	6-8 hr
Repaglinide (REPA, EUREPA)	0.5-4 mg BD-TID	4-5 hr
Nateglinide (GLINATE)	60-120 mg BD-TID	3-4 hr
Pioglitazone (GLITA, PIOZONE)	15-45 mg OD	12-24 hr
Rosiglitazone (ROSS, ROSICON)	2-8 OD	24 hr
Acarbose (DIABOSE, ACRAB)	25-100 mg before each meal	-
Miglitol	25-100 mg before each meal	-

TABLE 67.3: Dose and duration of action of oral hypoglycaemics

extensively bound to plasma proteins, metabolised in the liver and some are excreted in the urine. Hence they should be avoided in patients with renal or liver dysfunction. Dose - Table 67.3.

Adverse effects

Second generation agents have fewer adverse effects. Hypoglycaemia is the most common adverse effect, least with tolbutamide due to short t½ and low potency.

Nausea, vomiting, jaundice, and allergic reactions can occur (Table 67.4). Patients on sulfonylureas may have an increase in the rate of cardiovascular death. However this is still controversial and sulfonylureas continue to be used.

Sulfonylureas can precipitate a disulfirawm like reaction on consumption of alcohol. Patients should be warned to abstain from alcohol while on sulfonyureas.

Drug interactions

I. *Drugs that augment hypoglycaemic effect.*

- NSAIDs, warfarin, sulfonamides - displace sulfonylureas from protein binding sites.
- Alcohol, chloramphenicol, cimetidine - inhibit metabolism

II. *Drugs that decrease the action of sulfonylureas*

- Diuretics and corticosteroids - increase blood glucose levels.

BIGUANIDES

Biguanides lower blood glucose level by insulin-like effects on the tissues. Mechanism of action is not clear. They

- Suppress hepatic gluconeogenesis.
- Inhibit glucose absorption from the intestines.
- Stimulate peripheral uptake of glucose in tissues in the presence of insulin.

Phenformin is not used therapeutically as it causes lactic acidosis. **Metformin** is safer with lower incidence of lactic acidosis. It does not cause hypoglycaemia since it is an euglycaemic agent.

Adverse effects

Nausea, diarrhoea, and metallic taste are self-limiting. Rarely lactic acidosis can occur. Anorexia is advantageous as it helps in reducing body weight. Long term use may interfere with vitamin B_{12} absorption.

MEGLITINIDES

Repaglinide and nateglinide are insulin secretogogues. Like sulphonylureas, meglitinides enhance the release of insulin by blocking the ATP dependent K^+ channels in the pancreatic cells.

Both repaglinide and nateglinide are rapidly absorbed from the gut; repaglinide has a t½ of 1 hour. Both drugs can cause hypersensitivity reactions and hypoglycaemia – but the incidence is relatively lower with nateglinide. Gastrointestinal disturbances are common with repaglinide.

Meglitinides can be used in type 2 diabetes mellitus either alone or with biguanides. They can also be used as alternatives to sulfonylureas in patients allergic to sulfonylureas. Meglitinides enhance insulin release *in presence of glucose* - therefore the incidence of hypoglycemia is least with their use. For the same reason they are indicated mainly in patients who have significant postprandial hyperglycemia but the basal insulin secretion is not altered by meglitinides.

Keybox 67.1
Biguanides
• Have insulin-like effects
• Do not cause hypoglycaemia
• Weight reduction - due to anorexia
• Nausea, diarrhoea, metallic taste are transient
• Preferred in obese diabetics either alone or with sulfonylureas
• Contraindicated in renal, hepatic and cardiac diseases

Nateglinide is safe in patients with renal impairment and also causes least hypoglycemia.

THIAZOLIDINEDIONES (TZDS)

Thiazolidinediones or glitazones are agonists at the PPAR γ receptors (gamma subtype of Peroxisome proliferator - activated receptors). These are nuclear receptors present mostly in adipose tissue and also in muscle, liver and other tissues. TZDs activate the PPARγ receptors and modulate the expression of insulin sensitive genes. *ie.,* they induce the synthesis of genes which enhance insulin action.

TZDs increase insulin-mediated glucose transport into muscle and adipose tissue. They also promote glucose utilization.

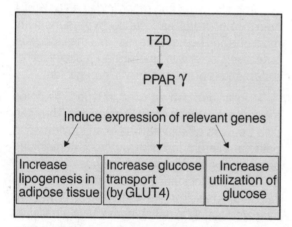

Advantages

- Reduce hepatic gluconeogenesis
- Once a day administration
- Low potential for hypoglycaemia
- Increase HDL cholesterol
- No clinically significant drug interactions known so far.

Disadvantages

- 6-12 weeks of treatment is required to establish maximum therapeutic effect.
- May cause weight gain and anaemia.

- May cause edema and precipitate or worsen CCF.
- Liver function should be monitored regularly.
- Troglitazone causes severe hepatotoxicity and therefore is not used now.

Uses

TZDs are used as adjuvants to sulfonylureas or biguanides in Type II diabetes mellitus. Though they can also be used as monotherapy in mild cases of type II diabetes, further studies are needed to prove their long term benefits.

α - GLUCOSIDASE INHIBITORS

Acarbose an oligosaccharide and **miglitol** competitively inhibit the enzymes α – glucosidases present in the intestinal brush border and thereby prevent the absorption of carbohydrates. Monosaccharides like glucose and fructose are absorbed from the intestines while disaccharides and oligosaccharides are broken down into monosaccharides before being absorbed. This 'breaking down' is done by the enzymes α-glucosidases (eg: sucrase, maltase, glycoamylase) and α - amylase present in the intestinal wall. Alpha glucosidase inhibitors inhibit the hydrolysis of disaccharides and decrease carbohydrate absorption.

- Alpha glucosidase inhibitors reduce the glucose absorption from upper intestines thereby reducing post prandial blood glucose levels.
- Alpha glucosidase inhibitors do not cause hypoglycaemia. But when used with other antidiabetics if hypoglycaemia occurs, glucose should be given and not sucrose because sucrase is inhibited.
- They may cause gastrointestinal disturbances including abdominal distention, flatulence and diarrhoea because of undigested carbohydrates reaching the colon and then getting fermented.

They can be used alone in patients with

predominantly postprandial hyperglycaemia or in combination with other oral antidiabetics or insulin.

TREATMENT OF DIABETES MELLITUS

The aim of treatment is to keep the blood sugar within normal limits and prevent complications of diabetes. For patients with IDDM, insulin is the only treatment as there is insulin deficiency due to destruction of pancreatic β cells. Sulfonylureas need functional β cells for their action and therefore are not useful in IDDM.

Mild NIDDM may be controlled by diet, exercise and weight reduction. When not controlled, an oral hypoglycaemic should be given. Most NIDDM patients may require insulin sometime later in life.

Status of oral antidiabetics

Uncomplicated NIDDM patients not controlled by diet and exercise are given oral hypoglycaemics. Mild NIDDM patients with recent onset diabetes, age above 40 years at the onset of diabetes, obese with fasting blood sugar < 200 mg/dl are candidates for oral hypoglycaemics. They are convenient to use. Sulfonylureas are preferred, but when not adequately controlled, metformin can be added. Metformin has the advantages of reducing appetite and being euglycaemic. In conditions like stress, surgery or complications of diabetes, insulin should be used. TZDs, meglitinides or a - glucosidase inhibitors may be used as monotherapy in mild NIDDM patients or as adjuvants along with sulfonylureas or biguanides.

Therapeutic failure

If patients are not responding to OAD from the very beginning, it is called primary failure and is rare. Secondary failure of sulfonylureas may result from poor diet control, progression of the disease, or from desensitization of the receptors. In such cases, change over to another sulfonylurea or add metformin and if still not controlled, switch over to insulin. In some patients, insulin may be supplemented with sulfonylureas as the latter increase the tissue sensitivity to insulin.

Insulin

Insulin is effective in all types of diabetes mellitus. The dose should be adjusted as per the needs of

TABLE 67.4: Mechanism of action and adverse effects of oral antidiabetics

Oral antidiabetics	Major Mechanism	Adverse effects
Sulfonylureas (eg: Tolbutamide, glibenclamide)	↑ insulin release from pancreas ↑ tissue sensitivity to insulin	Hypoglycaemia, cholestatic jaundice
Biguanides (Metformin)	↓ hepatic gluconeogenesis ↑ tissue sensitivity to insulin	Diarrhoea, metallic taste, rarely lactic acidosis.
Meglitinides (Repaglinide, nateglinide)	↑insulin release	Hypoglycaemia from pancreas
Thiazolidinediones (Rosiglitazone, pioglitazone)	PPAR γ agonist ↑ glucose transport into tissues ↓ hepatic gluconeogenesis	Weight gain, edema, may ppt CCF, Risk of hepatotoxicity
α glucosidase inhibitors (Acarbose, Miglitol)	↓ glucose absorption ↓ hydrolysis of disaccharides	Flatulence, diarrhoea, abdominal distension

each patient - guided by blood sugar levels.

Insulin resistance is said to be present when the insulin requirement is increased to > 200 U/day. Many consider requirement of > 100 U/day insulin as resistance. Insulin resistance is due to the antibodies to insulin which partly neutralise it. This is rare with purified preparations and human insulin. Antibodies may also develop to contaminants and other added constituents like protamine. Hence in presence of resistance, it is necessary to change over to highly purified/human insulin. In some patients immunosuppression with corticosteroids like prednisolone may help.

Diabetic ketoacidosis

Diabetic ketoacidosis is a medical emergency and can be life threatening. It is more common in patients with IDDM. Ketoacidosis may be precipitated by infection, trauma or stress. Insulin deficiency results in severe hyperglycemia (600-800mg / dl) and excessive production of ketone bodies.

Clinical features include metabolic acidosis, dehydration with loss of sodium and potassium in the urine causing electrolyte imbalance, impaired consciousness and hyperventilation - may proceed to coma.

Treatment

- *Correction of hyperglycaemia* - Intravenous regular (plane) insulin 0.1U/kg bolus followed by 0.1 U/kg/hour by continuous IV infusion till the patient recovers. Once the patient has fully recovered, SC insulin should be administered 30 minutes before stopping the infusion.
- *Correction of dehydration* - Fluid and electrolyte replacement are important. Normal saline infusion 1 litre in the first hour and then 1 litre over the next 4 hours and then the dose can be titrated based on the severity of dehydration.

Keybox 67.2
Drugs that can cause hyperglycemia
• Diazoxide, phenytoin, thiazides • Hormones - Adrenaline, glucagon, glucocorticoids, thyroid hormones.
Drugs that can cause hypoglycemia
• Quinine   • Lithium   • Glucogon • Alcohol   • Pentamidine

- *Correction of acidosis* - Sodium bicarbonate may be needed in some patients with severe acidosis.
- *Potassium* - Rapid correction of hyperglycaemia may result in the movement of potassium into the cells resulting in hypokalemia. 10-20 mEq/hour potassium chloride is added to the drip. When serum phosphate is also low, potassium biphosphate may be given to supplement both potassium and phosphorus.
- *Blood glucose* - may come down to normal but ketosis requires a longer time to be corrected and requires adequate insulin. Hence when the blood glucose comes down to about 300mg/dl it may be needed to administer glucose with insulin while we wait for the clearance of ketone bodies.

Hyperglycemic, hyperosmolar, nonketotic, coma - Severe hyperglycaemia and glycosuria result in severe dehydration and increased plasma osmolarity leading to coma and has a high mortality rate.

The treatment is similar to ketoacidosis with correction of fluid and electrolyte balance and plane insulin.

GLUCAGON

Glucagon is synthesized in the alpha (A) cells of the pancreatic islets of Langerhans; like insulin, the secretion of glucagon is regulated by nutrients - chiefly glucose, paracrine hormones and autonomic nervous system. Fasting stimulates glucagon secretion. It is degraded in the liver, kidney and plasma.

Actions

Glucagon increases blood glucose level by glycogenolysis and gluconeogenesis in the liver. It evokes insulin release. It mobilises stored fat and carbohydrates. Glucagon increases heart rate and force of contraction. It also relaxes the intestinal smooth muscles.

Uses

1. Severe hypoglycaemia - glucagon can be used in the emergency treatment of severe hypoglycaemia due to insulin.

2. Diagnostic uses - for diagnosis of IDDM.

3. Radiology of the bowel - as glucagon relaxes intestines.

68 Oxytocin and Drugs acting on the Uterus

- Uterine stimulants
  - Oxytocin
  - Ergometrine
  - Prostaglandins
- Uterine relaxants

UTERINE STIMULANTS

Drugs which stimulate the uterine contractions are **oxytocin, ergometrine** and **prostaglandins.** They are also called **oxytocics** or **ecbolics.** These drugs are useful in obstetrics.

Oxytocin

Oxytocin is a peptide hormone secreted by the posterior pituitary along with ADH. It is synthesized in the supraoptic and paraventricular nuclei of the hypothalamus, transported along the axon and stored in the neurohypophysis. It is released by stimuli such as suckling, coitus and parturition.

Actions

Uterus Oxytocin contracts the uterus. The fundus and the body contract, while the lower segment is relaxed. Both force and frequency of contractions are enhanced and there is full relaxation in between the contractions. This relaxation allows adequate blood supply to the foetus. At full term, the uterus is highly sensitive to the effects of oxytocin as there is an increase in the number of oxytocin receptors. Estrogen enhances the synthesis of oxytocin receptors and sensitizes the uterus to the effects of oxytocin. The effects are dose dependent. High doses produce sustained contractions with no relaxation in between, resulting in reduced blood flow to the foetus, foetal distress and death. Synthetic oxytocin is used for therapeutic purpose.

Mammary gland Oxytocin facilitates milk ejection by contraction of the myoepithelium in the mammary alveoli. Suckling stimulates the release of oxytocin.

Other actions Oxytocin has mild antidiuretic effects

Pharmacokinetics Oxytocin is given as IV infusion. It is metabolised by the liver and kidneys by the enzyme oxytocinase.

Adverse Effects Large doses cause water intoxication and very powerful contractions.

Uses

- **Induction of labour** Oxytocin is used to induce or augment labour when uterine contractions are inadequate.

- **PPH** Oxytocin can be used as an alternative to ergometrine.

- **Milk ejection** When milk ejection is impaired in nursing mothers, intranasal oxytocin spray can be used.

- **Abortion** As an alternative to induce midtrimester abortion.

Ergometrine

Ergometrine and its derivative methylergometrine are used as uterine stimulants. Ergot has been used by midwives to quicken labour since centuries. Ergot alkaloids - (See page 270).

Actions on the Uterus

Ergometrine is a powerful uterine stimulant. The force and frequency of uterine contractions are enhanced. All parts of the uterus including the fundus, body and the lower segment to contract. There is no relaxation in between contractions. Full term uterus is more sensitive to the actions of ergometrine. Ergometrine also causes some vasoconstriction which helps to reduce bleeding from the uterus in post partal state. It brings about its effects by binding to serotonin receptors.

Pharmacokinetics Ergometrine is rapid and short acting. It can be given orally, IM or IV.

Adverse Effects Adverse effects include nausea, vomiting and, rarely, hypertension

Uses

1. Postpartum haemorrhage - ergometrine is used to control and prevent PPH.

2. To hasten uterine involution ergometrine is given for 7 days.

3. To prevent uterine atony - after caesarean section.

	Oxytocin	**Ergometrine**
Source	Synthetic - (for commercial use)	Natural *(Claviceps purpurea)*
Chemistry	Peptide	Alkaloid
Acts on:	Oxytocin receptors	5HT receptors
Occurence	Produced in the body (Endogenous)	Exogenous
Administration	• Not effective orally	• Effective orally
	• Given as IV drip	• Both IM and IV
Duration of action	Short	Longer
$t\frac{1}{2}$	15 minutes	1-2 hours
Action on uterus	• Contracts body and fundus	• Contracts whole ulerus
	• Relaxes lower segment	• No relaxation
		• Tone increased.
Uses	• Induction of labour	• PPH
	• Milk ejection	• To ensure uterine involution after delivery

Table 68.1 Comparison between oxytocin and ergometrine.

Prostaglandins

Prostaglandins (See page 274)are synthesized by the uterus and play a significant role in menstruation as well as parturition. PGE_2 and $PGF_{2\alpha}$ stimulate the contraction of both pregnant and nonpregnant uterus though sensitivity is higher during pregnancy. They also soften the cervix and hasten dilatation (cervical ripening). PGs produced by foetal tissues mediate initiation and progression of labour.

PGs used in obstetrics are

- Dinoprostone (PGE_2) - intravaginal or extraamniotic
- Carboprost (15 methyl $PGF_{2\alpha}$) - deep IM
- Misoprostol (Gemeprost, PGE_1) - intravaginal

Prostaglandins are also involved in the pathogenesis of dysmenorrhoea and menorrhagia. Hence NSAIDs are useful in relieving dysmenorrhoea and probably menorrhagia

Adverse effects include nausea, vomiting, headache, fever and diarrhoea.

Uses

1. *Abortion:* PGs are used as vaginal suppositories to induce mid-trimester abortion. Dinoprostone is given intravaginally or by the extra amniotic route. PGs are also used with mifepristone in the termination of pregnancy upto 9 weeks. Gemeprost is given as vaginal pessary following mifepristone.

2. *PPH* - as an alternative to ergometrine carboprost can be used

3. *Cervical priming* - gels are used intravaginally to soften the cervix and for cervical ripening prior to induction of labour.

4. *Induction of labour* – PGs are used as alternatives to oxytocin.

UTERINE RELAXANTS (Tocolytics)

Tocolytics are drugs that reduce uterine motility and relax the uterus.
They are:

- β_2-adrenergic agonists -
  Salbutamol, terbutaline and isoxsuprine.

- **Miscellaneous** -
  Ethylalcohol, calcium channel blockers, aspirin, magnesium sulfate.

Salbutamol IV infusion is started 10mg per minute and the dose may be gradually increased upto 40mg per minute. Alternatively ritodrine IV infusion may be started - 50mg per minute and gradually increased to 100 mg per minute till the contractions stop.

Intravenous magnesium sulfate is used as an alternative when β_2 agonists are contraindicated. But high doses can cause significant CNS and respiratory depression.

Calcium channel blockers like nifedipine relax the uterus but can reduce placental perfusion and hence are not preferred. Alcohol given IV is a tocolytic but produces marked CNS depression. Similarly aspirin is not preferred as a tocolytic because of the risk of closure of ductus arteriosus and other adverse effects.

Uses of tocolytics

1. To delay premature labour
2. In threatened abortion to inhibit uterine contractions
3. Dysmenorrhoea.

69

Agents Affecting Bone Mineral Turnover

- **Calcium**
- **Phosphorus**
- **Parathormone**
- **Vitamin D**
- **Calcitonin**
- **Drugs used in the disorders of bone**

Calcium and phosphorus are the most important minerals of the bone with 1-2 kg of calcium and 1 kg of phosphorus stored in it. Calcium and phosphorus metabolism are chiefly regulated by vitamin D and parathormone. Other hormones that also influence calcium and phosphorus metabolism are calcitonin, growth hormone, insulin, thyroid hormone, prolactin, glucocorticoids and sex hormones.

CALCIUM

Calcium is essential for tissue excitability, muscular excitation-contraction coupling,

secretion from glands, myocardial contractility and formation of bone and teeth. It also maintains the integrity of mucous membranes and cell membrane. Calcium is essential for normal blood coagulation.

Calcium is absorbed from the small intestine by a carrier mediated active transport. Normally about 30% of the dietary calcium is absorbed, while in Ca++ deficiency, the absorption increases under the control of vitamin D (Fig. 69.1). The normal plasma calcium level is 9-11 mg/dl. It is excreted in faeces, urine and sweat.

Adverse effects

Oral calcium can produce constipation.

Uses

1. To prevent and treat calcium deficiency. Calcium supplements are given orally in children, pregnant and lactating women and in postmenopausal osteoporosis to prevent calcium deficiency.

501

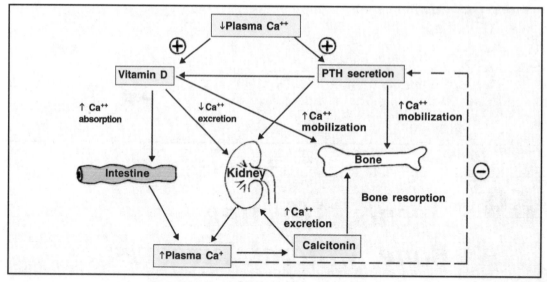

Fig. 69.1 Regulation of plasma calcium level

Tetany: 5-10 ml IV calcium gluconate followed by 50-100 ml slow IV infusion promptly reverses the muscular spasm. The injection produces a sense of warmth. This is followed by oral calcium 1.5 g daily for several weeks.

2. Vitamin D deficiency rickets - calcium is given along with vitamin D.

3. As an antacid - calcium carbonate is used.

4. For placebo effect - IV calcium is used in weakness, pruritus and some dermatoses. The feeling of warmth produced by the injection could afford psychological benefit.

PHOSPHOROUS

Phosphorus is present in many food items - including milk, cereals, fish, meat, pulses and nuts.

Daily requirement of phosphorus is about 900 to 1000mg in adults. Human body contains about 500 - 600 grams of phosphorus of which 75% is present in bones. In bones and teeth phosphorus is in the form of orthophosphates while in soft tissues it is in the form of organic esters. When plasma phosphate is measured it is nothing but the plasma inorganic phosphate measured. Phosphorus is absorbed by the small intestine. Excretion of phosphorus is under the control of paratharmone. The renal excretion of phosphorus is increased by paratharmone.

Physiological functions:

1. Phosphorus is necessary for the formation of bones and teeth.

2. Phosphorus is essential for phosphorylation reactions

3. Phosphorus is present in the nuclei and cytoplasm

4. Phosphorus is important in maintaining the acid - base balance in the plasma and the cells - phosphates are buffers.

5. Phosphates play a vital role in various enzymatic reactions and are important for the structure and function of the cells.

Hypophosphatemia
Causes

1. Dietary phosphorus deficiency

2. Long term intake of aluminium containing antacids

3. Vitamin D deficiency

4. Hyperparathyroidism

5. Chronic alcoholism

6. Diabetic ketoacidosis

Signs & symptoms - Anorexia, muscular weakness and pain, abnormal bone mineralization, haemolysis, decreased myocardial contractility and respiratory failure.

Hyperphosphatemia

Causes Hypoparathyroidism, acromegaly and renal failure.

Clinical features Hypocalcemia, bone resorption and calcification of soft tissues.

Uses of phosphorus:

1. Phosphorus deficiency

2. Chronic hypercalcemia (without hyper-phosphatemia)

PARATHYROID HORMONE (PARATHORMONE, PTH)

Parathormone is a peptide secreted by the parathyroid gland. Secretion of PTH is regulated by plasma Ca^{++} concentration - low plasma Ca^{++} stimulates PTH release, while high levels inhibit secretion (see Fig. 69.1). Parathormone maintains plasma calcium concentration by mobilising calcium from the bone, promoting reabsorption of Ca^{++} from the kidneys and by stimulating the synthesis of calcitriol which in turn enhances calcium absorption from the intestines. PTH also promotes phosphate excretion.

Hypoparathyroidism is characterised by low plasma calcium levels with its associated manifestations. Hyperparathyroidism which is most commonly due to parathyroid tumour produces hypercalcaemia and deformities of the bone.

Keybox 69.1

Hormones that influence bone metabolism

- Vitamin D
- Glucocorticoids
- Parathormone
- Estrogens
- Calcitonin

PTH is not therapeutically used. It is used for the diagnosis of pseudohypoparathyroidism.

VITAMIN D

Vitamin D a fat-soluble vitamin, is a prehormone produced in the skin from 7-dehydrocholesterol under the influence of ultraviolet rays. It is converted to active metabolites in the body which regulate plasma calcium levels and various functions of the cells.

Source

- Diet as ergocalciferol (vitamin D_2) from plants.

- Fish, liver, fish liver oils - (cod, shark liver oil); milk.

- Cholecalciferol (vitamin D_3) is synthesized in the skin from 7-dehydrocholesterol.

Cholecalciferol (vitamin D_3) is converted to $25\text{-}OHD_3$ (calcifediol) in the liver (Fig. 69.2) which is in turn converted to 1,25-dihydroxycholecalciferol (calcitriol) in the kidneys. Calcitriol is the active form of vitamin D while calcifediol is the main metabolite in circulation. Convertion of calcifediol to calcitriol is influenced by PTH and plasma phosphate concentration.

Actions

The chief actions of calcitriol are:

- It stimulates calcium and phosphate absorption in the intestine

- Mobilises calcium from bone by promoting osteoclastic activity

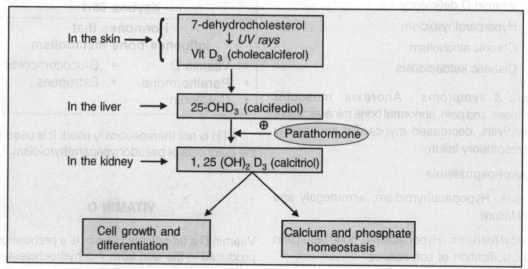

Fig. 69.2 Synthesis and functions of vitamin D

- Increases reabsorption of Ca^{++} from kidney tubules.

Calcitriol is essential for normal bone mineralization. It is essential for skeletal muscles as well as cellular growth and differentiation.

Vitamin D deficiency results in low plasma calcium and phosphate levels with abnormal mineralization of the bone; causes rickets in children and osteomalacia in adults.

Daily requirement - 400 IU (10 mg).

Pharmacokinetics

Given orally, vit D is well-absorbed from the small intestines in the presence of bile salts. It is converted to 25-OHD$_3$ in the liver and circulates in the plasma, bound to a protein and is stored in the adipose tissue. Vitamin D is also degraded in the liver and the metabolites are excreted in the bile.

Preparations

- Calciferol capsules 25000; 50,000 IU.
- Cholecalciferol granules - oral 60,000 IU in

IG; 3,00,000 IU/ml; 6,00,000 IU/ml inj.

- Shark liver oil with vit D - 1000 IU/ml, vit A - 6000 IU/ml.

Calcifediol (25(OH)D$_3$), alfa calcidiol (1-a(OH)D$_3$) and calcitriol(1,25(OH)$_2$D$_3$) are synthetic Vitamin D analogs available for use.

Adverse reactions

High doses of vitamin D used for long periods result in hypervitaminosis D manifesting as generalised decalcification of the bones, hypercalcaemia, hyperphosphataemia resulting in weakness, drowsiness, nausea, abdominal pain, thirst, renal stones and hypertension. Hypervitaminosis D in children is most often due to unnecessary vitamin D supplementation by parents.

Uses

1. Prophylaxis - 400 IU daily or 3,00,000 IU every 3-6 months IM prevents vit D deficiency. Adequate dietary calcium and phosphate intake is necessary. In the breastfed infants, from the first month onwards oral vit D supplements are needed.

In obstructive jaundice, prophylactic 6,00,000 units vit D given IM prevents deficiency.

2. **Nutritional rickets and osteomalacia** 6,00,000 units IM repeated after 4-6 weeks is needed in rickets and osteomalacia along with calcium supplements.

3. **Vitamin D resistant rickets** is a hereditary disorder with abnormality in renal phosphate reabsorption. Phosphate with vitamin D is found to be useful.

4. **Vitamin D dependent rickets** is due to calcitriol deficiency (inability to convert calcifediol to calcitriol) and is treated with calcitriol.

5. **Senile osteoporosis** Oral vitamin D supplements with calcium may be tried.

6. **Hypoparathyroidism** Calcitriol with Ca^{++} supplements are beneficial.

CALCITONIN

Calcitonin is a peptide hormone secreted by the parafollicular 'C' cells of the thyroid gland. Secretion is regulated by plasma Ca^{++} concentration - high plasma Ca^{++} stimulates calcitonin release.

Actions

The chief effects of calcitonin are to lower serum calcium and phosphate by its actions on the bone and kidney. It inhibits osteoclastic bone resorption and in the kidney, it reduces both calcium and phosphate reabsorption.

In general the effects are opposite to that of PTH. Calcitonin is used to control hypercalcaemia, Paget's disease, metastatic bone cancer and osteoporosis and to increase bone mineral density.

Other hormones that regulate bone turnover are glucocorticoids and oestrogens. Glucocorticoids antagonise vitamin D stimulated intestinal calcium absorption and enhance renal Ca^{++} excretion. Oestrogens reduce bone

resorption by PTH and also enhance calcitriol levels. Estrogen receptors are found in bone which suggests that they may also have a direct effect on bone remodeling.

DRUGS USED IN THE DISORDERS OF BONE

Drugs used in disorders of bone are

- Bisphosphonates -
  Alendronate   etidronate
  Pamidronate   residronate
- Raloxifene (selective estrogen receptor modulator)
- Vitamin D

Bisphosphonates

Bisphosphonates are analogs of pyrophosphate; they inhibit bone resorption. Bisphosphonates get incorporated into bone matrix, are imbibed by osteoclasts and then incapacitate the osteoclasts resulting in reduced bone resorption. They also slow the formation and dissolution of hydroxyapatite crystals.

Fever, esophagitis, gastritis and hypocalcaemia can occur. Long-term use can lead to osteomalacia due to inhibition of bone mineralization.

Uses

Bisphosphonates are used in Paget's disease of the bone, hypercalcaemia and are tried in postmenopausal osteoporosis.

1. Paget's disease - Bisphosphonates relieve pain and induce remission

2. Hypercalcaemia malignancies - Some malignancies are associated with hypercalcaemia. Intravenous Pamidronate is useful in reducing plasma ca^{++} levels.

3. Osteoporosis - Alendronate and residronate

are tried with calcium and vitamin D for the prevention if postmenopausal osteoporosis.

Raloxifene is a SERM useful in women for the prevention of postmenopausal osteoporosis.

AGENTS USED IN THE PREVENTION AND TREATMENT OF OSTEOPOROSIS

Drugs may be used either to prevent bone resorption or promote bone formation or a combination of both in the prevention and treatment of osteoporosis. These agents reduce the risk of fractures in patients with osteoporosis.

Drugs that prevent bone resorption

- Calcium ($\uparrow$BMD)*

- Vitamin D ($\uparrow$ absorption of calcium)
- Estrogen (prevents osteoporosis)
- Raloxifene – a SERM ($\uparrow$ BMD)
- Calcitonin (prevents bone resorption, ($\uparrow$BMD)
- Bisphosphonates - $\downarrow$bone resorption, ($\uparrow$BMD)
  *(BMD – Bone mineral density.)

Drugs that promote bone formation

- Fluoride (in small doses - osteoblastic activity - $\uparrow$bone mass - but generally not preferred).
- Testosterone (in hypogonadal men)
- Anabolic steroids (in postmenopausal women).
- PTH analogs (are being tried).

MISCELLANEOUS DRUGS

- ◆ Gene therapy
- ◆ Antiseptics and disinfectants
- ◆ Vaccines and antisera
- ◆ Chelating agents
- ◆ Vitamins & Minerals
- ◆ Enzymes in therapy
- ◆ Treatment of Poisoning
- ◆ Geriatric Pharmocology

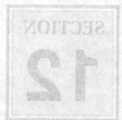

SECTION

12

MISCELLANEOUS DRUGS

70   *Gene Therapy*

- **Vectors**
- **Therapeutic applications**

Gene therapy is the replacement of defective gene by the insertion of a normal, functional gene. It is the genetic modification of cells for the prevention or treatment of a disease. Gene transfer may be done to replace a missing or defective gene or provide extra-copies of a normally expressed gene. Gene therapy is aimed at genetically correcting the defect in the affected part of the body. Unlike all other drugs which only alter the rate of normal cell functions, gene therapy can confer new functions to the cell.

VECTORS

Gene transfer requires the use of vectors to deliver the DNA material. An ideal vector should be safe and effective in inserting the therapeutic gene into the target cells. Physical, chemical and biological vectors have been tried.

- Physical vectors - DNA is complexed with substances like lipids and administered.
- Chemical vectors - liposomes are used to carry genes into the cells.
- Biological vectors - The most important biological vectors are viral vectors - Viruses invade cells and use the metabolic processes of these host cell for replication. This property of viruses helps to deliver the gene - adenoviruses and retroviruses are used.

THERAPEUTIC APPLICATIONS

Gene therapy is at present a developing area. Though originally it was seen as a remedy for inherited single gene defects, gene therapy has now been found to be useful in several acquired disorders. The principle applications are in single gene defects like thalassemia, cystic fibrosis and haemoglobinopathies and in the treatment of cancer, cardiovascular diseases, atherosclerosis, immunodeficiency disorders - particularly AIDS; anaemia, Alzheimer's disease and many infectious diseases. Some examples are-

1. *Growth hormone deficiency* - Growth hormone gene is transferred to myoblasts and these are implanted in patients.

2. *Familial hypercholesterolemia* - LDL receptor gene is introduced into liver cells.

3. *Cancer -*
   - Introducing genes which make the malignant cells sensitive to drugs.
   - Inactivating the expression of oncogenes.
   - Introducing genes that attach to cancer cells and make them susceptible to host defence cells.
   - Introducing genes to healthy cells to protect them from cytotoxic drugs.

4. *HIV infections*
   - Introducing genes coding for CD_4 cells that could inactivate HIV before entering the cell itself.
   - Introducing genes that enhance immunity against HIV.

5. *Diabetes mellitus* - Introducing insulin gene into the liver which can produce insulin.

6. *Coronary atherosclerosis* - Prevention of restenosis and ischemia in coronary vessels by genes which inhibit the growth of vascular endothelial cells.

71 *Antiseptics and Disinfectants*

- Mechanism of action
- Classification
- Acids
- Alcohols
- Aldehydes
- Surfactants
- Phenol derivatives
- Halogens
- Oxidizing agents
- Dyes
- Metals

Disinfection is destruction of all pathogenic organisms but not spores. If spores are also killed, it is called *sterilization*. A *disinfectant* is used on **inanimate objects**.

Antiseptic is an agent that destroys microorganisms and can be used on *living tissues*. The term **germicide** can be used for either drugs. Germicides are widely used in domestic products

like soaps, tooth pastes and after-shave lotions.

MECHANISM OF ACTION

Germicides may act by the following mechanisms:

1. Oxidation of bacterial protoplasm

2. Denaturation of bacterial proteins

3. Detergent like action

4. Competition with essential substrates for the important enzymes in the bacterial cell.

An ideal germicide should have a wide antibacterial spectrum, should be chemically stable, should have rapid action, non-irritating to the tissues, not interfere with wound healing activity even in presence of pus, exudates and tissue degradation products; it should not be absorbed into systemic circulation.

Classification

1. *Acids* — Boric acid, Benzoic acid
2. *Alcohols* — Ethanol, Isopropyl alcohol
3. *Aldehydes* — Formaldehyde, Glutaraldehyde
4. *Surfactants* — Soaps, Benzalkonium, Cetrimide, Cetylpyridinium chloride, Dequalinium chloride
5. *Phenol derivatives* — Phenol, Cresol, Resorcinal, Chlorhexidine, Chloroxylenol, Hexachlorophene
6. *Halogens* — Iodine, Iodophores, Chlorine, Chloramines
7. *Oxidizing agents* — Hydrogen peroxide, Potassium permanganate, Benzoyl peroxide
8. *Dyes* — Gentian violet, Methylene blue, Brilliant green, Acriflavine, Proflavine
9. *Metallic salts* — Mercurial compounds, Silver nitrate, Zinc compounds

Factors that influence the activity of germicidal agents

1. *Concentration of the drug and duration of contact* In general, higher the concentration of the antiseptic, greater is its effect. But alcohol is an exception to this and at 70% concentration maximum antiseptic effect is seen.
2. *Susceptibility of the organism* Spores and viruses are resistant to many antiseptics.

increase antiseptic activity.

ACIDS

Boric acid and sodium borate (borax) have weak bacteriostatic and fungistatic activity. Aqueous solutions of boric acid are used for irrigating eyes, bladder, vagina and large wounds.

Benzoic acid is an antibacterial (below pH 5) and antifungal agent used as a preservative in laboratory.

Salicylic acid has bacteriostatic, fungicidal and keratolytic properties. It is used as a dusting powder or 2% ointment for seborrhoeic dermatitis, warts and corns.

ALCOHOLS

Ethyl alcohol is employed as an antiseptic at 60-90% concentration. The antiseptic activity decreases above 90%. It rapidly denatures the bacterial proteins (see Chap 26).

Disadvantages

1. It has poor activity against spores, some viruses and fungi
2. Irritant - causes burning when applied on open wounds
3. Alcohols are flammable - should be allowed to evaporate before using cautery or laser surgery.

Uses Ethyl alcohol is used to clean the skin before injections and surgeries.

Isopropyl alcohol is more potent and more toxic than ethanol. It is used in 68-72% concentration

ALDEHYDES

Formaldehyde

Formaldehyde is a gas at room temperature used for fumigation; the 40% aqueous solution is noncorrosive and has a broad antimicrobial spectrum. It has a pungent odour and is an irritant - highly irritating to respiratory mucous membranes and eyes. Formaldehyde is also a carcinogen and OSHA has set standards to limit exposure of health care workers to formaldehyde.

Mechanism of action Aldehydes act by alkylation of chemical groups in proteins and nucleic acids.

Uses

Formaldehyde gas is used for fumigation and for sterilizing instruments which cannot be moistened with solution. Formaldehyde 40% solution (100% formalin) in water is used for disinfection of surgical instruments and gloves; embalming and preservation of tissues. Fibreoptic endoscopies, respiratory therapy equipment, haemodialysers and dental hand pieces which cannot withstand high temperatures of steam sterilisation are disinfected with formaldehyde.

Automatic circulating baths are used which increase penetration of aldehyde solution into the instruments and decrease operator exposure to the chemical. It's rapidity of action increases by making a solution in 70% propanol.

Glutaraldehyde

Glutaraldehyde is a dialdehyde used as a 2% solution. It is bactericidal, sporicidal, fungicidal and viricidal. pH should be between 7.4 and 8.5. It is less irritant than formaldehyde; has greater sporicidal activity; does not damage lenses and cementing material in endoscopes. Glutaraldehyde is superior to formaldehyde for sterilising rubber, plastic and metal appliances. Two per cent solution is used for local application in idiopathic hyperhidrosis of palms and soles.

SURFACTANTS

Surfactants are chemicals that lower the surface tension of solutions and are termed detergents. They may be anionic, cationic, ampholytic surfactants or polysorbates.

Anionic surfactants e.g. soaps.

- They dissociate in aqueous solutions to form a large and complex anion which lowers the surface tension.
- Effective for gram-positive and acid fast organisms.
- Microorganisms are enmeshed in the lather and washed away on rinsing.
- Anionic surfactants have a narrow spectrum; precipitate in hard water; cause drying of the skin.

Preparations

1. Potassium hydroxide or sodium hydroxide + vegetable oil.
2. Sodium lauryl sulphate - is effective in hard water.

Cationic surfactants - e.g. Benzalkonium chloride, Cetrimide, Cetylpyridinium chloride, Dequalinium chloride. Cationic surfactants dissociate into large cations.

They are:

- active against gram-positive and gram-negative organisms (less active against spores, viruses and fungi)
- most effective in neutral solution
- non-irritating and safe
- incompatible with anionic surfactants
- absorbed by cotton and rubber
- one of the most commonly used germicidal agents.

Benzalkonium chloride *(ZEPHIRAN)* has an aromatic odour and is soluble in water.

- 1:2000 for mucous membranes and denuded skin
- 1:20,000 for irrigation of the bladder and urethra
- It is also used for (1: 1000-4000) storing sterilised surgical instruments. But instruments should be thoroughly washed before use.

Cetrimide *(CETAVLON)* 1% solution is used like above. It is also used as a cream. It is very effective for cleaning wounds. In combination with chlorhexidine is one of the most popular antiseptics. SAVLON is cetrimide 3% + chlorhexidine.

Dequalinium chloride is used in gum paints and lozenges.

Cetylpyridinium chloride is used in mouthwashes and lozenges.

PHENOL DERIVATIVES

Phenol is one of the oldest antiseptics introduced by Lord Lister in 1867. It is bactericidal and fungicidal but has poor action against spores and viruses. It acts by denaturing the bacterial proteins. It also has a mild local anaesthetic action. Phenol rapidly penetrates even intact skin and mucous membrane. It is a protoplasmic poison.

Phenol is extremely irritant to exposed tissues (corrosive) - when swallowed, it burns buccal, oesophagal and gastric mucous membrane.

Uses Phenol is used to disinfect urine, faeces, sputum of patients and is sometimes used as antipruritic because of its local anaesthetic action.

Cresol is methylphenol, which is as toxic as phenol but is more active. It is used as a disinfectant for utensils and excreta.

Lysol is cresol with soap solution. It has higher antiseptic activity and is an useful disinfectant for hospital and domestic use.

Chloroxylenol *(DETTOL)* is a less toxic chlorinated phenol, effective against gram-positive and gram-negative organisms. Surgical dettol contains 1.4% of chloroxylenol for skin; 6.25% for instruments and 1 to 3% in antiseptic cream.

Hexachlorophene This chlorinated phenol acts by inhibiting bacterial enzymes and causing lysis. It is effective mainly against gram-positive organisms and has weak action against gram-negative organisms. It is odourless and non-irritating to use on skin. It is used in soaps for surgical scrubbing, for cleaning the skin in obstetrics, carbuncles and seborrhoeic dermatitis. It may cause allergic reactions. It also reduces body odour by preventing bacterial decomposition of organic material and therefore is used as a deodorant. In USA, hexachlorophene was used to wash newborn babies which resulted in brain damage in such babies and therefore use of >3% hexachlorophene is banned.

Chlorhexidine *(HIBITANE)* is effective against gram-positive, gram-negative organisms and fungi. It is rapid acting and non-irritating. SAVLON - chlorhexidine + cetrimide.

HALOGENS

Iodine is one of the oldest antiseptics. It has a broad spectrum of activity, is a powerful bactericidal, sporicidal, fungicidal and viricidal agent. The activity is inhibited by organic material but enhanced by alcohol.

Disadvantages It is irritating, painful, stains the area, and may delay wound healing. Rashes, fever and generalised skin eruptions may develop in some patients who are sensitive to iodine. Prolonged systemic use causes iodism.

Uses of iodine

1. *Tincture iodine (I_2 in KI + alcohol)* - is used to clean skin before surgery. Iodine crystals are used to sterilize water for soaking

vegetables and cleaning before use.

2. *Mandl's paint (Compound Iodide paint)* is used in the treatment of tonsillitis and pharyngitis.

3. Iodine ointment - as fungicide in ringworm. Iodides have no antibacterial action.

Iodophors are soluble complexes of iodine with surfactants like detergents. The detergents serve as carriers and slowly release iodine, e.g. Povidone iodine (BETADINE) - 5% solution; Piodine - 10% solution.

Advantages

Iodophors are non-irritating, non-staining, water-soluble, less toxic and non-sensitizing to the skin.

Uses

Used for preoperative scrubbing, skin preparation, disinfection of instruments, as local antiseptic in boils, furunculosis, burns, ulcers, ringworm and in oral/vaginal moniliasis.

Chlorine

Chlorine is a potent germicide and is bactericidal against several gram-positive and gram-negative organisms in a very low concentration (0.1 PPM in 30 seconds). It also destroys protozoa and viruses. The antibacterial activity of chlorine is reduced in presence of organic matter since they bind chlorine and therefore need higher concentration of free chlorine. Chloramines are compounds that release chlorine slowly.

1. *Chlorinated lime* (bleaching powder) is obtained by the action of chlorine on lime. It is used for disinfection of water in swimming pools and water for drinking.

2. *Chloramine* is an organic chloride. The freshly prepared solution is used for mouthwash, irrigating bladder and urethra.

3. *Eusol* is a solution of chlorinated lime with boric acid.

OXIDIZING AGENTS

Hydrogen peroxide

Hydrogen peroxide is a colourless and odourless liquid. It liberates nascent oxygen when applied to tissues and then oxidizes bacteria and necrotic tissue. On application, there is effervescence and this helps in removing tissue debris, ear wax, etc. Hydrogen peroxide has poor penetrability and the action is of short duration. On keeping, it loses its potency. It is also a deodorant.

Uses Hydrogen peroxide is used for cleansing wounds, abscesses and for irrigation. In dentistry, it is used to clean septic sockets and root canals and also as a mouthwash and deodorant gargle. It is used as ear drops while removing ear wax.

Potassium permanganate

Potassium Permanganate is an oxidizing agent and an astringent. The purple crystals are water-soluble. It acts by liberating oxygen which oxidizes bacterial protoplasm. Organic matter reduces its activity and the solution gets decolourised. It promotes rusting; concentrated solution is caustic and causes burns and blistering.

Uses

- 1:4000-1: 10000 solution of potassium permanganate is used for gargling, irrigating cavities, urethra and wounds.

- For stomach wash in alkaloidal poisoning (except atropine and cocaine as these are not efficiently oxidized).

- 1% solution in mycotic infections like athletes foot.

- 5% solution as a styptic.

- Topically to oxidise venom in case of snake and scorpion bite.

- To purify well water.

- To disinfect vegetables and fruits.

DYES

Gentian violet

Gentian violet (aniline dye, crystal violet or medicinal gentian violet) is effective against gram-positive organisms and fungi. Staining is the only disadvantage. It is a non-irritant and potent antiseptic. 0.5-1% solution is used topically on furunculosis, burns, boils, chronic ulcers, infected eczema, thrush, ringworm and mycotic infections of the skin and mucous membranes.

Brilliant green

Actions are similar to gentian violet. It is used as a 0.5-1% solution in the treatment of burns, impetigo and infected wounds like gentian violet.

Methylene blue

Methylene blue is used systemically in cyanide poisoning as it converts methaemoglobin to haemoglobin.

Acriflavine and proflavine

Acriflavine and proflavine are acridine dyes active against gram-positive bacteria and gonococci (proflavine is better). They are non - irritant; efficacy is unaffected by organic matter but is increased in alkaline medium; 1: 1000 solution is used in infected wounds and burns, 2% pessary in vaginitis and cervicitis.

Triple dye lotion

Tripe dye lotion contains gentian violet 0.25% + brilliant green 0.25% + acriflavine or proflavine 0.1% - it is used in burns dressing.

METALS

Silver compounds

Silver compounds have antiseptic, astringent and caustic properties. Silver nitrate kills microbes rapidly and the action is prolonged due to slow release of silver ions from silver proteinate that is formed by an interaction with tissue proteins. The reduced silver gets deposited and stains the tissues black.

Silver nitrate is used for the prophylaxis of ophthalmia neonatorum.

Silver sulfadiazine is active against *pseudo monas* and is used in burn wounds.

Colloidal silver compounds slowly release silver. They are non-corrosive, non-irritant, non-astringent and have better penetrability used as nasal and eye drops.

Zinc salts

Zinc salts like zinc oxide have astringent and mild antiseptic properties. Zinc oxide is used as an ointment or lotion in eczema, impetigo and psoriasis.

Mercury compounds

Mercury compounds act by inhibiting sulphydryl enzymes of bacteria. They are bacteriostatic and are poor antiseptics - not commonly used.

72 *Vaccines and Antisera*

- Vaccines
- Toxoids
- Antisera
- Immunoglobulins
- Active immunisation
- Passive immunisation
- Primary immunisation
- Secondary immunisation

Vaccines are suspensions of micro-organisms (dead or live attenuated) which stimulate the immunological defence of the host by developing antibodies.

Toxoids Bacterial exotoxins modified to remove toxicity but retain antigenicity are toxoids.

Antisera contain antibodies against a particular microorganism - they provide passive immunity. Antisera like tetanus antitoxin, gas gangrene antitoxin, diphtheria and antirabies sera are obtained from sera of horses which are actively

immunised against the specific organism. Sensitivity tests should be done before giving antisera. Allergic reactions may occur because of the animal source.

Immunoglobulins (Ig) are human gammaglobulins that carry the antibodies - like normal human gammaglobulin, tetanus Ig, rabies Ig, antidiphtheria Ig and hepatitis-B Ig. Allergic reactions including serum sickness & anaphylaxis can occur with antisera, while it is uncommon with Igs.

Active immunisation is the administration of antigen to the host in order to induce antibody production. Vaccines are used for active immunisation. They impart active immunity, which takes sometime to develop and are therefore used prophylactically. The antibodies so developed destroy the specific micro-organism when it enters the body. Some commonly used vaccines are given in Table 72.1. Vaccines for Japanese encephalitis, Kyasnur forest disease (KFD) & epidemic typhus are also available now.

Passive immunisation is imparting immunity to a host passively by the transfer of antibodies, e.g. antisera and immunoglobulins (Ig). This affords immediate protection because ready-made antibodies are available.

Primary immunisation provides primary immunity and is usually given in children, e.g. DPT (Triple antigen given to infants).

Secondary immunisation

Secondary immunization is done to reinforce the primary immunity by giving booster doses.

Vaccines in common use and their recommended schedules are given in Table 72.1. Preparations for passive immunization are given in Tables 72.2 and 72.3

Immunizing agents may be classified as :

CLASSIFICATION:

1. Vaccines

	Bacterial	Viral	Rickettsial
Live attenuated vaccines	BCG Plague Typhoid oral	Oral polio Measles Mumps Rubella Influenza Yellow fever	Epidemic typhus
Inactivated or killed vaccines	Cholera Typhoid Pertussis Plague Meningococcal H. influenzae type b Pneumococcal	Rabies Polio Influenza Hepatitis B Japanese encephalitis KFD	
Toxoids	Diphtheria Tetanus		

2. Antisera and Immunoglobulins

	Bacterial	Viral	Others
Antisera	Diphtheria Tetanus Gas gangrene Botulism	Rabies	
Human Ig	Diphtheria Tetanus	Measles Varicella Mumps Hepatitis A Hepatitis B Rabies	Rh (D)

TABLE 72.1: Vaccines in common use and their recommended schedules					
Vaccine	Type of agent	ROA immunisation	Primary	Booster	Indication
Bacterial vaccines					
BCG	Live attenuated	ID/SC	At Birth	7 and 14 years	In all children
Cholera	Inactivated	SC/IM	Adults: two doses 1 month apart	Every 6 months	People living in endemic areas
	Killed	Oral	2 doses 10-14 days apart		
	Live attinuated	Oral	Single dose		Risk of exposure
Diphtheria	Toxoid	IM of age	6, 10,14 weeks at 4-6 years	18 months and	For all children
Pertussis	Inactivated	IM	6, 10,14 weeks of age	18 months and at 4-6 years	For all children
Tetanus	Toxoid	IM	6, 10,14 weeks of age	18 months and at 4-6 years	For all children; Adults: Postexposure prophylaxis if > 5 years has passed since last dose
Typhoid/ Parathyroid	Inactivated	SC	After 3 years at any age: two doses 4 weeks apart	Every 3 years	Risk of exposure to typhoid fever
Typhoid (TYPHORAL)	Live inactivated	Oral (capsules) fever 3 doses on	Above 6 years at any age: alternate days 1 hr before food	Every 3 years to typhoid	Risk of exposure
Meningococcal	Bacterial poly- saccharides	SC	One dose	–	1. Travellers to areas with meningococcal epidemics 2. Control of out- break in closed population
Plague	Inactivated	IM	One dose	–	In an epidemic
Haemophillus influenzae (type B)	Bacterial Polysaccharide	IM	One dose	-	1. For all children 2. Patients at risk
Pneumococcal	Bacterial Polysaccharides	SC	One dose	every 3-5 years- If there is high risk of exposure	1. Travellers to areas with apidemics 2. Control of epidemics in closed population. 3 Military recruits

Note: Diphtheria, Pertussis and Tetanus are bracketed together as TRIPLE ANTIGEN

Contd...

Contd...

Vaccine	Type of agent	ROA	Primary	Booster immunisation	Indication
Viral Vaccines					
Poliomyelitis (OPV)	Live virus	Oral	6, 10 and 14 weeks of age	18 months;again at 4-6 years	For all children
Measles, mumps, rubella (MMR) (MORUPAR)	Live virus	SC	12-15 months	11-12 years	For all children
Hepatitis A	Inactivated virus	IM	1 dose (2-4 weeks before travelling to endemic areas)	After 6-12 months	1. Travellers to endemic areas 2. Homosexual men 3. Persons at occupational risk
Hepatitis B	Inactive viral antigen	IM	At birth, 1 month, 6-18 months	After 5 yrs but not routinely recommended	1. For all children 2. Persons at occupational risk 3. Haemophiliacs 4. Postexposure prophylaxis
Influenza	Inactivated virus	IM	One dose	Yearly	1. High risk people like elderly, asthmatics
Rabies (RABIPUR)	Inactivated virus	IM/ID	**Pre-exposure** 3 doses at days 0,7 and 21 **Postexposure:** 6 doses IM 0,3,7,14,30 and 90	After 1 year then at 2-5 years	1. Postexposure treatment 2. Pre-exposure prophylaxis in persons at risk for contact with rabies virus
Varicella	Live virus	SC	2 doses 4-8 weeks apart at 18 months	--	All children from 18 months to 13 years with no history of varicella infection
Yellow fever	Live virus	SC	1 dose	every 10 years	1. Travellers to areas where yellow fever is seen 2. Laboratory personnel at risk of exposure
Japanese Encephalitis	Killed	SC	2 Doses 7-14 days apart	Before 1 Year	Population at risk

ID - intradermal, SC - subcutaneous, IM - intramuscular ROA - Route of Administration

TABLE 72..2: Passive immunisation

Preparation with source	Dose and Route	Indication
Diphtheria antitoxin (horse)	IV or IM 20,000-1,20,000 units	*Diphtheria* Clinical diphtheria - to be given immediately
Tetanus immuneglobulin (human)	IM Prophylaxis : 2500 Units Treatment : 3,000 - 6,000 Units	*Tetanus* Treatment and post exposure prophylaxis of unclean wounds in inadequately immunized persons
Tetanus antitoxin (ATS) (horse) (If tetanus Ig is not available)	IM/SC Prophylaxis 1500-3000 IU Treatment: 50,000-1,00,000 IU	*Tetanus* Treatment and Postexposure prophylaxis of unclean wounds in inadequately immunised persons
Botulinum antitoxin	IM/IV 10,000 IU	Treatment and Postexposure prophylaxis of botulism
Rabies immunoglobulin (human)	20 IU/kg; half the dose infiltrated around the wound; remaining IM	*Rabies* Postexposure prophylaxis combined with rabies vaccine
Antirabies serum (ARS) (horse)	IM 40 IU/ kg	Used if rabies Ig is not available but is inferior to it
Gas gangrene antitoxin (AGS) (horse)	IM/SC/IV Prophylaxis: 10,000 IU Treatment: 30,000-75,000 IU	*Gas gangrene* Postexposure prophylaxis and treatment
Hepatitis B immunoglobulin (HBIG)	IM 0.06 ml/kg	Postexposure prophylaxis in nonimmune persons; Hepatitis B vaccine shall also be given.
Antisnake venom polyvalent (horse)	IV 20-30 ml to be given within 4 hr after the bite; additional doses may be required	Snake bite- Cobra, vipers, krait
Human gammaglobulin		Gammaglobulin deficiency; prophylaxis of hepatitis A, measles, mumps, rubella
Anti RhD Ig	IM 300 mcg	To the Rh -ve mother after the birth of Rh +ve baby or after uncompleted pregnancy with Rh +ve father

TABLE 72..3: Conditions for which passive immunization is available

Infections		Others
Botulism	Vaccinia	Snake bite
Diphtheria	Varicella	Black widow spider bite
Measles	Hepatitis A	Chronic lymphocytic leukemia
Rabies	Hepatitis B	Idiopathic thrombocytopenic
Rubella	Cytomegalovirus	purpura
Tetanus	HIV-infected children	Bone marrow transplantation
Respiratory syncytial virus		Anti-D (Rh) Ig

73 *Chelating Agents*

- • **Calcium disodium edetate**
- • **Dimercaprol**
- • **Succimer**
- • **Unithiol**
- • **d-Penicillamine**
- • **Desferrioxamine**
- • **Deferiprone**

Heavy metals bind to and inactivate the functional groups (ligands) of essential tissue enzymes. By this they interfere with normal cell functions which require these ligands. Heavy metals cannot be metabolised in the body.

Chelating agents or heavy metal antagonists bind the heavy metal ions and make them non-toxic. The chemical complex formed is called chelate (*Chele* = claw; in Greek). The process of complex formation is chelation. The complex so formed is water-soluble and is eliminated by the kidneys.

The clinically useful chelating agents are $CaNa_2$ EDTA, dimercaprol, d-penicillamine and desferrioxamine. Chelating agents are more effective in preventing the utilization of ligands than in reactivating them - hence, the earlier they are given, the better.

Calcium disodium edetate (CaNa₂ EDTA)

Chelates many divalent and trivalent metals like zinc, manganese, iron and lead. It is used in the treatment of lead poisoning. Given parenterally, lead deposits in the bone are mobilised, chelated and excreted through kidneys.

Adverse effects include nephrotoxicity, fatigue, fever, myalgia and dermatitis.

Uses $CaNa_2$ EDTA is mainly used in lead poisoning. It can also be used in zinc, manganese and iron poisoning. Sodium edetate is used in severe hypercalcaemia.

Dimercaprol

Dimercaprol is a colourless, oily liquid developed by the British during World war II as an antidote to lewisite - an arsenical war gas. Hence it is also known as British Anti-lewisite or BAL. Dimercaprol chelates arsenic, mercury, lead and other heavy metals. It is given IM; appropriate plasma concentrations should be maintained.

Adverse effects are dose related and include hypertension, tachycardia, vomiting, sweating, burning sensation in the lips and mouth and headache.

Uses Dimercaprol is used in arsenic and mercury poisoning; also used in lead poisoning with $CaNa_2$ EDTA.

Unithiol

Unithiol is a water soluble analog of dimercaprol that can be given both orally and parenterally. It enhances the excretion of mercury, arsenic and lead. Adverse effects are mild and include allergic reactions. Unthiol may be used in mercury, lead and arsenic poisoning.

Succimer

Succimer is a water soluble analog of dimercaprol. It protects against acute arsenic poisoning and it also effective in lead and mercury poisoning. It can be given both orally and intravenously. Succimer is used in the treatment of chronic lead poisoning and in mercury and arsenic poising. Anorexia, nausea, vomiting, diarrhoea and skin rashes can occur.

d-Penicillamine

d-Penicillamine is prepared by degradation of penicillin but has no antibacterial activity. It chelates copper, mercury, zinc and lead. It is orally effective (See page 238).

Toxicity Patients allergic to penicillin may develop anaphylaxis; dermatitis may occur in some. On long - term use renal, haematological, dermatological and other toxicities can occur.

Uses

1. Treatment of copper, mercury and lead poisoning.

2. Wilson's disease (hepatolenticular degeneration) - copper is deposited in the liver and brain causing degeneration.

3. Rheumatoid arthritis

4. Cystinuria - promotes excretion of cysteine by forming soluble complexes and prevents formation of cysteine stones.

Desferrioxamine

Desferrioxamine isolated from *Streptomyces pilosus,* chelates iron. It has a high affinity for iron, forms stable complexes and removes iron from haemosiderin and ferritin. It does not chelate the iron in haemoglobin and cytochromes. It is given parenterally (See page 297).

Toxicity Allergic reactions range from rashes to anaphylaxis (rare), diarrhoea, muscle cramps and blurred vision.

Uses

1. Acute iron poisoning - desferrioxamine is the drug of choice.

2. Chronic iron poisoning - as in thalassaemia patients who receive repeated blood transfusion.

Deferiprone chelates iron and is orally effective. It is used in thalassemia major to chelate iron as an alternative to desferrioxamine.

74 *Vitamins & Minerals*

- Fat- soluble vitamins
- Water-soluble vitamins
- Minerals
    - Sodium
    - Potassium
    - Magnesium
    - Zinc
    - Manganese

Vitamins are organic compounds essential for normal metabolism in the body. They are supplied by the diet. A balanced diet supplies adequate amounts of vitamins to fulfill the daily require ment. The requirement is increased during periods of rapid growth, pregnancy and lactation. Vitamin deficiencies result in characteristic signs and symptoms.

Vitamins are grouped into fat-soluble and water-soluble vitamins (Table 74.1).

FAT-SOLUBLE VITAMINS

Vitamin A

Vitamin A is present in the diet as retinol, dehydroretinol or as carotenoids. Carotenoids are pigments present in green yellow vegetables and fruits and are converted in the body to retinol.

Source Green leafy vegetables, carrots, mango, papaya, eggs, milk, butter, cheese, liver and fish liver oils. Maximum content is in Halibut liver oil - 9,00,000 mcg/100 g.

Physiological functions Vitamin A has an important role in dark adaptation. It is essential for the synthesis of rhodopsin, the photosensitive pigment of rods. Vitamin A is also essential for maintenance of the integrity of epithelial cells, for growth and cell-mediated immunity.

Signs and symptoms of deficiency Xerophthalmia (dryness of eyes), Bitot's spots in the conjunctiva, night blindness, diarrhoea, dry and rough skin are seen in early stages. In the later stages, keratomalacia, perforation of the cornea, necrosis and blindness can occur.

Daily requirement - 3000-5000 IU/day.

Uses

In the prophylaxis and treatment of vitamin A deficiency.

1. Prophylaxis - 3000-5000 IU/day in presence of increased requirement.

2. Treatment - 50,000-1,00,000 IU intramuscularly or orally for 1-3 days followed by oral supplementation.

3. Acne - Retinoic acid or synthetic analogs of vitamin A like tretinoin or isotretinoin are used.

Hypervitaminosis A

Since vitamin A is a fat-soluble vitamin, it accumulates in the body on prolonged administration. The symptoms are dry skin (hyperkeratosis), anorexia, fever, alopecia, anaemia, oedema, headache, skin ulcers and tenderness over the bones.

Vitamin D See Page 502

Vitamin K See Page 309

Vitamin E

Vitamin E or Alpha tocopherol is present in wheat germ oil, rice germ oil and soya been oil.

Physiological role Vitamin E acts as an antioxidant. It prevents the damage due to free radicals in normal metabolic reactions. Vitamin E is essential for normal structure and function of the nervous system. It is also required to maintain the integrity of the biological membranes. Vitamin E deficiency in animals result in reproductive and haemopoietic system abnormalities, degenerative changes in the spinal cord and heart. Daily requirement is 10-15 mg.

Uses

Clinically vitamin E deficiency in human beings is not known. It has been tried in G-6-PD deficiency, sterility, menopausal syndrome and other conditions with no definite evidence of obvious benefit.

WATER-SOLUBLE VITAMINS

Vitamin B-complex

B-complex group of vitamins includes thiamine, riboflavin, nicotinic acid, pyridoxine, pantothenic acid, biotin and cyanocobalamin.

Thiamine (Vitamin B_1, Aneurine)

Sources Pulses, outer layers of cereals, rice polishings, peas, nuts, green vegetables, egg and meat.

Physiological role Thiamine is converted to thiamine pyrophosphate which acts as a coenzyme in carbohydrate metabolism.

Daily requirement 1-2 mg.

Symptoms of deficiency Thiamine deficiency produces *Beriberi*.

Dry beriberi is characterised by peripheral neuritis and muscular atrophy.

Wet beriberi The characteristic features are dependent oedema and high output cardiac failure. Wernicke's encephalopathy and Korsakoff's psychosis are also thought to be due to thiamine deficiency.

Uses

1. Prophylactically in presence of increased demand as in pregnancy, lactation and in infants.

2. Beriberi - 50 mg daily parenterally. Once the

patient recovers, maintenance dose of 10 mg/day is given orally.

3. Chronic alcoholics - 50 mg daily.

4. Empirical use - Thiamine is tried in several neurological and cardiovascular disorders and morning sickness.

Riboflavin (Vitamin B$_2$)

Sources Milk, egg, liver, meat, grains and green leafy vegetables.

Physiological function Flavin mononucleotide (FMN) and flavin adenine dinucleotide (FAD) containing the active form of riboflavin are coenzymes in various oxidation-reduction reactions.

Symptoms of deficiency Angular stomatitis, glossitis, seborrhoeic keratosis of the nose, ulcers in the mouth, dry skin, burning sensation in the plantar surface of the feet, vascularization of the cornea and alopecia.

Uses

Riboflavin is used for the prevention and treatment (2-10 mg) of riboflavin deficiency.

Nicotinic Acid and Nicotinamide (Vitamin B$_3$)

Nicotinic acid and nicotinamide are together known as *niacin.*

Sources Rice polishings, liver, fish, milk, eggs, nuts and pulses.

Physiological functions Nicotinic acid is converted to nicotinamide. Nicotinamide adenine nucleotide (NAD) and its phosphate (NADP) are coenzymes involved in several oxidation-reduction reactions.

Nicotinic acid is also a lipid-lowering agent.

Symptoms of deficiency Niacin deficiency results in Pellagra characterised by dermatitis, diarrhoea and dementia. Other symptoms include:

pigmentation of the skin, stomatitis, glossitis, headache, insomnia, hallucinations, confusion and megaloblastic anaemia. Chronic alcoholics, people living on maize as the staple diet, patients with malabsorption and cirrhosis develop pellagra.

Uses

1. Prophylaxis and treatment of pellagra (50-500 mg).

2. Nicotinic acid is used in hyperlipopro teinaemia (See page 313).

Pyridoxine (Vitamin B$_6$)

Sources Cereals, legumes, liver, milk, meat and eggs.

Physiological functions Pyridoxal phosphate is a coenzyme involved in the synthesis of several amino acids, biogenic amines and other compounds like GABA.

Symptoms of deficiency Glossitis, peripheral neuritis, anaemia, dermatitis and low seizure threshold due to decreased GABA levels in the brain.

Uses

1. Prophylaxis and treatment of pyridoxine deficiency.

2. INH induced peripheral neuritis - pyridoxine is used both for prophylaxis and treatment.

3. Convulsions in infants due to pyridoxine deficiency.

4. 'Morning sickness' in pregnancy - pyridoxine may reduce vomiting by an unknown mechanism.

Pantothenic Acid

Sources Wheat, cereals, milk, peanuts, liver, egg yolk and vegetables.

Physiological role Pantothenic acid is converted to coenzyme A which is involved in several

TABLE 74.1: Sources, Recommended daily allowances and Deficiency symptoms of various vitamins in the diet (for adults)

Vitamin	Important dietary sources	Daily allowance	Deficiency symptoms
Fat soluble vitamins			
Vitamin A	Green leafy vegetables carrots, mango, papaya, eggs, milk, butter, cheese, liver and fish liver oils.	3000-4000 IU	Night blindness, xerophthalamia, hyperkeratosis of skin and epithelial tissues.
Vitamin D	liver, egg yolk, fish liver oils, milk, butter	200-400 IU	Rickets, osteomalacia
Vitamin E	wheat germ, nuts, cereals, eggs, green leafy vegetables	10-15 mg	Not known
Vitamin K	Green leafy vegetables, liver, meat, cheese, egg yolk and tomatoes.	50-100 mg	hypoprothrombinemia, haemeorrhage
Water soluble vitamins			
Vitamin B complex			
Thiamine (B_1)	Cereals, rice polishing, liver, egg yolk	1.2-1.4mg	Beriberi, peripheral neuritis, anorexia
Riboflavin (B_2)	Milk, cereals, pulses, leafy vegetables, eggs, and meat.	1.5-2 mg	Stomatitis, glossitis, cheilosis, vascularisation of cornea.
Nicotinic acid (Niacin B_3)	Rice polishings, cereals, pulses, groundnut, liver, meat, fish.	20 mg	Pellagra - diarrhoea, dermatitis, dementia; glossitis, stomatitis, delusions, confusion.
Pantothenic acid	Rice polishings, whole grains, meat, egg yolk	4-7 mg	Weakness, fatigue, burning sensation in the feet.
Pyridoxine (B_6)	Whole grains, pulses, green vegetables, milk, glossitis, stomatitis liver, egg yolk	2 mg	Peripheral neuritis
Biotin		0.1-0.2 mg	
Folic acid	Leafy vegetables, milk, liver, meat, cereals	100-200 mcg	Megaloblastic anaemia, glossitis, g.i. disturbances
Vitamin B_{12}	Milk, egg yolk, liver, meat, fish	1-2 mg	Megaloblastic anaemia, demyelinating, neurological disorders of the spinal cord.
Vitamin C	Goose berry (amla), citrus fruits, green vegetables and tomatoes germinating pulses	50 mg	Scurvy - petichiae, bleeding gums, easy bruising, delayed wound healing, anemia, weakness.

metabolic reactions. Pantothenic acid deficiency in human beings is not known. Experimentally induced deficiency results in fatigue and paraesthesia. Calcium pantothenate is a component of multivitamin preparations.

Biotin

Biotin is an organic acid found in liver, nuts, egg yolk and other foods. Biotin deficiency in humans is not known. Experimentally induced deficiency results in dermatitis, anorexia, alopecia and glossitis. Biotin is a coenzyme in several metabolic reactions. It is present in many multi-vitamin preparations. Avidin, a protein present in egg white prevents the absorption of biotin.

Vitamin B$_{12}$, Folic acid (See page 297)

Vitamin C (Ascorbic acid)

Sources Citrus fruits, tomatoes, gooseberry, green vegetables and potatoes are rich in vitamin C.

Physiological role Ascorbic acid is involved in several metabolic reactions including oxidation reduction reactions and in cellular respiration. It is essential for the integrity of connective tissue, for the development of cartilage, bone and teeth and for wound healing.

Symptoms of deficiency Vitamin C deficiency results in scurvy characterised by connective tissue defects resulting in haemorrhages in subcutaneous tissues, petechiae, ecchymoses, impaired wound healing, tender bleeding gums, deformed teeth, brittle bones, anaemia and growth retardation.

Uses

1. Prevention of vitamin C deficiency - 50-100 mg daily.

2. Scurvy - 500-1000 mg daily.

3. Common cold - large doses (0.5-1.5 g) of vitamin C has been tried as a prophylactic against common cold with controversial benefits.

4. To acidify urine.

MINERALS

Minerals are natural compounds/elements. About 5% of human body is made up of minerals. Minerals are essential for the normal body functions. Some minerals are needed in large quantities while others are in small quantities (trace elements).

Minerals needed in large quantities:

Calcium, sodium, potassium, magnesium, phosphorus, chloride, sulphur

Minerals needed in small quantities:

Iron, zinc, manganese, copper, iodine, fluoride, cobalt.

CALCIUM (See page 500)

SODIUM

Distribution in the body - Sodium is mainly present in extracellular fluid and bone. It is present as a salt with chloride, phosphate, bicarbonate and lactase.

Daily requirement - of sodium varies from 5 to 15 grams. In tropical countries and in the coastal areas, lot of sodium is lost in the sweat and the sodium requirement is more in such places.

Metabolism Sodium is excreted mainly by the kidneys. It is also lost in the sweat and in stools in patients with diarrhoea.

Absorption of sodium is increased both directly and indirectly by glucose. Absorption of glucose increases water absorption and sodium follows. Aldosterone enhances the sodium reabsorption by the kidneys. Sodium depletion increases plasma renin levels.

Hyponatremia

Causes - excessive sweating, diarrhoea, burns, diuretics, starvation.

Signs and symptoms - anorexia, lethargy, muscle cramps, hypotension and shock.

Treatment - intravenous infusion of normal saline.

Hypernatremia

Common causes: Acute nephritis, aldosteronism, CCF, drugs like NSAIDs.

Signs and symptoms: Edema and increased blood pressure.

Treatment: Restricting dietary sodium intake, diuretics (frusemide) to promote sodium excretion in urine.

POTASSIUM

Potassium, a cation, is mainly present inside the cells. The total body content of potassium in an adult male is about 45mEq/Kg of which 70% is present in the muscles.

Sources: Coconut water, vegetables, fruits, nuts, meat and liver.

Daily requirement: 3 - 5 g in adults.

Physiological functions: Potassium is the chief cation in the cells (400mg/dl) while plasma potassium is about 20 mg/ml. Potassium has an important role in regulating muscular activity, maintaining water and electrolyte balance and acid base balance; potassium is also essential for neuronal activity. (Table 74.2)

MAGNESIUM

Source: Vegetables, grains, nuts, cocoa, fish, meat.

Daily requirement: 300 mg in adults. Plasma magnesium levels - 1.8 to 2.4mg/dl. The total body content of magnesium in an adult male is 20 to 30 g of which about 50 to 60% is present in bones and 25% in the muscles. Parathormone is essential for absorption of magnesium. It also helps in renal tubular reabsorption of magnesium.

Physiological role

- Magnesium is a CNS depressant.
- Magnesium depresses neuromuscular transmission by inhibiting the release of acetylcholine as well as antagonizing its

TABLE 74.2: Causes, Clinical features and treatment of Hypo and Hyperkalemia

CAUSES	CLINICAL FEATURES	TREATMENT
HYPOKALEMIA		
Dietary deficiency, excessive loss in sweating, vomiting, diarrhoea; diabetic ketoacidosis, diuretic overdosage, Fanconi's syndrome, nephrotic syndrome	Fatigue, muscle weakness, mental confusion, thirst, hypotension, bradycardia, cardiac arrhythmias, renal imparement, neuro-muscular paralysis	Mild - oral Potassium chloride Severe - KCl-Slow IV Drip (rapid potassium infusion can cause sudden death due to cardiac arrest)
HYPERKALEMIA		
Drug induced (ACE inhibitors, spironolactone); Addison's disease,	Cardiac arrhythmias, skeletal muscle & respiratory paralysis, cardiac arrest	↑urinary K^+ excretion by dialysis and diuretics (Frusemide + a thiazide) Cation exchange resin, Promoting K^+ shift into cells using plain insulin 5-10 units with 50 ml of 50% glucose IV over 5 min.

depolarising activity at the motor end plate.

- Magnesium depresses the myocardium to some extent and also causes peripheral vasodilation resulting in flushing and hypotension.
- Magnesium is a cofactor in several enzyme mediated reactions.

Therapeutic uses:

1. Magnesium deficiency - Magnesium hydroxide is given orally in mild cases and magnesium sulphate is given slow IV. In severe deficiency - 5 ml of 50% magnesium is given slow IV.

2. As antacids - magnesium hydroxide and magnesium trisilicate are used as antacids.

3. Osmotic purgative - Magnesium sulphate is used as osmotic purgative.

4. As anticonvulsant - Magnesium sulfate is used IV (or IM) to control seizures in toxaemia of pregnancy.

5. Tocolytic - IV Magnesium sulphate may be used as an alternative to relax the uterus in preterm labour.

6. Cardiac arrhythmias - Magnesium chloride may be used in the treatment of arrhythmias that may follow myocardial infarction.

7. In raised intracranial tension - Rectal administration of Magnesium sulphate solution may help to reduce intracranial tension.

8. Topical - 25 - 50% Magnesium sulphate in glycerin (Mag sulf poultice) is used topically to relieve local edema. Magnesium sulphate exerts osmotic effect (while glycerin is hygroscopic) and reduces local inflammation.

Defeciency:

Magnesium deficiency may occur in severe diarrhoea, malabsorption, diuretic therapy, hyperthyroidism, hyperparathyroidism, aldosteronism and renal dysfunction. It is characterized by neuromuscular irritability, tremors, nystagmus, difficulty in swallowing, cardiac disturbances, restlessness, altered behaviour and convulsions. Treatment is with magnesium sulfate (or any other magnesium salt) 10 ml of 25% solution IM or slow IV.

PHOSPHORUS (See page 501)

IRON (See page 295)

ZINC

Source:

Vegetables, fruits, nuts, pulses, egg, milk, liver and meat.

Functions:

Zinc is a cofactor of many enzymes like carbonic anhydrase, alkaline phosphatase.

Dificiency:

Dificiency of zinc results in impaired wound healing, decreased acuity of taste and smell, alopecia, dermatitis and decreased growth in children.

Zinc is component of several multivitamin preparations.

MANGANESE

Manganese acts as co-factor certain enzymes like decarboxylase. It also plays role in glycoprotiene synthesis.

Sources Cereals, nuts, whole grains, fruits and vegetables are rich in manganese. It is stored in the liver.

Deficiency symptoms are not known.

75

Enzymes In Therapy

- Mammalian enzymes
- Bacterial enzymes
- Plant enzymes

Enzymes are proteins produced by the living cells. They catalyse several biochemical reactions. Some substances act with specific enzymes and are called coenzymes.

Enzymes used in therapeutics are:

Mammalian enzymes
Hyaluronidase, Trypsin, Chymotrypsin, Alpha chymotrypsin, Pancreatic dornase.

Bacterial enzymes
Streptokinase, Streptodornase, Collagenase, Serratiopeptidase, L-asparaginase.

Plant enzymes
Papain (Papase).

MAMMALIAN ENZYMES

Hyaluronidase is obtained from mammalian testes. It depolymerizes hyaluronic acid of connective tissue. Given subcutaneously, it increases the tissue permeability and enhances the rate of absorption of subcutaneously administered fluids and drugs.

Hyaluronidase can produce allergic reactions. It should not be injected around an infected site to avoid the spread of infection.
It is available as dry powder.
Uses

1. Hyaluronidase is used for hypodermoclysis in infants and children in whom, large volumes of fluids are given subcutaneously.

2. To hasten resorption of fluids and blood in haematoma.

3. Along with local anaesthetics - to increase the effectiveness of local anaesthesia.

4. Radiography - hyaluronidase enhances

absorption of the radio-opaque substances.

Trypsin

Trypsin is obtained from bovine pancreas. It is a proteolytic enzyme which directly hydrolyses natural proteins. It digests dead tissue, bacteria and debris. Trypsin may be used topically, sublingually or intramuscularly.

Adverse effects Allergic reactions can occur.

Uses

1. Trypsin (freshly prepared solution) is used topically for debridement of necrotic tissues.

2. Used topically for liquefaction of coagulated blood and exudates.

3. Trypsin containing gelatin capsules are inserted into sinuses and fistulae that cannot be adequately irrigated.

4. It can also be used for irrigation of nasal cavities.

5. Used sublingually for thrombophlebitis, deep contusions and skin ulcers.

Chymotrypsin

Chymotrypsin is an endopeptidase obtained from bovine pancreas. Like trypsin, it hydrolyses natural proteins. It is used in several skin conditions including abscesses and ulcers and postoperatively to reduce inflammation and oedema. It is also used following tooth extraction and tooth impaction.

Alpha chymotrypsin

Alpha chymotrypsin has proteolytic activity like chymotrypsin. It is used in cataract operations to dissolve the suspensory ligament of the lens (enzymatic zonulolysis). This makes it easy to remove the lens.

Pancreatic dornase

Pancreatic dornase is a deoxyribonuclease. It acts extracellularly and makes the secretions thin by degrading deoxyribnucleoprotein. It is obtained from pancreas of cattle and is used as an aerosol. It can cause allergic reactions. See mucolytics (See page 290).

BACTERIAL ENZYMES

Streptokinase

Streptokinase obtained from beta haemolytic streptococci causes fibrinolysis (See page 306).

Streptodornase

Streptodornase is a group of proteolytic enzymes which catalyse depolymerization of nucleoproteins like deoxyribonucleic acid that is present in dead cells of the pus. Thus streptodornase liquifies viscous and purulent material. It has no effect on living cells.

Streptokinase and streptodornase are used in combination both topically and for instillation into body cavities.

Adverse effects Allergic reactions may occur.

Streptokinase and streptodornase are contraindicated in presence of bleeding. They should not be used around a local infected area.

Streptokinase and streptodornase are used topically to liquify clotted blood, pus and to clear the debris in chronic ulcers, osteomyelitis and other wounds and lesions.

Collagenase

Collagenase obtained from *Clostridium histolyticum* is used topically for the debridement of dermal ulcers and burns. It also promotes the growth of granulation tissue.

Serratiopeptidase

Serratiopeptidase is a proteolytic enzyme obtained from the serratia species.

It is administered orally to relieve inflammatory edema in the soft tissues. It is claimed to digest necrotic tissue, exudates and clots which are cleared faster from the site of trauma. However, adequate evidence to prove its efficacy is currently not available.

Serratiopeptidase is tried as an adjuvant in a wide variety of conditions associated with inflammation like rheumatoid arthritis, osteoarthritis, cervical spondylosis, ankylosing spondylitis, fractures and other musculoskeletal disorders; sinusitis, otitis, bronchitis, bronchial asthma and pulmonary tuberculosis to facilitate expectoration; subconjunctival haemorrhage and pulmonary tuberculosis to facilitate expectoration; subconjunctical haemorrhage and hyphaema;

Post operative patients, traumatic injury, following tonsillectomy, episiotomy, perineal laceration; dental infections, pericoronitis and alveolar abcess.

L-asparaginase - is obtained from *E.coli* cultures for commercial use (See page 443).

PLANT ENZYMES

Papain is obtained from the unripe fruit of *Cacira papaya.* It is a proteolytic enzyme used topically for debriding wound surfaces.

76 *Treatment of Poisoning*

CHAPTER

- **Symptoms & signs**
- **General management**
- **Treatment of snake bite**
- **Food poisoning**

Toxicology is the science that deals with the study of poisons, their source, properties, actions, detection and treatment of poisoning.

A **poison** may be defined as any substance, which if administered or comes in contact with a living being produces, ill-health, disease or death

Every drug in a high dose can cause poisoning. Poisoning could be accidental, suicidal or homicidal. Millions of poisoning cases are seen every year with several hundreds dying but several more are unreported. Mortality rate varies from country to country. In India, it is around 35% while in America it is 2%! When treated on time with appropriate drugs, treatment of poisoning can be successful.

Sources - venom, toxins and poisons may be originating from animals, microorganisms, plants or chemicals.

Poisoning may be -

• **Acute** - a single large dose or multiple small doses repeated at short intervals result in acute poisoning. Onset of signs and symptoms are abrupt.

• **Chronic** - small doses repeated over a long period result in chronic poisoning. Signs and symptoms appear gradually.

Symptoms and signs - Acute poisoning can be rapidly fatal. Awareness of the symptoms of poisoning, mechanisms involved in death due to poisoning and early, appropriate treatment are all important to reduce the morbidity and mortality from poisoning. Clinical assessment of the patient for vital signs should be done immediately. Respiration, heart rate, blood pressure, pupillary size, body temperature, neurological status and level of consciousness are assessed. Generally, symptoms like hypotension and dehydration due to vomiting and diarrhoea are common; cardiac arrhythmias can occur particularly from drugs like digitalis, theophylline, amphetamines, ephedrine and some antiarrhythmic drugs. Bronchospasm and respiratory depression need immediate attention. In a comatose patient, airway obstruction and aspiration of stomach contents into the respiratory tract may result in death. CNS depressants can cause stupor and coma.

No time should be lost in identifying the exact poison. Treatment should be started immediately with supportive measures.

Steps in the treatment of poisoning include:

1. Stop the source of poison - the patient should be shifted away from the source of poison.

2. Limit the absorption of poison - This depends on the route of entry. If taken orally, vomiting may be induced or stomach wash may be given to prevent further absorption of the poison. Cathartics or bowel irrigation may also be tried. In case of poisoning through skin eg: by organophosphorus compounds, the clothing should be changed and the skin should be washed with soap and water.

3. Supportive therapy - emergency stabilization of the cardiovascular and respiratory system is needed - ABC (Airway, Breathing, Circulation) of poisoning

   i) Airway should be cleared of any mucous or vomitus that may be present. Suction of the air passages may be needed and if required an endotracheal tube may be inserted. Patient should be put in lateral position.

   ii) If breathing is depressed, artificial ventilation should be given. Oxygen may be needed.

   iii) Circulation - Circulatory status should be assessed by pulse rate, blood pressure and urine output. Suitable IV fluids should be given. Generally 1 litre of normal saline with 1 litre of dextrose is injected in the first 24 hours. If hypotension is present, the foot end of the bed should be raised.

   iv) If the patient is in coma, nothing should be given orally. Blood glucose should be estimated to rule out hypoglycemic coma. In all comatose patients, with signs of CNS depression, administration of *'coma cock tail'* is routinely recommended - it includes -

   > 1. Naloxone - 2mg
   > 2. Thiamine - 100 mg
   > 3. Dextrose - (50 ml of 50% solution)
   >
   > All are given intravenously

   These are given with the intention that - if the poison is an opioid, naloxone overcomes the respiratory and CNS depression. Naloxone also overcomes the effects of opioids released in the body in pain; dextrose helps if the coma is due to hypoglycemia. Thiamine helps to prevent Wernickes encephalopathy in alcoholics.

4. Specific therapy - specific antidotes, antivenoms and antitoxins should be used whenever available. For some poisons specific therapies may be available though we don't call them antidotes. For example ethanol in methanol poisoning, nitrites in cyanide poisoning. These can often be life saving.

5. Other measures - like forced diuresis, peritoneal dialysis, hemodialysis, hemoperfusion, exchange transfusion etc., are carried out in certain cases of poisoning only if indicated. Excretion of acidic drugs like salicylates can be enhanced by **forced alkaline diuresis -** using frusemide, sodium bicarbonate and IV fluids. Excretion of basic drugs like amphetamines may be enhanced by **forced acid diuresis** using frusemide, ascorbic acid and IV fluids.

However, these procedures may lead to volume overload and also expose the kidneys to a high dose of the toxin. Excretion of drugs like amphetamines, barbiturates, ethyl and methyl alcohol, phenytoin, salicylates, theophylline, and lithium can be effectively carried out by **haemodialysis. Haemoperfusion** can be carried out in some poisons particularly the fat soluble drugs.

GENERAL MANAGEMENT

1.Gut decontamination

Vomiting may be induced or stomach wash (gastric lavage) may be given to clear the stomach of the unabsorbed poison.

Emesis: Vomiting can be induced with 20-30 ml of syrup of ipecac. It acts within 15 minutes. Alternatively freshly prepared mustard powder solution (1 teaspoon mustard powder in water) can be used. Vomiting may also be induced by mechanical stimulation of the pharynx with fingertips or by using strong salt solution (1 tablespoonful in half a glass of warm water) - but both these are considered dangerous. Because salt solution can cause severe hypernatraemia, it is generally not recommended. However, salt solution is the most easily available household remedy. Hence in acute poisoning, it may be worthwhile trying induction of emesis with salt solution as an alternative because sometimes this could be time saving and therefore life saving. Moreover, most of the excess salt is lost in vomiting. Adequate fluid intake should be ensured. Induction of vomiting is helpful in clearing the poison, which may be present in the stomach and also in duodenum.

Vomiting should not be induced -

- if the poison is a corrosive agent or a petroleum product

- if the patient is unconscious

Stomach Wash - washing the stomach with large amounts of water removes unabsorbed poison. Stomach wash can be carried out only in a conscious patient. Warm water or saline may be used for lavage. Cold lavage solutions can result in hypothermia. In alkaloidal poisons, tannic acid or potassium permangenate solution can be used. An orogastric tube of approximately ½ inch diameter and 150 cm in length may be employed. The patient is put in left lateral position and the tube inserted orally. Wash has to be carried out till the returning fluid becomes clear. Once this is achieved, a slurry of activated charcoal (1 g/kg) in water (10:1) is to be left in the stomach and the tube should be removed. The first returning fluid should be retained for chemical analysis.

There is some controversy regarding the time limit for stomach wash. Though generally stomach decontamination is recommended to be done up to 1 hour of poison ingestion, it is worth trying it upto days in all suitable cases. There are reports of poisons being detected in the stomach even after 5-6 days of poisoning. Moreover, certain poisons (some basic drugs) may diffuse into the stomach from blood vessels even when given intravenously. Hence it is worth giving a stomach wash in all suitable cases unless contraindicated.

Contraindications - Stomach wash should not be given in poisoning with corrosives (except carbolic acid), petroleum products, foreign body ingestion and in poisoning with convulsants .

Activated charcoal is obtained by destructive distillation of wood and then treating it with an activating agent like steam, carbon dioxide etc. Activated charcoal can adsorb (attract particles on to its surface) several drugs and thereby prevent their absorption. Activated charcoal has multiple microscopic pores which enhance its surface area ($1000\text{-}2000\ M^2/gram$). This enables it to adsorb drugs and chemicals. It is administered as a solution of 4 parts of water mixed with one part of activated charcoal (dose 1 gram/kg body weight). It is a safe and useful measure except that it is unpalatable. In western countries, a palatable preparation is available called *medicoal.*

Activated charcoal is useful in several cases of poisoning including that of barbiturates, salicylates, paracetamol, antidepressants, phenytoin, carbamazepine, theophylline and many other organic and inorganic compounds. It is not effective in poisoning by heavy metals, alcohol and corrosives.

Purgatives - purgatives may help to speed up the excretion of drugs from the gut. If a purgative is needed, saline purgatives are generally used. Magnesium sulfate 20-30 grams or sodium sulfate also 20-30 g may be given orally. Adequate fluid intake is needed. Irrigation of the gut with a balanced solution of polyethylene glycol and electrolytes may help in poisoning particularly due to sustained release preparations like that of iron.

2. Management of respiratory failure

It is necessary to maintain a clear airway. Patient should be placed in a semiprone position, secretions should be aspirated regularly and tongue should be drawn forward. An oropharyngeal airway of suitable size may be inserted if required. In comatose patients air way can be kept clear with a cuffed endotracheal tube. Respiratory stimulants like doxapram or nikethamide may help some patients - but the benefit is not proved and therefore are not preferred. **Oxygen** may be given if there is hypoxia or increased carbondioxide (hypercapnoea) on blood gas analysis.

In profound respiratory depression, mechanical ventilation is needed.

Pulmonary edema and increased bronchial secretions may be caused by volatile irritant poisons and organophosphates. Pulmonary edema should be relieved immediately as it can interfere with gaseous exchange. The patient should be in the sitting position. Secretions in the throat should be removed by suction. If there is cyanosis, oxygen (60-100%) may be administered using a face mask .Oxygen may be saturated with ethyl alcohol vapour by bubbling it through a bottle of alcohol. This causes collapse of the foam in the alveoli and allows better gas exchange. Intravenous frusemide (40mg) relieves pulmonary edema by shifting the blood from pulmonary to systemic circulation.

3. Management of circulatory failure

In presence of hypotension, foot end of the bed should be elevated. Plasma expanders like dextran or whole blood itself may be needed in hypovolemic shock. Vasopressors like dopamine (2-10µg/kg), phenylephrine (5-20µg/kg), methoxamine or mephenteramine may be used intravenously in profound hypotension.

4. Management of fluid and electrolyte imbalance

Hyponatremia (plasma sodium <130mEq/L) can cause salt and water retention . It is treated with normal saline infusion.

Hypernatremia (plasma sodium >150mEq/L) may be treated with a loop diuretic like frusemide. Half normal saline or infusion of 0.2% sodium chloride solution helps to dilute plasma sodium levels.

Hypokalemia: (Plasma potassium <3.5mEq/L) can cause dangerous arrhythmias. Potassium chloride 4-6 mEq/L to a maximum of 40-80 mEq/day is administered orally in divided doses or as a **very slow** intravenous infusion. Potassium should never be pushed rapidly into the vein because it can cause cardiac arrest and sudden death.

Hyperkalemia - (Plasma potassium >5.5 mEq/L). In mild hyperkalemia diuretics like frusemide (1 mg/ kg IV) and thiazide may be used to enhance excretion of potassium.

Severe hyperkalemia is a medical emergency and requires immediate treatment. 10% calcium gluconate given slow IV minimizes membrane excitability. Dialysis is indicated in patients with chronic renal failure.

Hypocalcemia (plasma calcium <4 mEq/L) - 10% Calcium gluconate given IV helps to raise the plasma calcium level.

5. Metabolic acidosis - sodium bicarbonate 1-2mEq/L intravenously over 30 minutes helps to overcome acidosis.

6. Convulsions - Diazepam 10 mg given slowly intravenously is the drug of choice. The same IV preparation of diazepam may be given rectally if getting an IV line is difficult. Phenytoin 10mg/kg IV or phenobarbitone 10mg/kg are other alternatives. If seizures do not respond to these, a skeletal muscle relaxant (pancuronium) or IV anaesthetic thiopental sodium may be given.

7. Antidotes - An antidote is a substance which antagonizes and overcomes the effects of a poison. The right antidote used at the right time in right dose can reverse the effects of the corresponding poison and can be life saving. Unfortunately specific antidotes are available only for a few toxins. Therefore, in majority of the poisoning cases treatment is only supportive and symptomatic.

Antidotes may be classified based on the mode of action into 3 groups as follows -

1. **Physical antidotes** - act by reducing the absorption of the poison.

   Eg: activated charcoal adsorbs alkaloids.

2. **Chemical antidotes** - act by forming a complex with the poison.

   Eg: acetic acid reacts with alkalies. Potassium permangenate oxidizes compounds like barbiturates, phosphorus, alkalies; chelating agents bind heavy metals like lead, arsenic, copper, mercury etc.

3. **Pharmacological antidotes** - The antidotes compete for binding to the same receptors or sites where the toxin binds. Eg: Naloxone for morphine, Flumazenil for diazepam and atropine for organophosphorus poisoning.

Universal antidote consists of

(i) 1 part tannic acid (to precipitate alkaloids, glycosides and heavy metals)

(ii) 1 part milk of magnesia (to neutralize acids)

(iii) 2 parts burnt toast (to adsorb alkaloid)

This was earlier used with the hope of preventing absorption and overcoming the toxic effects of most of the poisons. We now know that actually *it does not serve any purpose and is no more recommended.*

TREATMENT OF SNAKE BITE

There are more than 3000 species of snakes in the world of which about 216 are found in India. 52 types of the snakes in India are poisonous. All over the world snake bites are responsible for 30,000 to 40,000 deaths every year. In India about 2 lakh people are bitten by snakes every year of which abovt 16,000 die. Vipers, cobras and kraits are the common poisonous snakes.

Signs and symptoms: In all cases of snake bite the patient is in great fear and is in a stage of neurogenic shock. The patient is in a semiconscious state with cold, clammy skin, feeble pulse, rapid and shallow breathing. Other symptoms vary according to the type of snake.

The signs and symptoms of systemic toxicity appear in about half an hour.

1. Elapid bite (cobra, krait etc - neurotoxic)

Local reactions - Pain, burning, swelling, discolouration of the site, oozing of blood stained fluid are seen in 1-3 hours. Blisters and local necrosis may occur. Systemic effects include vomiting headache, loss of consciousness, ptosis, ophthalmoplegia (eyes become fixed in central position) convulsions followed by flaccid paralysis.

2. Viper bite - Haemotoxic

Local reactions are prominent with swelling, discolouration, blister formation and bleeding from the site. Bleeding from the gums, haematuria, disseminated intravascular coagulation are seen.

3. Sea snakes (Hydrophids - Myotoxic)

Local reactions are mild swelling and pain.

TABLE 76.1 SOME SPECIFIC ANTIDOTES FOR DRUGS AND CHEMICALS

	AGENT CAUSING TOXICITY	ANTIDOTE	DOSE
1.	Paracetamol	N-acetyl cysteine	Oral140mg/kg followed by 70mg/kg every 4 hrs, or IV 150mg/kg infusion over 15 min. repeated as required.
2.	Morphine and other opioids	Naloxone	1-2 mg IV repeated every 10-15 minutes.
3.	Heparin	Protamine Sulphate	1mg IV for every 100 units of heparin.
4.	Cyanide	Sodium nitrate + Sodium thiosulfate	10 ml of 3% solution IV 50 ml of 25% solution IV
5.	Organophosphates	Atropine, Oximes	2mg IV repeated every 10 minutes Pralidoxime 1 gram IV every 3-4hrs 3 doses
6.	Theophylline, caffeine	Esmolol	25-50µg/kg/min- IV
7.	Atropine	Physostigmine	1-2mg IV slowly (or SC) may be repeated if symptoms reappear
8.	Curare and other non depolarizing skeletal muscle relaxants	Neostigmine	2mg IV repeated as required.
9.	Copper	d-penicillamine	100mg/kg/day orally in 4 divided doses for 3-7 days.
10.	Iron	Desferrioxamine	15mg/kg/hour IV (100mg desferrioxamine binds 8.5mg of iron)
11.	Arsenic	Dimercaprol	Ist day 400-800mg deep IM in divided doses; 2nd& 3rd day 200-400 mg. 4th day onwards. - 100-200mg
12.	Lead	Calcium disodium edetate	1 gram in 250 ml saline infusion twice a day.
13.	Streptokinase and other fibrinolytics	Epsilon amino caproic acid	5gm oral or IV followed by1gm hourly till bleeding stops (Max 30 gm in 24hrs)
14.	Insu1lin	Glucose	50ml of 50% solution.
15.	Digitalis	Digoxin specific antibody fragments	one vial for every 500mg of digoxin.
16.	Methanol, ethylene glycol	Ethanol or Fomepizole	10%ethanol is given orally -0.7mg/kg loading dose; 0.15ml/kg infusion. loading dose 15mg/kg repeated every 12 hours.
17.	Carbon monoxide	Oxygen	100% by high-flow non-rebreathing mask.
18.	Nitrites	Methylene blue	0.1% solution slow IV in the dose of 1-2mg/kg body weight.
19.	Warfarin	Vitamin K1 oxide, Fresh blood.	10mg IM followed by 5mg 4 hrly As required.
20.	Benzodiazepines	Flumazenil	0.2mg IV repeated as required (Max. 3mg)

Systemic myotoxic effects include muscle pain, stiffness, renal and hepatic necrosis.

Treatment

First aid -

- Reassurance
- Immobilise the bitten part Measures like local incision, suction, application of ice are all found to be **harmful** and no more recommended.

Supportive therapy: Blood pressure, respiration, and urine output are to be menitored. ECG and blood gas analysis are needed. Fresh blood transfusion may be needed to correct coagulation parameters. Analgesics like paracetamol for pain, prophylactic antibiotics as required and tetanus toxoid injection are to be given in all cases.

Specific therapy: Antisnake venom (ASV) is indicated in presence of signs of systemic envenomisation. Dose of antivenom varies.

Mild envenomisation	3 -5 vials
Moderate envenomisation	5 -10 vials
Severe envenomisation	10 - 20 vials

Infusion should be done after test dose.

Watch for reactions to ASV. Hypersensitivity reactions including anaphylaxis can occur. Clean the bite site with providone iodine.

FOOD POISONING

Food poisoning can occur on consumption of food that is contaminated with microorganisms, toxins or chemicals.

Nausea, vomiting, abdominal pain, fever, weakness and diarrhoea are the common symptoms of food poisoning. Other symptoms depend on the causative agent.

Causes for food poisoning

1. Microorganisms
   - Bacteria
   - Protozoa
   - Viruses
2. Toxins- present in certain fish, plants and mushrooms.
3. Chemicals

Food poisoning due to microorganisms

Consumption of food contaminated with microorganisms is the most common cause of food poisoning. The incubation period varies from a few (1-2) hours to a few days.

Microorganisms - Bacteria including *Staphylococcus aureus, Salmonella typhi, Shigella, Vibrio cholerae, Vibrio parahemolyticus, Bacillus cercus, Clostridium botulinum, (Clostridium perfeingenes), Streptococcus, Campylobacter* and *E-coli* can cause food poisoning.

Viral gastroenteritis may be caused by rotavirus, parvovirus and adenovirus. Treatment is symptomatic.

Fungi: The spores of moulds grow on food & can release mycotoxin. These mycotoxins are heat stable. *Aspergillus flavens* can produce aftlatoxins, *Penicillium islandicum* can produce islanditoxin.

Others- Protozoa like *Entamoeba histolytica* amoibiasis) and *Giardia lamblia* (giardiasis) are common causes of food poisoning. Metronidazole is the drug of choice in both.

Mushrooms Of the large variety of mushrooms only about 5% are poisonous. Consumption of such mushrooms can cause a variety of toxic effects depending on the toxin - they can cause cellular destruction, affect central or autonomic nervous system, gastrointestinal system or the kidney.

Treatment however is symptomatic in all these cases except when autonomic nervous system is involved. Inocybe, clitocybe and some species of amanita contain muscarine which stimulates the cholinergic muscarinic receptors. Symptoms include salivation, sweating, diarrhoea, constricted pupils, dyspnoea, bradycardia and hypotension. The specific antidote is atropine (Img IV repeated as required).

Chemicals - Contamination of food with chemicals like arsenic, mercury, antimony or insecticides in fruits and vegetables can cause poisoning. Monosodium glutamate is a food additive commonly used in chinese food. Dose more than 1 gram can cause troublesome symptoms including burning and numbness of face and neck, chest pain, headache, vomiting and vertigo. In children convulsions can sometimes occur.

Treatment is supportive and symptomatic.

TABLE 76.2 DRUGS USED IN FOOD POISONING DUE TO BACTERIA			
Bacteria	**Incubation Period**	**Mode of action**	**Treatment**
Staph.aureus	2-4 hours	• Enterotoxin	• Symptomatic
Shigella	1-3 days	• enterotoxin+neurotoxin • destruction of intestinal mucosa	• Ciprofloxacin
Salmonella	12 hours to 2 days (1 week in case of enteric fever)	• Destruction of intestinal mucosa	Ciprofloxacin Supportive measures
Bacillus cereus	3-8 hours	Enterotoxin	Symptomatic
Vibrio cholerae	Few hours to 5 days	Enterotoxin	• Symptomatic - Fluid replacement, Electrolyte replacement
Vibrio para hemolyticus	6 hrs- 4 days	• Invasion of intestinal mucosa; • Enterotoxin	Symptomatic
Clostridium botulinum	6 hrs- 7 days	Neurotoxin	• Antitoxin, • Symptomatic
Campylobacter	1-8 days	• Enterotoxin, • Invasion of intestinal mucosa	Erythromycin
E. coli	1-3 days	• Enterotoxin • Invasion of intestinal mucosa	• Ciprofloxacin

77 *Geriatric Pharmacology*

- • **Drug Prescription in Geriatric patients**
- • **Pharmacokinetic changes**
- • **Pharmacodynamic aspects**

Drug Prescription in Geriatric patients

People above 65 years of age are called 'elderly'. They form a good percentage of the population and there has been a steady increase in their number. This is the age group which requires medical care as a large percentage of diseases affect the elderly than the young. Several factors influence treatment in the geriatric age group including social and economic conditions and changes in the pharmacokinetics and pharmacodynamic aspects with advanced age. A medical practitioner should be aware of these changes and consider them in drug usage in the elderly. Though people above 65 years are considered elderly, most changes could occur only above 75 years of age. Geriatric medicine infact has evovled as a separate discipline.

Pharmacokinetic changes

There are no significant changes though absorption in the elderly may be slower and less complete. Decreased body water and muscle mass and a higher amount of total body fat are some important variations in the elderly. Moreover the plasma albumin levels are low but the α_1 acid glycoprotein levels are high - this may alter the protein binding of drugs.

Decrease in the activity of the hepatic enzymes and reduced blood flow to the liver may slow down the metabolism of some drugs. Excretion of drugs through the kidneys may be slower because of decreased blood flow to the kidneys and reduced renal function in general.

542

This affects excretion of drugs which are mainly eliminated by the kidneys.

Pharmacodynamic aspects

Elderly respond better to some drugs like analgesics. They are more likely to experience adverse effects to drugs. They may also be receiving other drugs. Hence drug interactions should be considered. However there are no significant pharmacodynamic variations in the elderly.

Decreased income, multiple diseases, emotional stress and a decreased capacity to tolerate pain and suffering in general - all make elderly - a group that requires good attention and medical care.

APPENDICES

Appendices

APPENDIX-1

Important Drug Interactions

Interacting drugs	Consequence	Pharmacological basis
1. β-blockers + hydralazine/frusemide	↑ β blocking effect	↓ metabolism of propranolol
2. β-blockers + insulin	i. β-blockers mask palpitation, the most important warning symptom of hypoglycaemia	• Blockade of cardiac β receptors
	ii. They prolong recovery from hypoglycaemia	• Block hepatic glycogenolysis mediated by β_2 receptors; homoeostatic mechanisms are blocked
3. Propranolol + ephedrine	↑ BP	As β receptors are blocked, unopposed stimulation of α receptors by ephedrine elevates BP
4. Propranolol + verapamil	May cause heart block resulting in cardiac arrest	Both drugs depress conducting tissues of the heart and have negative inotropic effects

Contd...

Contd...

Interacting drugs	Consequence	Pharmacological basis
5. Calcium channel blockers + phenytoin/rifampicin	↓ effects of calcium channel blockers	Both increase metabolism of calcium channel blockers by enzyme induction
6. Digoxin + hydrochlorothiazide	Digoxin toxicity	Thiazides cause hypokalaemia which in turn aggravates digoxin toxicity
7. Digoxin + quinidine	Digoxin toxicity	Quinidine displaces digoxin from tissue binding sites and inhibits digoxin excretion
8. Digoxin + antacids/ sucralfate/metoclopramide	↓ bioavailability of digoxin	Reduce absorption of digoxin
9. Bile acid-binding resins + Frusemide/ thiazides/thyroid hormones	↓ bioavailability	Bind and prevent absorption of orally administered drugs
10. Anticoagulants + phenylbutazone	Anticoagulant toxicity	Inhibit anticoagulant metabolism
11. Warfarin + aspirin	i. Anticoagulant toxicity	• Aspirin displaces warfarin from binding sites
	ii. Bleeding from aspirin induced peptic ulcer	• Inhibition of platelet aggregation by aspirin potentiates anticoagulant effect • Aspirin induced gastric erosion and ulcers may bleed more due to anticoagulant effects
12. Alcohol + disulfiram *Other drugs that produce disulfiram like effects* cephalosporins, metronidazole, sulfonylureas	Antabuse reaction	Disulfiram inhibits aldehyde dehydrogenase resulting in accumulation of acetaldehyde
13. Alcohol + CNS depressants like opioids/antidepressants /antihistamines/hypnotics	Profound CNS depression	CNS depressant effect gets added up
14. Carbamazepine + haloperidol/oral contra- ceptives/corticosteroids	Decreased efficacy of interacting drugs	Carbamazepine is an enzyme inducer - enhances metabolism of interacting drugs
15. Carbamazepine + cimetidine/erythromycin/ INH/ketoconazole	Decreased carbamazepine metabolism	Inhibition of drug metabolising enzymes by interacting drugs
16. Phenytoin + carbamazepine	Decreased effects of both	Phenytoin and carbamazepine increase each other's metabolism
17. Phenytoin + chloramphe- nicol/cimetidine/warfarin	Phenytoin toxicity	The interacting drugs inhibit phenytoin metabolism
18. Phenytoin + steroids/ doxycycline/theophylline	Phenytoin increases meta- bolism of interacting drugs	Phenytoin is an enzyme inducer

Contd...

Interacting drugs	Consequence	Pharmacological basis
19. Barbiturates + other CNS depressants	Profound CNS depression	CNS depression gets added up
20. Barbiturates + calcium channel blockers/cortico-steroids/ketoconazole/ estrogen/chloramphenicol/ tricyclic antidepressants	Decreased efficacy of interacting drugs	Barbiturates are enzyme inducers. They enhance the metabolism of drugs metabolised by microsomal enzymes
21. Tricyclic and related antidepressants + carbamazapine/rifampicin	Increased metabolism of antidepressants	Carbamazepine and rifampicin are enzyme inducers
22. Tricyclic antidepressants + SSRIs like fluoxetine and paroxetine	Decreased metabolism of antidepressants	SSRIs inhibit metabolising enzymes
23. Tricyclic antidepressants + MAO inhibitors	Hypertensive crisis	Uninhibited action of catecholamines due to inhibition of MAO
24. Levodopa + phenothiazines	Decreased anti-parkinsonian effect	Phenothiazines block dopamine receptors
25. Levodopa + pyridoxine	Inhibits antiparkinsonian effect	Pyridoxine enhances peripheral decarboxylation of levodopa
26. Lithium + diuretics	Lithium toxicity	Decreased excretion of lithium
27. NSAIDs + frusemide	Blunting of diuretic effect	PG inhibition may result in salt and water retention
28. Aspirin + warfarin/ phenytoin/ sulfonylureas	Toxicity of co-administered drugs	Aspirin displaces these drugs from protein binding sites
29. Quinolone antibiotics + sucralfate/antacids	↓ bioavailability	Reduced gastrointestinal absorption of quinolones
30. Quinolones + theophylline/caffeine	Toxicity due to theophylline/caffeine	Quinolones inhibit the metabo-lism of theophylline/caffeine
31. Chloramphenicol + phenytoin/sulfonylureas	Toxicity due to phenytoin/sulfonylureas	Chloramphenicol decreases metabolism of these drugs
32. Rifampicin + oestrogens/ corticosteroids/sulfonylureas/ theophylline	Therapeutic failure	Rifampicin is an enzyme inducer and increases the metabolism of other drugs
33. Antacids + quinolones/ salicylates/tetracycline	↓ bioavailability	Antacids may adsorb drugs and reduce their absorption
34. Antacids + sucralfate	Therapeutic failure of sucralfate	Sucralfate acts in acidic pH while antacids make the gastric pH alkaline
35. Allopurinol + 6-mercaptopurine	6-mercaptopurine toxicity	Allopurinol inhibits xanthine oxidase which metabolises 6-mercaptopurine
36. Piperazine citrate + pyrantel pamoate	Therapeutic failure	Piperazine causes hyperpolari-zation while pyrantel causes depolarization. They antagonise each others effects

APPENDIX - 2

MODEL LIST OF ESSENTIAL DRUGS

1. **Anaesthetics**
   1.1 *General anaesthetics and oxygen*
       ether anaesthetic
       halothane
       ketamine
       nitrous oxide
       oxygen
       thiopental
   1.2 *Local anaesthetics*
       bupivacaine
       lidocaine
       Complementary drug
       ephedrine (C)
   1.3 *Preoperative medication and sedation for short-term procedures*
       atropine
       chloral hydrate
       morphine
       promethazine
       diazepam

2. **Analgesics, antipyretics, nonsteroidal anti-inflammatory drugs, drugs used to treat gout and disease-modifying agents used in rheumatic disorders**
   2.1 *Non-opioid analgesics and nonsteroidal anti-inflammatory drugs*
       acetylsalicylic acid
       ibuprofen
       paracetamol
   2.2 *Opioid analgesics*
       codeine
       morphine
       Complementary drug
       pethidine
   2.3 *Drugs used to treat gout*
       allopurinol
       colchicine
   2.4 *Disease-modifying agents used in rheumatic disorders*
       azathioprine
       methotrexate
       chloroquine
       penicillamine
       cyclophosphamide
       sulfasalazine

3. **Antiallergics and drugs used in anaphylaxis**
       chlorpheniramine
       hydrocortisone
       dexamethasone
       prednisolone
       epinephrine

4. **Antidotes and other substances used in poisonings**
   4.1 *Non-specific*
       charcoal, activated
       ipecacuanha
   4.2 *Specific*
       atropine
       calcium gluconate
       deferoxamine
       dimercaprol
       DL-methionine
       methylthioninium chloride (methylene blue)
       naloxone
       penicillamine
       potassium ferric hexacyanoferrate (II $2H_2O$ (Prussian blue)
       sodium calcium edetate
       sodium nitrite
       sodium thiosulfate

5. **Anticonvulsants/antiepileptics**
       carbamazepine
       diazepam
       ethosuximide
       phenobarbital
       phenytoin
       valproic acid
       Complementary drugs
       clonazepam
       magnesium sulfate

6. **Anti-infective drugs**
   6.1 *Anthelminthics*
       6.1.1 Intestinal anthelminthics
           albendazole
           levamisole
           mebendazole
           niclosamide
           praziquantel
           pyrantel

6.1.2 Antifilarials
    diethylcarbamazine
    ivermectin
    Complementary drug
    suramin sodium
6.1.3 Antischistosomals and other
antitrematode drugs
    praziquantel
    triclabendazole
    Complementary drug
    oxamniquine
6.2 *Antibacterials*
    6.2.1 β-*lactam drugs*
        amoxicillin
        ampicillin
        benzathine
          benzylpenicillin
        benzylpenicillin
        cloxacillin
        phenoxymethyl-
          penicillin
        procaine benzylpenicillin
      Restricted indications
        amoxicillin + clavulanic
              acid
        ceftazidime
        ceftraxone
        imipenem + cilastatin
    6.2.2 Other antibacterials
        chloramphenicol
        ciprofloxacin
        doxycycline
        erythromycin
        gentamicin
        metronidazole
        nalidixic acid
        nitrofurantoin
        spectinomycin
        sulfadiazine
        sulfamethoxazole +
          trimethoprim
        trimethoprim
      Complementary drugs
        chloramphenicol
        clindamycin
      Restricted indications
        vancomycin
    6.2.3 *Antileprosy drugs*
        clofazimine
        dapsone
        rifampicin

6.2.4 *Antituberculosis drugs*
    ethambutol
    isoniazid
    isoniazid + ethambutol
    pyrazinamide
    rifampicin
    rifampicin + isoniazid
    rifampicin + isoniazid +
      pyrazinamide
    streptomycin
    Complementary drug
    thioacetazone + isoniazid
6.3 *Antifungal drugs*
    amphotericin B
    griseofulvin
    ketoconazole
    nystatin
    Complementary drugs
    flucytosine
    potassium iodide
6.4 *Antiviral drugs*
    6.4.1 Antiherpes drugs
        acyclovir
    6.4.2 *Antiretroviral drugs*
        zidovudine
6.5 *Antiprotozoal drugs*
    6.5.1 Antiamoebic and antigiardiasis
    drugs
        diloxanide
        metronidazole
    6.5.2 *Antileishmaniasis drugs*
        meglumine antimoniate
        pentamidine
      Complementary drug
        amphotericin B
    6.5.3 *Antimalarial drugs*
    (a) *For curative treatment*
        chloroquine
        primaquine
        quinine
      Complementary drugs
        doxycycline
        mefloquine
        sulfadoxine +
          pyrimethamine
      Restricted indications
        artemether
    (b) *For prophylaxis*
        chloroquine
        mefloquine
        proguanil

hydralazine
hydrochlorothiazide
methyldopa
nifedipine
reserpine
Complementary drugs
doxazosin
sodium nitroprusside

12.4 *Drugs used in heart failure*
captopril
digoxin
dopamine
hydrochlorothiazide

12.5 *Antithrombotic drugs*
acetylsalicylic acid
Complementary drug
streptokinase

12.6 *Lipid-lowering agents*
choice of drugs to be
dicided at the national level

13. **Dermatological drugs (topical)**

13.1 *Antifungal drugs*
benzoic acid + salicylic acid
miconazole
sodium thiosulfate
Complementary drug
selenium sulfide

13.2 *Anti-infective drugs*
methylrosanilinium chloride
(gentian violet)
neomycin + bacitracin
potassium permanganate
silver sulfadiazine

13.3 *Anti-inflammatory and antipruritic drugs*
betamethasone
calamine lotion
hydrocortisone

13.4 *Astringent drugs*
aluminium diacetate

13.5 *Drugs affecting skin differentiation and proliferation*
benzoyl peroxide
coal tar
dithranol
fluorouracil
podophyllum resin
salicylic acid
urea

13.6 *Scabicides and pediculicides*
benzyl benzoate
permethrin

13.7 *Ultraviolet-blocking agents*
Complementary drug
topical sun protection agent
with activity against
ultraviolet A and ultraviolet B

14. **Diagnostic agents**

14.1 *Ophthalmic drugs*
fluorescein
tropicamide

14.2 *Radiocontrast media*
amidotrizoate
barium sulfate
iopanoic acid
propyliodone
complementary drug
meglumine iotroxate

15. **Disinfectants and antiseptics**

15.1 *Antiseptics*
chlorhexidine
polyvidone iodine

15.2 *Disinfectants*
chlorine base compound
chloroxylenol
glutaral

16. **Diuretics**
amiloride
furosemide
hydrochlorothiazide
spironolactone
Complementary drug
mannitol

17. **Gastrointestinal drugs**

17.1 *Antacids and other antiulcer drugs*
aluminium hydroxide
cimetidine
magnesium hydroxide

17.2 *Antiemetic drugs*
metoclopramide
promethazine

17.3 *Antihaemorrhoidal drugs*
local anaesthetic, astringent and anti-inflammatory drug

17.4 *Anti-inflammatory drugs*
hydrocortisone
sulfasalazine

17.5   *Antispasmodic drugs*
    atropine
17.6   *Laxatives*
    senna
17.7   *Drugs used in diarrhoea*
   17.7.1 Oral rehydration
    oral rehydration salts
   17.7.2 Antidiarrhoeal drugs
    codeine

18. **Hormones, other endocrine drugs and contraceptives**
18.1   *Adrenal hormones and synthetic substitutes*
    dexamethasone
    hydrocortisone
    prednisolone
   Complementary drugs
    fludrocortisone
18.2   *Androgens*
   Complementary drug
    testosterone
18.3   *Contraceptives*
   18.3.1 Hormonal contraceptives
    ethinylestradiol
      + levonorgestrel
    ethinylestradiol
      + norethisterone
   Complementary drugs
    ethinylestradiol
      + levonorgestrel
    levonorgestrel
    medroxyprogesterone
      acetate
    norethisterone exantate
   18.3.2 Intrauterine devices
    copper-containing device
   18.3.3 Barrier methods
    condoms with or without
      spermicide (nonoxinol)
    diaphragms with spermicide
18.4   *Oestrogens*
    ethinylestradiol
18.5   *Insulins and other antidiabetic agents*
    glibenclamide
    insulin injection (soluble)
    intermediate-acting insulin
    metfomin
18.6   *Ovulation inducers*
    clomifene (2,8)

18.7   *Progestogens*
    norethisterone
   Complementary drug
    medroxyprogesterone acetate (B)
18.8   *Thyroid hormones and antithyroid drugs*
    levothyroxine
    potassium iodide
    propylthiouracil

19. **Immunologicals**
19.1   *Diagnostic agents*
    tuberculin, purified protein
      derivative (PPD)
19.2   *Sera and immunoglobulins*
    anti-D immunoglobulin (human)
    antiscorpion sera
    antitetanus immunoglobulin
      (human)
    antivenom sera
    diptheria antitoxin
    immunoglobulin, human normal
    rabies immunoglobulin
19.3   *Vaccines*
   19.3.1 For universal immunization
    BCG vaccine (dried)
    diphtheria-pertussis-tetanus vaccine
    diphtheria-tetanus vaccine
    hepatitis B vaccine
    measles-mumps-rubella vaccine
    measles vaccine
    poliomyelitis vaccine (inactivated)
    poliomyelitis vaccine
      (live attenuated)
    tetanus vaccine
    tetanus-diphtheria (Td) vaccine
   19.3.2 For specific groups of individuals
    influenza vaccine
    meningococcal vaccine
    rabies vaccine (inactivated)
      (prepared in cell culture)
    rubella vaccine
    typhoid vaccine
    yellow fever vaccine

20. **Muscle relaxants (peripherally acting) and cholinesterase inhibitors**
    alcuronium
    neostigmine
    pyridostigmine (2,8)

suxamethonium (2)
Complementary drug
vecuronium (C)

21. **Ophthalmological preparations**
21.1   *Anti-infective agents*
gentamicin
idoxurdine
silver nitrate
tetracycline
21.2   *Anti-inflammatory agents*
prednisolone
21.3   *Local anaesthetics*
tetracaine
21.4   *Miotics and antiglaucoma drugs*
acetazolamide
pilocarpine
timolol
21.5   *Mydriatics*
atropine
Complementary drug
epinephrine (A)

22. **Oxytocics and antioxytocics**
22.1   *Oxytocics*
ergometrine (1c)
oxytocin
22.2   *Antioxytocics*
salbutamol (2)

23. **Peritoneal dialysis solution**
23.1   Intraperitoneal dialysis solution
(of appropriate composition)

24. **Drugs used in psychotic disorders**
24.1   *Drugs used in psychotic disorders*
Chlorpromazine
fluphenazine
haloperidol
24.2   *Drugs used in mood disorders*
24.2.1 *Drugs used in depressive disorders*
amitriptyline
24.2.2 *Drugs used in bipolar disorders*
carbamazepine
lithium carbonate
valproic acid

24.3   *Drugs used in generalized anxiety and sleep disorders*
diazepam
24.4   *Drugs used in obsessive-compulsive disorders and panic attacks*
clomipramine

25. **Drugs used on the respiratory tract**
25.1   *Antiasthmatic drugs*
aminophylline
beclometasone
epinephrine
ipratropium bromide
salbutamol
theophylline
Complementary drug
cromoglicic acid
25.2   *Antitussives*
dextromethorphan

26. **Solutions correcting water, electrolyte and acid-base disturbances**
26.1   *Oral*
Oral rehydration salts
Potassium chloride
26.2   *Parenteral*
glucose
glucose with sodium chloride
potassium chloride
sodium chloride
sodium hydrogen carbonate
compound solution of sodium lactate
26.3   *Miscellaneous*
Water for injection

27. **Vitamins and minerals**
ascorbic acid
ergocalciferol
iodine
nicotinamide
pyridoxine
retinol
riboflavin
sodium fluoride
thiamine
Complementary drug
calcium gluconate

APPENDIX - 3

PRESCRIPTION WRITING

The Prescription is a written order by a physician to the pharmacist to prepare and/or dispense specific medication for a specific patient. A specific pattern should be followed in writing prescriptions, in order to avoid errors and to safeguard the interests of the patient. Moreover the fact that it is a medicolegal document makes it all the more important to be accurate and precise.

The following points should be remembered in writing a prescription:

1. The writing should be legible.

2. Indelible ink should be used in writing.

3. Abbreviations should be avoided.

4. In writing quantities - decimals should be avoided; when inevitable, zero should be used - 0.1 for .1.

5. Less than 1 gm - should be written as milligrams, e.g. 200 mg and not 0.2 g. No abbreviation should be used for micrograms and units.

6. Blank space should be avoided between direction and the signature of the doctor. If blank space is present, it should be striked off to avoid misuse of the space to obtain drugs illegally.

PARTS OF THE PRESCRIPTION

1. Date of writing the prescription.

2. Address of the prescriber - preferrably prescriptions are written on the letter pad with doctor's name and address printed at the top.

3. Name, age, sex and address of the patient.

4. Superscription - the symbol ℞ meaning 'take thou' is also considered as an invocation to the Greek gods of healing - Jupitor and Horus.

5. Drug name and strength. This is the body of the prescription - also called inscription. Abbreviations should never be used.

6. Directions to the pharmacist (subscription) - consists of instructions for compounding if any and the quantity to be supplied.

7. Directions to the patient - should be clear and should indicate the quantity, frequency, time, route of administration and other information relevant to the preparation. If a drug is meant only for external application or needs to be shaken well or mixed before using - such instructions should be mentioned.

8. Signature of the prescriber—the prescriber should sign along with registration number.

TYPES OF PRESCRIPTIONS

1. *Precompounded prescription* orders for a drug manufactured by a pharmaceutical company, has a trade name and is available for use.

2. *Compounded or extemporaneous prescription* - the physician directs the pharmacist to compound a preparation. The ingredients, their quantity and the form of preparation (like mixture, powder or ointment) is chosen by the physician and instructed accordingly.

MODEL PRESCRIPTION

Dr Vaidya   July 10, 2001
Highland
Mangalore   Tel No._____

Ramu   Male   Age: 35 years
No. 7, Kankanady
Mangalore

    R
Tab Roxithromycin 150 mg
Dispense 14 tablets
Label - Take 1 tab orally twice a day, 30 minutes before food for 7 days.

    Signature

    Regn. No.

SOME COMMONLY USED LATIN ABBREVIATIONS IN PRESCRIPTIONS

Abbreviation	Latin derivation	Meaning in English
o.d.	onus in die	once a day
b.d.	bis in die	twice a day
b.i.d.	bis in die	twice a day
t.i.d.	ter in die	three times a day
t.d.s.	ter die sumendum	three times a day
q.i.d.	quarter in die	four times a day
h.s.	hora somni	at bed time
stat	statim	at once
s.o.s.	si opus sit	if necessary
q.s.	quantum sufficit	A sufficient amount
p.o./po	per os	by mouth
ung	unguentum	ointment
caps	capsula	capsules
Tab	Tabella	Tablet
a.c.	ante cibum	before food

APPENDIX - 4

SYRINGES AND NEEDLES

Drugs are administered as injections using a needle and a syringe. A syringe consists of a barrel and a plunger. A type of syringe known as Luer - Lock syringe has the advantage that the needle can be locked in position. Intravenous injections are given with the help of an infusion set.

Sizes: Syringes are available in various sizes 1, 2, 5, 10, 20 and 50 ml. Syringes may be of two materials - Glass and plastic.

Glass Syringes

Advantages

- The markings are accurate and therefore exact quantity can be drawn.
- The fluid level can be clearly seen as the glass is transparent.
- They can be easily sterilized by boiling and reused
- Glass syringes are resistant to punctures.

Disadvantages

- Glass syringes can break
- They carry a greater risk of air embolism because they are rigid
- They are more expensive.

Glass syringes are no more preferred because of the risk of spreading dangerous diseases like AIDS when not properly sterilized.

Plastic Syringes

Advantages:

- Plastic syringes do not break easily
- Because they are collapsible, they allow proper emptying of the syringe - hence less risk of air embolism.
- They are cheaper
- They are disposable

Disadvantages

- Plastic syringes are not very accurate in scale.
- They cannot be easily sterilized.
- They cannot be reused.

Special Syringes

Insulin syringe has markings in units - (40 in 1ml (red) or 80 in 1ml (green) are suitable for administration of insulin.

Tuberculin syringe is a syringe of 1ml capacity with 0.01ml markings. It is useful for administration of very small volumes.

Disposable syringes and needles

Sterile disposable syringes are made of plastic and are packed with a needle to be fixed at the time of use. They have the following advantages
1. Need no sterilization
2. Injections are less painful as needle is sharp
3. Convenient to use.

Disadvantages

Works out costlier as they are not reusable.

Needles

Needles are made of stainless steel, which is rust proof. At the end of the shaft is the tip, which is bevelled. The bevelling may be short, very short or regular. Needle is available in different gauge thickness and length. The gauge numbers are from 13 (thickest) to 27 (finest). Depending on the route of administration, size of the patient and the thickness of the solution to be injected, the needle is selected.

Route		Preferred size
Subcutaneous	5/8 inch	25 gauge
IM, IV	1.5 inch	22-24 gauge
Intradermal	short	26 gauge

Further Reading

1. Katzung BG: *Basic and Clinical Pharmacology* (9th edn). Mc Graw Hill International Edition 2004.

2. Satoskar RS, Bhandarkar SD, Ainapure SS: *Pharmacology and Pharmacotherapeutics*. Revised eighteenth edition 2005.

3. Tripathi KD : *Essentials of Medical Pharmacology* (5th edn). Jaypee Brothers: New Delhi, 2003.

4. Barar FSK : *Essentials of Pharmacotherapeutics* (3rd edn.). S. Chand & Company Ltd. New Delhi, 2000.

5. Lawrence DR, Bennet PN, Brown MJ: *Clinical Pharmacology* (9th edn). Chruchill Livingstone: London, 2002.

6. Rang HP, Dale MM, Ritter JM: *Pharmacology* (5th edn). Churchill Livingstone: New York, 2003.

7. Hardman JG, Limbird LE *et al*: Goodman and Gilman's: *The Pharmacological Basis of Therapeutics* (10th edn). Mc Graw Hill: New York, 2001.

8. Craig CR; Robert E. Stitzel *Modern Pharmacology with Clinical Applications* (6th edn). Little Brown: Boston, 2003.

9.   Park K. Park's: Text book of Preventive and Social Medicine (17th edn.). M/s Bharanidas Bhanot, Jabalpur, 2002.

10. Page CP, Curtis MJ et al: *Integrated Pharmacology* (2nd edn) Mosby, London 2002.

11. Martindale: *The complete Drug Reference* (33rd edn.) Pharmaceutical Press, 2002.

12. Mary J. Mycek, Richard A. Harvey, Pamela C. Champe, Bruce D. Fisher, *Lippincott's illustrated Reviews* (2nd edn) Lippincot - Raven Publishers, 1992.

13. Harrison's Prnciples of Internal Medicine 14th edition, Mc Graw Hill: 1998. International edition.

14. Robert E. Rakel, Conn's Current therapy 2000 W.B. Saunders Company, Pennsylvania.

INDEX

D

F

M

U

V